MANUAL of
PERIOPERATIVE CARE in
ADULT CARDIAC SURGERY

Fourth Edition

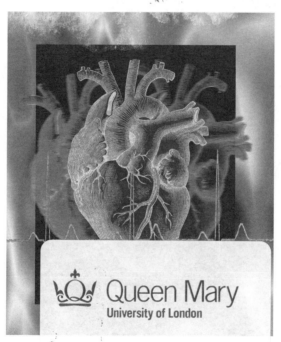

MANUAL of PERIOPERATIVE CARE in ADULT CARDIAC SURGERY

Fourth Edition

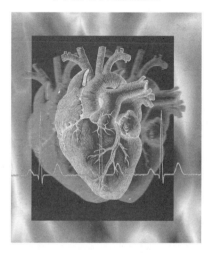

By

Robert M. Bojar, M.D.

Associate Professor of Cardiothoracic Surgery
Tufts University School of Medicine
Chief of Cardiothoracic Surgery
St. Vincent Hospital, Worcester, Massachusetts
Senior Cardiothoracic Surgeon
Tufts–New England Medical Center, Boston, Massachusetts

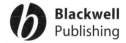

Blackwell
Publishing

Blackwell Publishing, Inc., 350 Main Street, Malden, Massachusetts 02148-5018, USA
Blackwell Publishing Ltd, 9600 Garsington Road, Oxford OX4 2DQ, UK
Blackwell Publishing Asia Pty Ltd, 550 Swanston Street, Carlton, Victoria 3053, Australia

04 05 06 07 5 4 3 2 1

ISBN: 1-4051-0439-2

Library of Congress Cataloging-in-Publication Data

Bojar, Robert M., 1951–
    Manual of perioperative care in adult cardiac surgery/by Robert M. Bojar.—4th ed.
    p. ; cm.
    Includes bibliographical references and index.
    ISBN 1-4051-0439-2 (pbk.)
    1. Heart—Surgery—Handbooks, manuals, etc. 2. Therapeuticsm Surgical—
Handbooks, manuals, etc.
    [DNLM: 1. Cardiac Surgical Procedures—Outlines. 2. Perioperative Care—
methods—Outlines. WG 18.2 B685m 2005] I. Bojar, Robert M., 1951–. Manual of
perioperative care in cardiac surgery. II. Title.

    RD598.B64 2005
    617.4'12—dc22

                                                        2004019487

A catalogue record for this title is available from the British Library

Acquisitions: Nancy Anastasi Duffy
Development: Kate Heinle
Production: Debra Murphy
Cover design: Eve Siegel
Interior design: Eve Siegel
Illustrations by Electronic Illustrators Group
Typesetter: International Typesetting and Composition
Printed and bound by Capital City Press in Berlin, VT

For further information on Blackwell Publishing, visit our website:
www.blackwellmedicine.com

The publisher's policy is to use permanent paper from mills that operate a sustainable forestry policy, and which has been manufactured from pulp processed using acid-free and elementary chlorine-free practices. Furthermore, the publisher ensures that the text paper and cover board used have met acceptable environmental accreditation standards.

Dedication

To my wife, Mercedes, for her patience and understanding as I deprived Alana and Rebecca of their bedtime stories—but not any longer!

Table of Contents

Preface

Technological advances in cardiovascular care have changed the patient population referred to cardiac surgeons. At a time when off-pump surgery and robotics are being utilized to offer the patient a less invasive and potentially more benign procedure, the advent of drug-eluting stents has dramatically decreased referrals for coronary bypass surgery. Saphenous vein graft disease, multivessel disease, and at times, left main disease have become "endovascular" problems to be approached by percutaneous coronary interventions (PCI) in the cath lab. Seemingly, coronary artery bypass surgery (CABG) has become reserved for patients with failed stents, unstentable disease, or such diffuse disease that even the most aggressive cardiologist admits defeat and refers the patient to surgery. The percentage of patients requiring valve or combined surgery has increased, although isolated coronary surgery still remains the most common procedure. Yet, despite these trends, surgical results, as tracked by the Society of Thoracic Surgeons database, continue to improve. So, we must be doing something right!

Improvements in intraoperative management have contributed to better patient outcomes. Excellence in cardiac anesthesia with protocols to achieve early extubation and routine use of intraoperative transesophageal echocardiography play a major role in optimizing surgical outcome. Surgeons have also become more technically proficient and recognize the importance of excellent myocardial protection. Despite improvements in cardiopulmonary bypass (CPB) technology, off-pump surgery (OPCAB) has been promoted as a means of minimizing the adverse effects of CPB, although its advantages over traditional on-pump CABG are somewhat controversial. Some surgeons reserve its use for patients with advanced comorbidities that might otherwise contraindicate on-pump CABG. However, no matter which technique of surgery is used and how well it is performed, excellence in perioperative care will affect the outcome in critically ill patients. That is why an update of the manual is timely, now 6 years since the last edition.

In an attempt to keep this manual at a reasonable length and not weigh down the pocket of the user, the decision was made to retain only the Adult Cardiac Surgery section of the book. Each chapter has been extensively updated and rereferenced to include the latest information on perioperative care. The outline format, which most readers have found quite beneficial in providing easy access to information, has been retained. It should be noted that the book is written in a chronological fashion from Chapters 2 to 8, covering diagnostic tests, then preoperative, intraoperative, and early postoperative care issues. Chapters 9–12 discuss bleeding, and the respiratory, cardiac, and renal subsystems in depth, and the final chapter covers additional problems and issues on the postoperative floor. Thus, there is no chapter devoted specifically to off-pump surgery, which is discussed primarily in the chapters on intraoperative and postoperative management (Chapters 4 and 8).

I am hopeful that this 4th edition will provide a timely update on perioperative care that will allow its readers to provide the best possible care to their adult cardiac surgical patients.

Robert M. Bojar, M.D.
December 2004

Acknowledgments

Close cooperation and communication among all members of the healthcare team are essential to provide the best possible care to patients undergoing cardiac surgical operations. This often involves consultation with specialty services which can offer their expertise in the management of difficult management problems. The breadth of knowledge and technology in the medical subspecialties has achieved such expansion that it is difficult to remain abreast of all the latest developments. Therefore, I am grateful to many individuals who set aside valuable time to review sections of this manuscript. I would like to acknowledge the assistance of Drs. Robert Black, George Gordon, Munther Homoud, Charles Zee, Timothy Hastings CRNA, and Wanda Reynolds CRT for their comments. I specifically would like to acknowledge the outstanding physician assistants with whom I work for their support and expertise in patient care. Those who reviewed sections of the manuscript to make sure everything was "just right" include Theresa Phillips, Jennifer Hardy, Jennifer Delhotal, Joshua Deisenroth, and Philip Carpino. The section on cardiopulmonary bypass and myocardial protection was reviewed by members of the outstanding perfusion team at St. Vincent Hospital, Bettina Alpert, Anne Oulton, and Mark Wante.

I would also like to acknowledge the comments of Eric H. Awtry, MD, FACC, Julie Pappalardo, MHS, PA-C, and Loisann Stapleton, RN, MSN, ACNP, CCRN, whose reviews and suggestions framed the content of the current edition.

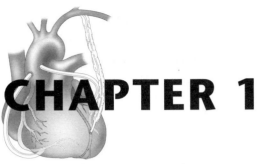

CHAPTER 1

Synopsis of Adult Cardiac Surgical Disease

Synopsis of Adult Cardiac Surgical Disease

It is essential that all individuals involved in the assessment and management of patients with cardiac surgical disease have a basic understanding of the disease processes that are being treated. This chapter presents the spectrum of adult cardiac surgical disease that is encountered in most cardiac surgical practices. The pathophysiology, indications for surgery, specific preoperative considerations, and surgical options for various diseases are presented. Diagnostic techniques and general preoperative considerations are presented in subsequent chapters, and postoperative issues specific to each type of surgical procedure are discussed in Chapter 8.

I. Coronary Artery Disease

A. Pathophysiology. Coronary artery disease (CAD) results from progressive blockage of the coronary arteries by atherosclerosis. Clinical syndromes result from an imbalance of oxygen supply and demand resulting in inadequate myocardial perfusion to meet metabolic demand (ischemia). Plaque rupture with superimposed thrombosis is responsible for most acute coronary syndromes.

B. Management strategies

1. Symptomatic coronary disease is initially treated with nitrates, β-adrenergic blockers, calcium channel blockers, and aspirin.[1] Angiotensin-converting enzyme (ACE) inhibitors are generally used for hypertension control, and "statins" are beneficial for hyperlipidemia and plaque stabilization.[2]

2. ST-segment infarctions should be treated by either primary angioplasty and stenting or thrombolytic therapy if the patient presents within 6 hours of the onset of chest pain.[3,4]

3. Patients presenting with acute coronary syndromes with non–ST-segment myocardial infarctions should be administered unfractionated or low-molecular-weight heparin, aspirin, and clopidogrel (Plavix).[5–10] The latter should not be given if urgent surgery is considered likely.

4. In patients with continuing ischemia and high-risk features (crescendo angina over 48 hours, rest pain, electrocardiographic changes at rest, congestive heart failure [CHF], or elevated troponins levels), platelet glycoprotein IIb/IIIa inhibitors, such as tirofiban or eptifibatide, should also be given with plans to proceed to an early invasive strategy of catheterization, at which time the appropriate means of intervention (angioplasty and stenting versus surgery) can be determined.[11]

C. Selection of an interventional procedure[12]

1. An assessment of the patient's clinical presentation, coronary anatomy, degree of inducible ischemia on stress testing, and status of ventricular function is taken into consideration in determining whether the patient is an appropriate candidate for an interventional procedure. The primary objective of any intervention is the relief of ischemia, and it should be considered for any patient with the appropriate

coronary anatomy in whom refractory angina is present or in whom the degree of ischemia, symptomatic or not, threatens to lead to myocardial infarction (MI). When the indications for an intervention are present, selection of the appropriate procedure depends on the extent and nature of the coronary disease.

2. Improvements in the technology of percutaneous coronary intervention (PCI) have altered the basic approach to patients with CAD. Use of balloon angioplasty and/or stenting is applicable to many patients with multivessel disease. Early results of the use of drug-eluting stents in reducing restenosis rates are encouraging, although the long-term results are not known because such devices only became available in early 2003.[13,14] There is still some limitation in the capacity of PCI to achieve complete and lasting revascularization in patients with diffuse multivessel disease, especially in diabetics, but data suggest that with careful follow-up and repeat interventions, comparable long-term results to coronary bypass surgery may be achieved.[15] Results in the precoated stent era were optimized by the administration of clopidogrel prior to the stenting procedure and continuing it for at least 1 month, and probably for as long as 1 year.[16]

D. **Indications for surgery.** If PCI is not feasible (e.g., tight left main disease, diffuse multivessel disease, or calcified coronaries) or if it is unsuccessful (e.g., inability to cross the lesion, in-stent stenosis), surgery is indicated in the following situations:

1. Patient has refractory angina or a large amount of myocardium in ischemic jeopardy:
   a. Class III–IV chronic stable angina refractory to medical therapy (Box 1.1).
   b. Unstable angina refractory to medical therapy. The term "acute coronary syndrome" applies to the overlapping presentations of unstable angina and MI of varying degrees. Measurement of troponin levels can differentiate unstable angina without MI from a non–ST-segment elevation infarction. An elevated troponin level is associated with an increased incidence of adverse cardiovascular events and is an indication for an early invasive strategy.
   c. Acute ischemia or hemodynamic instability following attempted coronary angioplasty or stenting (especially with dissection and compromised flow).
   d. Acute evolving infarction within 4–6 hours of the onset of chest pain or later if evidence of ongoing ischemia (early postinfarction ischemia).
   e. Markedly positive stress test prior to major intraabdominal or vascular surgery.
   f. Ischemic pulmonary edema, a common angina equivalent in elderly women.

Box 1.1 • New York Heart Association Functional Classification

Class

I. No limitation of physical activity

II. Slight limitation of physical activity. Ordinary activity results in fatigue, palpitation, dyspnea, or anginal pain

III. Marked limitation of physical activity. Less than ordinary activity causes fatigue, palpitation, dyspnea, or anginal pain

IV. Inability to carry out any physical activity without discomfort. Symptoms may be present even at rest

2. A second group of patients includes those without disabling angina or refractory ischemia in whom the extent of coronary disease, the status of ventricular function, and the degree of inducible ischemia on stress testing are such that surgery may improve long-term survival. This is presumed to occur by preventing infarction and preserving ventricular function. Surgery is especially beneficial for patients with impaired ventricular function and inducible ischemia in whom the medical prognosis is unfavorable.

   a. Left main stenosis > 50%.
   b. Three-vessel disease with ejection fraction (EF) < 50%.
   c. Three-vessel disease with EF > 50% and significant inducible ischemia.
   d. Two-vessel disease with involvement of proximal left anterior descending artery (LAD).
   e. One- and two-vessel disease with extensive myocardium in jeopardy but lesions not amenable to PCI.

3. A third group of patients should undergo bypass surgery when other open-heart procedures are indicated:

   a. Valvular operations, septal myectomy, and so forth with associated CAD.
   b. Concomitant surgery for postinfarction mechanical defects (left ventricular aneurysm, ventricular septal rupture, acute mitral regurgitation).
   c. Coronary artery anomalies with risk of sudden death (vessel passing between the aorta and pulmonary artery).

4. The American Heart Association/American College of Cardiology (AHA/ACC) publications on coronary artery bypass grafting (CABG) have provided indications for surgery according to class I–III evidence of efficacy, subdividing the indications initially by the clinical indication and then by coronary anatomy (Table 1.1).

E. **Preoperative considerations**

1. Preoperative autologous blood donation is feasible in patients with chronic stable angina to reduce the requirement for homologous transfusion.[17,18] However, with the use of antifibrinolytic drugs for on-pump surgery and the frequent performance of off-pump surgery, fewer than 50% of patients receive any blood products during their hospital stay. Thus, there is little benefit to autologous donation in the healthy elective patient. It is best avoided in patients with unstable ischemic syndromes and left main coronary disease, many of whom require urgent surgery soon after catheterization and often have low hematocrits.

2. Avoidance of myocardial ischemia is essential in the immediate preoperative period. All antianginal medications should be continued up to and including the morning of surgery. Several studies have demonstrated the benefit of preoperative β-blocker therapy on lowering perioperative mortality in cardiac surgery patients.[19,20] Patients being admitted the morning of surgery should be reminded to take their medications before coming to the hospital.

3. Aggressive management of ischemia is indicated in unstable patients to reduce the risk of surgery. This may include adequate sedation, heparin and antiplatelet therapy, antiischemic medications (intravenous nitrates and β-blockers) to control heart rate and blood pressure, and/or placement of an intraaortic balloon pump (IABP) for refractory ischemia. It cannot be overemphasized that just because a patient has been catheterized and accepted for surgery does not mean that his or her medical care should not be aggressive up to the time of surgery!

Table 1.1 • *ACC/AHA Guidelines for CABG Surgery: Indications for Surgery*

	Class I	Class IIA	Class IIB
ST-elevation MI	Persistent or recurrent ischemia or hemodynamic instability if PCI fails or patient is not a candidate for PCI Cardiogenic shock developing within 36 h of STEMI if CABG possible within 18 h of developing shock (< age 75) Life threatening ventricular arrhythmias with left main ≥ 50% or 3 VD	Noncandidates for PCI or fibrinolysis within 6–12 h of evolving STEMI Cardiogenic shock as noted in class I but age > 75	None
Unstable angina Non-STEMI	Left main ≥ 50% Left main equivalent* Refractory ischemia on maximal medical therapy	Proximal LAD with 1–2 VD	1–2 VD not involving LAD
Stable angina	Left main ≥ 50% Left main equivalent 3 VD 2 VD with > 70% proximal LAD and EF < 50% or + ETT 1–2 VD without proximal LAD but large area of viable ischemic myocardium Refractory angina with + ETT	Proximal LAD with 1 VD 1–2 VD without proximal LAD with moderate area of ischemic myocardium	None
Asymptomatic/mild angina	Left main ≥ 50% Left main equivalent 3 VD	Proximal LAD with 1–2 VD	1–2 VD not involving LAD

Poor LV function	Left main ≥ 50% Left main equivalent Proximal LAD with 2–3 VD	Significant viable, dysfunctional myocardium with CAD other than noted at left	None
Ventricular arrhythmias	Left main ≥ 50% 3 VD	Bypassable 1–2 VD Proximal LAD with 1–2 VD	None
Failed PCI	Ongoing ischemia or threatened occlusion Hemodynamic compromise	Foreign body in crucial position Hemodynamic compromise with coagulopathy if no previous sternotomy	Hemodynamic compromise with coagulopathy needing reoperation
Reoperation	Disabling angina on maximal medical therapy No patent grafts but class I indications for surgery for native vessel disease (left main, LM equivalent, 3 VD)	Bypassable arteries with large area of ischemia Atherosclerotic vein graft to LAD or a large area of myocardium	None

Class I: Procedure is useful and effective; class IIa: weight of opinion is in favor of usefulness/efficacy; class IIB: usefulness/efficacy is less well established.
* Left main equivalent is >70% in proximal LAD and circumflex.
CABG = coronary artery bypass grafting; LAD = left anterior descending artery; VD = vessel disease; Non-STEMI = non–ST-segment elevation myocardial infarction; MI = myocardial infarction; EF = ejection fraction; ETT = exercise tolerance test; LV = left ventricular; CAD = coronary artery disease; PCI = percutaneous coronary intervention; ITA = internal thoracic artery.

If the patient has persistent ischemia despite all of these measures, emergency surgery is mandatory.

4. Intravenous unfractionated **heparin** is often used in patients with unstable angina, left main coronary disease, or a preoperative IABP. The heparin should generally be continued up to the time of surgery to avoid the potential problem of precipitating ischemia in the prebypass period when the anticoagulant effect of heparin dissipates. Central lines can usually be placed safely while the patient is heparinized. Patients receiving heparin should have their platelet count rechecked daily to detect the development of heparin-induced thrombocytopenia, particularly within 24 hours of surgery. If low-molecular-weight heparin is used, it must be stopped at least 12 hours prior to surgery.[21]

5. Preoperative blood transfusions should be considered in patients with unstable angina and a hematocrit < 26%. This not only may improve the ischemic syndrome but will minimize hemodilution during surgery and the requirement for blood product transfusion. In addition to blood withdrawal for preoperative lab tests, it is not uncommon for the hematocrit to fall several points after a cardiac catheterization both from blood loss and hemodilution with hydration. One study showed that coronary angiography was associated with a fall in hemoglobin of 1.8 g/dL (equivalent to about a 5.4% fall in hematocrit).[22] The requirement for transfusions has been documented to increase perioperative mortality rates in the Society of Thoracic Surgeons (STS) database.[23]

6. Whether **aspirin** should be stopped preoperatively is controversial. Although several studies in the 1980s and early 1990s demonstrated increased perioperative bleeding in patients who remained on aspirin up to the time of surgery,[24,25] other studies failed to demonstrate this.[26,27] Despite the traditional recommendation that aspirin should be stopped 7 days prior to elective surgery, studies have shown that platelet function generally returns to normal without an increase in transfusion requirements if it is stopped just 3 days preoperatively.[28,29] Fueling this controversy even more is evidence that perioperative mortality is lower in patients in whom aspirin is continued up to the time of surgery.[30,31]

7. In contrast, the preoperative use of **clopidogrel** has been shown in many, but not all, studies to significantly increase the risk of bleeding and reexploration for bleeding.[32–35] Thus, it has been recommended that it be stopped 7–10 days before elective surgery.

   a. Many patients are given a 300-mg loading dose of clopidogrel upon arrival in the catheterization lab in anticipation of a stenting procedure, only to find that surgery is indicated on an urgent basis. Furthermore, stenting of culprit vessels may occasionally be performed on an emergency basis for an evolving infarction with subsequent referral for urgent surgery to achieve complete revascularization. Thus, it may not be possible to have the patient off clopidogrel for the recommended period of time.

   b. Surgeons must take additional steps, including platelet transfusions, to control bleeding caused by clopidogrel-induced platelet dysfunction. Unfortunately, the circulating active metabolite of clopidogrel may bind to transfused platelets and limit their effectiveness. It has been recommended that IIb/IIIa inhibitors should be used rather than clopidogrel in patients with acute coronary syndromes if there is any possibility that urgent surgery may be necessary.[35]

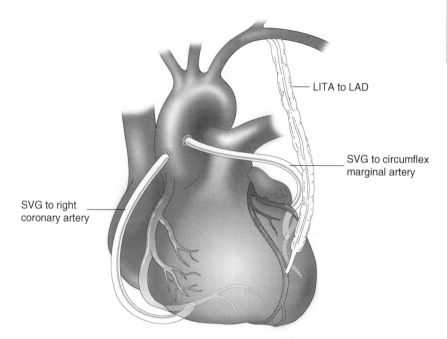

Figure 1.1 • Coronary artery bypass grafting. A left internal thoracic artery (LITA) has been placed to the left anterior descending artery (LAD) with aortocoronary saphenous vein grafts (SVG) to the circumflex marginal and right coronary arteries.

F. Surgical procedures

1. **Traditional coronary bypass grafting** is performed through a median sternotomy incision using cardiopulmonary bypass (CPB). Myocardial preservation is usually provided by cardioplegic arrest. The procedure involves bypassing the coronary blockages with a variety of conduits. The left internal thoracic (or mammary) artery (ITA) is usually used as a pedicled graft to the LAD and is supplemented by saphenous vein grafts interposed between the aorta and the coronary arteries (Figure 1.1).

   a. The saphenous vein should be harvested endoscopically or with skip incisions to minimize patient comfort, reduce the incidence of leg edema and wound healing problems, and optimize cosmesis.[36]

   b. Since improved event-free survival has been documented with use of arterial conduits, expanded use of the ITA (bilateral ITAs and sequential grafts)[37] and use of the radial artery have become more commonplace.[38,39] The radial artery usually is harvested through an open incision but can now be harvested endoscopically.[40] Intravenous diltiazem 0.1 mg/kg/h (usually 5–10 mg/h) or intravenous nitroglycerin 10–20 µg/kg/min is initiated during surgery and continued into the postoperative period to minimize spasm in radial artery conduits, although the necessity of using such pharmacologic management has not been proved necessary.

2. Concerns about the adverse effects of CPB spurred the development of technology to allow safe **"off-pump" coronary artery bypass (OPCAB)** during which complete

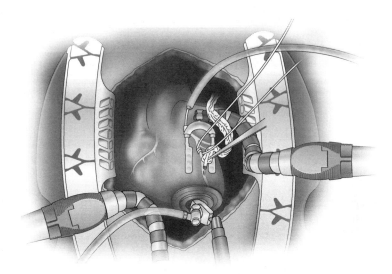

Figure 1.2 • Off-pump bypass grafting requires displacement of the heart using techniques to avoid hemodynamic compromise. These may include placement and elevation of deep pericardial sutures or use of an apical suction device. A stabilizing device is used to minimize motion and a proximal vessel loop is placed to minimize bleeding at the site of the anastomosis.

revascularization could be performed with the avoidance of CPB. Deep pericardial sutures are placed that, upon traction, allow for positioning of the heart without hemodynamic compromise. Various devices provide assistance in retracting the apex of the heart to improve lateral wall exposure. A stabilizing platform of various types (pressure, suction) minimizes movement at the site of the arteriotomy (Figure 1.2). Intracoronary or aortocoronary shunting can minimize ischemia after an arteriotomy is performed.

a. Conversion to on-pump surgery may be necessary in the following circumstances:

  i. Coronary arteries are very small, severely diseased, or intramyocardial.

  ii. LV function is very poor, or there is severe cardiomegaly or hypertrophy that precludes adequate cardiac translocation without hemodynamic compromise or arrhythmias.

  iii. Uncontrollable ischemia or arrhythmias develop with vessel occlusion that persist despite distal shunting.

  iv. Intractable bleeding occurs that cannot be controlled with vessel loops or an intracoronary shunt.

b. Several studies have reported that OPCABs lower mortality rates, reduce transfusion requirements, and arguably reduce the risk of neurocognitive dysfunction, renal dysfunction, and atrial fibrillation (AF). Despite these potential advantages, the wave of enthusiasm for this technique has partially waned, and many surgeons are reserving its use for patients with limited disease. Its major advantage may be in very high-risk patients with multiple comorbidities in whom it is critical to avoid CPB.[41–43]

c. In some patients with severe ventricular dysfunction, the heart will not tolerate the manipulation required during off-pump surgery. In this circumstance, right ventricular (RV) assist devices can be used to improve hemodynamics. Alternatively, surgery can be done on pump on an empty beating heart to avoid the period of cardioplegic arrest.

3. **Minimally invasive direct coronary artery bypass** (MIDCAB) was a procedure popularized in the late 1990s that involved bypassing the LAD with the ITA without use of CPB via a short left anterior thoracotomy incision. Although an additional incision could be used to bypass the right coronary artery, most surgeons abandoned this technique in favor of an off-pump procedure via a median sternotomy incision.

4. **Transmyocardial revascularization** (TMR) is a technique in which laser channels are drilled in the heart with CO_2 or holmium-YAG lasers to improve myocardial perfusion. Although the channels occlude within a few days, the inflammatory reaction created induces neoangiogenesis that may be associated with upregulation of various growth factors, such as vascular endothelial growth factor. This procedure can be used as a sole procedure performed through a left thoracotomy for patients with inoperable CAD in regions of viable myocardium. Alternatively, it can be used as an adjunct to CABG in viable regions of the heart where bypass grafts cannot be placed.[44–47]

II. Left Ventricular Aneurysm

A. **Pathophysiology**

1. An LV aneurysm results from the occlusion of a major coronary artery that produces an extensive transmural infarction. The damaged myocardium is converted to thin scar tissue that exhibits dyskinesia during ventricular systole.[48]

2. The two most common presentations are those of ischemic syndromes and CHF. Angina results from the presence of multivessel disease associated with the increased systolic wall stress of a dilated ventricle. CHF results from poor ventricular function and the reduction of stroke volume caused by geometric remodeling of the aneurysmal segment due to loss of contractile tissue and an increase in ventricular size.

3. Systemic thromboembolism may result from thrombus formation within the dyskinetic segment.

4. Malignant ventricular arrhythmias or sudden death may result from the development of a macroreentry circuit at the border zone between scar tissue and viable myocardium.

B. **Indications for surgery.** Surgery is usually not indicated for the patient with an asymptomatic aneurysm because of its favorable natural history. This is in contrast to the unpredictable prognosis and absolute indication for surgery in a patient with a false aneurysm, which is caused by a contained rupture of the ventricular muscle. Surgery may be beneficial in the patient with asymptomatic disease when an extremely large aneurysm is present or when extensive clot formation is present in the aneurysm. Surgery is most commonly indicated to improve symptoms and prolong survival when one of the four clinical syndromes noted above is present: angina, CHF, systemic thromboembolism, or malignant arrhythmias. In the past, the latter was treated by a map-guided endocardial resection, but the expensive equipment for intraoperative mapping is no longer manufactured. Therefore, it is treated by a nonguided endocardial resection through the aneurysm with or without cryosurgery along with subsequent placement of a transvenous implantable cardioverter-defibrillator (ICD).

C. Preoperative considerations

1. A biplane left ventriculogram is helpful in differentiating aneurysms from areas of akinesis and for evaluating the function of the nonaneurysmal ventricle. The thinning of the ventricle is best identified by echocardiography.

2. The patient should be maintained on heparin up to the time of surgery if LV thrombus is present. Thrombus is best delineated by echocardiography.

D. Surgical procedures[49,50]

1. Standard aneurysmectomy entails a ventriculotomy through the aneurysm, resection of the aneurysm wall, including part of the septum if involved, and linear closure over felt strips (Figure 1.3).[51,52]

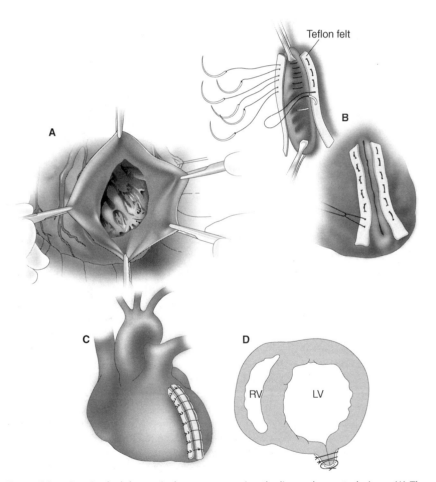

Figure 1.3 • Repair of a left ventricular aneurysm using the linear closure technique. (A) The thinned out scar tissue is opened and partially resected. Any left ventricular thrombus is removed. (B) The aneurysm is then closed with mattress sutures over felt strips. (C) An additional over-and-over suture is placed over a third felt strip. (D) Cross section of the final repair.

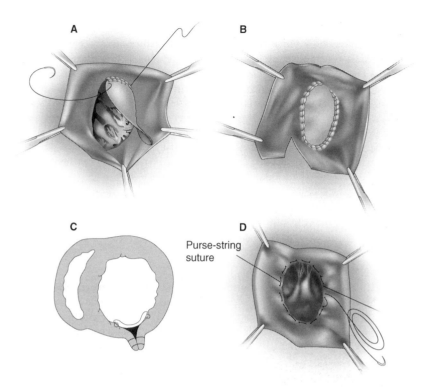

Figure 1.4 • Repair of a left ventricular aneurysm using the endoaneurysmorrhaphy technique. (A,B) A pericardial patch is sewn at the base of the defect at the junction of scar and normal myocardium to better preserve ventricular geometry. The left ventricle is closed in a similar fashion to the linear technique. (C) Cross section of the final repair. (D) The Dor procedure is a modification of this technique in which a circumferential pursestring suture is placed at the base of the defect to restore a normal orientation to the ventricle. A patch is then sewn over the defect.

2. The "endoaneurysmorrhaphy" technique is used for large aneurysms. A pericardial or Dacron patch is sewn to the edges of viable myocardium at the base of the aneurysm and the aneurysm wall is reapproximated over the patch (Figure 1.4). This preserves LV geometry and improves ventricular function to a greater degree than the linear closure method.[53]

3. Other methods of endoventricular repair involve tailoring of the residual muscle before patch closure (Jatene operation) and the endoventricular circular patch plasty technique of Dor that excludes the noncontracting segment with a patch (Figure 1.4D).[49,54,55] A slight modification of the Dor procedure called surgical anterior ventricular endocardial restoration (SAVER) produces an elliptical contour of the heart and results in significant improvement in ventricular size and function.[56]

4. Coronary bypass grafting of critically diseased vessels should be performed. Bypass of the LAD and diagonal arteries should be considered if septal reperfusion can be accomplished.

III. Ventricular Septal Defect

A. **Pathophysiology.** Extensive myocardial damage subsequent to occlusion of a major coronary vessel may result in septal necrosis and rupture. This usually occurs within the first week of an infarction, more commonly in the anteroapical region (from occlusion of the LAD) and less commonly in the inferior wall (usually from occlusion of the right coronary artery). It is noted in fewer than 1% of acute MIs, and the incidence has been reduced by use of early reperfusion therapy for ST-segment elevation infarctions. The presence of a ventricular septal defect (VSD) is suggested by the presence of a loud holosystolic murmur that reflects the left-to-right shunting across the ruptured septum. The patient usually develops acute pulmonary edema and cardiogenic shock from the left-to-right shunt.[57]

B. **Indications for surgery.** Surgery is indicated on an emergency basis for nearly all postinfarction VSDs to prevent the development of progressive multisystem organ failure. Occasionally, a small VSD with a shunt of < 2:1 can be managed medically, but it usually should be repaired after 6 weeks to prevent future hemodynamic problems.

C. **Preoperative considerations**

1. Prompt diagnosis can be made using a Swan-Ganz catheter, which detects a step-up of oxygen saturation in the right ventricle. Two-dimensional echocardiography can confirm the diagnosis of a VSD and differentiate it from acute mitral regurgitation, which can produce a similar clinical scenario.

2. Inotropic support and reduction of afterload, usually with an IABP, are indicated in all patients with VSDs in anticipation of emergent cardiac catheterization and surgery.

3. Cardiac catheterization with coronary angiography should be performed to confirm the severity of the shunt and to identify associated CAD.

D. **Surgical procedures**

1. The traditional surgical treatment for postinfarct VSDs had been performance of a ventriculotomy through the infarcted zone, resection of the area of septal necrosis, and Teflon felt or pericardial patching of the septum and free wall. This technique requires transmural suturing and is prone to recurrence.[58]

2. The preferred approach is to perform circumferential pericardial patching around the border of the infarcted ventricular muscle. This technique excludes the infarcted septum to eliminate the shunt and reduces recurrence rates because suturing is performed to viable myocardium away from the area of necrosis (Figure 1.5).[59]

3. Coronary bypass grafting of critically diseased vessels should be performed since it has been shown to improve long-term survival after surgery.[60]

IV. Aortic Stenosis

A. **Pathophysiology.** Aortic stenosis (AS) results from thickening, calcification, and/or fusion of the aortic valve leaflets, which produce an obstruction to LV outflow. In younger patients, AS usually develops on congenitally bicuspid valves, whereas in older patients, degenerative change in trileaflet valves is more common. The impairment to cusp opening leads to pressure overload, compensatory left ventricular hypertrophy (LVH), and reduced ventricular compliance.[61,62]

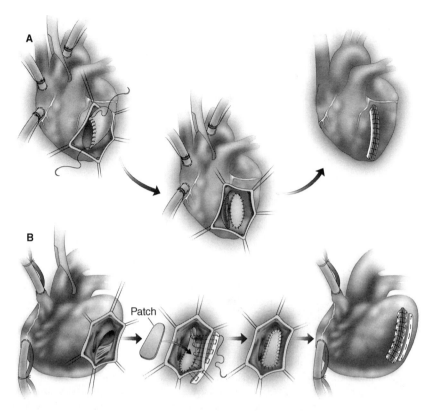

Figure 1.5 • Closure of a postinfarction ventricular septal defect using the exclusion technique. (A) Anterior VSD. (B) Inferior VSD. The pericardial patch is anchored to viable myocardium away from the site of the defect, thus eliminating shunt flow across the septal defect.

1. The development of LVH maintains normal wall stress and a normal EF. If the increase in wall thickness does not increase in proportion to the rise in intraventricular pressure, wall stress will increase and EF will fall. It is important to assess whether a reduced EF is the result of excessive afterload (i.e., inadequate hypertrophy to overcome the obstruction) or depressed contractility. If the latter is present, surgical risk is higher.

2. In patients with excessive LVH, wall stress is low and the heart will become hyperdynamic with a very high EF. This finding portends a worse prognosis after surgical correction.[63,64]

3. Angina may result from the increased myocardial oxygen demand caused by increased wall stress, from reduction in blood supply per gram of hypertrophied tissue, and/or from limited coronary vasodilator reserve. Thus it may occur with or without concomitant CAD. Symptoms of CHF result from elevation of filling pressures due to diastolic dysfunction and eventually by progressive decline in LV systolic function. Cardiac output is relatively fixed across the valve orifice and can lead to syncope in the face of peripheral vasodilatation. The development of AF

commonly causes symptoms due to the dependence of the hypertrophied ventricle on atrial "kick" to maintain a satisfactory stroke volume.

4. The degree of valve stenosis is determined by measuring the cardiac output and the peak or mean pressure gradient across the valve (pressures obtained from the left ventricle and aorta). A valve area is calculated from the ratio of the cardiac output to the square root of the valve gradient (the Gorlin formula).

$$AVA = \frac{CO/(SEP \times HR)}{44.5\sqrt{\text{mean gradient}}}$$

where:

SEP is systolic ejection period (per beat)

CO is cardiac output (mL/min)

HR is heart rate

AVA is aortic valve area in cm^2 (normal = 2.5–3.5 cm^2)

5. The severity of AS can be readily diagnosed by either echocardiography or cardiac catheterization. In patients with critically diseased valves, it is occasionally impossible to cross the valve with the catheter to measure the gradient. Furthermore, one study showed that the risk of embolic stroke was significant in patients in whom catheterization was used to assess the degree of AS, suggesting that confirmation by echocardiography should provide sufficient information and may be safer.[65]

6. Echocardiography can provide an assessment of valve area using the continuity equation, which examines the dimensions of the LV outflow tract and the flow velocities. It may also measure the valve area directly by planimetry in the short-axis view. A mean echocardiographic gradient >50 mm Hg with an AVA <0.75 cm^2 is consistent with severe AS.[66]

7. Aortic stenosis may be graded as mild (AVA > 1.5 cm^2), moderate (AVA = 1.0–1.5 cm^2), severe (AVA < 1.0 cm^2), or critical (AVA < 0.75 cm^2). More precisely, the valve area should be indexed to the patient's size, since a valve area of 1.0 cm^2 may not be significant in a small patient but may be very significant in a larger patient. Critical AS is present when the AVA index is less than 0.45 cm^2.

B. Indications for surgery

1. The average survival of the symptomatic patient with severe AS is less than 2–3 years, and thus the traditional indications for surgery have been the presence of angina, CHF, syncope, or resuscitation from an episode of sudden death. In contrast, surgery has not been considered for the patient with asymptomatic disease no matter how severe the degree of stenosis because the risk of sudden death is considered to be low. However, the majority of patients with critical AS will have symptoms in a short period of time and are at an increased risk of sudden death.[67] Furthermore, they can develop significant LVH, which is an adverse marker for long-term survival. Although the rate of progression of AS can be quite variable, analysis of Doppler outflow velocity and its rate of increase during serial studies can predict the rate of hemodynamic progression of the AS and the clinical outcome.[68,69] Thus, patients with severe or critical AS require very careful monitoring for the development of symptoms and progressive disease that warrant surgery.

2. Indications for surgery in the patient with asymptomatic disease are controversial, since the risk of sudden death is very low. However, the presence of LV systolic dysfunction, a hypotensive response to exercise, ventricular tachycardia (VT), or marked LVH (> 15 mm) are adverse prognostic signs that should prompt earlier surgery. Thus, these findings as well as an AVA < 0.6 cm^2 and a transvalvular peak gradient > 50 mm Hg can be considered indications for surgery in a patient with asymptomatic disease.[62]

3. If a patient requires coronary bypass grafting, an aortic valve with a valve area of 1.1 cm^2 or less should be replaced. Invariably, a native valve with this degree of stenosis will require surgery within a few years for progressive obstruction, thus mandating a reoperative procedure at higher risk. In this situation, one consideration is to place a valve with hemodynamics superior to the valve being replaced because there must be assurance that the benefits outweigh the risks of potential prosthetic valve complications. However, even if comparable hemodynamics are obtained, a prosthetic valve will not develop progressive stenosis as a native valve will, thus avoiding reoperation.

4. Assessing the degree of AS in a patient with a low gradient and poor ventricular function can be problematic. This combination may translate into a low calculated valve area, although the degree of AS may not be significant. Dobutamine stress echocardiography can be used in this circumstance to determine whether poor ventricular function is primarily related to afterload mismatch or contractile dysfunction. If the patient has an increase in cardiac output with little increase in gradient, the valve area will increase, indicating that the severity of valve stenosis was overestimated and surgery is not indicated. In contrast, if there is contractile reserve with an increase in cardiac output and gradient, valve area will remain the same, confirming true AS is present that will benefit from surgery.[70–72]

C. Preoperative considerations

1. Coronary angiography should be performed in any patient over the age of 40 years or in a younger patient with coronary risk factors, angina, or a positive stress test.

2. Ischemic syndromes in patients with AS require judicious management. Medications that should be avoided are those that can reduce preload (nitroglycerin), afterload (calcium channel blockers), or heart rate (β-blockers) because they may lower cardiac output and precipitate cardiac arrest in a patient with critical AS. The ventricular response to AF must be controlled, and cardioversion should be performed if this rhythm is poorly tolerated.

3. Dental work should be performed before surgery to minimize the risk of prosthetic valve endocarditis unless it is felt to be a prohibitive risk.

4. Selection of the appropriate procedure and valve type depends on a number of factors, including the patient's age, contraindications to long-term anticoagulation, and the patient's desire to avoid anticoagulation.

D. Surgical procedures

1. Aortic valve procedures are usually performed through a full median sternotomy incision, although an upper sternotomy with a "J" or "T" incision into the third or fourth intercostal space can provide adequate exposure.[73,74] Cannulation for CPB can be performed either through the incision or using the femoral vessels for minimally invasive approaches.

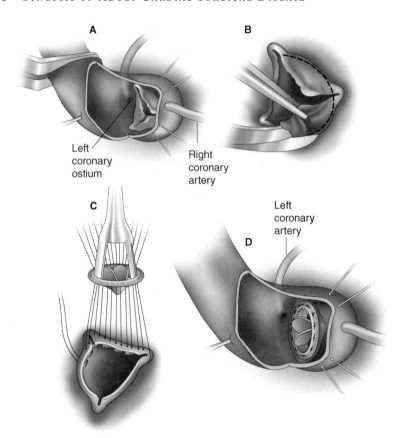

Left
coronary
ostium

Right
coronary
artery

Left
coronary
artery

Figure 1.6 • Aortic valve replacement. (A) A transverse aortotomy incision is made and hold-ing sutures are placed. (B) The valve is excised, and the annulus is debrided and sized. (C, D) Pledgetted mattress sutures are placed through the annulus and through the sewing ring of the valve, which is tied into position. The aortotomy is then closed.

2. Aortic valve replacement with either a tissue or mechanical valve is the standard treatment for AS (Figure 1.6). A stentless valve may provide a larger effective orifice area and may be placed in the subcoronary position or as a root replace-ment (Figure 1.7). The Ross procedure, in which the patient's own pulmonary valve is used to replace the aortic root, with the pulmonary valve replaced with a homograft, is a more complicated procedure generally reserved for patients younger than age 50 who wish to avoid anticoagulation (Figure 1.8).[75] Homografts are usually used for patients with aortic valve endocarditis.[76]

3. Reparative procedures, such as commissurotomy or debridement, have little role in the management of critical AS. However, debridement may be considered in the patient with moderate AS in whom the valve disease is not severe enough to warrant valve replacement but in whom decalcification may delay surgery for a number of years.

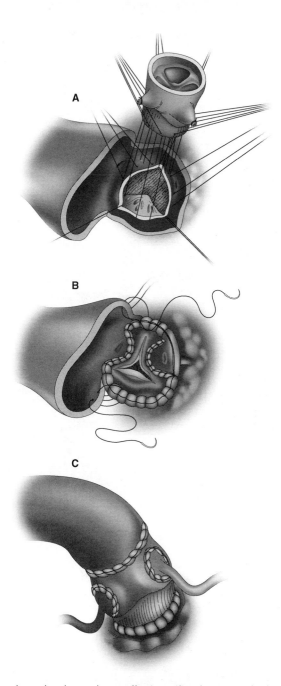

Figure 1.7 • Stentless valves have a larger effective orifice than stented valves that allows for more regression of LV hypertrophy. (A) The proximal suture line sews the lower Dacron skirt of the prosthesis to the aortic annulus. (B) Subcoronary implantation of a Medtronic Freestyle® valve. This requires scalloping of two sinuses with the distal suture line carried out below the coronary ostia. (C) A stentless valve can be used as a root replacement, requiring reimplantation of buttons of the coronary ostia. The distal suture line is an end-to-end anastomosis to the aortic wall.

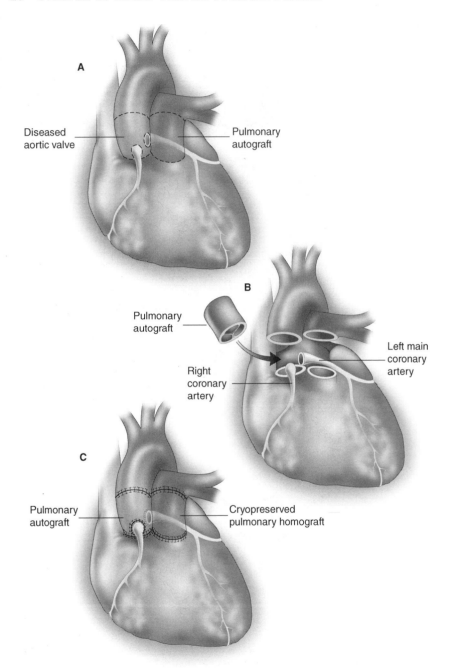

Figure 1.8 • Ross procedure. (A) The aorta is opened and the diseased aortic valve is removed. The pulmonic valve and main pulmonary artery are carefully excised and the coronary arteries are mobilized. (B) The pulmonary autograft is then transposed to the aortic root. (C) The coronary arteries are reimplanted and the RV outflow tract is reconstructed with a cryopreserved pulmonary valved homograft.

V. Aortic Regurgitation

A. **Pathophysiology.** Aortic regurgitation (AR) results from abnormalities in the aortic valve leaflets (postinflammatory deformity, bicuspid valve, destruction from endocarditis) or from aortic root dilatation that prevents leaflet coaptation (annuloaortic ectasia, aortic dissection with cusp prolapse). Acute AR from endocarditis or a type A dissection produces acute LV failure and pulmonary edema because the ventricle is unable to dilate acutely to handle the volume overload. Chronic AR produces pressure and volume overload of the left ventricle, resulting in progressive LV dilatation, increase in wall stress, progressive hypertrophy, and symptoms of left-sided failure. The increased stroke volume increases pulse pressure, increases systolic blood pressure, and produces peripheral manifestations of a hyperdynamic circulation. Eventually, increased afterload and impaired contractility lead to a fall in EF. Angina may also occur.[61,62,77]

B. **Indications for surgery**

1. Acute AR with congestive heart failure.

2. Endocarditis with hemodynamic compromise, persistent bacteremia or sepsis, conduction abnormalities, recurrent systemic embolization from vegetations, or annular abscess formation (see section IX).

3. The presence of symptoms is an indication for surgery as long as the AR is considered to be severe. If LV function is normal (EF > 50%), surgery is recommended for patients in New York Heart Association (NYHA) class III–IV. If the EF is < 50%, surgery is also recommended for patients in NYHA class II.

4. Patients with asymptomatic or minimally symptomatic disease must be followed closely for the development of symptoms or evidence of ventricular decompensation. Patients with impaired LV function will become symptomatic at a rate of about 25%/yr, whereas those with normal LV function have a 4% annual rate of development of symptoms or LV systolic dysfunction. Once there is evidence of ventricular decompensation, survival even with surgery may be compromised. Thus, surgery is recommended in the following patients whose disease is relatively asymptomatic:[62,77–79]

   a. EF < 50%

   b. EF > 50% but evidence of progressive LV dilatation (end-diastolic dimension > 75 mm or end-systolic dimension > 55 mm at rest) or decline in EF > 5% with exercise

5. Moderate to severe AR is an indication for valve replacement if present during surgery for another indication, whether symptomatic or not.

C. **Preoperative considerations**

1. Systemic hypertension should be controlled with vasodilators to reduce the degree of regurgitation. However, excessive afterload reduction may reduce diastolic coronary perfusion pressure and exacerbate ischemia.

2. β-blockers for control of ischemia must be used cautiously because a slow heart rate increases the amount of regurgitation.

3. Placement of an IABP for control of anginal symptoms is contraindicated.

4. As for all valve patients, dental work should be completed before surgery.

5. Contraindications to warfarin should be identified so that the appropriate valve can be chosen.

D. Surgical procedures

1. Aortic valve replacement has traditionally been the procedure of choice for adults with AR. This may involve use of a tissue or mechanical valve, the Ross procedure, or a cryopreserved homograft.

2. Aortic valve repair, involving resection of portions of the valve leaflets and reapproximation to improve leaflet coaptation (especially for bicuspid valves), often with a suture annuloplasty, has been performed successfully. This is valuable in the younger patient in whom a valve-sparing procedure is preferable to valve replacement.[80,81]

3. A valved conduit ("Bentall procedure") is placed if an ascending aortic aneurysm ("annuloaortic ectasia") is also present (Figure 1.9).

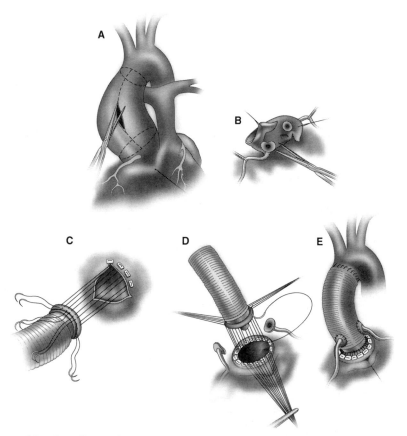

Figure 1.9 • Bentall procedure. (A) The aorta is opened longitudinally and then divided proximally and distally. (B) Coronary ostial buttons are mobilized. (C, D) A valve incorporated into the proximal end of the conduit is then sewn to the aortic annulus. (E) The coronary ostial buttons are reimplanted and the distal suture line is completed.

VI. Mitral Stenosis

A. **Pathophysiology.** Mitral stenosis (MS) occurs nearly exclusively as a consequence of rheumatic fever. Thickening of the valve leaflets with commissural fusion, and thickening and shortening of the chordae tendineae gradually reduce the size of the mitral valve orifice and the efficiency of LV filling. These changes decrease the forward output and increase the left atrial and pulmonary venous pressures, leading to CHF. The development of atrial fibrillation may further decrease ventricular filling and precipitate symptoms of CHF. The development of pulmonary hypertension may eventually lead to right-sided heart failure and functional tricuspid regurgitation (TR). The severity of MS is determined by measuring a transvalvular mean gradient (pulmonary capillary wedge pressure [PCWP] minus the LV mean diastolic pressure) and calculating a mitral valve area that relates the cardiac output to the gradient.

$$MVA = \frac{CO/(DFP \times HR)}{37.7\sqrt{\text{mean gradient}}}$$

where

DFP is diastolic filling period/beat

mean gradient is PCWP − LV mean diastolic pressure

MVA is mitral valve area in cm^2 (normal = 4–6 cm^2)

B. **Indications for interventions**

1. An interventional procedure is indicated for a patient in NYHA class III–IV with moderate or severe MS (MVA < 1.5 cm^2). It may also be considered for patients in class II when critical MS (MVA < 1 cm^2) is present.

2. Percutaneous balloon mitral valvuloplasty (PBMV) is the procedure of choice if valve morphology is favorable. This is determined by an echocardiographic assessment of valve thickness, leaflet pliability, commissural calcification, and subvalvular disease. The presence of left atrial thrombus or more than 2+ MR usually contraindicates this procedure. Thus, PBMV is recommended for symptomatic class II–IV patients and patients with asymptomatic disease who have pulmonary hypertension (> 50 mm Hg at rest or > 60 mm Hg with exercise) and perhaps those with new-onset AF. This technique generally results in a doubling of the valve area and a 50% reduction in the mean gradient with excellent long-term results.

3. Surgery is indicated when PBMV is contraindicated or not feasible. This includes symptomatic class III–IV patients with an MVA < 1.5 cm^2, unfavorable valve morphology for PBMV, left atrial thrombus, MR, or a history of systemic thromboembolism from left atrial thrombus despite adequate anticoagulation. Generally, surgery is not indicated in patients with NYHA class I–II symptoms unless there is critical MS (MVA < 1 cm^2) with severe pulmonary hypertension (pulmonary artery systolic pressure > 60 mm Hg).

C. **Preoperative considerations**

1. Many patients with long-standing MS are cachectic and at increased risk of respiratory failure. Aggressive preoperative diuresis and nutritional supplementation may reduce morbidity in the early postoperative period.

2. Warfarin may be used for AF or the presence of left atrial thrombus. It should be stopped 4 days before surgery and the patient placed on heparin when the international normalized ratio (INR) falls below the therapeutic range (generally < 1.8) until the morning of surgery.

3. There is often a delicate balance between fluid overload, which can precipitate pulmonary edema, and aggressive diuresis, which can compromise renal function when the cardiac output is marginal. Thus, preload must be adjusted judiciously to ensure adequate LV filling across the stenotic valve. The ventricular response to AF must be controlled to prolong the diastolic filling period. Most patients are on digoxin for rate control, and this should be given up to the morning of surgery.

D. **Surgical procedures**

1. Closed mitral commissurotomy has been supplanted by PBMV, which produces similar results. Either should be considered in the pregnant patient with critical MS in whom CPB should be avoided.[82,83]

2. Traditional mitral valve operations have been performed through a median sternotomy incision. Other "minimal access" approaches, such as an upper sternotomy incision (using the "superior" approach to the valve between the aorta and superior vena cava [SVC]), a right parasternal incision (using the biatrial transseptal approach), or a right anterolateral thoracotomy (using the posterior approach behind the interatrial septum), can also be considered. CPB can be established either directly through the chest or through the femoral vessels.

3. Open mitral commissurotomy is performed if PBMV is not considered feasible or there is evidence of left atrial thrombus. It produces better hemodynamics than either a PBMV or a closed commissurotomy.[83,84]

4. Mitral valve replacement is indicated if the valve leaflets are calcified and fibrotic or there is significant subvalvular fusion (Figure 1.10).

5. A Maze procedure should be considered in a patient with preoperative AF. Either a "cut and sew" Maze is performed or an energy source (cryo, microwave, radiofrequency) is delivered to well-defined areas to ablate this arrhythmia with fairly good success rates (see section XIV).[85,86]

6. A tricuspid valve ring should be considered for patients with 3–4+ TR, especially when the pulmonary vascular resistance is elevated. Although functional TR usually improves after left-sided surgery, a better clinical result will be obtained if a tricuspid annuloplasty is performed for significant TR.

VII. Mitral Regurgitation

A. **Pathophysiology.** Mitral regurgitation may result from abnormalities of the annulus (dilatation), valve leaflets (myxomatous change with redundancy and prolapse, leaflet defect or damage from endocarditis, leaflet shrinkage from rheumatic disease), chordae tendineae (rupture, elongation), or papillary muscles (rupture, ischemic dysfunction).

1. Acute MR usually results from myocardial ischemia or infarction with papillary muscle rupture, from endocarditis, or from idiopathic chordal rupture. Acute LV volume overload develops with a reduction in forward output and regurgitant flow into a small noncompliant left atrium. This may result in both cardiogenic shock and acute pulmonary edema.

2. Chronic MR is characterized by a progressive increase in compliance of the left atrium and ventricle, followed by progressive dilatation of the left ventricle. There is an increase in preload that increases overall stroke volume and maintains forward cardiac output. At the same time, there is a decrease in afterload due to ventricular unloading into the left atrium. Thus, ventricular function may be impaired despite a normal EF. Patients may remain asymptomatic well

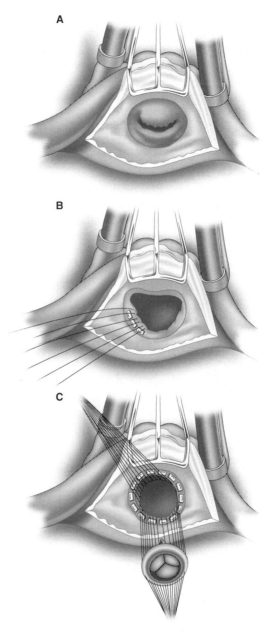

Figure 1.10 • Mitral valve replacement via the posterior approach. (A) The left atrium is opened behind the intraatrial groove and the retractor is positioned. Although both leaflets may be retained, the anterior leaflet is usually resected. (B) The posterior leaflet is retained and imbricated into the suture line. (C) Pledgetted mattress sutures are placed through the annulus, through or around the valve tissue, and into the sewing ring. The valve is then tied into position. The left atrial appendage may be sewn off from inside the left atrium.

after ventricular decompensation has occurred. Eventually, LV dysfunction becomes evident and is associated with progressive LV dilatation and elevated filling pressures. The progression of MR and assessment of LV dimensions and function should be followed by serial echocardiograms.

3. "Ischemic MR" may be acute or chronic. Acute MR may be the result of a mechanical complication, such as papillary muscle rupture, or it may be functional, due to ongoing ischemia. Chronic ischemic MR may develop following an MI from either annular dilatation caused by LV enlargement that prevents leaflet coaptation, or from papillary muscle displacement caused by LV remodeling that produces apical tethering of the leaflets.

B. Indications for surgery[62,77]

1. Acute MR associated with CHF or cardiogenic shock.

2. Acute endocarditis with hemodynamic compromise, persistent bacteremia or sepsis, annular abscess, recurrent systemic embolization from vegetations, or threatened embolization from large vegetations.

3. NYHA class II–IV symptoms with severe (3–4+) MR independent of EF (although high risk with EF < 25%).

4. Asymptomatic/class I patients should be considered for surgery in any of the following circumstances when severe MR is present:

   a. EF < 60%

   b. End-systolic dimension > 45 mm (even if EF > 60%)

   c. Preserved LV function with atrial fibrillation or pulmonary artery (PA) systolic pressure > 50 mm Hg at rest or > 60 mm Hg with exercise

   d. Subnormal right ventricular EF at rest

5. Earlier operation can be recommended when the likelihood of mitral valve repair is high. This is particularly true in patients with preserved LV function or recent-onset AF.

6. Mitral regurgitation present at the time of coronary surgery has been shown in some, but not all, studies to adversely affect long-term prognosis. However, it should generally be repaired if it is 2+ or greater.[87–89]

C. Preoperative considerations

1. Patients with acute MR are susceptible to pulmonary edema and multisystem organ failure from a reduced forward cardiac output. Use of inotropes, vasodilators, and the IABP can transiently improve myocardial function and forward flow in anticipation of urgent cardiac catheterization and surgery. Intubation and mechanical ventilation are frequently required for progressive hypoxia or hypercarbia. Diuretics must be used judiciously to improve pulmonary edema while not creating prerenal azotemia. Some patients with chordal rupture who present with acute pulmonary edema may stabilize and develop chronic MR that can be managed electively.

2. Patients with chronic MR are treated with digoxin, diuretics, and oral unloading agents, such as the ACE inhibitors. These medications should be continued up to the time of surgery.

3. Adequate preload must be maintained to ensure forward output while carefully monitoring the patient for evidence of CHF. Systemic hypertension should be avoided because it will increase the amount of regurgitant flow. If the patient has ischemic MR or a borderline cardiac output, use of systemic vasodilators or an IABP generally improves forward flow.

4. Left ventriculography may quantitate the degree of MR inaccurately, depending on catheter position, the amount and force of contrast injection, the size of the left atrium, and the presence of arrhythmias. Echocardiography, preferably by the transesophageal approach, should be used to better determine the degree and nature of MR. The latter is invaluable to the surgeon in helping to determine whether a valve can be repaired, what type of repair might be performed, or whether replacement is indicated from the outset.

5. There is often a discrepancy between the degree of mitral regurgitation identified preoperatively in the awake patient and that assessed under general anesthesia with an alteration in systemic resistance and loading conditions. Thus, preoperative transesophageal echocardiography (TEE) is essential to quantitate the degree of MR and define the precise anatomic mechanism for the MR.

D. Surgical procedures

1. Mitral valve reconstruction is applicable to more than 90% of patients with degenerative MR. Techniques include annuloplasty rings, leaflet repairs, and chordal transfers and replacement (Figure 1.11).[90–92] These reparative techniques can also be applied to patients with mitral valve endocarditis.[93] The decision to repair or

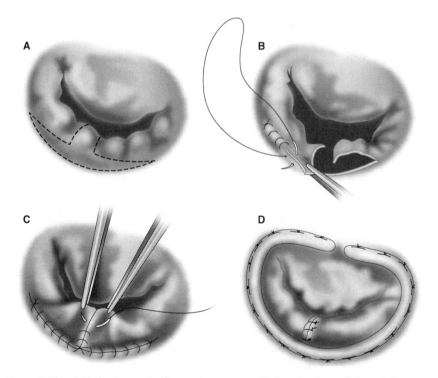

Figure 1.11 • Mitral valve repair. The most common pathology involves a flail posterior mitral leaflet. (A) A quadrangular excision is made as indicated by the dotted lines and the flail segment is resected. The remaining leaflet tissue may be incised along the annulus. (B) It is then advanced and reattached to the annulus ("sliding plasty"). (C) The leaflet tissue is then approximated, and (D) an annuloplasty ring is placed.

replace a valve for ischemic MR can be difficult and depends on an understanding of the pathophysiology of the MR and patient-related factors.[94-97]

2. Mitral valve replacement is indicated when satisfactory repair cannot be accomplished. Acute MR from papillary muscle rupture usually requires mitral valve replacement. Chordal preservation of at least the posterior leaflet should be considered for all mitral valve replacements performed for MR. This improves ventricular function and minimizes the risk of LV rupture.

VIII. Tricuspid Valve Disease

A. **Pathophysiology.** Isolated tricuspid stenosis (TS) is very rare, but tricuspid regurgitation (TR) is commonly seen on a functional basis secondary to mitral valve disease, which leads to pulmonary hypertension, RV dilatation, and tricuspid annular dilatation. RV systolic dysfunction contributes to elevated right atrial and systemic venous pressures, producing signs of right-sided heart failure. Atrial fibrillation is common. Forward output may also be reduced, resulting in fatigue and a low output state. TR may develop as a result of endocarditis, usually in association with intravenous drug abuse.

B. **Indications for surgery**

1. Repair of TS is indicated for class III–IV symptoms, including hepatic congestion, ascites, and peripheral edema that are refractory to salt restriction and diuretics.

2. Repair of TR is indicated for severe symptoms or when moderate to severe functional TR is present at the time of left-sided valve surgery. Repair is especially important if the pulmonary vascular resistance is elevated. It is indicated for severe TR if the mean PA pressure is less than 60 mm Hg and the patient is symptomatic after a trial of diuretic therapy.[62] Surgery is high risk if the mean PA pressure exceeds 60 mm Hg, especially in the absence of left-sided valvular disease.

3. Persistent sepsis or recurrent pulmonary embolization from tricuspid valve vegetations is an indication for surgery.

C. **Preoperative considerations**

1. Passive congestion of the liver frequently leads to coagulation abnormalities, which should be treated aggressively before and during surgery. Frequently, these patients have uncorrectable prothrombin times before surgery.

2. Salt restriction, digoxin, and diuretics may improve hepatic function, but significant improvement in liver function tests may not be possible until after surgery.

3. Maintenance of an elevated central venous pressure is essential to achieve satisfactory forward flow. A normal sinus mechanism provides better hemodynamics than AF, although the latter is frequently present. Slower heart rates are preferable for TS and faster heart rates for TR.

D. **Surgical procedures**

1. Tricuspid commissurotomy can be performed for rheumatic TS.

2. Tricuspid annuloplasty with a ring (Carpentier) or suture technique (DeVega or bicuspidization) is feasible for the majority of patients with annular dilatation (Figure 1.12).[98]

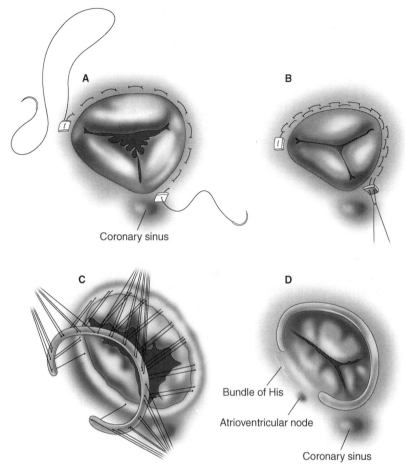

Figure 1.12 • Tricuspid valve repair involves reduction of annular dilatation to correct functional tricuspid regurgitation. (A, B) The circumferential suturing technique ("DeVega" repair). (C, D) Placement of an annuloplasty ring. Note the location of the coronary sinus and the proximity of the conduction system to the repair.

3. Tricuspid valve replacement is necessary when leaflet shrinkage and poor coaptation prevent an annuloplasty technique from eliminating the TR. Biologic valves are preferred, not just due to concerns about thromboembolism on mechanical valves in the right side of the heart, but also because long-term survival after tricuspid valve replacement is suboptimal, especially in patients with multivalvular disease (about 60% 5-year survival).[99,100]

4. Due to the necessity of placing sutures near the conduction system, patients are more prone to developing heart block after tricuspid valve surgery. If there are concerns that permanent pacing may be required, epicardial pacing leads should be placed on the right ventricle, pacing and sensing thresholds determined, and

the pacing leads buried in a subcutaneous pocket for later attachment to a permanent pacemaker.

5. The management of tricuspid valve endocarditis is noted below.

IX. Endocarditis

A. **Pathophysiology.** Endocarditis can result in destruction of valve leaflets, invasion of surrounding myocardial tissue, systemic embolization of valve vegetations, or persistent systemic sepsis. Tricuspid valve endocarditis is usually caused by intravenous drug abuse. The incidence of prosthetic valve endocarditis (PVE) is approximately 0.5% per patient-year for mechanical mitral valves and 1.0% per patient-year for all other valves except homografts.[101]

B. **Indications for surgery in native valve endocarditis**

1. Presence of moderate to severe CHF

2. Worsening renal or pulmonary function after initial improvement

3. Persistent bacteremia despite adequate antibiotic therapy

4. Evidence of local extension producing annular or myocardial abscesses, conduction disturbances, or intracardiac fistulas

5. Second episode of systemic embolization. Large (> 1.5 cm) or enlarging vegetations with threatened embolization may also be considered a relative indication for surgery.[102] It has been shown that vegetations caused by *Staphylococcus aureus* that are larger than 1 cm and involve the mitral valve tend to embolize.[103]

C. **Indications for surgery in PVE**[101,104]

1. All of the above

2. Fungal PVE

3. Valvular dysfunction or dehiscence (unstable prosthesis or perivalvular leak)

4. New onset of heart block

5. Relative indications: early-onset PVE, nonstreptococcal organism, relapse following completion of therapy, culture-negative PVE with persistent fever

D. **Preoperative considerations**

1. TEE is the gold standard for the diagnosis of endocarditis. It can be used to identify and quantify the size of vegetations, detect annular destruction, and identify valvular abnormalities.[105]

2. A 6-week course of antibiotics should ideally be completed before surgery to reduce the risk of PVE. However, surgery is more commonly indicated at an earlier phase due to one of the indications listed above. The appropriate antibiotics should then be continued for a total course of 6 weeks. The risk of PVE is significantly greater (around 10%) if surgery is performed during the phase of active endocarditis (i.e., prior to completing the 6-week course).

3. Attempts should be made to optimize hemodynamic and renal status before operation, but surgery should not be delayed if there is evidence of progressive organ system deterioration.

4. If the patient has developed a neurologic deficit from a cerebral embolism, surgery can be performed safely as long as a CT scan does not demonstrate a hemorrhagic infarction. However, an increase in cerebral edema in an area of extensive infarction could ensue if surgery is performed too soon after a stroke has occurred.

5. Patients with aortic valve endocarditis may have evidence of heart block from involvement of the conduction system by periannular infection. This may require preoperative placement of a transvenous pacing wire.

E. **Surgical procedures**

1. Surgery entails excision of all infected valve tissue, drainage and debridement of abscess cavities, and repair or replacement of the damaged valves. An aortic valve homograft is the valve of choice because of its increased resistance to infection and adaptability to disrupted tissue in the aortic root.[77] Homograft replacement is technically quite complex and many surgeons are not experienced in their placement. Furthermore, appropriately sized homografts may not be immediately available. Aortic valve replacement with either mechanical or tissue valves is a satisfactory alternative.[106,107] The risk of PVE on tissue or mechanical valves is fairly comparable.

2. Mitral endocarditis can frequently be repaired, especially if leaflet perforation is the primary pathology.[93] More advanced stages of endocarditis usually require valve replacement.

3. Tricuspid valve repair is recommended if there is single leaflet involvement.[108] If repair cannot be accomplished, tricuspid valvulectomy can be performed in patients without pulmonary hypertension with few adverse hemodynamic sequelae.[109] Otherwise, a tricuspid valve should be placed. The decision whether or not to place a prosthetic valve is controversial, especially in drug addicts. One must weigh the relative risks of hemodynamic compromise against the high risk of PVE if the patient continues intravenous drug abuse.

X. Hypertrophic Obstructive Cardiomyopathy

A. **Pathophysiology**. Septal hypertrophy and mitral septal-apposition (systolic anterior motion, or SAM) that produce dynamic LV outflow tract obstruction are present to varying degrees in patients with hypertrophic obstructive cardiomyopathy (HOCM). Symptoms of CHF are usually caused by diastolic dysfunction and may be present with or without outflow tract obstruction. Angina is usually related to abnormal coronary microvasculature and inadequate capillary density for the degree of hypertrophy. Atrial fibrillation may develop due to left atrial enlargement in 20–25% of patients. The risk of sudden death is estimated at 1%/yr but may be increased in patients with any of the following risk factors: a history of cardiac arrest, sustained ventricular tachycardia (VT) or repetitive prolonged bursts of nonsustained VT, a family history of premature HOCM-related death, syncope, a hypotensive blood pressure response to exercise, or extreme LVH with wall thickness greater than 30 mm.[110-112]

B. **Indications for intervention**

1. No pharmacologic regimen has been shown conclusively to reduce the risk of sudden death. Therefore, medications are used to alleviate symptoms, usually those of CHF. β-blockers should be initiated along with disopyramide (if outflow tract obstruction) or verapamil (if no obstruction). β-blockers will mitigate the gradient and alleviate symptoms in most patients.

2. ICD placement should be considered in patients at high risk for sudden death (as noted above).

3. Biventricular pacing with a short atrioventricular delay to ensure complete ventricular-paced activation is effective in reducing the gradient by approximately

50% and in improving symptoms. It may be beneficial in elderly patients, but symptomatic relief in younger patients has not been shown to correlate with documented improvement in exercise tolerance.

4. Further intervention is indicated in patients with a peak gradient > 50 mm Hg and persistent symptoms despite medications. It may also be considered in patients with asymptomatic disease who are considered to be at high risk for sudden death, including younger patients and those with a peak gradient > 80 mm Hg.

5. Alcohol septal ablation may prove to be an alternative for patients with medically refractory symptoms. It has been demonstrated to initially reduce LV ejection acceleration, and subsequently to reduce basal septal thickness, enlarge the LV outflow tract, and decrease SAM. It is associated with a number of complications, especially the need for a permanent pacemaker, and the long-term results are not known.

C. Preoperative considerations

1. Measures that produce hypovolemia or vasodilatation must be avoided because they increase the outflow tract gradient. Volume infusions should be used to maintain preload with the use of α-agonists to maintain systemic resistance.

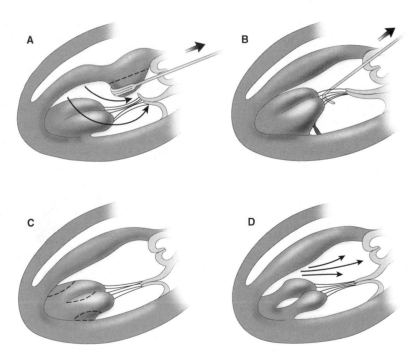

Figure 1.13 • (A) Hypertrophic obstructive cardiomyopathy is characterized by septal hypertrophy which orients the outflow jet into the anterior leaflet of the mitral valve, producing systolic anterior motion (SAM). An extensive septal myectomy is performed, often requiring a midventricular resection. (B, C) Using a nerve hook to provide traction, the atypical attachments of hypertrophied anomalous papillary muscles are partially detached from the ventricular wall and trimmed. (D) After this procedure, the outflow jet is directed more anteriorly.

2. Use of β-blockers and calcium channel blockers to reduce heart rate and contractility are the mainstay of medical management of HOCM and should be continued up to the time of surgery.

D. **Surgical procedures**

1. The traditional surgical approach of an LV myotomy-myomectomy entailed resection of a 1.5 × 4 cm wedge of septum below the right coronary aortic leaflet through an aortotomy incision.

2. With further understanding of the mechanism of SAM, the current operation of choice is an extended septal myectomy to the base of the papillary muscles, mobilization and partial excision of the papillary muscles off the ventricular wall to allow the papillary muscles to assume a more posterior position in the left ventricle, and anterior mitral leaflet plication if there is any redundancy. This reduces chordal and leaflet slack that can produce SAM (Figure 1.13).

3. Mitral valve replacement is indicated if the septal thickness is less than 18 mm, if there is atypical septal morphology, if there is significant MR, or if other procedures fail to relieve the outflow tract gradient.

XI. Aortic Dissections

A. **Pathophysiology.** An aortic dissection results from an intimal tear that allows passage of blood into the media, creating a false channel. This channel is contained externally by the outer medial and adventitial layers of the aorta. With each cardiac contraction, the dissected channel can extend proximally or distally. Depending on the location of the intimal tear and the extent of the dissection, potential complications include cardiac tamponade from hemopericardium (the most common cause of death), aortic regurgitation, myocardial infarction, stroke, intrapleural rupture, or branch artery compromise. The latter may involve the brachiocephalic vessels, causing stroke or discrepancy in upper extremity blood pressures, the intercostal vessels causing paraplegia, mesenteric or renal vessels compromising blood flow to the bowel or kidneys, or iliofemoral vessels reducing distal blood flow to the legs. Dissections involving the ascending aorta are classified as Stanford type A (DeBakey type I–II, or proximal), whereas those not involving the ascending aorta are called Stanford type B (DeBakey type III, or distal) dissections (Figure 1.14).[113–115] The dissection is termed acute when it is diagnosed within 2 weeks of onset; otherwise, it is termed chronic.

B. **Indications for surgery**

1. **Type A dissection**: Surgery is indicated for all patients unless it is considered to carry a prohibitive risk because of medical debility; extensive renal, myocardial, or bowel infarction; or massive stroke. Surgery is also indicated for virtually all patients with chronic type A dissections.

2. **Type B dissections**: Patients with uncomplicated type B dissections are usually treated medically, with surgery reserved for complicated dissections (i.e., patients with persistent pain, uncontrollable hypertension, evidence of aneurysmal expansion or rupture, or visceral, renal, or lower extremity vascular compromise). Centers with extensive experience in thoracic aortic surgery are operating more routinely on low-risk candidates with acute type B dissections with low mortality and excellent long-term results. Chronic type B dissections should be operated upon when they reach 6–6.5 cm in diameter.[116]

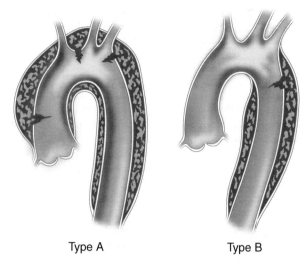

Type A   Type B

Figure 1.14 • Classification of aortic dissection. Type A dissections involve the ascending aorta. Type B dissections usually originate distal to the left subclavian artery and do not involve the ascending aorta. If they do extend retrograde, they are then considered type A dissections.

C. Preoperative considerations

1. Upon suspicion of the diagnosis, all patients must be treated pharmacologically to reduce the blood pressure (to about 110 mm Hg systolic), the force of cardiac ejection (dp/dt) and the heart rate (to 60–70/min). The patient should be carefully monitored and must undergo diagnostic testing as soon as possible to establish or exclude the diagnosis.

2. Recommended antihypertensive regimens include sodium nitroprusside with a β-blocker (esmolol or metoprolol), or just a β-blocker (esmolol, metoprolol, or labetalol) (see Table 11.7 for dosages). Aggressive management up to the time of surgery is essential to prevent rupture.

3. A careful pulse examination may indicate the extent of the dissection. Particular attention should be paid to the carotid, radial, and femoral pulses. Differential upper extremity blood pressures in a young patient with chest pain is a strong clue to the presence of a dissection.

4. A detailed preoperative neurologic examination is essential because a deficit recognized postoperatively may have been present at the time of presentation. A change in neurologic status may indicate progressive compromise of cerebral perfusion that can resolve with emergency surgery. Evidence of renal dysfunction (rising BUN or creatinine, oliguria) or bowel ischemia (abdominal pain, acidosis) may necessitate modification of the surgical approach. Recurrent chest or back pain usually indicates extension, expansion, or rupture of the dissection.

5. Dissections can be diagnosed by a variety of techniques.

   a. TEE has become the gold standard for identifying intimal flaps, evidence of tamponade, and aortic insufficiency. However, this must be performed **very**

cautiously because sedation may lead to hypotension in a patient with a pericardial effusion, and acute hypertension due to inadequate sedation could precipitate rupture. Transthoracic echocardiography may be valuable in ruling out a significant effusion before proceeding with a TEE.

  b. When TEE is not immediately available, CT scanning with contrast should be performed first. It is the most commonly performed screening test for aortic dissection in smaller hospitals to which many patients present before being transferred to an open-heart surgery center.

  c. Magnetic resonance imaging (MRI) may be the most sensitive and specific diagnostic technique to identify a dissection, but only rarely can it be obtained on an emergency basis. Furthermore, there are usually limitations to its performance in a patient requiring careful monitoring and intravenous drug infusions.

  d. Due to the availability and reliability of echocardiography and CT as initial tests for the diagnosis of aortic dissection, there is currently little role for aortography in the evaluation of an acute dissection unless there is a need to define branch vessel perfusion in the abdomen.

  e. Because of the surgical urgency of an acute type A dissection, coronary arteriography is rarely done.[117] Furthermore, catheter manipulation in the proximal ascending aorta is fraught with danger. A confusing picture that may lead to coronary angiography is myocardial ischemia due to compromise of the coronary ostia by the dissection. In contrast, coronary angiography and aortography are helpful in planning surgical strategy in patients with chronic dissections.

D. Surgical procedures

  1. Type A dissection. Repair involves resuspension or replacement of the aortic valve (if AR is present), resection of the intimal tear, and interposition graft replacement to reapproximate the aortic wall (Figure 1.15).[118] Biologic glue (preferably BioGlue) can be used to improve tissue integrity for grafting.[119] If the root is destroyed and cannot be reconstructed, a Bentall procedure (valved conduit) is performed. Repair of type A dissections is usually performed during a period of deep hypothermic circulatory arrest (see section XII.E). The complex situation of the type A dissection with a tear in the descending aorta can be managed by an initial repair via a median sternotomy leaving an elephant trunk for repair of the descending aorta.[120]

  2. Type B dissection. Repair involves resection of the intimal tear and interposition graft replacement to reapproximate the aortic wall.[121] The risk of paraplegia is greater in patients with dissections than with atherosclerotic aneurysms because less collateral flow is present. Thus, measures to reduce spinal cord ischemia by maintaining distal perfusion should be taken (see section XII.E). Visceral malperfusion may improve with restoration of flow into the true lumen. Otherwise a fenestration procedure should be performed to produce a communication between the true and false lumens in an attempt to improve organ system perfusion.[122] Percutaneous fenestration is a newer means of accomplishing this and may be beneficial in a patient with significant life-threatening malperfusion, thus obviating the need for thoracotomy and grafting. Endovascular stenting has become more common in the management of type B dissections.[123]

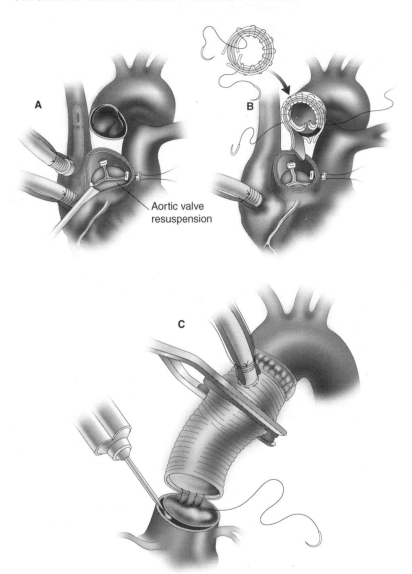

Figure 1.15 • Repair of a type A aortic dissection. (A) During circulatory arrest without aortic crossclamping, the aorta is opened and the entry site is resected. The aortic valve is resuspended. (B) The proximal and distal suture lines are fragile and are reinforced. Two felt strips are shown for the distal suture line, being placed inside the true lumen and outside the adventitia. (C) After the distal suture line is completed, the graft is cannulated to reestablish antegrade cardiopulmonary bypass flow with proximal application of a cross-clamp. BioGlue is injected to stabilize the proximal suture line, and the proximal graft anastomosis is performed.

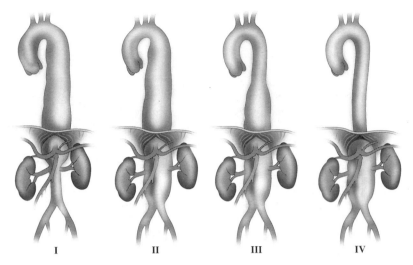

Figure 1.16 • Crawford classification of thoracoabdominal aneurysms.

XII. Thoracic Aortic Aneurysms

  A. Pathophysiology. Ascending aortic aneurysms usually result from medial degeneration, whereas those in the distal arch, descending thoracic aorta, and thoracoabdominal aorta are generally atherosclerotic in nature (Figure 1.16).[124] Aneurysms in any location may result from expansion of chronic dissections. Although progressive enlargement may result in compression of adjacent structures, most deaths result from aneurysmal rupture or dissection. Natural history studies have attempted to correlate the rupture rate of aneurysms based on their size so as to provide objective data on when surgery should be performed.[125–127]

  B. Indications for surgery

   1. Ascending aortic aneurysms

    a. Symptomatic, expanding, > 5 cm in diameter with Marfan's syndrome, or > 5.5 cm without Marfan's syndrome.[125,126]

    b. Aneurysms > 4.5–5 cm if operation is indicated for AS or AR ("annuloaortic ectasia"). Studies have shown that the risk of subsequent dissection is more than 20% if the aortic size exceeds 5 cm at the time of aortic valve replacement.[128] Resecting aneurysms that exceed 4 cm in diameter may be considered in patients undergoing surgery with bicuspid aortic valves.

    c. All acute type A dissections (as noted above)

    d. Mycotic aneurysms

   2. Transverse arch aneurysms

    a. Ascending aortic aneurysms that require replacement that also extend into the arch

    b. Acute arch dissections with an intimal tear in the arch or evidence of arch expansion or rupture

    c. Aneurysms > 5–6 cm in diameter

   3. **Descending thoracic and thoracoabdominal aneurysms** (see Figure 1.16 for classification)
      a. Symptomatic aneurysms
      b. Aneurysms > 6.5 cm in diameter (atherosclerotic or chronic dissections)
      c. Complicated acute type B dissections (uncomplicated if low risk patient)

C. **Preoperative considerations**
   1. Coronary angiography is required before surgery for ascending aortic and proximal arch aneurysms (not acute dissections). If significant coronary disease is present, it is bypassed at the time of the aneurysm resection.
   2. Myocardial perfusion stress imaging (dipyridamole-thallium or sestamibi) is indicated in patients with descending thoracic aneurysms because of the likelihood of coexistent CAD. If the scan is positive, coronary angiography should be performed. The presence of significant coronary disease usually warrants some form of intervention (PCI or CABG) to reduce the risk of cardiac complications associated with repair of the aneurysm.
   3. A careful preoperative baseline neurologic evaluation is important because of the risks associated with circulatory arrest (stroke, seizures) and aortic cross-clamping (paraplegia). A detailed informed consent discussion with the patient about these devastating complications is essential and must be documented.
   4. Pulmonary status must be optimized prior to surgery. Many patients with aneurysmal disease have concomitant chronic obstructive pulmonary disease, and the use of a thoracotomy incision, lung manipulation during surgery, anticoagulation, and multiple blood transfusions may have a detrimental effect on pulmonary function.
   5. Renal function must be monitored carefully after angiography, especially in diabetic patients. The creatinine should be allowed to return to baseline before surgery to reduce the risk of renal dysfunction associated with aortic cross-clamping.

D. **Surgical procedures**
   1. **Ascending aortic aneurysms**
      a. Supracoronary interposition graft placement is performed if the aneurysm does not involve the sinuses.
      b. A valved conduit (Bentall procedure) is placed in the patient with Marfan's syndrome, if the sinuses are involved, or for annuloaortic ectasia (see Figure 1.9).
      c. An aortic valve–sparing operation can be performed for ascending aneurysms even if aortic insufficiency is present. The design of this procedure depends on the exact location of the aneurysm (whether it involves the sinuses or not) and the pathophysiology of aortic insufficiency.[129,130]
      d. CPB is required for repair of ascending aortic aneurysms. Depending on the site of the distal anastomosis, simple aortic cross-clamping or a period of deep hypothermic circulatory arrest may be necessary. Arterial access for CPB can be achieved through the femoral artery or the axillary artery if significant descending aortic atherosclerosis is present. For an arch repair, antegrade cerebral perfusion can be achieved through an axillary artery cannula after the arch vessels are attached.
      e. Adjuncts to improve cerebral protection during a period of circulatory arrest include thiopental or pentobarbital 5–10 mg/kg, methylprednisolone 30 mg/kg, packing the head in ice, and continuous retrograde perfusion of

the SVC or antegrade perfusion of the cerebral vessels.[131–133] The central core temperature should be lowered to 18°C at which time there is presumed to be electroencephalographic silence; this should provide 45–60 minutes of safe arrest with minimal risk of neurologic insult.

f. Profound hypothermia and warming are associated with a coagulopathy. Platelets, fresh frozen plasma, and cryoprecipitate are helpful in achieving hemostasis. Aprotinin is arguably helpful in reducing intraoperative bleeding in patients undergoing surgery with deep hypothermia, although there have been reports of adverse neurologic sequelae. Proponents of aprotinin believe it is safe as long as certain measures are taken. These include ensuring an adequate activated clotting time (ACT) (> 750–1000 seconds by kaolin ACT), giving additional heparin (1 mg/kg just prior to period of circulatory arrest), and stopping the infusion of aprotinin during the arrest period.[134,135] Alternatively, aprotinin may be started during the rewarming phase.

2. Transverse arch aneurysms

a. Hemiarch repair is performed if the ascending aorta and proximal arch are involved. A graft is sewn to the undersurface of the arch leaving the brachiocephalic vessels attached to the native aorta.

b. Extended arch repair involves placement of an interposition graft and reimplantation of a brachiocephalic island during a period of circulatory arrest. Alternatively, a trifurcation graft can be placed with individual anastomoses to the arch vessels. Retrograde or antegrade cerebral perfusion can be used to minimize the risk of cerebral complications during the period of deep hypothermic circulatory arrest.[131–133]

c. Distal arch repair can be performed via a left thoracotomy without CPB. Use of CPB and a period of circulatory arrest (through either a sternotomy or a thoracotomy incision) may be useful when additional exposure is required for the proximal anastomosis or when a difficult dissection is anticipated (reoperations).

d. If it is anticipated that a descending aortic repair may be necessary in the future, a piece of graft material is left dangling from the distal anastomosis and can be retrieved at a subsequent operation through the left chest (the "elephant trunk" procedure).[136]

3. Descending thoracic aorta

a. Graft replacement of the diseased aorta is performed with reimplantation of intercostals vessels at the level of T8–T12 for more extensive aneurysms. This is performed through a left thoracotomy or thoracoabdominal incision with use of one-lung anesthesia.

b. Consideration should be given to the use of adjuncts (medications, cerebrospinal fluid drainage, shunting) to prevent spinal cord ischemia during the period of aortic cross-clamping.[137,138] Shunting can be accomplished by draining blood from a site proximal to the aortic cross-clamp (inferior pulmonary vein/left atrium/proximal aorta) and returning it distally (distal aorta/femoral artery) to perfuse the spinal cord and kidneys. A Biomedicus centrifugal pump, which actively returns blood to the patient at a designated rate, can be used with or without oxygenation

c. Left-heart bypass alone has been shown to reduce the incidence of paraplegia during surgery for thoracoabdominal aneurysms, but not necessarily more limited descending thoracic aneurysms.[139,140] Alternatively, partial femorofemoral bypass can be used. Circulatory arrest using femorofemoral bypass is an excellent alternative to the above techniques when clamping is not possible due to extensive disease or calcification. This technique also provides visceral and spinal cord protection.[141]

d. Arterial monitoring lines are inserted in the right radial and the femoral artery to monitor proximal and distal pressures during the period of aortic cross-clamping, especially if left-heart bypass is used.

XIII. Ventricular Tachycardia and Sudden Death

A. Pathophysiology

1. Nonidiopathic ventricular tachycardia (VT) occurs in association with structural heart disease. It may be subdivided into ischemic and nonischemic etiologies.[142,143]

   a. Ischemic VT refers to VT that is caused by active ischemia, usually from a ruptured plaque, or from a previous MI. The latter results from heterogeneous myocardial damage that produces the electrophysiologic substrate for the development of a reentrant rhythm. This commonly occurs at the border zone of an LV aneurysm between dense subendocardial scar tissue and normal myocardium. Premature stimuli delivered during electrophysiologic testing may initiate an impulse that triggers the reentrant circuit of monomorphic VT ("inducible VT").

   b. Nonischemic VT may be the result of reentrant circuits or triggered automaticity. It is most commonly noted in patients with dilated cardiomyopathies and markedly depressed ventricular function, as well as less common entities such as arrhythmogenic RV dysplasia. In these conditions, the arrhythmogenic focus frequently cannot be adequately mapped and is difficult to ablate with catheter intervention.

2. Idiopathic VT occurs in the absence of structural heart disease and may arise along the RV outflow tract or in the left posterior fascicle of the left ventricle. It is usually caused by triggered activity related to a high adrenergic state. As such, it can be treated by medical therapy or, if that fails, by radiofrequency catheter ablation.

3. Out-of-hospital cardiac arrest (so-called sudden cardiac death) is estimated to be the first manifestation of coronary disease in 40% of patients, usually as a result of rupture of an unstable plaque. Other patients have no identifiable cause for such an event and may or may not have inducible arrhythmias. Numerous secondary-prevention studies have been carried out to identify the proper treatment for these patients.[144]

B. Interventional procedures and their indications[144,145]

1. ICD implantation is indicated in patients with:

   a. Cardiac arrest due to ventricular fibrillation (VF) or VT not due to a transient or reversible cause, such as documented myocardial ischemia that should initially be treated by CABG. Three secondary prevention trials (Antiarrhythmics Versus Implantable Defibrillator [AVID], Cardiac Arrest Study Hamburg [CASH], and Canadian Implantable Defibrillator Study [CIDS]) have shown reduction in mortality with ICDs compared with medical therapy, usually with amiodarone.

b. Spontaneous sustained VT with structural heart disease (usually a dilated cardiomyopathy with depressed ventricular function).

c. Syncope of undetermined origin if hemodynamically significant sustained VT or VF is inducible and drug therapy is ineffective, not tolerated, or not preferred.

d. Nonsustained VT in patients with coronary disease, previous MI, LV dysfunction (EF < 35%), and inducible VF or sustained VT at electrophysiologic study that is not suppressible with procainamide (Multicenter Automatic Defibrillator Implantation Trial [MADIT]). Note that patients were excluded from this trial if they were candidates for surgical revascularization.

e. Spontaneous sustained VT without structural heart disease (idiopathic VT) that is not amenable to medications or catheter ablation (which generally is 90% successful).

f. Patients with EF < 30% at least 1 month after MI and 3 months after CABG (MADIT II).[146] Note that these patients benefit from ICD without any electrophysiologic testing to assess for inducibility.

g. Note: There are no trials that have studied whether ICD placement is of benefit in patients with poor LV function who develop nonsustained VT within the first few weeks after a CABG, even if VT is inducible. However, it is intuitive, based on an understanding of the mechanism of reentrant circuits, that an ICD should benefit patients who are inducible for VT (extrapolation of the MADIT and MUSTT [Multicenter Unsustained Tachycardia Trial] results). The unresolved question is whether ICD implantation is indicated without electrophysiologic study in patients developing nonsustained VT within a few weeks of surgery.

h. Two additional indications are cardiac arrest presumed to be on the basis of VF when electrophysiologic testing cannot be performed and the development of severe symptoms (such as syncope) that may be attributable to ventricular tachyarrhythmias in a patient awaiting cardiac transplantation.

2. Blind endocardial resection should be performed when ischemic VT is present in a patient undergoing resection of an LV aneurysm. This has supplanted the map-guided surgery used through the mid-1990s that achieved success rates greater than 75% and reached 90% with the addition of medications. In high-risk patients with depressed ventricular function, one study showed that long-term survival was fairly similar with direct VT surgery or placement of an ICD, often with associated CABG.[147]

C. Preoperative considerations

1. A thorough preoperative evaluation should be undertaken to determine whether structural heart disease is present. Preliminary cardiac catheterization should be performed to ascertain whether myocardial revascularization is indicated. This may lower the risk of ICD implantation, and may also reduce the risk of recurrent VT if it was occurring on an ischemic basis.

2. Many patients with cardiomyopathies are maintained on warfarin, which must be held for several days to prevent bleeding into the ICD pocket. Infection developing in the pocket implies infection of the entire lead system and mandates its removal.[148] Prophylactic antibiotics are indicated.

3. Careful monitoring and provisions for cardiac resuscitation (trained personnel and equipment) are essential during ICD implantation.

D. Surgical procedures

1. Myocardial revascularization should be performed in the patient with reversible ischemia and bypassable anatomy. The role of PCI in such patients is undefined. Standard indications for ICD implantation, including electrophysiologic testing for inducibility, should then be followed.

2. The equipment for map-guided endocardial resection is no longer available, but blind endocardial resection should be performed at the time of aneurysm surgery. Aggressive resection of scar tissue, including that on the septum, with cryoablation at the periphery of the scar tissue and reconstruction of the ventricle by geometric remodeling (Dor procedure or SAVER, see page 13), which may also reduce inducibility, should be performed.[149]

3. ICD implantation is usually performed in the electrophysiology lab. The single chamber system consists of one RV lead that contains shocking coils that lie within the SVC and the right ventricle and bipolar sensing and pacing electrodes that lie within the ventricle. Dual-chamber systems provide ports for additional atrial or LV electrodes which can be used to perform atrioventricular sequential pacing, biventricular pacing, and antitachycardia pacing. The device is implanted in a prepectoral pocket. Testing of the leads for sensing and defibrillation thresholds is performed. The generator is then connected to the leads and the system is retested (Figure 1.17).

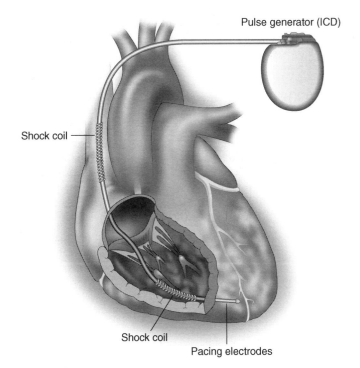

Pulse generator (ICD)

Shock coil

Shock coil

Pacing electrodes

Figure 1.17 • Transvenous ICD system. The single chamber system consists of one right ventricular lead that contains shocking coils that lie within the SVC and the right ventricle and bipolar sensing and pacing electrodes that lie within the ventricle.

4. Prior to the development of transvenous systems, ICD implantation was performed through left thoracotomy, median sternotomy, subcostal or subxiphoid approaches. Device replacement and removal of infected lead systems mandate an understanding of their implantation methods. These systems usually involved two rate-sensing electrodes placed into the right or left ventricular epicardium and two titanium mesh patches for defibrillation placed over the ventricles, either inside or outside the pericardium.

XIV. Atrial Fibrillation

A. Pathophysiology

1. Atrial fibrillation (AF) results from the presence of multiple reentrant circuits that prevent the synchronous activation of adequate atrial tissue to generate mechanical contraction. It is perpetuated by the variable refractoriness of atrial tissue to the generation of these circuits. Atrial distention may predispose to this arrhythmia, which then promotes progressive atrial dilatation and remodeling, leading to chronic AF. AF can lead to:

   a. Loss of atrioventricular (AV) synchrony, which reduces ventricular filling and stroke volume. This can produce dizziness, fatigue, and shortness of breath, especially when the ventricular rate is high.

   b. Thrombus formation in the left atrium with a predisposition to thromboembolism and stroke.

   c. Symptoms of an irregular heartbeat (palpitations).

   d. Cardiomyopathy if the rate is not controlled.

2. AF may occur as an isolated entity ("lone AF") in patients with no structural heart disease, in which case it may be chronic or paroxysmal. The latter usually lasts less than 48 hours in duration and the atrial foci that serve as the trigger are usually located in the tissue surrounding the pulmonary veins as they enter the left atrium. However, AF is more common in patients with hypertension or valvular heart disease, in whom the AF tends to be chronic rather than paroxysmal. The reentrant circuits usually originate from the left atrium.[150]

B. Management considerations

1. AF is managed with medications to control the ventricular rate (β-blockers, calcium channel blockers, digoxin) and to prevent thromboembolism (warfarin). When the rate cannot be controlled, symptoms are disabling, thromboembolism occurs on anticoagulation, or anticoagulation cannot be tolerated or is not desirable, surgery should be considered.

2. AF present when surgery is performed for other indications can be treated during the same operation.

3. In the absence of the above indications, surgery for AF is generally not indicated, although with the use of thoracoscopic approaches and advances in catheter ablation technology, the indications may expand to include patients with lone AF or those in whom the indications noted above are not present.

4. Paroxysmal AF arising from the pulmonary veins can be ablated successfully by transcatheter intervention in about 80% of cases.

C. Preoperative considerations

1. Procedures to correct AF may not be successful for several months. Therefore, medications used for rate control or for AF prophylaxis can be continued up to the time of surgery.

    2. Other considerations pertain to the specific lesion for which surgery is indicated if the AF surgery is being performed as an additional procedure.

D. Surgical procedures

    1. In 1986, Cox designed an operation called the "Maze" procedure, which was used to ablate AF, restore AV synchrony, and preserve atrial transport function. Early results of this technically complex procedure were encouraging with success rates of 90%, although 40% of patients required atrial pacemakers.[151]

    2. Because the original Maze operation was technically difficult, frequently associated with the inability to generate a sinus tachycardia in response to exercise, and associated with left atrial dysfunction, a modification called the Cox-Maze III operation was designed to address these issues.[152] The incisions not only interrupted the microreentrant circuits, but also allowed the sinus node to function and directed propagation of the sinus impulse through both atria. Sinus rhythm occurred more commonly than with previous operations, but 10% of patients still required pacemakers. Although this operation simplified the original Maze operation, it still was not widely adopted because the "cut and sew" technique was complex and time consuming.

    3. Various ablation technologies have now been developed to mimic the suture lines of the Cox-Maze III operation, including cryo-, radiofrequency, laser, and microwave ablation, all with fairly comparable results.[153–157] To achieve success, the lesions created must achieve transmurality. Since the left atrium is usually the primary focus of reentry, a left-sided Maze is most commonly performed.

    a. A left-sided Maze operation is usually performed in conjunction with mitral valve surgery (Figure 1.18). This procedure produces ablation lines that encircle and connect the right and left pulmonary veins, and one that

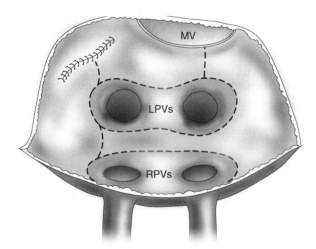

Figure 1.18 • The left-sided Maze involves ablation lines that encircle and connect the right and left pulmonary veins and one that extends from the left inferior pulmonary vein to the mitral valve annulus. The left atrial appendage is amputated and an additional ablation line extended from the base of the appendage to the left pulmonary veins.

extends from the inferior pulmonary vein to the mitral valve annulus. The left atrial appendage is usually amputated and an ablation line carried from the base of the appendage to the left pulmonary vein encircling line.

b. The right-sided Maze includes one incision extending from the base of the amputated right atrial appendage about 4 cm toward the IVC and another posterior longitudinal incision extending from just caudad to the SVC cannulation site toward the atrioventricular groove reaching the interatrial septum. Through this incision, the endocardium between the SVC and IVC is ablated (Figure 1.19A). Additional ablation lines extend from the base of the excised right atrial appendage to the anterior tricuspid valve leaflet, from the end of the longitudinal incision to the posterior tricuspid valve annulus, and from the middle of right atriotomy across the fossa ovalis up to the coronary sinus, down to the IVC, and then back to the tricuspid valve (Figure 1.19B).[156]

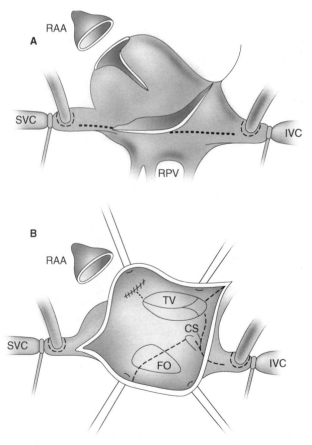

Figure 1.19 • (A) The right-sided Maze involves two incisions in the right atrial wall with an ablation line between the SVC and IVC cannulation sites. (B) Sites for endocardial ablation are shown by the dotted lines (see text).

XV. End-Stage Heart Failure

A. Pathophysiology

1. End-stage heart failure develops due to progressive deterioration in LV function associated with LV remodeling. The left ventricle dilates and changes from an elliptical to a spherical shape. This increases wall stress, which increases oxygen requirements, causes pathologic cardiomyocyte hypertrophy that further compromises contractile function, and induces functional MR. These changes lead to intractable heart failure. In addition, ventricular remodeling increases the tendency to develop ventricular arrhythmias.[158]

2. The prognosis for end-stage heart failure is very poor, with a markedly impaired quality of life and a limited life span. Clinical improvement and improved survival have been noted with use of ACE inhibitors, β-blockers, and spironolactone, but in the absence of revascularization, annual mortality rates exceed 12%/year.[159,160] Thus, alternative strategies are essential to treat this growing segment of the population.

B. Indications for surgery and surgical procedures. A variety of surgical procedures can be utilized to treat patients with end-stage heart failure, depending on the pathophysiology of their disease.

1. Coronary bypass surgery should be performed in patients with ischemic hibernating myocardium. This can improve anginal symptoms, in many cases improve ventricular function, lower the risk of sudden cardiac death, and improve survival.[160,161]

2. Mitral valve repair with a small annuloplasty ring can be offered to patients with severe MR to promote reverse remodeling, restore normal geometric relationships, and alleviate symptoms of CHF.[162]

3. Cardiac resynchronization (atrial-synchronized biventricular pacing) has been demonstrated to improve heart failure symptoms and exercise tolerance, and to promote reverse remodeling. It increases LV filling time, decreases septal dyskinesis, and may reduce MR.[163,164]

4. Procedures that reduce the size of the left ventricle or limit its expansion may reduce wall stress with the expectation that alleviation of CHF symptoms will result.

   a. LV reconstructive procedures can be used for patients with areas of akinesis or dyskinesis subsequent to an MI. Myocardial revascularization, resection of nonfunctioning tissue, and restoration of more normal size and shape result in a decrease in ventricular volume and an improvement in EF and apical geometry. These procedures, including the Dor and SAVER procedures noted in section II.D, can be performed with moderately low risk, producing symptomatic improvement and an increase in long-term survival.[52]

   b. The Batista operation or left ventriculectomy was popularized in the late 1990s but has since been abandoned. However, it conceptually brought to light the concept of improving ventricular contractile efficiency by reducing ventricular volume.

   c. Techniques and devices that prevent ventricular dilatation, such as a cardiomyoplasty, the Acorn restraint device, and the Myocor myosplint, which tethers the anterior and posterior walls together, are being investigated as means of improving symptoms of CHF. These have been shown to reduce end-diastolic dimensions, reduce wall stress, improve EF, and reduce MR.[158,165–167]

5. When the patient has advanced heart failure and is not a candidate for any of the above procedures, cardiac transplantation should be considered. Patients with end-stage heart failure with an EF < 15% and MvO_2 < 10 mL/min/m² are generally considered to be candidates for transplantation.

    a. Insertion of a left ventricular assist device (LVAD) should be considered when a patient develops progressive hemodynamic deterioration despite use of maximal pharmacologic therapy and an IABP. This can provide adequate bridging to transplantation.[168–171]

    b. An LVAD may be used as destination therapy when a patient is not considered to be a transplantation candidate.[172] As of late 2004, only the Thoratec VE HeartMate device was approved for this use, but centrifugal pumps and several devices using axial flow technology have been under investigation for years for bridging and potential destination therapy (see pages 383–387).

6. Muscle and stem cell transplantation into areas of infarcted myocardium are being investigated as a means of improving ventricular function.[173,174]

XVI. Pericardial Disease

A. **Pathophysiology.** The pericardium may become involved in a variety of systemic disease processes that produce either pericardial effusions or constriction. The most common causes of effusions are idiopathic (probably viral), malignant, uremic, pyogenic, and tuberculous. The most common causes of constriction are idiopathic, radiation, and tuberculous. Early and late postoperative cardiac tamponade due to hemopericardium are discussed on pages 283 and 524.

1. Large effusions result in tamponade physiology with progressive low output states.[175] They are best documented by two-dimensional echocardiography, which delineates their size and provides hemodynamic evidence of tamponade. Findings include right atrial and ventricular diastolic collapse, increased reversal of flow in the hepatic veins during atrial systole, a dilated IVC with lack of inspiratory collapse, and decreased SVC flow during diastole.[176] Equilibration of intracardiac pressures (RVEDP = PCWP = LVEDP) will be detected by cardiac catheterization.

2. Constriction can also produce a low output state despite preserved systolic function. Cardiac catheterization will demonstrate a "square-root sign" in the RV tracing, indicating rapid early filling and a diastolic plateau caused by severe impairment of RV filling (see Figure 1.20). CT scanning can be done to assess the thickness of the pericardium. The differentiation of constriction, which is surgically correctable, from restriction, which is not, can be difficult because they have many findings in common. Although restrictive pathology is associated with diastolic dysfunction, it may or may not be associated with systolic dysfunction. However, the presence of significant pulmonary hypertension suggests a restrictive process, since it is rarely seen with constriction.[177,178]

B. **Indications for surgery[179]**

1. Large effusions that fail to respond to noninvasive measures (dialysis for uremia, antibiotics for infection, radiation or chemotherapy for malignancy, thyroid replacement for myxedema) may be treated by pericardiocentesis and percutaneous catheter drainage or by percutaneous balloon pericardiostomy.[180]

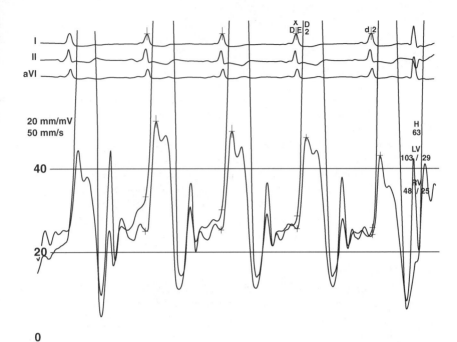

Figure 1.20 • Simultaneous right and left ventricular pressure tracings in constrictive pericarditis. Note the "dip-and-plateau" pattern as diastolic filling of the ventricular chambers is abruptly truncated by the constriction. Not also the equilibration of diastolic ventricular pressures. *(Reproduced with permission from Myers RBH, Spodick DH. Constrictive pericarditis: clinical and pathophysiologic characteristics. Am Heart J 1999;138:219–32.)*

    If these measures cannot be performed or the effusion recurs, a surgical drainage procedure should be performed.

  2. Constriction that produces a refractory low output state, hepatomegaly, or peripheral edema should be treated by a pericardiectomy. Lesser degrees of constriction may resolve spontaneously or respond to a course of nonsteroidal antiinflammatory medications or steroids.

C. Preoperative considerations

  1. The progressive development of cardiac tamponade frequently leads to renal dysfunction and hepatic congestion, and neither problem will improve until drainage is accomplished. Fresh frozen plasma should be available if there is a preexisting coagulopathy.

  2. Tamponade and constriction are associated with low cardiac output states. Intrinsic compensatory mechanisms to maintain blood pressure and cardiac output include a tachycardia and increased sympathetic tone. Maintenance of adequate preload is essential to increase cardiac output. Use of β-blockers and vasodilators must be avoided.

  3. Patients with low output states from severe constriction may benefit from a few days of inotropic support prior to surgery.[181]

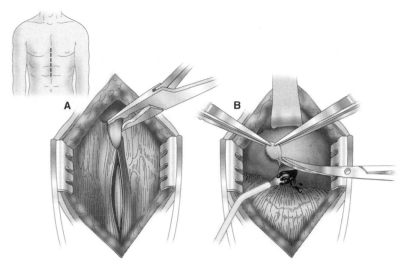

Figure 1.21 • The subxiphoid approach to pericardial disease. (A) An incision is made over the xiphisternal junction extending inferiorly for 5 cm. The rectus fascia is incised and the xiphoid process is removed. (B) With upward traction on the distal sternum, the preperitoneal fat is swept away. The pericardium is grasped and incised and a small specimen may be removed. A finger is insinuated to break up any loculations, and pericardial fluid is aspirated with a suction catheter. One or two chest tubes are then placed within the pericardium.

4. Preliminary pericardiocentesis for very large effusions improves the safety of anesthetic induction, which can produce vasodilatation, a fall in filling pressures, and profound hypotension.

D. Surgical procedures

1. Percutaneous catheter drainage with a pigtail catheter should be the initial procedure for a large pericardial effusion. Echocardiography is helpful in localizing the effusion and determining whether it is easily accessible to a percutaneous needle or not.[182–184] If the effusion recurs, especially in patients with malignant effusions, consideration may be given to instilling a sclerosing agent into the pericardium to prevent reaccumulation of fluid (doxycycline, bleomycin, thiotepa).[185,186]

2. A subxiphoid pericardiostomy opens the pericardium, drains the pericardial space, allows for obtaining a small biopsy specimen, and obliterates the pericardial space by promoting the formation of adhesions with several days of chest tube drainage (Figure 1.21). It is the safest surgical approach in the unstable patient and the best for patients with malignancies and a limited life span. Studies have shown that the recurrence rate for an effusion is significantly less with this procedure than with percutaneous catheter drainage.[183,184] A modification of this technique may allow for drainage of pericardial fluid into the peritoneal cavity.[187]

3. A pericardial window, created with a balloon technique,[180] limited thoracotomy, or a thoracoscopic approach[188] can be used to drain the effusion into the pleural space and obtain a biopsy specimen. The latter two procedures require general

anesthesia and are best utilized when there is suspicion of underlying pleuropulmonary pathology. Although recurrence rates are low, the pericardial window may seal as the adjacent lung becomes adherent to the surrounding tissues.

4. Pericardiectomy is best performed through a median sternotomy approach with pump standby.[181,189] The pericardium is removed to within 2 cm of the phrenic nerves on either side, or at least as far as exposure allows. Dissection of the aorta and pulmonary arteries should be performed first, followed by the left and then the right ventricle to avoid pulmonary edema. If severe epicardial constriction is present with no dissection plane, a "waffle" procedure is performed, which entails multiple criss-crossing incisions in the scar tissue to optimize ventricular expansion and filling. When dense, calcific adhesions are present without a cleavage plane, use of CPB may allow for a safer dissection, although bleeding may be increased due to the need for systemic heparinization. It is frequently prudent to leave heavily calcified areas adherent to the heart to minimize bleeding and pericardial damage.

References

1. Yeghiazarians Y, Braunstein JB, Askari A, Stone PH. Unstable angina pectoris. N Engl J Med 2000;342:101–14.
2. Foody JM, Nissen SE. Effectiveness of statins in acute coronary syndromes. Am J Cardiol 2001;88(suppl):31F–5.
3. Antman EM, Anbe DT, Armstrong PW, et al. ACC/AHA guidelines for the management of patients with ST-elevation myocardial infarction—executive summary. A report of the American College of Cardiology/American Heart Association task force on practice guidelines (writing committee to revise the 1999 guidelines for the management of patients with acute myocardial infarction. J Am Coll Cardiol 2004;44:671–719.
4. Andersen HR, Nielsen TT, Rasmussen K, et al. A comparison of coronary angioplasty with fibrinolytic therapy in acute myocardial infarction. N Engl J Med 2003;349:733–42.
5. Braunwald E, Antman EM, Beasley JW et al. ACC/AHA 2002 guideline update for the management of patients with unstable angina and non–ST-segment elevation myocardial infarction–summary article. A report of the American College of Cardiology/American Heart Association task force on practice guidelines (Committee on the management of patients with unstable angina). J Am Coll Cardiol 2002;40:1366–74 and Circulation 2002;106:1893–1900.
6. Roe MT, Staman KL, Pollack C, Teaff R, French PA, Peterson ED. A practical guide to understanding the 2002 ACC/AHA guidelines for the management of patients with non–ST segment elevation acute coronary syndromes. Crit Path Cardiol 2002;1:129–49.
7. Topol EJ. A guide to therapeutic decision-making in patients with non–ST-segment elevation acute coronary syndromes. J Am Coll Cardiol 2003;41:123S–9.
8. Jneid H, Bhatt DL, Corti R, Badimon JJ, Fuster V, Francis CS. Aspirin and clopidogrel in acute coronary syndromes: therapeutic insights from the CURE trial. Arch Intern Med 2003;26:1145–53.
9. Cohen M, Demers C, Gurfinkel EP, et al. A comparison of low-molecular weight heparin with unfractionated heparin for unstable coronary artery disease. N Engl J Med 1997;337:447–52.
10. Wong GC, Giugliano RP, Antman EM. Use of low-molecular weight heparins in the management of acute coronary syndromes and percutaneous coronary intervention. JAMA 2003;289:331–42.
11. Mahoney EM, Jurkoitz C, Chu N, et al. Cost and cost-effectiveness of an early invasive vs. conservative strategy for the treatment of unstable angina and non–ST-segment elevation myocardial infarction. JAMA 2002;288:1851–58.
12. Eagle KA, Guyton RA, Davidoff R, et al. ACC/AHA guidelines for coronary artery bypass graft surgery. A report of the American College of Cardiology/American Heart Association Task Force on Practice Guidelines (Committee to revise the 1991 guidelines for coronary artery bypass graft surgery). J Am Coll Cardiol 1999;34:1262–347.
13. Moses JW, Leon MB, Popma JJ, et al. Sirolimus-eluting stents versus standard stents in patients with stenosis in a native coronary artery. N Engl J Med 2003;349:1315–23.
14. Stone GW, Ellis SG, Cox DA, et al. A polymer-based, paclitaxel-eluting stent in patients with coronary artery disease. N Engl J Med 2004;350:221–31.
15. Serruys PA, Unger F, Sousa JE, et al. Comparison of coronary-artery bypass surgery and stenting for the treatment of multivessel disease. N Engl J Med 2001;314:1117–24.
16. Steinhubl ST, Berger PB, Mann III JT, et al. Early and sustained dual oral antiplatelet therapy following percutaneous coronary intervention. A randomized controlled trial. JAMA 2002; 288:2411–20.
17. Kiyama H, Ohshima N, Imazeki T, Yamada T. Autologous blood donation with recombinant human erythropoietin in anemic patients. Ann Thorac Surg 1999;68:1652–6.
18. Karkouti KM, McClusky S. Pro: preoperative autologous blood donation has a role in cardiac surgery. J Cardiothorac Vasc Anesth 2003;17:121–5.
19. ten Broecke PW, De Hert SG, Mertens E, Adriaensen HF. Effect of preoperative beta-blockade on perioperative mortality in coronary surgery. Br J Anaesth 2003;90:27–31.
20. Ferguson TB, Coombs LP, Peterson ED. Preoperative beta-blocker use and mortality and morbidity following CABG surgery in North America. JAMA 2002;287:2221–7.
21. Kincaid EH, Monroe ML, Saliba DL, Kon ND, Byerly WG, Richert MG. Effects of preoperative enoxaparin versus unfractionated heparin on bleeding indices in patients undergoing coronary artery bypass grafting. Ann Thorac Surg 2003;76:124–8.

22. Ereth MH, Nuttall GA, Orszulak TA, Santrach PJ, Cooney WP IV, Oliver WC Jr. Blood loss from coronary angiography increases transfusion requirements for coronary artery bypass graft surgery. J Cardiothorac Vasc Anesth 2000;14:177–81.

23. www.STS.org/database.

24. Sethi GK, Copeland JG, Goldman S, Moritz T, Zadina K, Henderson WG. Implications of preoperative administration of aspirin in patients undergoing coronary artery bypass grafting. J Am Coll Cardiol 1990;15:15–20.

25. Ferraris VA, Ferraris SP, Lough FC, Berry WR. Preoperative aspirin ingestion increases operative blood loss after coronary artery bypass grafting. Ann Thorac Surg 1988;45:71–4.

26. Tuman KJ, McCarthy RJ, O'Connor CJ, McCarthy WE, Ivankovich AD. Aspirin does not increase allogeneic blood transfusions in reoperative coronary artery surgery. Anesth Analg 1996;83:1178–84.

27. Reich DL, Patel GC, Vela-Cantos F, Bodian C, Lansman S. Aspirin does not increase homologous blood requirements in elective coronary bypass surgery. Anesth Analg 1994;79:4–8.

28. Gibbs NM, Weightman WM, Thackray NM, Michalopoulos N, Weidmann C. The effects of recent aspirin ingestion on platelet function in cardiac surgical patients. J Cardiothorac Vasc Anesth 2001;15:55–9.

29. Weightman WM, Gibbs NM, Weidmann CR, et al. The effect of preoperative aspirin-free interval on red blood cell transfusion requirements in cardiac surgical patients. J Cardiothorac Vasc Anesth 2002;16:54–8.

30. Dacey LJ, Munoz JJ, Johnson ER, et al. Effects of preoperative aspirin use on mortality in coronary artery bypass grafting patients. Ann Thorac Surg 2000;70:1986–90.

31. Mangano DT for the multicenter study of perioperative ischemia research group. Aspirin and mortality from coronary bypass surgery. N Engl J Med 2002;347:1309–17.

32. Hongo RH, Ley J, Dick SE, Yee RR. The effect of clopidogrel in combination with aspirin when given before coronary artery bypass grafting. J Am Coll Cardiol 2002;40:231–7.

33. Ray JG, Deniz S, Olivieri A, et al. Increased blood product use among coronary artery bypass patients prescribed preoperative aspirin and clopidogrel. BMC Cardiovasc Discord 2003;3:3.

34. Karabulut H, Toraman F, Evrenkaya S, Goksel O, Taarcan S, Alban C. Clopidogrel does not increase bleeding and allogenic blood transfusion in coronary artery surgery. Eur J Cardiothorac Surg 2004;25:419–23.

35. Genoni M, Tavakoli R, Hofer C, Bertel O, Turina M. Clopidogrel before urgent coronary artery bypass graft. J Thorac Cardiovasc Surg 2003;126:288–9.

36. Bitondo JM, Daggett WM, Torchiana DF, et al. Endoscopic versus open saphenous vein harvest: a comparison of postoperative wound infections. Ann Thorac Surg 2002;73:523–8.

37. Lytle BW, Blackstone EH, Loop FD, et al. Two internal thoracic artery grafts are better than one. J Thorac Cardiovasc Surg 1999;117:855–72.

38. Dietl CA, Benoit CH. Radial artery graft for coronary revascularization: technical considerations. Ann Thorac Surg 1995;60:102–10.

39. Reyes AT, Frame R, Brodman RF. Technique for harvesting the radial artery as a coronary artery bypass graft. Ann Thorac Surg 1995;59:118–26.

40. Connolly MW, Torillo LD, Stauder MJ, et al. Endoscopic radial artery harvesting: results of the first 300 patients. Ann Thorac Surg 2002;74:502–5.

41. Ascione R, Caputo M, Angelini GD. Off-pump coronary artery bypass grafting: not a flash in the pan. Ann Thorac Surg 2003;75:306–13.

42. Reston JT, Tregear SJ, Turkelson CM. Meta-analysis of short-term and mid-term outcomes following off-pump coronary artery bypass grafting. Ann Thorac Surg 2003;76:1510–5.

43. Mack MJ. Beating heart surgery: does it make a difference? Am Heart Hosp J 2003;1:149–57.

44. Allen KB, Dowling RD, Angell WW, et al. Transmyocardial revascularization: 5-year follow-up of a prospective, randomized multicenter trial. Ann Thorac Surg 2004;77:1228–34.

45. Peterson ED, Kaul P, Kaczmarek RG, et al. From controlled trials to clinical practice: monitoring transmyocardial revascularization use and outcomes. J Am Coll Cardiol 2004;42:1611–6.

46. Allen KB, Dowling RD, Schuch DR, et al. Adjunctive transmyocardial revascularization: five-year follow-up of a prospective, randomized trial. Ann Thorac Surg 2004;78:458–65.

47. Bridges CR, Horvath KA, Nugent WC, et al. The Society of Thoracic Surgeons practice guideline series: transmyocardial laser revascularization. Ann Thorac Surg 2004;77:1494–1502.

48. Ba'albaki HA, Clements SD Jr. Left ventricular aneurysm: a review. Clin Cardiol 1989;12:5–13.

49. Dor V, ed. Ventricular aneurysm surgery. Semin Thorac Cardiovasc Surg 1997;9:112–55.

50. Mills NL, Everson CT, Hockmuth DR. Technical advances in the treatment of left ventricular aneurysm. Ann Thorac Surg 1993;55:792–800.

51. Mickelborough LL, Carson S, Ivanov J. Repair of dyskinetic or akinetic left ventricular aneurysm: results obtained with a modified linear closure. J Thorac Cardiovasc Surg 2001;121:675–82.

52. Mickleborough LL, Merchant N, Provost Y, Carson S, Ivanov J. Ventricular reconstruction for ischemic cardiomyopathy. Ann Thorac Surg 2003;75:S6–12.

53. Shapira OM, Davidoff R, Hilkert RJ, Aldea GS, Fitzgerald CA, Shemin RJ. Repair of left ventricular aneurysm: long-term results of linear repair versus endoaneurysmorrhaphy. Ann Thorac Surg 1997;63:701–5.

54. Dor V, Di Donato M, Sabatier M, Montiglio F, Civaia F. Left ventricular reconstruction by endoventricular circular patch plasty repair: a 17-year experience. Semin Thorac Cardiovasc Surg 2001;13:435–7.

55. Di Donato M, Sabatier M, Dor V, et al. Effects of the Dor procedure on left ventricular dimension and shape and geometric correlates of mitral regurgitation one year after surgery. J Thorac Cardiovasc Surg 2001;121:91–6.

56. Athanasuleas CL, Stanley AWH Jr, Buckberg GD, Dor V, DiDonato M, Blackstone EH and the RESTORE group. Surgical anterior ventricular endocardial restoration (SAVER) in the dilated remodeled ventricle after anterior myocardial infarction. J Am Coll Cardiol 2001;37:1199–209.

57. Birnbaum Y, Fishbein MC, Blanche C, Siegel RJ. Ventricular septal rupture after acute myocardial infarction. N Engl J Med 2002;347:1426–32.

58. Heitmiller R, Jacobs ML, Daggett WM. Surgical management of postinfarction ventricular septal rupture. Ann Thorac Surg 1986;41:683–91.

59. David TE, Dale L, Sun Z. Postinfarction ventricular septal rupture: repair by endocardial patch with infarct exclusion. J Thorac Cardiovasc Surg 1995;110:1315–22.

60. Muehrcke DD, Daggett WM Jr, Buckley MJ, Akins CW, Hilgenberg AD, Austen WG. Postinfarct ventricular septal defect repair: effect of coronary artery bypass grafting. Ann Thorac Surg 1992;54:876–83.

61. Carabello BA, Crawford FA Jr. Valvular heart disease. N Engl J Med 1997;337:32–41.

62. Bonow RO, Carabello B, de Leon AC Jr, et al. ACC/AHA guidelines for the management of patients with valvular heart disease. Executive summary. A report of the American College of Cardiology/American Heart Association task force on practice guidelines (Committee on management of patients with valvular heart disease). Circulation 1998;98:1949–84.

63. Aurigemma G, Battista S, Orsinelli D, Sweeney A, Pape L, Cuenoud H. Abnormal left ventricular intracavity flow acceleration in patients undergoing aortic valve replacement for aortic stenosis. A marker for high postoperative morbidity and mortality. Circulation. 1992;86:926–36.

64. Bartunek J, Sys SU, Rodrigues AC, Scheurbeeck EV, Mortier L, de Bruyne B. Abnormal systolic intracavity flow velocities after valve replacement for aortic stenosis. Mechanisms, predictive factors, and prognostic significance. Circulation 1996;93:712–9.

65. Omran H, Schmidt H, Hackenbroch M, et al. Silent and apparent cerebral embolism after retrograde catheterization of the aortic valve in valvular stenosis: a prospective, randomized study. Lancet 2003;361:1241–6.

66. Mochizuki Y, Pandian NG. Role of echocardiography in the diagnosis and treatment of patients with aortic stenosis. Curr Opin Cardiol 2003;18:327–33.

67. Pellika PA, Nishimura RA, Bailey KR, Tajik AJ. The natural history of adults with asymptomatic, hemodynamically significant aortic stenosis. J Am Coll Cardiol 1990;15:1012–7.

68. Otto CM, Burwash IG, Legget ME, et al. Prospective study of asymptomatic valvular aortic stenosis. Clinical, echocardiographic, and exercise predictors of outcome. Circulation 1997;95:2262–70.

69. Lester SJ, Heilbron B, Gin K, Dodek A, Jue J. The natural history and rate of progression of aortic stenosis. Chest 1998;113:1109–14.

70. Monin JL, Monchi M, Gest V, Duval-Moulin AM, Dubois-Rande JL, Gueret P. Aortic stenosis with severe left ventricular dysfunction and low transvalvular pressure gradients. Risk stratification by low-dose dobutamine echocardiography. J Am Coll Cardiol 2001;37:2101–7.

71. Perreira JJ, Lauer MS, Bashir M, et al. Survival after aortic valve replacement for severe aortic stenosis with low transvalvular gradients and severe left ventricular dysfunction. J Am Coll Cardiol 2002;39:1356–63.

72. Nishimura RA, Grantham JA, Connolly HM, Schaff HV, Higano ST, Holmes DR Jr. Low-output, low-gradient aortic stenosis in patients with depressed left ventricular systolic function: the clinical utility of the dobutamine challenge in the catheterization laboratory. Circulation 2002;106:809–13.

73. Dogan S, Dzemali O, Winzer-Greinecker G, et al. Minimally invasive versus conventional aortic valve replacement: a prospective randomized trial. J Heart Valve Dis 2003;12:76–80.

74. Corbi P, Rahmati M, Donal E, et al. Prospective evaluation of minimally invasive and standard techniques for aortic valve replacement: initial experience in the first hundred patients. J Card Surg 2003;18:113–9.

75. Elkins RC. The Ross operation: a 12-year experience. Ann Thorac Surg 1999;68:S14–8.

76. Sabik JF, Lytle BW, Blackstone EH, Marullo AGM, Pettersson GB, Cosgrove DM. Aortic root replacement with cryopreserved allograft for prosthetic valve endocarditis. Ann Thorac Surg 2002;74:650–9.

77. Borer JS, Bonow RO. Contemporary approach to aortic and mitral regurgitation. Circulation 2003;108:2432–8.

78. Klodas E, Enriquez-Sarano M, Tajik AJ, Mullany CJ, Bailey KR, Seward JB. Optimizing timing of surgical correction in patients with severe aortic regurgitation: role of symptoms. J Am Coll Cardiol 1997;30:746–52.

79. Borer JS, Herrold EM, Hochreiter CA, et al. Aortic regurgitation: selection of asymptomatic patients for valve surgery. Adv Cardiol 2002;39:74–85.

80. Fraser CD Jr, Cosgrove DM III. Surgical techniques for aortic valvuloplasty. Texas Heart Inst J 1994;21:305–9.

81. Schafers HJ, Langer F, Aicher D, Graeter TP, Wendler O. Remodeling of the aortic root and reconstruction of the bicuspid aortic valve. Ann Thorac Surg 2000;70:542–6.

82. Turi ZG, Reyes VP, Raju BS, et al. Percutaneous balloon versus surgical closed commissurotomy for mitral stenosis. A prospective, randomized trial. Circulation 1991;83:1179–85.

83. Farhet MB, Boussadia H, Gandjbakhch I, et al. Closed versus open mitral commissurotomy in pure noncalcific mitral stenosis: hemodynamic studies before and after operation. J Thorac Cardiovasc Surg 1990;99:639–44.

84. Choudhary SK, Dhareshwar J, Govil A, Airan B, Kumar AS. Open mitral commissurotomy in the current era: indications, technique, and results. Ann Thorac Surg 2003;75:41–6.

85. Kondo N, Takahashi K, Minakawa M, Daitoku K. Left atrial Maze procedure: a useful addition to other corrective operations. Ann Thorac Surg 2003;75:1490–4.

86. Sie HT, Beukema WP, Elvan A, Misier ARR. Long-term results of irrigated radiofrequency modified Maze procedure in 200 patients with concomitant cardiac surgery: six years experience. Ann Thorac Surg 2004;77:512–7.

87. Di Donato M, Frigiola A, Menicanti L, et al. Moderate ischemic mitral regurgitation and coronary artery bypass surgery: effect of mitral repair on clinical outcome. J Heart Valve Dis 2003;12:272–9.

88. Trichon BH, Glower DD, Shaw LK, et al. Survival after coronary revascularization, with and without mitral valve surgery, in patients with ischemic mitral regurgitation. Circulation 2003;108 (suppl I):II-103–10.

89. Paparella D, Mickleborough LL, Carson S, Ivanov J. Mild to moderate mitral regurgitation in patients undergoing coronary bypass grafting: effects on operative mortality and long-term significance. Ann Thorac Surg 2003;76:1094–100.

90. Gillinov AM Cosgrove DM. Mitral valve repair for degenerative disease. J Heart Valve Dis 2002;11(suppl 1):S15–20.

91. Gillinov AM, Cosgrove DM. Current status of mitral valve repair. Am Heart Hosp J 2003;1:47–54.

92. Phillips MR, Daly RC, Schaff HV, Dearani JA, Mullany CJ, Orzulak T. Repair of anterior leaflet mitral valve prolapse: chordal replacement versus chordal shortening. Ann Thorac Surg 2000;69:25–9.

93. Dreyfus G, Serraf A, Jebara VA, et al. Valve repair in acute endocarditis. Ann Thorac Surg 1990;49:706–13.

94. Gillinov AM, Wierup PN, Blackstone EH, et al. Is repair preferable to replacement for ischemic mitral regurgitation? J Thorac Cardiovasc Surg 2001;122:1125–41.

95. Gillinov AM, Faber C, Houghtaling PL, et al. Repair versus replacement for degenerative mitral valve disease with coexisting ischemic heart disease. J Thorac Cardiovasc Surg 2003;125:1350–62.

96. Miller DC. Ischemic mitral regurgitation redux: to repair or to replace? J Thorac Cardiovasc Surg 2001;122:1059–62.

97. Grossi EA, Goldberg JD, LaPietra A, et al. Ischemic mitral valve reconstruction and replacement: comparison of long-term survival and complications. J Thorac Cardiovasc Surg 2001;122:1107–24.

98. McCarthy PM, Bhudia SK, Rajeswaran J, et al. Tricuspid valve repair: durability and risk factors for failure. J Thorac Cardiovasc Surg 2004;127:674–85.

99. McGrath LB, Gonzalez-Lavin L, Bailey BM, Grunkemeier GL, Fernandez J, Laub GW. Tricuspid valve operations in 530 patients. Twenty-five-year assessment of early and late phase events. J Thorac Cardiovasc Surg 1990;99:124–33.

100. Carrier M, Hebert Y, Pellerin M, et al. Tricuspid valve replacement: analysis of 25 years of experience at a single center. Ann Thorac Surg 2003;75:47–50.

101. Vlessis AA, Khaki A, Grunkemeier GL, Li HH, Starr A. Risk, diagnosis, and management of prosthetic valve endocarditis: a review. J Heart Valve Disease 1997;6:443–65.

102. Di Salvo G, Habib G, Pergola V, et al. Echocardiography predicts embolic events in infective endocarditis. J Am Coll Cardiol 2001;37:1069–76.

103. Vilacosta I, Graupner C, San Roman JA, et al. Risk of embolization after institution of antibiotic therapy for infective endocarditis. J Am Coll Cardiol 2002;39:1489–95.

104. Cowgill LD, Addonizio VP, Hopeman AR, Harken AH. A practical approach to prosthetic valve endocarditis. Ann Thorac Surg 1987;43:450–7.

105. Lindner JR. Role of echocardiographic imaging in infective endocarditis. ACC Current Journal Review Mar/Apr 2002.

106. Moon MR, Miller DC, Moore KA, et al. Treatment of endocarditis with valve replacement: the question of tissue versus mechanical prosthesis. Ann Thorac Surg 2001;71:1164–71.

107. Hagl C, Galla JD, Lansman SL, et al. Replacing the ascending aorta and aortic valve for acute prosthetic valve endocarditis: is using prosthetic material contraindicated? Ann Thorac Surg 2002;74:S1781–5.

108. Carozza A, Renzulli A, de Feo M, et al. Tricuspid repair for infective endocarditis. Clinical and echocardiographic results. Tex Heart Inst J 2001;28:96–101.

109. Arbulu A, Holmes RJ, Asfaw I. Tricuspid valvulectomy without replacement. Twenty years' clinical experience. J Thorac Cardiovasc Surg 1991;102:917–22.

110. Maron BJ. Hypertrophic cardiomyopathy. A systematic review. JAMA 2002;287:1308–20.

111. Sherrid MV, Chaudhry FA, Swistel DG. Obstructive hypertrophic cardiomyopathy: echocardiography, pathophysiology, and the continuing evolution of surgery for obstruction. Ann Thorac Surg 2003;75:620–32.

112. Maron BJ, McKenna WJ, Danielson GK, et al. American College of Cardiology/European Society of Cardiology Clinical Expert Consensus Document on Hypertrophic Cardiomyopathy. A report of the American College of Cardiology Foundation Task Force on Clinical Expert Consensus Documents and the European Society of Cardiology Committee for Practice Guidelines. J Am Coll Cardiol 2003;42:1687–713.

113. Crawford ES. The diagnosis and management of aortic dissection. JAMA 1990;264:2537–41.

114. Khan IA, Nair CK. Clinical, diagnostic, and management perspectives of aortic dissection. Chest 2002;122:311–28.

115. Hagan PG, Nienaber CA, Isselbacher EM, et al. The international registry of acute aortic dissection (IRAD). New insights into an old disease. JAMA 2000;283:897–903.

116. Hata M, Shiono M, Inoue T, et al. Optimal treatment of type B acute aortic dissection: long-term medical follow-up results. Ann Thorac Surg 2003;75:1781–4.

117. Motallebzadeh R, Batas D, Valencia O, et al. The role of coronary angiography in acute type A aortic dissection. Eur J Cardiothorac Surg 2004;25:231–5.

118. Bavaria JE, Brinster DR, Gorman RC, Woo YJ, Gleason T, Pochettino A. Advances in the treatment of acute type A dissection: an integrated approach. Ann Thorac Surg 2002;74:S1848–52.

119. Passage J, Jalali H, Tam RKW, Harrocks S, O'Brien MF. BioGlue surgical adhesive: an appraisal of its indications in cardiac surgery. Ann Thorac Surg 2002;74:432–7.

120. Hanafusa Y, Ogino H, Sasaki H, et al. Total arch replacement with elephant trunk procedure for retrograde dissection. Ann Thorac Surg 2002;74:S1836–9.

121. Lansman SL, Hagl C, Fink D, et al. Acute type B aortic dissection: surgical therapy. Ann Thorac Surg 2002;74:S1833–5.

122. Elefteriades JA, Hartleroad J, Gusberg RJ, et al. Long-term experience with descending aortic dissection: the complication-specific approach. Ann Thorac Surg 1992;53:11–21.

123. Buffolo E, da Fonseca JHP, de Souza JAM, Alves CMR. Revolutionary treatment of aneurysms and dissections of the descending aorta: the endovascular approach. Ann Thorac Surg 2002;74:S1815–7.

124. Kouchoukos NT, Dougenis D. Surgery of the thoracic aorta. N Engl J Med 1997;336:1876–88.

125. Elefteriades JA. Natural history of thoracic aortic aneurysms: indications for surgery, and surgical versus nonsurgical risks. Ann Thorac Surg 2002;74:S1877–80.

126. Pitt MPI, Bonser RS. The natural history of thoracic aortic aneurysm disease: an overview. J Cardiac Surg 1997;12:270–8.

127. Coady MA, Rizzo JA, Hammond GL, et al. What is the appropriate size criterion for resection of thoracic aortic aneurysms? J Thorac Cardiovasc Surg 1997;113:476–91.

128. Pieters FAA, Widdershoven JW, Gerardy AC, Geskes G, Cheriex EC, Wellens HJ. Risk of aortic dissection after aortic valve replacement. Am J Cardiol 1993;72:1043–7.

129. Westaby S, Saito S, Anastasiadis K, Moorjani N, Jin XY. Aortic root remodeling in atheromatous aneurysms: the role of selected sinus repair. Eur J Cardiothorac Surg 2002;21:459–64.

130. David TE, Ivanov J, Armstrong S, Feindel CM, Webb GD. Aortic valve sparing operations in patients with aneurysms of the aortic root or ascending aorta. Ann Thorac Surg 2002;74: S1758–61.

131. Griepp RB. Cerebral protection during aortic arch surgery. J Thorac Cardiovasc Surg 2001;121:425–7.

132. Reich DL, Uysal S, Ergin MA, Griepp RB. Retrograde cerebral perfusion as a method of neuroprotection during thoracic aortic surgery. Ann Thorac Surg 2001;72:1774–82.

133. Di Eusanio M, Schepens AAM, Morshuis WJ, et al. Brain protection using antegrade selective cerebral perfusion: a multicenter study. Ann Thorac Surg 2003;76:1181–9.

134. Royston D. Pro: aprotinin should be used in patients undergoing hypothermic circulatory arrest. J Cardiothorac Vasc Anesth 2001;15:121–5.

135. Smith CR, Spanier TB. Aprotinin in deep hypothermic circulatory arrest. Ann Thorac Surg 1999;68:278–86.

136. Safi HJ, Miller CC III, Estrera AL, et al. Staged repair of extensive aortic aneurysm: morbidity and mortality in the elephant trunk technique. Circulation 2001;104:2938–42.

137. Estrera AL, Rubenstein FS, Miller CC III, Huynh TTT, Letsou GV, Safi HJ. Descending thoracic aortic aneurysm: surgical approach and treatment using the adjuncts cerebrospinal fluid drainage and distal aortic perfusion. Ann Thorac Surg 2001;72:481–6.

138. Plestis KA, Nair DG, Russo M, Gold JP. Left atrial femoral bypass and cerebrospinal fluid drainage decreases neurologic complications in repair of descending and thoracoabdominal aortic aneurysms. Ann Vasc Surg 2001;15:49–52.

139. Coselli JS, LeMaire SA, Conklin LD, Adams GJ. Left heart bypass during descending thoracic aortic aneurysm repair does not reduce the incidence of paraplegia. Ann Thorac Surg 2004;77:1298–303.

140. Coselli JS, LeMaire SA. Left heart bypass reduces paraplegia rates following thoracoabdominal aortic aneurysm repair. Ann Thorac Surg 1999;67:1931–4.

141. Kouchoukos NT, Masetti P, Rokkas CK, Murphy SF, Blackstone EH. Safety and efficacy of hypothermic cardiopulmonary bypass and circulatory arrest for operations on the descending thoracic and thoracoabdominal aorta. Ann Thorac Surg 2001;72:699–708.

142. Angkeow P, Calkins H. Radiofrequency catheter ablation of ventricular tachycardia. Am Coll Cardiol Curr J Rev Nov/Dec 2001.

143. Bhatia A, Cooley R, Berger M, et al. The implantable cardioverter defibrillator: technology, indications, and impact on cardiovascular survival. Curr Probl Cardiol 2004;29:303–56.

144. DiMarco JP. Implantable cardioverters-defibrillators. N Engl J Med 2003;349:1836–47.

145. Gregoratos G, Abrams J, Epstein AE. et al. ACC/AHA/NASPE 2002 Guideline update for implantation of cardiac pacemakers and antiarrhythmia devices: summary article. A report of the American College of Cardiology/American Heart Association task force on practice guidelines (ACC/AHA/NASPE committee to update the 1998 pacemaker guidelines). Circulation 2002;106:2145–61 or J Am Coll Cardiol 2002;40:1703–19.

146. Moss AJ, Zareba W, Hall WJ, et al. Prophylactic implantation of a defibrillator in patients with myocardial infarction and reduced ejection fraction. N Engl J Med 2002;346:877–83.

147. Ferguson TB Jr, Smith JM, Cox JL, Cain ME, Lindsay BD. Direct operation versus ICD therapy for ischemic ventricular tachycardia. Ann Thorac Surg 1994;58:1291–6.

148. del Rio A, Anguera I, Miro JM, et al. Surgical treatment of pacemaker and defibrillator lead endocarditis: the impact of electrode lead extraction on outcome. Chest 2003;124:1451–9.

149. Mickleborough LL, Merchant N, Provost Y, Carson S, Ivanov J. Ventricular reconstruction for ischemic cardiomyopathy. Ann Thorac Surg 2003;75:S6–12.

150. Yamauchi S, Ogasawara H, Saji Y, Bessho R, Miyagi Y, Fujii M. Efficacy of intraoperative mapping to optimize surgical ablation of atrial fibrillation in cardiac surgery. Ann Thorac Surg 2002;74:450–7.

151. Cox JL, Boineau, JP, Schuessler RB, Kater KM, Lappas DG. Five-year experience with the Maze procedure for atrial fibrillation. J Thorac Cardiovasc Surg 1993;56:814–24.

152. Cox JL, Jaquiss RDB, Schuessler RB, Boineau JP. Modification of the Maze procedure for atrial flutter and atrial fibrillation. II. Surgical technique of the Maze III procedure. Rationale and surgical results. J Thorac Cardiovasc Surg 1995;110:485–95.

153. Gillinov AM, McCarthy PM. Atricure bipolar radiofrequency clamp for intraoperative ablation of atrial fibrillation. Ann Thorac Surg 2002;74:2165–8.

154. Gillinov AM, Smedira NG, Cosgrove III DM. Microwave ablation of atrial fibrillation during mitral valve operations. Ann Thorac Surg 2002;74:1259–61.

155. Guden M, Akpinar B, Sanisoglu I, Sagbas E, Bayindir O. Intraoperative saline-irrigated radiofrequency modified Maze procedure for atrial fibrillation. Ann Thorac Surg 2002;74:S1301–6.

156. Williams MR, Stewart JR, Bolling SF, et al. Surgical treatment of atrial fibrillation using radiofrequency energy. Ann Thorac Surg 2001;71:1939–44.

157. Chiappini B, Martin-Suarez S, LoForte A, Arpesella G, Di Bartolomeo R, Marinelli G. Cox/Maze operation versus radiofrequency ablation for the surgical treatment of atrial fibrillation: a comparative study. Ann Thorac Surg 2004;77:87–92.

158. Sabbah HN. The cardiac support device and the Myosplint: treating heart failure by targeting left ventricular size and shape. Ann Thorac Surg 2003;75:S13–9.

159. Hunt SA, Baker DW, Chin MH, et al. ACC/AHA guidelines for the evaluation and management of chronic heart failure in the adult: executive summary. A report of the American College of Cardiology/American Heart Association Task Force on Practice Guidelines (Committee to Revise the 1995 guidelines for the evaluation and management of heart failure. J Am Coll Cardiol 2001;38:2101-13, J Heart Lung Transplant 2002;21:189-203, Circulation 2001;104:2496–3007.

160. Lytle BW. The role of coronary revascularization in the treatment of ischemic cardiomyopathy. Ann Thorac Surg 2003;75:S2–5.

161. Allman KC, Shaw LJ, Hachamovitch R. Udelson JE. Myocardial viability testing and impact of revascularization on prognosis in patients with coronary artery disease and left ventricular dysfunction: a meta-analysis. J Am Coll Cardiol 2002;39:1151–8.

162. Romano MA, Bolling SF. Mitral valve repair as an alternative treatment for heart failure patients. Heart Fail Monit 2003;4:7–12.

163. Abraham WT. Cardiac resynchronization therapy for the management of chronic heart failure. Am Heart Hosp J 2003;1:55–61.

164. Abraham WT, Hayes DL. Cardiac resynchronization therapy for heart failure. Circulation 2003;108:2596–603.

165. Raman JS, Byrne MJ, Power JM, Alferness CA. Ventricular constraint in severe heart failure halts decline in cardiovascular function associated with experimental dilated cardiomyopathy. Ann Thorac Surg 2003;76:141–7.

166. Oz MC, Konertz WF, Kleber FX, et al. Global surgical experience with the Acorn cardiac support device. J Thorac Cardiovasc Surg 2003;126:983–91.

167. Schenk S, Reichenspurner H. Ventricular reshaping with devices. Heart Surg Forum 2003;6:237–43.

168. Aaronson KD, Patel H, Pagani FD. Patient selection for left ventricular assist device therapy. Ann Thorac Surg 2003;75:S29–35.

169. Rao V, Oz MC, Flannery MA, Catanese KA, Argenziano M, Naka Y. Revised screening scale to predict survival after insertion of a left ventricular assist device. J Thorac Cardiovasc Surg 2003;125:855–62.

170. Holman WL, Davies JE, Rayburn BK, et al. Treatment of end-stage heart disease with outpatient ventricular assist devices. Ann Thorac Surg 2002;73:1489–94.

171. Frazier OH, Rose EA, Oz MC, et al. Multicenter clinical evaluation of the HeartMate vented electric left ventricular assist system in patients awaiting heart transplantation. J Thorac Cardiovasc Surg 2001;122:1186–95.

172. Rose EA, Gelijns AC, Moskowitz AJ, for the REMATCH Study Group. Long-term use of a left ventricular assist device for end-stage heart failure. N Engl J Med 2001;345:1435–43.

173. Hassink RJ, de la Riviere AB, Mummery CL, Doevendans PA. Transplantation of cells for cardiac repair. J Am Coll Cardiol 2003;41:711–7.

174. Menasche P. Cell transplantation in myocardium. Ann Thorac Surg 2003;75:S20–8.

175. Spodick DH. Acute cardiac tamponade. N Engl J Med 2003;349:684–90.

176. Tsang TSM, Oh JK, Seward JB. Diagnosis and management of cardiac tamponade in the era of echocardiography. Clin Cardiol 1999;22:446–52.

177. Garcia MJ. Constriction vs. restriction: how to evaluate? Am Coll Cardiol Curr J Rev Jul/Aug 2003.

178. Hoit BD. Management of effusive and constrictive pericardial heart disease. Circulation 2002:105:2939–42.

179. Myers RB, Spodick DH. Constrictive pericarditis: clinical and pathophysiologic characteristics. Am Heart J 1999;138:219–32.

180. Galli M, Politi A, Pedretti F, Castiglioni B, Zerboni S. Percutaneous balloon pericardiotomy for malignant pericardial tamponade. Chest 1995;108:1499–1501.

181. Yetkin U, Kestelli M, Yilik L, et al. Recent surgical experience in chronic constrictive pericarditis. Tex Heart Inst J 2003;30:27–30.

182. Buchanan CL, Sullivan VV, Lampman R, Kulkarni MG. Pericardiocentesis with extended catheter drainage: an effective therapy. Ann Thorac Surg 2003;76:817–20.

183. McDonald JM, Meyers BF, Guthrie TJ, Battafarano RJ, Cooper JD, Patterson GA. Comparison of open subxiphoid pericardial drainage with percutaneous catheter drainage for symptomatic pericardial effusion. Ann Thorac Surg 2003;76:811–6.

184. Allen KB, Faber LP, Warren WH, Shaar CJ. Pericardial effusion: subxiphoid pericardiostomy versus percutaneous catheter drainage. Ann Thorac Surg 1999;67:437–40.

185. Maher EA, Shepherd FA, Todd TJR. Pericardial sclerosis as the primary management of malignant pericardial effusion and cardiac tamponade. J Thorac Cardiovasc Surg 1996;112:637–43.

186. Girardi LN, Ginsberg RJ, Burt ME. Pericardiocentesis and intrapericardial sclerosis: effective therapy for malignant pericardial effusions. Ann Thorac Surg 1997;64:1422–8.

187. Ancalmo N, Ocshner JL. Pericardioperitoneal window. Ann Thorac Surg 1993;55:541–2.

188. Liu HP, Chang CH, Lin PJ, Hsieh HC, Chang JP, Hsieh MJ. Thoracoscopic management of effusive pericardial disease: indications and technique. Ann Thorac Surg 1994;58:1695–7.

189. DeValeria PA, Baumgartner WA, Casale AS, et al. Current indications, risks, and outcome after pericardiectomy. Ann Thorac Surg 1991;52:219–24.

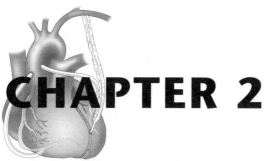

CHAPTER 2

Diagnostic Techniques in Cardiac Surgery

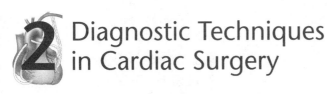

Diagnostic Techniques in Cardiac Surgery

Although the general nature of a patient's cardiac disease can usually be ascertained from a thorough history and physical examination, diagnostic tests are essential to define the pathology and extent of cardiac disease more precisely. Both noninvasive and invasive modalities are available to obtain this information and should be chosen selectively. Various techniques may provide unique or complementary data, while others may provide comparable information and need not be performed. This chapter will briefly review the basic types of diagnostic modalities available to the clinician and define their role in preoperative evaluation. Updated detailed discussions of the indications, uses, and results of several diagnostic tests can be found in the American College of Cardiology/American Heart Association (ACC/AHA) guidelines section at www.acc.org.

I. Chest Radiography

A. A PA and lateral chest x-ray should be obtained on all patients before surgery. It should be consistent with the patient's cardiac diagnosis and can provide a wealth of potential information to the surgeon (Figure 2.1).

1. Compatibility with the diagnosis: Left ventricular (LV) enlargement in patients with a dilated cardiomyopathy or volume overload (aortic insufficiency/mitral regurgitation), left ventricular hypertrophy (LVH) in aortic stenosis, large left atrium in mitral valve disease, calcified mitral valve or annulus, enlarged cardiac silhouette with a large pericardial effusion, wide mediastinum with an aortic dissection.

2. Identify complications of cardiac disease: congestive heart failure (CHF) or pulmonary vascular redistribution that should be treated by preoperative diuresis.

3. Identify other potentially relevant abnormalities:

   a. Pulmonary: emphysema, pneumonia, parenchymal nodules, interstitial disease, previous pulmonary resection

   b. Pleural: effusions, pneumothorax

   c. Mediastinum: tumors or widened mediastinum consistent with aortic disease

   d. Bone: pectus excavatum, rib resection from a previous thoracotomy

   e. Foreign bodies: sternal wires from a previous sternotomy, pacemaker wires, central venous catheters, position of an intraaortic balloon pump (IABP), type of prosthetic heart valve

B. The chest x-ray also provides specific information of importance to the surgeon during an operative procedure.

1. Calcification of the ascending aorta or arch may influence the techniques of cannulation and clamping in order to reduce the risk of stroke. Calcification of the aortic knob is fairly common but of little significance. In contrast, suspicion of ascending aortic calcification (usually noted at the time of coronary angiography) is very important and may be further defined by noncontrast computed tomography (CT).

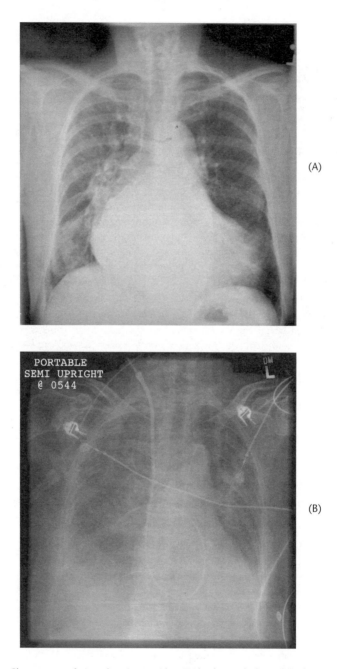

(A)

(B)

Figure 2.1 • Chest x-rays of several patients with mitral valve pathology. (A) Chest x-ray of a patient with advanced mitral stenosis that shows marked enlargement of the left atrium projecting to the right of the cardiac silhouette. (B) Acute pulmonary edema caused by acute mitral regurgitation from papillary muscle dysfunction due to acute myocardial infarction.

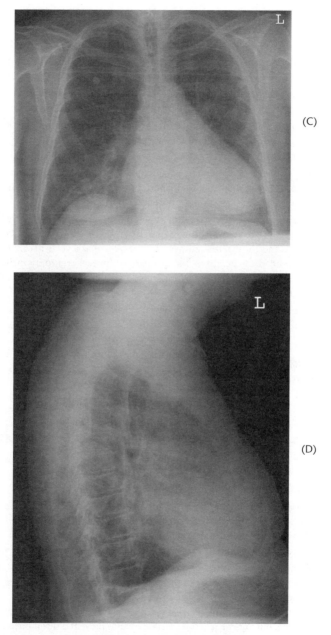

Figure 2.1 • (*Continued*) (C) Left ventricular enlargement from volume overload in a patient with chronic mitral insufficiency. (D) Lateral film of a patient with a prior coronary bypass operation with chronic mitral regurgitation. Note the proximity of the enlarged ventricle to the posterior table of the sternum. A lateral coronary angiogram may id proximity of the internal thoracic artery pedicle to the sternum.

Epiaortic echocardiographic imaging may be indicated during surgery to evaluate for ascending aortic atherosclerosis.[1]

2. An elevated hemidiaphragm on one side might deter the surgeon from using the contralateral internal thoracic artery (ITA), especially in diabetic patients who are more prone to phrenic nerve paresis.[2]

3. Mitral annular calcification in patients with MR makes mitral valve repair, as well as replacement, much more difficult and may necessitate creative surgical techniques.

4. For patients undergoing reoperation, the PA film will identify the proximity of the ITA pedicle to the midline. The lateral film will determine the proximity of the cardiac structures and the ITA pedicle clips to the posterior sternal table.

5. For patients with ascending aortic aneurysms, especially in reoperations, close proximity of the aneurysm to the posterior sternal table may necessitate groin cannulation for bypass prior to sternotomy.

6. The location and orientation of the heart should be considered when selecting the appropriate incision for minimally invasive surgery. For example, in thin patients and those with emphysema, the heart has a vertical orientation and lies quite caudad in the chest. Thus, a partial upper sternotomy incision for aortic valve surgery may require a transverse incision in the fourth rather than the third interspace.

7. The patient in profound CHF may benefit from aggressive diuresis or hemofiltration during bypass.

II. Electrocardiography

A. A 12-lead electrocardiogram must be reviewed prior to surgery because it can yield valuable information about the nature of the patient's disease, the urgency of surgery, the appropriate management of arrhythmias, and other considerations in perioperative management.

B. Disorders of rate and rhythm

1. The presence of sinus tachycardia in a patient with coronary disease suggests that the patient is inadequately β-blocked. These patients are more prone to the development of atrial fibrillation (AF) after surgery.

2. Patients with sinus bradycardia tend to require temporary postoperative pacing and may not tolerate β-blockers used prophylactically to prevent postoperative AF. Patients with known sick sinus or tachycardia/bradycardia syndrome are more likely to require a permanent pacemaker system postoperatively.

3. A rapid ventricular response to AF must be controlled medically. It can precipitate myocardial ischemia in the patient with coronary artery disease (CAD) and can compromise the cardiac output. If chronic AF is present preoperatively, there
i· l·ttl· h·n·fit to using medications postoperatively to convert the patient to sinus
nticoagulation must be used to prevent a thromboembolic stroke. A
re may be considered as an adjunct to other cardiac operations in
th either paroxysmal or chronic AF.

:hyarrhythmias may be present on the basis of ischemia or infarction.
:vascularization is indicated, a postoperative electrophysiology study
formed. An implantable defibrillator should be inserted in patients
d ventricular tachycardia and depressed LV function.

C. Conduction problems

   1. The presence of bifascicular block raises the risk of asystole during insertion of a Swan-Ganz pulmonary artery catheter. This should be deferred until after the sternotomy has been performed so that immediate epicardial pacing can be achieved.

   2. Ischemic ECG changes are difficult to assess in the patient with a bundle branch block, which may alter the aggressiveness of evaluation for the patient presenting with chest pain.

   3. The presence of conduction abnormalities in a patient with aortic valve endocarditis suggests annular extension of the infection, which is an indication for urgent surgery.

   4. Patients sustaining inferior infarctions may develop heart block and require temporary pacing preoperatively.

D. Evidence of ischemia and infarction

   1. ST and T wave changes consistent with ischemia require aggressive management. This may entail use of intravenous nitrates, antiplatelet agents, heparin, and/or placement of an IABP. An early invasive strategy with urgent percutaneous coronary intervention or surgery may be indicated. Evidence of recent infarction may influence the timing and risk of surgery.

   2. The presence of Q waves suggests myocardial damage in the distribution of specific coronary arteries and may dictate the appropriateness and selection of an interventional approach.

   3. The absence of Q waves in a patient with depressed LV function suggests that the myocardium may be chronically ischemic and hibernating, rather than infarcted. Further evaluation with viability studies may be indicated to determine whether surgery will prove beneficial.

E. Pacemaker issues

   1. The function of a permanent transvenous pacing system can be disrupted by use of electrocautery at the time of surgery. A magnet must be available to convert the pacemaker to a fixed mode.

   2. Because the right atrial lead may be displaced during surgery and because the pulse generator may be damaged by electrocautery, all permanent pacemaker systems must be interrogated immediately after surgery to ensure appropriate sensing and pacing.

III. Myocardial Perfusion Imaging

A. Rest and stress imaging play a major role in the evaluation of patients with coronary disease. Their primary role is to identify viable and ischemic myocardium that will benefit from an interventional procedure. The technology of stress imaging and radionuclide testing has become very sophisticated and only the salient features are presented.

B. Types of stress testing

   1. In its simplest form, an exercise tolerance test is performed with a graded protocol on a treadmill (Figure 2.2).[3–5] The following findings are consistent with multivessel coronary disease and an adverse prognosis, especially when they occur at a low workload (< 6 metabolic equivalents [mets]).

     a. Development of anginal symptoms

     b. > 2 mm ST depression in multiple leads and persisting > 5 minutes into recovery

     c. ST segment elevation

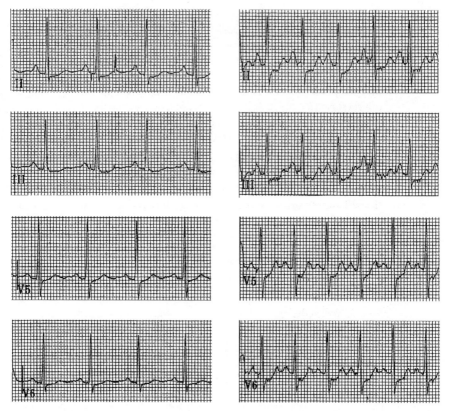

Figure 2.2 • Positive exercise stress test. (Left) Baseline ECG before exercise (leads II, III, V₅, V₆. (Right) Exercise ECG after 4 minutes of stage 2. At a heart rate of 157 beats/min, note the presence of 4 mm of ST depression in these leads, reflecting inferolateral ischemia.

    d. Failure to increase blood pressure to higher than 120 mm Hg, or a sustained decrease in blood pressure greater than 10 mm Hg or below rest levels

    e. Sustained ventricular tachycardia

2. More commonly, **myocardial perfusion imaging** is performed with planar images or single-proton emission computed tomography (SPECT) scanning. Thallium-201, technetium-99m sestamibi (Cardiolite), and technetium-99m tetrofosmin (Myoview) are the most commonly used tracers.[6,7] At peak exercise, the tracer is injected and scintigraphy is performed. These agents are taken up by viable myocardium and "light up" whereas they are not taken up by irreversibly infarcted muscle, which appears as a "cold spot." Ischemic muscle lights up on a delayed basis due to redistribution (Figure 2.3). In some patients, stress redistribution imaging may underestimate the degree of ischemic and viable

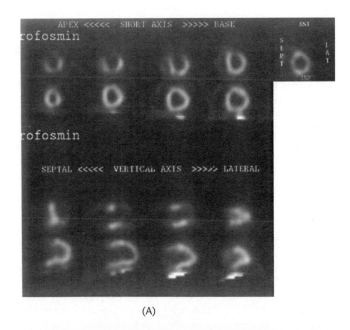

(A)

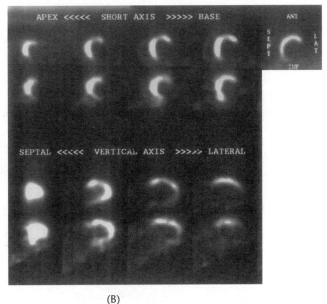

(B)

Figure 2.3 • Stress imaging studies with ^{99m}Tc-tetrofosmin. (A) The short-axis (upper two rows) and vertical long-axis views (lower two rows) at stress (top images of each pair) and redistribution (lower images of each pair). The stress images demonstrate reduced tracer uptake in the anteroapical region that improves during the redistribution phase, consistent with anteroapical ischemia. (B) Similar views demonstrating a defect in the inferolateral region in the stress images that does not improve with redistribution. This is consistent with infarction. *(Image courtesy of Dr. David Bader, Department of Radiology, St. Vincent Hospital, Worcester, MA.)*

myocardium, but reinjection will improve sensitivity.[8] If the patient cannot exercise, adenosine or dipyridamole (Persantine) is given to mimic the effect of exercise on the distribution of blood flow. Pharmacologic imaging produces fairly comparable results to exercise-induced ischemia.

3. **Exercise radionuclide angiography** can be used to identify myocardial ischemia. The development of a regional wall motion abnormality or fall in ejection fraction with exercise is indicative of ischemia. The use of technetium-labeled tracers can be used to assess both myocardial perfusion and ventricular function.[7]

4. **Exercise echocardiography** is based on the principle that stress-induced ischemia caused by coronary artery stenosis will produce regional wall motion abnormalities. These tests may be performed using bicycle or treadmill exercise. An alternative to exercise is the use of **dobutamine** to increase myocardial oxygen demand (dobutamine stress echocardiography [DSE]). If this cannot be met by an increase in blood flow, ischemia will produce regional wall motion abnormalities in the distribution of the stenotic coronary artery. These tests have provided comparable results to those of thallium imaging.[9,10]

C. **Viability studies.** Myocardial viability studies are useful in patients with severe LV dysfunction to identify "hibernating myocardium" that may recover function after revascularization. Studies that assess cell membrane integrity, metabolic activity, or contractile reserve have documented improved patient survival after myocardial revascularization when there is evidence of dysfunctional yet viable myocardium.[11–13] In contrast, survival is usually not improved if there is no demonstrable viability in these zones.[14] In patients with CHF, improvement in regional and global LV function usually improves symptoms and increases survival, with the degree of functional improvement correlating with the number of viable zones.[15] In patients with angina and in some patients with CHF, symptomatic improvement may be related to reperfusion of zones that demonstrate stress-induced ischemia, and thus may occur without any improvement in global or regional function. Consequently, increased survival may not necessarily be associated with improvement in LV function.

1. **Rest redistribution imaging with thallium** is the most basic means of assessing viability, using either planar imaging or SPECT. Thallium uptake reflects cell membrane integrity, so that viable zones, whether ischemic or not, will perfuse and retain thallium at rest. This is in contrast to stress imaging, during which ischemic zones only light up from reinjection or redistribution on delayed imaging.

2. **^{18}F-deoxyglucose (FDG) uptake** using positron emission tomography (PET) or SPECT imaging is a very sensitive test of viability. FDG is a marker of glucose uptake by the myocardium, thus assessing metabolism and cell viability. An assessment is made of perfusion with ^{13}N-ammonia, and then ^{18}FDG is injected to assess metabolism. Zones with matching perfusion and metabolism are not ischemic or are infarcted. Evidence of preserved metabolic activity in zones of reduced perfusion indicates viable, hibernating myocardium. These studies may detect viability in zones considered nonviable by thallium imaging.

3. **Dobutamine stress echo (DSE)** can be used to identify contractile reserve, which suggests viability.[9,10] Low doses of dobutamine are administered during echocardiography to assess any change in global and regional wall motion. A biphasic response during dobutamine echocardiography (improvement in function at low dose and worsening of function at peak stress from high doses of dobutamine) is highly predictive of recovery of regional contractile function in

patients with LV dysfunction.[16] Another use for this test is in patients with low-output, low-gradient aortic stenosis, in whom an improvement in LV function and an increase in the gradient with dobutamine suggests that the patient will benefit from an aortic valve replacement.[17]

4. **Contrast-enhanced magnetic resonance imaging (MRI)** holds promise as a means of assessing viability. MRI-defined diastolic wall thickness > 5.5 mm and dobutamine-induced systolic wall thickening > 2 mm are predictive of contractile recovery after coronary artery bypass grafting. MRI provides excellent image quality with precise identification of epicardial and endocardial borders to allow for assessment of wall motion and thickening.[18-21]

5. In a meta-analysis of PET, SPECT, and DSE in patients with LV dysfunction, all three tests showed relatively comparable efficacy in demonstrating the association between viability and improved survival after myocardial revascularization. PET and SPECT scanning were more sensitive, but DSE was more specific in predicting functional improvement.[11]

IV. Cardiac Catheterization

A. The gold standard for the diagnosis of most forms of cardiac disease remains cardiac catheterization.[22,23] It is indicated in most patients for whom an interventional procedure is contemplated based on a review of the history, examination, and stress test results. The exceptions are acute type A aortic dissections and patients with aortic valve endocarditis and vegetations, in whom the risk of catheter manipulation in the root is significant.

B. **Techniques** (Tables 2.1 and 2.2; Figures 2.4 and 2.5)

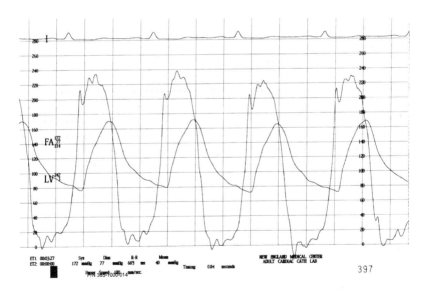

Figure 2.4 • Left heart catheterization of aortic stenosis. Comparison of the simultaneous peak left ventricular and femoral artery pressures demonstrates a peak gradient of 60 mm Hg. If there is a discrepancy between the central aortic and femoral artery pressures, the pullback gradient is calculated as the catheter is withdrawn from the left ventricle into the aorta. *(Image courtesy of Dr. John J. Smith, MD, PhD, Division of Cardiology, New England Medical Center.)*

Table 2.1 • Information Obtained from Right and Left Heart Catheterization

Elevated RA pressures	Tricuspid stenosis (large "a" wave) Tricuspid regurgitation (large "v" wave) RV dysfunction (pulmonary hypertension, RV infarction) Constrictive pericarditis/tamponade
Elevated RV pressures	RV dysfunction (pulmonary hypertension, RV infarction) Constrictive pericarditis (square root sign; rapid x and y descent) Cardiac tamponade (absent y descent)
Elevated PA pressures	Mitral stenosis/regurgitation LV systolic or diastolic dysfunction (ischemic, dilated cardiomyopathy, aortic stenosis/regurgitation) Pulmonary hypertension of other causes Constrictive pericarditis/tamponade
Elevated PCWP	Mitral stenosis (large "a" wave if sinus rhythm) Mitral regurgitation (large "v" wave) LV systolic or diastolic dysfunction (ischemic, dilated cardiomyopathy, aortic stenosis/regurgitation) Constrictive pericarditis/tamponade
Elevated LVEDP	LV systolic or diastolic dysfunction (ischemic, dilated cardiomyopathy, aortic stenosis/regurgitation) Constrictive pericarditis/tamponade

RA = right atrial; RV = right ventricular; LV = left ventricular; PA = pulmonary artery; PCWP = pulmonary capillary wedge pressure; LVEDP = left ventricular end-diastolic pressure.

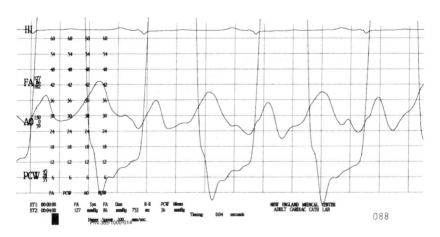

Figure 2.5 • Left heart catheterization of mitral stenosis. There is a pressure difference (gradient) of approximately 20 mm Hg between the pulmonary capillary wedge pressure and the mean left ventricular end-diastolic pressure. (*Image courtesy of Dr. John J. Smith, MD, PhD, Division of Cardiology, New England Medical Center.*)

Table 2.2 • Hemodynamic Norms During Cardiac Catheterization	
Location	**Pressures (mm Hg)**
Right atrium	Mean 3–8
Right ventricle	Systolic 15–30 Diastolic 3–8
Pulmonary artery	Systolic 15–30 Diastolic 5–12 Mean 9–16
PCW position	5–12
Left atrium	5–12
Left ventricle	Systolic 90–140 End-diastolic 5–12
Aorta	Systolic 90–140 Diastolic 60–90 Mean 70–105
PCW = pulmonary capillary wedge.	

1. **Right heart catheterization** is performed in patients with valve disease and those with coronary disease and LV dysfunction. It involves placement of a Swan-Ganz catheter through the venous system into the pulmonary artery. Intracardiac pressure measurements and pressure waves are obtained. In addition, oxygen saturations are obtained from each chamber and can detect intracardiac shunts (atrial or ventricular septal defects). Measurement of the mixed venous oxygen saturation from the PA port indirectly reflects the cardiac output. A thermodilution cardiac output is obtained and can be used along with pressure gradients obtained from right and left heart catheterization to calculate valve areas using the Gorlin formula (see Chapter 1).

2. **Left heart catheterization** involves placing a catheter from the aorta through the aortic valve into the left ventricle. This allows for the measurement of the left ventricular end-diastolic pressure, assessment of ejection fraction by **a left ventriculogram** (end-diastolic volume minus end-systolic volume) (Figure 2.6), identification of MR, and measurement of the gradient across the aortic valve during pullback of the catheter. A Fick cardiac output can be calculated. One study showed that there is an increased risk of cerebral embolization when attempts are made to cross a stenotic aortic valve to measure LV pressure. Consequently, if echocardiography identifies severe aortic stenosis, confirmation in the catheterization laboratory should not be necessary.[24]

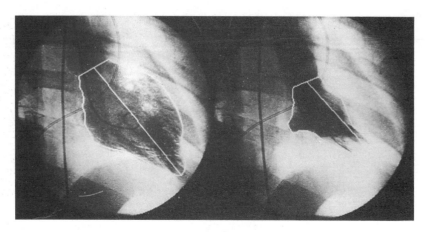

Figure 2.6 • Digital left ventriculogram. The ejection fraction is calculated from the end-diastolic volume (**left**) minus the end-systolic volume (**right**).

3. **Aortography** ("root shot") is usually performed in patients with aortic valve disease to assess the degree of aortic regurgitation (Figure 2.7). Both an aortogram and a left ventriculogram will give an estimate of aortic size that might necessitate replacement of the ascending aorta. Excessive whip of an angiographic catheter may also suggest the presence of a dilated aortic root. A CT scan or echocardiogram may be needed to further assess the size of the aorta, since magnification of the aorta is very common during aortography.

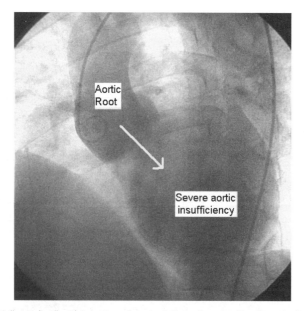

Figure 2.7 • A "root shot" with injection of contrast through a pigtail catheter in the proximal aorta demonstrating severe aortic insufficiency. This injection can also provide a relative assessment of the size of the ascending aorta, but magnification factors must be taken into consideration.

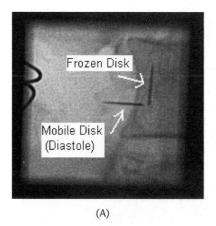
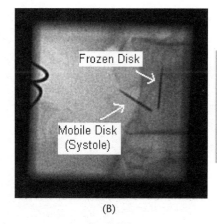

(A)   (B)

Figure 2.8 • Fluoroscopy of a patient with a St. Jude Medical Center bileaflet valve in the aortic position, which was noted to have a high gradient by echocardiography. Note that one leaflet is frozen open while the other one has limited excursion. Severe pannus ingrowth with minimal thrombus was noted at surgery.

4. **Fluoroscopy** can yield valuable information. This may demonstrate:
   a. Calcification of the ascending aorta (and the coronary arteries) that may necessitate further evaluation by CT scanning.
   b. The location of intravascular catheters or position of an IABP.
   c. "Rocking" of a prosthetic valve suggestive of endocarditis with annular invasion and possible dehiscence.
   d. Failure of movement of prosthetic valve disks, consistent with valve thrombosis or restriction by pannus ingrowth (Figure 2.8).

V. Coronary Angiography

A. Coronary angiography is performed as part of the cardiac catheterization procedure by placing special preformed catheters directly into the coronary ostia and injecting dye into the coronary arteries (Figures 2.9 and 2.10). Angiography will define whether the circulation is right or left dominant (*i.e.*, whether the posterior descending artery arises from the right or left system), and it will define the location, extent, and degree of coronary stenoses. It will also identify the quality and bypassability of the target vessels based on their size and the extent of distal disease. Anteroposterior, right anterior oblique, and left anterior oblique views are obtained at varying degrees of cranial and caudal angulation to optimally visualize each of the coronary arteries. Based on the clinical picture, the results of the stress test and angiogram, and an assessment of LV function, an informed decision can be made as to whether continued medical therapy, a percutaneous coronary intervention, or surgery is indicated.

B. Important indications for coronary angiography include:[22,23]
   1. Any patient with suspected CAD in whom an interventional procedure might be indicated on a clinical basis. Most prominently, this includes patients with ST segment elevation and non–ST-segment elevation myocardial infarctions, progressive or unstable angina, positive stress tests, and ischemic pulmonary edema.

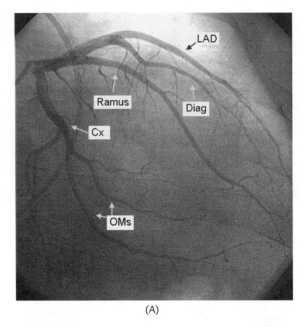

(A)

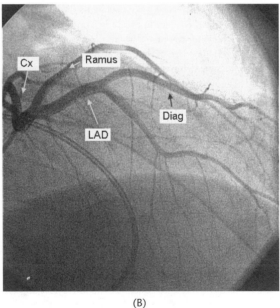

(B)

Figure 2.9 • Left coronary angiograms in four projections. (A) Right anterior oblique (RAO) nicely demonstrates the circumflex (Cx) marginal system. (B) RAO with cranial angulation best demonstrates the left anterior descending (LAD) and the origin of its diagonal branches. (C) Left anterior oblique (LAO) provides a good view of the LAD system and the origin of the circumflex. (D) LAO caudal "spider view" shows the left main giving rise to three vessels, including a large ramus intermedius.

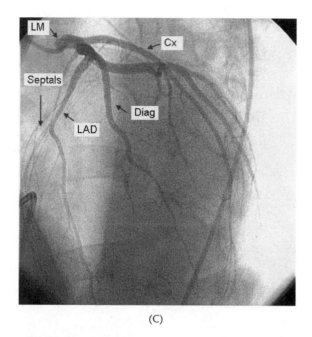

(C)

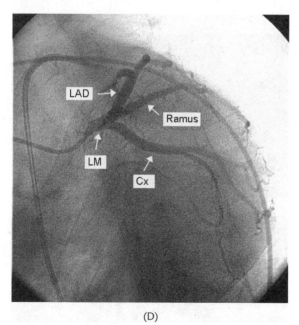

(D)

Figure 2.9 • (*Continued*)

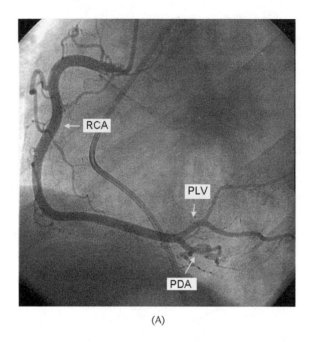

(A)

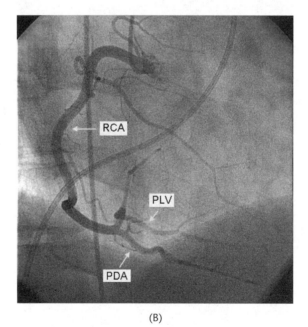

(B)

Figure 2.10 • Right coronary angiograms in the (A) LAO and (B) RAO projections. The right coronary artery (RCA) divides at the crux into the posterior descending artery (PDA), best seen in the RAO view and the posterior left ventricular branch (PLV), best seen in the LAO view.

2. Patients > age 40 who require open-heart surgery for other reasons. Angiography should also be considered in younger patients with multiple risk factors for premature CAD.

3. Annual follow-up of the cardiac transplantation patient to detect the development of silent allograft CAD.

C. The risk of sustaining a complication from cardiac catheterization and coronary angiography is 1–2%. To a great degree, the risks are dependent on the clinical status of the patient at the time of the study and on preexisting comorbidities, specifically renal dysfunction. Patients with left main disease carry the highest risks of myocardial infarction, arrhythmias, hemodynamic compromise, and death. In patients with renal dysfunction, use of nonionic contrast and *N*-acetylcysteine may reduce the risk of contrast-induced nephropathy.[25] Fenoldopam, a dopaminergic agonist, has also been used successfully in reducing the risk of renal dysfunction in patients at high risk.[26] Patients taking metformin for diabetes should withhold this medication for 1–2 days before and after catheterization to prevent the development of lactic acidosis after the use of ionic dyes.[27]

VI. Echocardiography

A. Echocardiography provides real-time two-dimensional (and recently three-dimensional) imaging of the thoracic aorta and cardiac structures. It is an invaluable noninvasive means of evaluating ventricular and valvular function before, during, and after surgery.[28–32] Although a transthoracic study is usually the initial study performed in the preoperative patient, transesophageal echocardiography (TEE) provides superior imaging because of the proximity of the probe to the heart. Routine evaluation includes multiplane two-dimensional imaging, pulsed wave Doppler, and color flow Doppler analysis. TEE is very important in the preoperative evaluation of the patient with mitral valve pathology (Figure 2.11). In patients with MR, it provides an assessment of the nature and degree of MR that may be different during intraoperative evaluation due to altered loading conditions. TEE has become the gold standard for the diagnosis of aortic dissections (Figure 2.12).[33,34] It is the best technique to identify the location and site of attachment of cardiac tumors (Figure 2.13A).

B. Dobutamine stress echocardiograms can be used to identify ischemia and myocardial viability as noted in section II.C above.[9,10,16]

C. Examples of information that can be derived from preoperative and postoperative echocardiography are noted in Tables 2.3 and 2.4. The utility of TEE in the operating room is noted in Table 4.1.

VII. Computed Tomography

A. CT is indicated primarily for the evaluation of thoracic aortic disease and has few applications in the assessment of cardiac disease. Specific indications for obtaining a CT scan in a cardiac surgical patient include:

1. Identification of an aortic dissection in a patient with unexplained chest pain (if echocardiography is not available or not interpretable). The scan must be performed with contrast (Figure 2.14). It can also be used for follow-up evaluation after repair of aortic dissections to identify distal aneurysmal disease, although MRI may be preferable.

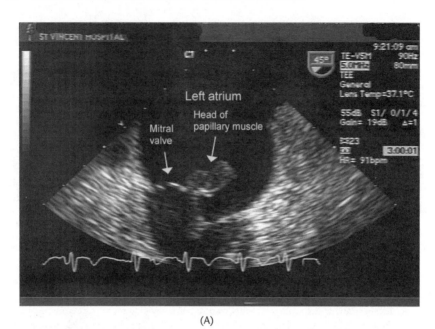

(A)

(B)

Figure 2.11 • Transesophageal echocardiograms of mitral valve pathology. (A) Papillary muscle rupture and acute mitral regurgitation. Note the flail anterior leaflet with the attached papillary muscle head. Color flow Doppler showed a severe degree of mitral regurgitation. (B) Vegetation on the anterior mitral valve leaflet in a patient with endocarditis.

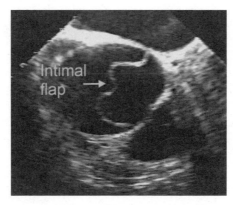

Figure 2.12 • Transesophageal echocardiogram of a type A aortic dissection. Note the intimal flap separating the true and false lumen.

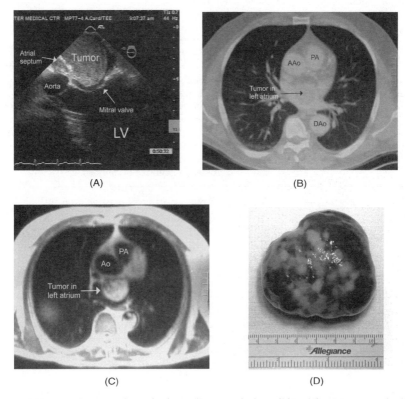

(A)

(B)

(C)

(D)

Figure 2.13 • (A) Transesophageal echocardiogram of a large left atrial myxoma attached to the superior aspect of the atrial septum. This mass was initially detected on a CT scan (B), and MRI (C) was also performed before the TEE was performed. (D) Photograph of the resected myxoma.

Table 2.3 • Information Obtained from Preoperative Echocardiography

All patients	Global and regional wall motion abnormalities Valve function Aortic atherosclerosis Pericardial fluid and thickening Presence of an intracardiac shunt
Coronary artery disease	Global and regional wall motion abnormalities LV mural thrombus Presence of mitral regurgitation Stress imaging for ischemic zones
Mitral stenosis	Size of left atrium Diastolic gradient Planimetry of valve area Presence of left atrial thrombus
Mitral regurgitation	Size of left atrium Degree of regurgitation Nature of pathology (annular dilatation, anterior or posterior leaflet prolapse, elongated or torn chords, papillary muscle rupture)
Aortic stenosis	Gradient calculation from flow velocity Planimetry of valve area Annular diameter (root enlargement, selection of homograft size) and root size (aortic replacement) Presence of mitral regurgitation
Aortic regurgitation	Degree of regurgitation Annular diameter (selection of homograft size)
Tricuspid valve disease	Calculation of pulmonary artery pressure from TR jet velocity ($4V^2$) Gradient (TS) or degree of regurgitation (TR)
Endocarditis	Vegetations Annular abscesses Valvular regurgitation
Aortic dissection	Location of intimal flap Detection of aortic regurgitation Presence of pericardial effusion
Cardiac masses	Location and relationship to cardiac structures of tumors, thrombus, vegetations
Pericardial tamponade	Diastolic collapse of atrial or ventricular chambers Location of fluid around heart

TR = tricuspid regurgitation; TS = tricuspid stenosis.

Table 2.4 • *Indications for Postoperative Echocardiography*

Low output states	LV systolic or diastolic dysfunction Cardiac tamponade Hypovolemia RV dysfunction
New/persistent murmur (recurrent CHF)	Paravalvular leak Inadequate valve repair Outflow tract gradient from small valve or systolic anterior motion of mitral valve leaflet (SAM) Recurrent ventricular septal defect
Evaluation of ventricular recovery after assist device insertion	LV or RV systolic function

    2. Assessment of aortic size

       a. When the standard angiogram (left ventriculogram or root shot) suggests ascending aortic enlargement, noncontrast CT can provide an exact measurement of dimensions in a transverse section (Figure 2.15). One has to be careful in interpreting these studies because an obliquely coursing structure (such as a tortuous or ectatic segment of aorta) may appear enlarged on a transverse section and this may not represent the true diameter of the aorta.

       b. Descending thoracic aneurysms (Figure 2.16A)

    3. Evaluation of ascending aortic calcification suggested by chest x-ray or angiogram (Figure 2.17). This may require alternative techniques of cannulation and clamping.

    4. Identification of the thickness of the pericardium in cases of constrictive pericarditis or the presence of pericardial effusions.

    5. Identification of intracardiac masses (see Figure 2.13B).

    6. Identification of pulmonary or mediastinal abnormalities on preoperative chest x-ray. Obtaining a baseline CT scan prior to cardiac surgery eliminates the potential distortion of pulmonary pathology by postoperative changes.

  B. With advancements in technology, several other modifications of CT have found application in cardiac disease.

    1. Electron beam CT (EBCT) with ultrafast scanning can provide an assessment of coronary artery calcification that assesses the atherosclerotic plaque burden. Its primary use is to screen asymptomatic patients with coronary risk factors for possible coronary disease and for assessing the progression or regression of disease in patients with modifiable risk factors.[35]

    2. Contrast-enhanced EBCT and multidetector-row (or multislice) CT angiography (MDCTA) may be useful in identifying coronary stenosis, but remain investigational.[35–40]

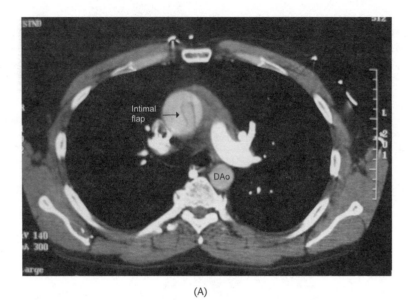

(A)

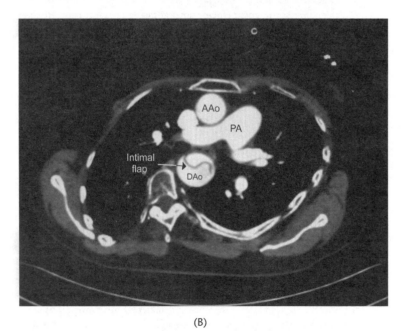

(B)

Figure 2.14 • CT scan with contrast of aortic dissections. (A) Type A involving only the ascending aorta. (B) Type B starting just distal to the left subclavian artery without any involvement of the ascending aorta. Note the intimal flap separating the true and false lumens. AAo, ascending aorta; DAo, descending aorta; PA, pulmonary artery.

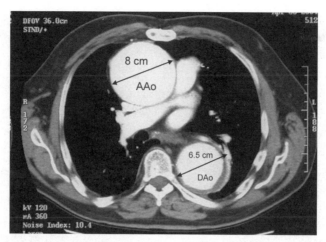

Figure 2.15 • CT scan demonstrating an enlarged ascending aorta to 8 cm that will need to be replaced at the time of aortic valve surgery by a valved conduit. Note the enlarged descending thoracic aorta with intraluminal thrombus.

VIII. Magnetic Resonance Imaging (MRI) and Angiography (MRA)

A. MR scanning can provide excellent images of the cardiac structures and aorta in multiple planes and does not require radiation. Tremendous advances in MR technology are now finding application in cardiovascular diagnoses.[41]

1. The primary indication for MRI is the evaluation of aortic disease.

   a. MRI is the most sensitive and specific test for detection of an aortic dissection (Figure 2.18), but it generally cannot be performed in an unstable patient who requires careful monitoring and often intravenous infusions. However, it should be considered when the clinical suspicion of a dissection is very high but the results of other tests have been inconclusive. Most commonly, it is used in the follow-up of patients who have had repair of an aortic dissection to assess the status of the false channel or distal aneurysmal expansion.[42]

   b. MRI can detect intracardiac masses and delineate any extension into the cardiac muscle (see Figure 2.13C).

   c. MRI is helpful in identifying the thickness of the pericardium in cases of constrictive pericarditis.

   d. MRA has virtually replaced routine arteriography for the evaluation of cerebrovascular, aortic, and peripheral vascular disease.

   e. MR scanning is useful in the evaluation of inflammatory aneurysms or in identifying fluid collections around aortic grafts when infection is suspected.

2. Myocardial viability may be evaluated using myocardial contrast-enhanced MRI or dobutamine MRI.[18–21,43,44]

3. Three-dimensional MRA has been used to identify stenoses in the proximal portion of the coronary arteries and is quite sensitive in identifying stenoses in

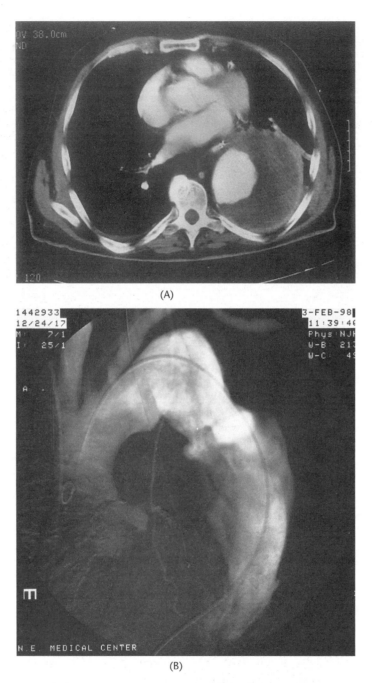

(A)

(B)

Figure 2.16 • (A) CT scan of a large descending thoracic aortic aneurysm. Note the large amount of thrombus surrounding the vascular channel. (B) A digital aortogram of the same patient. Although this gives a better appreciation of the proximal and distal extent of the aneurysm and its relationship to side branches, it significantly underestimates the overall size of the aneurysm.

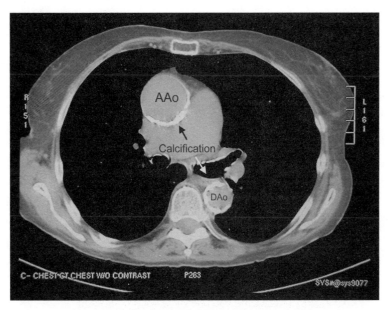

Figure 2.17 • A CT scan demonstrating severe calcification of the posterior wall of the ascending aorta and the entire circumference of the descending aorta. Because the anterior wall was normal, the patient could be cannulated for bypass. However, this patient required an aortic valve replacement, which was performed under circulatory arrest because the aorta could not be safely clamped.

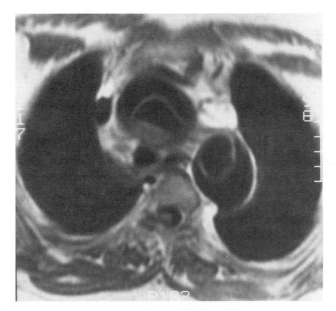

Figure 2.18 • MRI demonstrating the intimal flap separating the true and false lumens in a patient with an extensive aortic dissection involving both the ascending and descending thoracic aorta.

saphenous vein or internal thoracic artery grafts. At present, its usefulness seems to be in ruling out proximal left main or three-vessel disease in patients with atypical chest pain or equivocal stress tests.[36,39,45,46]

4. MRI may also identify coronary plaques with indications similar to those noted for EBCT.[36,47]

B. MRI cannot be performed in patients with pacemakers, implantable defibrillators, and early-generation (Starr-Edwards) valves. However, it can be performed safely in patients with St. Jude valves or retained epicardial pacing wires.[48] Although manufacturers of coronary stents recommend postponing MRI for 8 weeks after stent implantation to prevent thrombosis from dislodgment, one clinical study reported that early MRI scanning (at an average of 18 days) was safe.[49] The www.radiology.upmc.edu/MRsafety/ website provides additional information on these issues.

IX. Aortography

A. Once considered the gold standard for the diagnosis of aortic dissections, aortography is now reserved for the evaluation of aortic aneurysms, traumatic aortic tears, and chronic dissections. It images only the vascular lumen and can underestimate the overall size of an aneurysm (see Figure 2.16B). It does provide an appreciation of the extent of an aneurysm and its relationship to the aortic branches, especially using three-dimensional digital reconstruction of the aorta.

B. Advances in angiographic imaging have reduced some of the complications of angiography. One of the major drawbacks was dye-induced renal dysfunction, noted in a study from the 1980s to have an incidence of 10% overall but nearly 50% in patients with preexisting renal insufficiency.[50] Current technology uses digital acquisition, allowing for use of more dilute contrast in smaller amounts. Embolization of atheromatous material, aortic dissection, and puncture site complications (bleeding, false aneurysms) can still occur with intraarterial injections.

References

1. Wilson MJ, Boyd SY, Lisagor PG, Rubal BJ, Cohen DJ. Ascending aortic atheroma assessed intra-operatively by epiaortic and transesophageal echocardiography. Ann Thorac Surg 2000;70:25–30.

2. Yamazaki K, Kato H, Tsujimoto S, Kitamura R. Diabetes mellitus, internal thoracic artery grafting, and the risk of an elevated hemidiaphragm after coronary artery bypass surgery. J Cardiothorac Vasc Anesth 1994;8:437–40.

3. Gibbons RJ, Balady GJ, Bricker JT, et al. ACC/AHA Guidelines for exercise testing: summary article. A report of the American College of Cardiology/American Heart Association Task Force on Practice Guidelines (Committee to Update the 1997 Exercise Testing Guidelines. J Am Coll Cardiol 2002;40:1531–40.

4. Tavel ME. Stress testing in cardiac evaluation. Current concepts with emphasis on the ECG. Chest 2001;119:907–25.

5. Lee TH, Boucher CA. Noninvasive tests in patients with stable coronary artery disease. N Engl J Med 2001;344:1840–5.

6. Soman P, Taillefer R, DePuey EG, Udelson JE, Lahiri A. Enhanced detection of reversible perfusion defects by Tc-99m sestamibi compared to Tc-99m tetrofosmin during vasodilator stress SPECT imaging in mild-to-moderate coronary artery disease. J Am Coll Cardiol 2001;37:458–62.

7. Klocke FJ, Baird MG, Lorell BH, et al. ACC/AHA/ASNC Guidelines for the clinical use of cardiac radionuclide imaging—executive summary. A report of the American College of Cardiology/American Heart Association Task Force on Practice Guidelines (ACC/AHA/ASNC Committee to Revise the 1995 Guidelines for the Clinical Use of Cardiac Radionuclide Imaging). J Am Coll Cardiol 2003;42:1318–33.

8. Dilsizian V, Rocco TP, Freedman NM, Leon MB, Bonow RO. Enhanced detection of ischemic but viable myocardium by the reinjection of thallium after stress-redistribution imaging. N Engl J Med 1990;323:141–6.

9. Geleijnse ML, Fioretti PM, Roelandt JRTC. Methodology, feasibility, safety, and diagnostic accuracy of dobutamine stress echocardiography. J Am Coll Cardiol 1997;30:595–606.

10. Pellikka PA, Roger VL, Oh JK, Miller FA, Seward JB, Tajik AJ. Part II. Dobutamine stress echocardiography: techniques, implementation, clinical applications, and correlations. Mayo Clin Proc 1995;70:16–27.

11. Allman KC, Shaw LJ, Hachamovitch R. Udelson JE. Myocardial viability testing and impact of revascularization on prognosis in patients with coronary artery disease and left ventricular dysfunction: a meta-analysis. J Am Coll Cardiol 2002;39:1151–8.

12. Pagano D, Townend JN, Littler WA, Horton R, Camici PG, Bonser RS. Coronary artery bypass surgery as treatment for ischemic heart failure: the predictive value of viability assessment with quantitative positron emission tomography for symptomatic and functional outcome. J Thorac Cardiovasc Surg 1998;115:791–9.

13. DiCarli MF, Maddahi J, Rokhsar S, et al. Long-term survival of patients with coronary artery disease and left ventricular dysfunction: implications for the role of myocardial viability assessment in management decisions. J Thorac Cardiovasc Surg 1998;116:997–1004.

14. DiCarli MF, Hachamovitch R, Berman DS. The art and science of predicting postrevascularization improvement in left ventricular (LV) function in patients with severely depressed LV function. J Am Coll Cardiol 2002;40:1744–7.

15. Bax JJ, Poldermans D, Elhendy A, et al. Improvement of left ventricular ejection fraction, heart failure symptoms, and prognosis after revascularization in patients with chronic coronary artery disease and viable myocardium detected by dobutamine stress echocardiography. J Am Coll Cardiol 1999;34:163–9.

16. Cornel JH, Bax JJ, Elhendy A, et al. Biphasic response to dobutamine predicts improvement of global left ventricular function after surgical revascularization in patients with stable coronary artery disease. Implications of time course of recovery on diagnostic accuracy. J Am Coll Cardiol 1998;31:1002–10.

17. Nishimura RA, Grantham JA, Connolly HM, Schaff HV, Higano ST, Holmes DR Jr. Low-output, low-gradient aortic stenosis in patients with depressed left ventricular systolic function: the clinical utility of the dobutamine challenge in the catheterization laboratory. Circulation 2002;106:809–13.

18. Kim RJ, Wu E, Rafael A, et al. The use of contrast-enhanced magnetic resonance imaging to identify reversible myocardial dysfunction. N Engl J Med 2000;343:1445–53.

19. Nagel E, Lehmkuhl HB, Bocksch W, et al. Noninvasive diagnosis of ischemia-induced wall motion abnormalities with the use of high-dose dobutamine stress magnetic resonance imaging: comparison with dobutamine stress echocardiography. Circulation 1999;99:763–70.

20. Shan K, Constantine G, Sivananthan M, Flamm SD. Role of cardiac magnetic resonance imaging in the assessment of myocardial viability. Circulation 2004; 109:1328–34.

21. Zoghbi WA, Barasch E. Dobutamine MRI: a serious contender in pharmacological stress imaging. Circulation 1999;99:730–2.

22. Baim DS, Grossman W. Grossman's Cardiac catheterization, angiography, and intervention, 6th edition. Philadelphia: Lippincott Williams & Wilkins, 2000.

23. Scanlon PJ, Faxon DP, Audet AM, et al. ACC/AHA guidelines for coronary angiography. A report of the American College of Cardiology/American Heart Association Task Force on Practice Guidelines (Committee on Coronary Angiography). J Am Coll Cardiol 1999;33:1756–824.

24. Meine TJ, Harrison JK. Should we cross the valve: the risk of retrograde catheterization of the left ventricle in patients with aortic stenosis. Am Heart J 2004;148:41–2.

25. Kay J, Chow WH, Chan TM, et al. Acetylcysteine for prevention of acute deterioration of renal function following elective coronary angiography and intervention. A randomized controlled trial. JAMA 2003;289:553–8.

26. Kini AA, Sharma SK. Managing the high-risk patient: experience with fenoldopam, a selective dopamine receptor agonist, in prevention of radiocontrast nephropathy during percutaneous coronary intervention. Rev Cardiovasc Med 2001;2(suppl 1):S19–25.

27. Gupta R. Use of intravenous contrast agents in patients receiving metformin. Radiology 2002;225:311–2.

28. Seward JB, Khandheria BK, Freeman WK, et al. Multiplane transesophageal echocardiography: image orientation, examination technique, anatomic correlations, and clinical applications. Mayo Clin Proc 1993;68:523–51.

29. Schneider AT, Hsu TL, Schwartz SL, Pandian NG. Single, biplane, multiplane, and three-dimensional transesophageal echocardiography. Echocardiographic-anatomic correlations. Cardiol Clinics 1993;11:361–387.

30. Forrest AP, Lovelock ND, Hu JM, Fletcher SN. The impact of intraoperative echocardiography on an unselected cardiac surgical population: a review of 2343 cases. Anaesth Crit Care 2002;30:734–41.

31. Al-Tabbaa A, Gonzalez BM, Lee D. The role of state-of-the-art echocardiography in the assessment of myocardial injury during and following cardiac surgery. Ann Thorac Surg 2001;72:S2214–8.

32. Cicek S, Dermirkilic U, Kuralay E, Tatar H, Ozturk O. Transesophageal echocardiography in cardiac surgical emergencies. J Cardiac Surg 1995;10:236–44.

33. Willens JH, Kessler KM. Transesophageal echocardiography in the diagnosis of diseases of the thoracic aorta. Part 1. Aortic dissection, aortic intramural hematoma, and penetrating atherosclerotic ulcer of the aorta. Chest 1999;116:1772–9.

34. Willens JH, Kessler KM. Transesophageal echocardiography in the diagnosis of diseases of the thoracic aorta. Part II—Atherosclerotic and traumatic diseases of the aorta. Chest 2000;117:233–43.

35. O'Rourke RA, Brundage BH, Froelicher VF, et al. American College of Cardiology/American Heart Association expert consensus document on electron-beam computed tomography for the diagnosis and prognosis of coronary artery disease. J Am Coll Cardiol 2000;36:326–40.

36. Fayad ZA, Fuster V, Nikolaou K, Becker C. Computed tomography and magnetic resonance imaging for noninvasive coronary angiography and plaque imaging. Current and potential future concepts. Circulation 2002;106:2026–34.

37. Budoff MJ, Oudiz RJ, Zalace CP, et al. Intravenous three-dimensional coronary angiography using contrast enhanced electron beam computed tomography. Am J Cardiol 1999;83:840–5.

38. Mollett NR, Cademartiri F, Nieman K, et al. Multislice spiral computed tomography coronary angiography in patients with stable angina pectoris. J Am Coll Cardiol 2004;43:2265–70.

39. Budoff MJ, Achenbach S, Duerinckx A. Clinical utility of computed tomography and magnetic resonance techniques for noninvasive coronary angiography. J Am Coll Cardiol 2003;42:1867–78.

40. Kuettner A, Kopp AF, Schroeder S, et al. Diagnostic accuracy of multidetector computed tomography coronary angiography in patients with angiographically proven coronary artery disease. J Am Coll Cardiol 2004;43:831–9.

41. Carrol CL, Higgins CB, Caputo GR. Magnetic resonance imaging of acquired cardiac disease. Tex Heart Inst J 1996;23:144–54.

42. Barron DJ, Livesey SA, Brown IW, Delaney DJ, Lamb RK, Monro JL. Twenty-year follow-up of acute type A dissection: the incidence and extent of distal aortic disease using magnetic resonance imaging. J Cardiac Surg 1997;12:147–59.

43. Rogers WJ Jr, Kramer CM, Geskin G, et al. Early contrast-enhanced MRI predicts late functional recovery after reperfused myocardial infarction. Circulation 1999;99:744–50.

44. Baer FM, Voth E, LaRosee K, et al. Comparison of dobutamine transesophageal echocardiography and dobutamine magnetic resonance imaging for detection of residual myocardial viability. Am J Cardiol 1996;78:415–9.

45. Yang TP, Pohost GM. Magnetic resonance coronary angiography. Am Heart Hosp J 2003;1:141–8.

46. Kim WY, Danias PG, Stuber M, et al. Three-dimensional coronary magnetic resonance angiography for the detection of coronary stenosis. N Engl J Med 2001;345:1863–9.

47. Botnar TM, Stuber M, Kissinger KV, Kim WY, Spuentrup E, Manning WJ. Noninvasive coronary vessel wall and plaque imaging with magnetic resonance imaging. Circulation 2000;102:2582–7.

48. Hartnell GG, Spence L, Hughes LA, Cohen MC, Saouaf R, Buff B. Safety of MR imaging in patients who have retained metallic materials after cardiac surgery. Am J Roentgenol 1997;168:1157–9.

49. Gerber TC, Fasseas P, Lennon RJ, et al. Clinical safety of magnetic resonance imaging early after coronary artery stent placement. J Am Coll Cardiol 2003;42:1295–8.

50. Martin-Paredero V, Dixon SM, Baker JD, et al. Risk of renal failure after major angiography. Arch Surg 1983;118:1417–20.

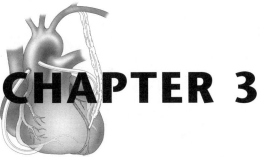

CHAPTER 3

Preoperative Considerations and Risk Assessment

Preoperative Considerations and Risk Assessment

I. General Considerations

A. Once a patient is considered a candidate for cardiac surgery, a comprehensive evaluation of the patient's overall medical condition and comorbidities is essential. This includes a detailed history and physical examination that should confirm the patient's cardiac diagnosis. It should also identify noncardiac problems that might have to be addressed perioperatively to minimize postoperative morbidity (Box 3.1). On occasion, the severity of comorbidities and an assessment of the patient's quality of life may contraindicate a surgical procedure that might otherwise seem to be indicated. Attention should also be paid to identifying new cardiac abnormalities that may have arisen since the initial cardiac catheterization that may warrant further workup. Baseline laboratory tests, if not recently performed, are also obtained, and further evaluation and consultation are performed, if indicated.

B. Evaluation of demographic factors, cardiac disease, and noncardiac comorbidities can afford both the surgeon and the patient an insight into the risk of surgery (see section VIII). Use of software that is compatible with the Society of Thoracic Surgeons (STS) database (see www.STS.org) is invaluable in allowing surgeons to compare their results not only with national norms but also, through sophisticated risk modeling, with the "expected" results for their own patient population (Table 3.1).

C. A cardiac anesthesiologist should interview the patient and discuss issues related to cessation or modification of preoperative medications (specifically insulin or oral hypoglycemic medications and any anticoagulant medications). Issues related to sedation, monitoring lines, awakening from anesthesia, and mechanical ventilation should also be discussed to make the patient aware of various aspects of the immediate perioperative period and hopefully to put his or her mind at ease (see Chapter 4).

D. Nurses with experience and an understanding of postoperative care should discuss a simplified critical pathway so that the patient has a realistic expectation of what will transpire during the hospital stay. Informing the patient of what procedures will take place and when, what is expected of him or her on each day, when discharge should be anticipated, and what the options are for post–hospital discharge care (skilled nursing facility, rehabilitation facility, home health care) are extremely beneficial in promoting prompt recovery from surgery and early hospital discharge. The patient should be provided with antiseptic scrub solution to be used during a shower at home prior to surgery.

Box 3.1 • Preoperative Evaluation for Open-Heart Surgery

History

1. Bleeding issues: antiplatelet or anticoagulant medications, bleeding history
2. Smoking (COPD, bronchospasm)
3. Alcohol (cirrhosis, DTs)
4. Diabetes (protamine reactions, wound infections)
5. Neurologic symptoms (transient ischemic attack, remote stroke, previous carotid endarterectomy)
6. Vein stripping (alternative conduits)
7. Distal vascular reconstruction (alternative conduits)
8. Urologic symptoms
9. Ulcer disease/GI bleeding (stress prophylaxis)
10. Active infections (urinary tract)
11. Current medications
12. Drug allergies

Physical Examination

1. Skin infections/rash
2. Dental caries (valve surgery)
3. Vascular examination—carotid bruits (stroke), abdominal aneurysm and peripheral pulses (IABP placement)
4. Differential arm blood pressures (pedicled ITA graft)
5. Heart/lungs (congestive heart failure, new murmur)
6. Varicose veins (alternative conduits)

Laboratory Data

1. Hematology: CBC, PT, PTT, platelet count
2. Chemistry: electrolytes, BUN, creatinine, blood sugar, liver function tests
3. Urinalysis
4. Chest x-ray PA and lateral
5. Electrocardiogram

Table 3.1 • Risk Factors for Operative Mortality in the STS Database (2004)

Demographics	Cardiac Disease
Age	History of MI < 24 h
Gender	Left main disease
BSA	Ejection fraction
Race	No. diseased vessels
	Associated valve disease

Comorbidities	Preoperative Status
Renal failure/dialysis	Salvage status
Cerebrovascular disease	Cardiogenic shock
COPD	Preop IABP
Diabetes	Reoperation
PVD	NYHA class
Hypertension	Failed PTCA < 6 h
Hypercholesterolemia	
Immunosuppressive therapy	

Factors are listed in order of their relative risk ratio for operative mortality within each category (i.e., the factor associated with the highest mortality is noted first and achieves greater weighting in the risk assessment model). A partial list of definitions from the 2004 STS specification publication is noted in Appendix 10.

BSA = body surface area; PTCA = percutaneous transluminal coronary angioplasty.

II. History

A. The nature, duration, and pattern of the patient's cardiac symptoms should be briefly summarized to allow for symptomatic classification using either the Canadian Classification System (for angina) or the New York Heart Association (NYHA) system (for both angina and heart failure symptoms). Adequate information must be provided to determine the patient's estimated operative risk of morbidity and mortality.[1] The results of diagnostic tests already performed should be noted.

B. Review of the patient's previous and current medications is important. Particular attention should be paid to anti-ischemic and antiplatelet/anticoagulant medications, which may need to be maintained or discontinued prior to surgery (Table 3.2).

   1. The recent use of **aspirin** has been shown in most studies to be associated with increased perioperative blood loss by superimposing impaired platelet function on the numerous derangements in the clotting mechanism caused by cardiopulmonary bypass (CPB).[2-4] Aspirin irreversibly acetylates platelet cyclooxygenase, impairing thromboxane A_2 formation and inhibiting platelet aggregation for the life span of the platelet (7-10 days). Although the traditional

Table 3.2 • Platelet Inhibitors to Be Stopped Prior to Surgery

Drug	Mechanism of Action	Duration of Effect	Discontinue
Aspirin	Cyclooxygenase inhibition	7 days (life span of platelet)	3–7 days preop
Clopidogrel	Inhibits ADP–mediated aggregation	7 days (life span of platelet)	5–7 days preop
Abciximab	Inhibits IIb/IIIa receptors	>12 h	12–24 h preop
Epitifibatide	Inhibits IIb/IIIa receptors	4–6 h	2–4 h preop
Tirofiban	Inhibits IIb/IIIa receptors	4–6 h	2–4 h preop

recommendation has been that aspirin should be stopped 7 days prior to surgery, newer studies have shown that a preoperative aspirin-free interval of only 3 days significantly improves platelet function and reduces transfusion requirements.[5-7] Other studies have documented reduced perioperative myocardial infarction (MI) rates and improved survival when aspirin is continued up to the time of surgery, so the concept of stopping aspirin prior to surgery has become more controversial.[8,9]

a. Some patients are aspirin resistant and appear to have inadequate inhibition of platelet function. This may account for why some patients on aspirin tend to bleed perioperatively, whereas others do not.[10]

b. A bleeding tendency is more likely in patients who are aspirin responders or have other conditions associated with platelet dysfunction, such as uremia and von Willebrand's disease. In these patients, the possibility of platelet dysfunction should prompt consideration of additional steps to optimize platelet function during surgery (use of aprotinin)[11,12] or lower the threshold for giving platelet transfusions at the conclusion of surgery if the patient is bleeding. In general, aspirin does not pose a significant perioperative bleeding problem and with careful attention to hemostasis and occasional use of platelets, perioperative hemorrhage is usually not a problem.

2. **Clopidogrel (Plavix)** is a thienopyridine that is biotransformed into an active metabolite that inhibits platelet function by irreversibly modifying the platelet adenosine diphosphate (ADP) receptor, thus inhibiting ADP-mediated activation of the platelet glycoprotein IIb/IIIa receptor. It is commonly administered to patients with acute coronary syndromes (CURE trial) and to those in whom stent placement is contemplated.[13] Given in a standard dose of 75 mg daily, it takes about 5 days to achieve 50% inhibition of platelet function. However, given in a 300-mg loading dose, as is commonly done prior to percutaneous coronary intervention, it produces significant platelet inhibition within 2–6 hours. This effect

lasts for the life span of the platelet. Most patients receiving clopidogrel also receive aspirin, which increases antiplatelet activity.

  a. For patients undergoing elective surgery, clopidogrel should be discontinued 5–7 days preoperatively.

  b. For patients receiving clopidogrel who require urgent surgery, the surgeon should be aware of the potential for increased bleeding. Several, but not all, studies have documented a significantly increased rate of bleeding and reexploration for bleeding in patients receiving clopidogrel.[14–18] Since clopidogrel has a half-life of 6–8 hours, recently administered doses may also inhibit exogenously administered platelets. Point-of-care testing can be used to determine whether significant inhibition of platelet function is present which will benefit from platelet transfusion. Aprotinin might potentially attenuate some of the platelet dysfunction noted with clopidogrel, but this has not been well studied.

3. **Heparin** is given to patients with acute coronary syndromes and is usually continued if critical coronary disease warranting surgical intervention is recommended. It is also used in patients with preoperative intraaortic balloon pumps (IABPs).

  a. **Unfractionated heparin** is given using a weight-based protocol (see Appendix 5) and requires monitoring by a partial thromboplastin time (PTT) to ensure a therapeutic range of approximately 50–60 seconds. There is usually little risk in continuing this up to the time of surgery as long as the anesthesiologist feels comfortable inserting neck lines with the patient heparinized. When heparin is used preoperatively, the platelet count should be checked on a daily basis to assess for the development of heparin-induced thrombocytopenia (HIT) (see pages 154–156).[19]

  b. A **low-molecular-weight heparin (LMWH)** (enoxaparin, dalteparin) 1 mg/kg SC twice a day is commonly used in patients with acute coronary syndromes due to its simplicity of use and the fact that it does not require blood monitoring. LMWHs have demonstrated comparable efficacy to unfractionated heparin and may be in fact be more effective, since they not only inhibit the conversion of prothrombin to thrombin, but also inhibit activated factor X (factor Xa).[20] Since only 60–80% of LMWH is neutralized by protamine, it should be stopped at least 12 hours prior to surgery to minimize perioperative bleeding.[21–23]

4. Patients taking **warfarin**, usually for atrial fibrillation (AF), a previous mechanical valve replacement, or a prior stroke, should stop their warfarin 4 days before surgery. Consideration may be given to using heparin when the international normalized ratio (INR) falls below the therapeutic range, although the risk of thromboembolism is considered to be very low during the brief period of subtherapeutic anticoagulation.[24–26]

  a. If there are concerns about an increased risk of thromboembolism, patients may be admitted the day before surgery and given unfractionated heparin IV or 5000 units SC. Alternatively, the latter may be given on an outpatient basis to provide protection when the INR becomes subtherapeutic.

  b. If the patient requires urgent surgery, administration of 5 mg of vitamin K (given intravenously over 30 minutes) should significantly reduce the INR within 12–24 hours, but fresh frozen plasma may be necessary if more emergent surgery is indicated.[27] Oral vitamin K is safer than parenteral administration (which has a risk of an anaphylactic reaction), although it takes longer to reverse the INR. It can be used in less urgent situations or when only partial reversal of the INR is desired, usually before an operation not requiring CPB.[28] Subcutaneous vitamin K has unpredictable and delayed absorption.[24]

5. **Glycoprotein IIb/IIIa inhibitors** are commonly used in patients with acute coronary syndromes and non–ST-segment myocardial infarctions in whom an early invasive strategy and possible percutaneous coronary intervention is planned.[29,30] As of late 2004, three drugs were available, one long-acting (abciximab) and two short-acting (eptifibatide [Integrilin] and tirofiban [Aggrastat]).

   a. **Abciximab (Reopro)** is the Fab fragment of a monoclonal antibody that binds to the IIb/IIIa receptor on the surface of platelets. Platelet aggregation is significantly inhibited by preventing the binding of fibrinogen and von Willebrand's factor to this receptor site on activated platelets.

      i. Reopro is usually given as a bolus dose of 0.25 mg/kg followed by a continuous infusion of 0.125 µg/kg/min for 12 hours. This achieves 80% saturation of the receptor sites, which is considered essential to render a damaged blood vessel nonreactive to platelets. Free abciximab is rapidly cleared from the circulation, although it has a half-life of at least 12 hours.

      ii. After the infusion is stopped, low levels of blockade persist for up to 10 days, but platelet function usually recovers within 48 hours. Elevated bleeding times and abnormal platelet aggregation tests are still noted in up to 25% of patients after 48 hours, but there is little hemostatic compromise when receptor blockade levels are less than 50%.

      iii. Ideally, surgery should be delayed for at least 12–24 hours after a patient has received Reopro. However, a patient should not be denied emergency surgery if it is indicated. Platelet transfusions are effective in producing hemostasis by reducing the overall number of platelet receptors bound to abciximab.[31] A hemoconcentrator can remove some of the residual free abciximab, allowing platelets to function more for hemostasis than binding free antibody.[32]

   b. **Eptifibatide** (Integrilin) and **tirofiban** (Aggrastat) are short-acting reversible antagonists of fibrinogen binding to the IIb/IIIa receptor.

      i. Eptifibatide is given in a 180-µg bolus followed by an infusion of 2.0 µg/kg/min for 72–96 hours. Tirofiban is given at a dosage of 0.4 µg/kg/min for 30 minutes followed by an infusion of 0.1 µg/kg/min for 48–96 hours.

      ii. The time course of platelet inhibition parallels their plasma level. It is estimated that platelet aggregation returns to 90% of normal within 4–8 hours after stopping tirofiban and to 50–80% of normal within 4 hours of stopping eptifibatide. It is recommended that these medications be stopped approximately 4 hours prior to surgery (see Table 3.2). It is noteworthy, however, that their use is not associated with increased post-bypass bleeding even if stopped 2 hours preoperatively or even as late as the time of skin incision. This may be attributable to their transient "platelet anesthesia" effects offsetting the adverse influence of CPB on platelet number and function.[33–35]

6. Surgery should be delayed at least 24 hours, if possible, in patients receiving **thrombolytic therapy** for an acute evolving infarction. Increased perioperative bleeding may result from the persistent systemic hemostatic defects of thrombolytic agents that outlive their short half-lives (less than 30 minutes for most recombinant tissue plasminogen activator preparations). These effects include

depletion of fibrinogen; reduction in factor II, V, and VIII levels; impairment of platelet aggregation; and the appearance of fibrin split products. When surgery must be performed on an emergency basis, the antifibrinolytic agents noted in Chapter 4 and a variety of clotting factors are usually necessary to control mediastinal hemorrhage.

7. Nonsteroidal antiinflammatory drugs have a reversible effect on platelet function and need to be stopped only a few days before surgery. Omega-3 fatty acids (fish oils), garlic, vitamin E, and gingko preparations all have antiplatelet activity and should be stopped as soon as possible before surgery.[36-38] Even flavonoids in purple grape juice have been shown to inhibit platelet function.[39] All of these vitamins and herbal remedies may be of benefit to patients with coronary artery disease but can contribute to significant perioperative bleeding if not recognized and stopped prior to surgery.

C. Inquiry should be made about any known clinical bleeding disorder or hypercoagulable state. This may direct perioperative anticoagulant management or provide direction in the management of bleeding problems.

1. **Antiphospholipid syndrome** is usually seen in patients with valvular heart disease and is associated with a hypercoagulable state due to the presence of antiphospholipid antibodies (anticardiolipin antibodies and/or lupus anticoagulant), even though thrombocytopenia is commonly present. In these patients, the baseline PTT or activated clotting time (ACT) is elevated, and the ACT is unreliable in assessing the degree of heparinization during surgery. Thus, it is recommended that the heparin-protamine titration test be used, aiming for a heparin level of 3.4 U/mL.[40]

2. Other hypercoagulable states, such as factor V Leiden or protein C or S deficiency, are usually not recognized until the patient sustains a postoperative thrombotic event. However, if these syndromes are known to be present and the patient was taking preoperative warfarin, aggressive anticoagulant measures should be taken to reduce the risk of postoperative thrombosis. Admission for preoperative heparinization should be considered when the INR is subtherapeutic. If the patient has an antithrombin III deficiency, which is also a hypercoagulable condition, either fresh frozen plasma or antithrombin III concentrate (Thrombate) may be required to achieve adequate heparinization during CPB.[41-43]

D. **Chronic obstructive pulmonary disease** (COPD) is a term often applied to patients with a significant smoking history independent of the degree of respiratory impairment. However, the degree of COPD is best defined by pulmonary function testing. Although mild to moderate COPD usually does not increase postoperative morbidity, significant COPD, especially that in elderly patients and those on steroids, is associated with an increased incidence of pulmonary and sternal wound complications, longer intensive care unit (ICU) stays, and increased operative mortality.[44-46]

1. The definitions of chronic lung disease in the 2004 STS database specifications distribution are as follows:

a. Mild: Forced expiratory volume in the first second (FEV_1) 60–75% of predicted and/or on chronic inhaled or oral bronchodilator therapy

b. Moderate: FEV_1 50–59% of predicted and/or on chronic steroid therapy

c. Severe: FEV_1 < 50% predicted and/or room air PO_2 < 60 torr or PCO_2 > 50 torr

2. Pulmonary complications are more common in patients who actively smoke, especially those with advanced age, obesity, diabetes, preoperative cardiac instability, a

productive cough, and lower respiratory tract colonization.[47–52] Actively smoking patients should be advised to terminate smoking at least 4 weeks (and preferably 2 months) before surgery to decrease the volume of airway secretions and improve mucociliary transport.[53–55] Of course, this is rarely feasible since most patients who continue to smoke are addicted to nicotine and have extreme difficulty stopping smoking. Not smoking for just a few days before surgery is probably of little benefit and may increase airway secretions.

3. An active pulmonary or bronchitic process (evidenced by a productive cough) should be resolved before surgery using antibiotics. Bronchospastic disease should be treated with bronchodilators and, if severe, with steroids. Pulmonary consultation may be indicated in this situation. Short-term pulmonary rehabilitation is effective in improving perioperative pulmonary function in patients with significant COPD and can reduce the risk of pulmonary complications.[56]

4. The patient's functional status, including the ability to walk up a flight of stairs or several hundred feet on a level surface, is at least as important as, if not more important than, spirometric studies in determining whether a patient can tolerate a surgical procedure. Although one study showed that a severe reduction in expiratory flow parameters (FEV_1, forced vital capacity [FVC], or maximal midexpiratory flow in the first 50–75 seconds [$MMEF_{50-75}$] less than 50% of predicted) was associated with the need for prolonged intubation and an increased risk of pulmonary complications,[50] other studies have not shown any correlation of pulmonary function tests (PFTs) with surgical outcome.[57] However, in patients with significant respiratory impairment, PFTs might identify patients at such high pulmonary risk that surgery may be contraindicated (generally an FEV_1 <0.6). Even then, it may be difficult to determine the contribution of a cardiac problem, such as advanced heart failure, to abnormal PFTs or diffusion capacity (<20% of predicted is an ominous sign of impaired ability to oxygenate). In this situation, careful clinical judgment must be used in deciding whether surgery will improve the patient's pulmonary status or will leave the patient a pulmonary cripple.

5. B-type natriuretic peptide (BNP) can be used as a diagnostic test to ascertain whether dyspnea is primarily of cardiac or pulmonary origin. BNP is secreted by the atria and ventricles in patients with systolic or diastolic dysfunction. A BNP level <100 pg/mL indicates that a patient's dyspnea is most likely related to a primary pulmonary process, such as exacerbation of COPD. In contrast, dyspnea in a patient with a BNP level >500 pg/mL is usually caused by decompensated heart failure. Intermediate values may be associated with LV dysfunction without decompensation, but a pulmonary process must also be considered in the differential diagnosis.[58,59]

6. Baseline pulse oximetry on room air should be obtained on every patient. If the patient has significant COPD, arterial blood gases can be valuable for comparison with postoperative values when weaning the patient from the ventilator. An elevated PCO_2 has been found to be the most significant marker for postoperative pulmonary morbidity and mortality.[51] Patients on home oxygen or with a baseline PO_2<60 torr are extremely borderline operative candidates.

7. Some patients on chronic amiodarone therapy are prone to the development of postoperative pulmonary toxicity and adult respiratory distress syndrome after surgery. This is manifested by dyspnea, hypoxia, radiographic infiltrates, and a

decrease in diffusion capacity, and carries a very high mortality rate.[60–62] The exact mechanism of pulmonary toxicity is not known, but it is more common in patients who have been on high doses of amiodarone for a long period of time. It is also more common in those with a documented preoperative decrease in diffusion capacity or prior history of pulmonary toxicity. Evidence of advanced pulmonary toxicity may contraindicate a cardiac surgical procedure. Avoidance of potential contributing causes, such as a high inspired oxygen fraction, long duration of bypass, and fluid overload, is critical. On rare occasions, this syndrome may occur after a very short course of amiodarone and appears to be an idiosyncratic or hypersensitivity reaction.[63]

E. A history of heavy **alcohol** abuse identifies potential problems with intraoperative bleeding and postoperative hepatic dysfunction, agitation, and alcohol withdrawal. Prevention of postoperative delirium tremens (DTs) with thiamine, folate, and benzodiazepines should be considered. Bioprosthetic valves should be selected to avoid postoperative anticoagulation.

1. Mildly elevated liver function tests are often of unclear significance and usually do not require further evaluation. However, in a patient with a drinking history, they may suggest the presence of alcoholic hepatitis or cirrhosis. A gastrointestinal (GI) evaluation is indicated and surgery should be deferred. A common cause of mildly elevated liver function tests is use of a "statin" medication for hypercholesterolemia.

2. A history of GI bleeding, an elevated prothrombin time (PT), or a low serum albumin, indicating impaired synthetic function or malnutrition, or a low platelet count may suggest the presence of severe cirrhosis with portal hypertension and/or hypersplenism. A liver biopsy may be indicated to evaluate the risk of surgery and the potential for postoperative hepatic failure.

3. Patients in Child-Pugh class A cirrhosis with a bilirubin < 2 mg/dL and albumin > 3.5 g/dL will usually tolerate CPB, but may have a higher risk of postoperative complications, including infections, bleeding, GI complications, respiratory and renal failure.[64–68] Patients with advanced alcoholic cirrhosis (class B or C) are generally not candidates for cardiac surgery.[64–68] The mortality rate for these patients is very high, with two studies showing a 50% mortality for class B and 100% for class C patients.[67,68] However, off-pump bypass surgery can be performed successfully in patients with advanced liver disease if their lifestyle and life span are compromised primarily by their heart disease.[68,69]

F. There is a higher incidence of stroke, infection, renal dysfunction, and operative mortality in patients with **diabetes mellitus** than in nondiabetics.[70,71] Insulin-dependent diabetics have higher rates of respiratory and renal failure than non–insulin-dependent diabetics.[71] Diabetes is a relative contraindication to bilateral internal thoracic artery (ITA) bypass grafting. Some studies have shown the risk of infection is significantly greater, although others have not.[72,73] Skeletonizing the ITA pedicle may reduce the risk of infection, although it remains significant in obese, diabetic women.[74] Diabetics are also more prone to phrenic nerve dysfunction after ITA harvesting.[75,76] Patients taking NPH insulin are at increased risk of experiencing a protamine reaction.[77]

G. **Neurologic symptoms**, whether active (transient ischemic attack) or remote (history of stroke), increase the risk of perioperative stroke and warrant evaluation.[78] Generally, a carotid noninvasive study with ultrasound imaging and measurement of flow velocities should be performed in the patient with neurologic symptoms, history of a carotid endarterectomy (CEA), or asymptomatic carotid bruits to assess for significant stenoses or flow-limiting lesions. It should also be considered as a screening test for patients with significant peripheral vascular disease or calcified aortas.[79] Further evaluation by carotid arteriography (usually magnetic resonance angiography) may be considered if noninvasive studies are inconclusive or more precise visualization of the carotid vessels is desired.

1. Actively symptomatic carotid disease always warrants CEA either prior to or at the time of cardiac surgery. Combined coronary artery bypass grafting (CABG)–CEA should be performed in the patient with unstable angina or significant myocardium at risk if neurologic symptoms are present.[80]

2. The management of asymptomatic carotid lesions in patients requiring cardiac surgery is controversial and is noted below in the discussion of carotid bruits.

H. A history of **saphenous vein strippings and/or ligation** or **distal vascular reconstructive procedures** using saphenous vein alerts the surgeon to potential problems in obtaining satisfactory conduits for bypass grafting. Noninvasive venous mapping of the lower extremities may identify satisfactory greater or lesser saphenous veins for use. Doppler assessment of the palmar arch should be performed to assess the feasibility of using the radial artery as a bypass conduit (i.e., confirming that the arm is ulnar dominant). Informing the patient of potential complications of radial artery harvesting (specifically numbness of the dorsum of the thumb and part of the thenar eminence from trauma to the superficial radial nerve) is essential.[81] Venipunctures and intravenous catheters should be avoided in the arm from which the radial artery will be harvested. The anesthesiologist should also be alerted to avoid placing a radial artery line or intravenous catheter in that arm in the operating room!

I. **Urologic symptoms** in women suggest the presence of an active urinary tract infection that must be treated before surgery. In men, a history of prostatic cancer treated by irradiation, a prior transurethral resection, or other urinary symptoms consistent with prostatic hypertrophy identify potential problems with Foley catheter placement in the operating room. Use of a Coudé catheter may be necessary. Urologic consultation should be obtained if a catheter cannot be passed. Either a catheter may be placed after dilating the urethra or a suprapubic tube may be inserted. Prolonged postoperative urinary drainage should be anticipated until the patient is fully ambulatory or until further urologic evaluation is performed.

J. A history of significant **ulcer disease** or **GI bleeding** may necessitate further evaluation by endoscopy, especially if the patient will require postoperative anticoagulation. However, invasive diagnostic tests might have to be deferred in patients with significant coronary disease. Use of postoperative proton pump inhibitors, H_2 blockers, or sucralfate should be considered in these patients.[82,83]

K. The risk of **infection** is increased if another infectious source is present in the body (commonly a urinary tract or skin infection). Concurrent infections must be identified and treated before surgery. An upper respiratory infection may increase the risk of pulmonary complications, and bacterial infections may increase the risk of a hematogenous sternal wound infection and can seed a prosthetic heart valve.

L. The patient's **medications and allergies** should be reviewed. Most cardiac medications should be continued up to the time of surgery; some must be stopped in advance (warfarin, antiplatelet drugs, metformin); and others may require specific attention during anesthesia and the early postoperative course (steroids, insulin, monoamine oxidase inhibitors, alternative antibiotics for antibiotic allergies)

M. Other significant medical history, such as previous chest wall irradiation for cancer, endocrine conditions, or psychiatric history, should be detailed in the medical record. A thorough review of systems will assist in identifying other comorbid conditions likely to affect the outcome of surgery.

III. Physical Examination

A. The patient's general appearance, mental status, and affect should be evaluated and noted in the medical record as a baseline for comparison with the postoperative period.

B. An active **skin infection or rash** that might be secondarily infected must be treated before surgery to minimize the risk of sternal wound infection.

C. **Dental caries** must be treated before operations during which prosthetic material (valves, grafts) will be placed.[84] Dental extractions, however, should be recommended cautiously to patients with severe ischemic heart disease or critical aortic stenosis. Cardiac complications may occur even if dental procedures are performed under local anesthesia.

D. **Carotid bruits** are a marker, although an insensitive one, of carotid disease, which is present in about 10% of patients with significant coronary disease. Carotid noninvasive studies are warranted in virtually all patients with bruits to assess for high-grade unilateral or bilateral disease.[85]

   1. The management of an asymptomatic carotid lesion in a patient requiring open-heart surgery is controversial. The risk of stroke with a high-grade unilateral stenotic lesion during an isolated CABG is increased.[86] Thus, if the patient presents with an acute coronary syndrome or has a large degree of myocardium at risk, most surgeons would perform a combined CABG-CEA for a unilateral stenosis > 90%. The risk of stroke in a combined operation for unilateral asymptomatic disease is very low, and this approach reduces the subsequent risk of stroke and is cost effective.[87–90] In contrast, preliminary CEA is the preferred approach in patients with stable angina and may result in a lower overall risk of stroke, MI, and death.[91]

   2. The risk of stroke with bilateral disease (> 75% bilaterally) is significant during isolated CABG (as high as 10–15%), especially in patients with unilateral stenosis with contralateral occlusion.[86] However, it remains quite significant even with a combined operation. Thus, the operations should be staged with the CEA performed first if cardiac disease permits. If this is not possible because of unstable angina, left main or severe three-vessel disease with a large amount of "myocardium in jeopardy," a combined operation should be performed, with the understanding that the risk of stroke is increased.

E. **Bilateral arm blood pressures** should be measured. Differential pressures may identify possible subclavian artery stenosis, a contraindication to use of a pedicled ITA graft. This finding is also noted in some patients presenting with an acute aortic dissection.

F. The presence of a **heart murmur** may warrant a pre- or intraoperative echocardiogram if no valvular abnormality had been identified at the time of catheterization. Occasionally, new-onset ischemic mitral regurgitation or unsuspected aortic valve disease will be detected.

G. An **abdominal aortic aneurysm** detected upon palpation should be evaluated by ultrasound. IABP placement through the femoral artery should be avoided to prevent distal atheroembolism.

H. Severe **peripheral vascular disease** (PVD) must be assessed by a careful pulse examination. It is often associated with cerebrovascular disease and may prompt a preoperative carotid noninvasive study. In several studies, PVD has been shown to be a risk factor for operative mortality.

1. Weak femoral pulses may be indicative of "inflow" aortoiliac disease. This may dictate the unsuitability of the femoral arteries for cannulation or placement of an IABP. If the ascending aorta is also significantly diseased and an alternative cannulation site must be utilized, the axillary artery should be considered.[92]

2. PVD may contribute to poor wound healing. Generally, the saphenous vein should be harvested from the leg with the best circulation to improve wound healing. This will also leave venous conduit for future peripheral vascular reconstruction. "Minimally invasive" vein harvesting using endoscopic equipment or through short "skip incisions" under direct vision is preferable to one long incision in the leg.[93]

I. The presence of **varicose veins** identifies potential problems with conduits for CABG. The distribution of varicosities may indicate whether or not the greater saphenous vein is involved. Noninvasive venous mapping may identify a normal greater saphenous vein despite significant varicosities. The lesser saphenous vein distribution should be inspected to determine whether it might serve as a potential conduit. Assessment of the radial artery, as noted above, should be considered.

IV. Laboratory Assessment

A. **Complete blood count (CBC), PT, PTT, and platelet count**

1. An elevated WBC may be associated with an infectious process that should be identified before surgery. However, it may also be a generalized marker of inflammation. One large study showed that the operative mortality for CABG was 2.8 times greater if the preoperative WBC exceeded 12,000.[94]

2. It is important to check a daily platelet count in a patient maintained on heparin because HIT may develop. If HIT is suspected based on a falling platelet count, further workup is indicated with testing for heparin-induced platelet aggregation (usually by the serotonin release assay) or by serologic testing for heparin antibodies.[19] If these tests are positive, an alternative means of anticoagulation during bypass may be necessary (see pages 154–156). The significance of serologic positivity for HIT in the absence of thrombocytopenia is unclear but should not contraindicate use of heparin during surgery.

3. Patients with unstable ischemic syndromes should be transfused to a hematocrit of at least 28%. This is beneficial in reducing potential cardiac ischemia as well as blood transfusion requirements at the time of surgery (a risk factor for increased mortality). It is noteworthy that many patients experience a significant fall in hematocrit following cardiac catheterization, approximating 5.4% on the average, either from hydration, external blood loss, groin hematomas, or retroperitoneal bleeding.[95] This may be lessened by the use of collagen plugs following sheath withdrawal from the femoral artery.

4. Some groups perform bleeding times on patients taking aspirin, but this test is generally of limited value. Although bleeding times are commonly elevated in

patients maintained on antiplatelet therapy, they are inconsistently reproducible, correlate poorly with the extent of intraoperative bleeding, and generally are not necessary.[96,97] The availability of point-of-care qualitative platelet function testing during surgery can dictate whether platelets are necessary to control bleeding in patients taking antiplatelet medications.

B. **Electrolytes, BUN, creatinine, blood sugar.** Patients with elevated creatinine (> 1.5 mg/dL) are more prone to progressive renal dysfunction after surgery and have a higher operative mortality.[98,99] The 2004 STS definition of preoperative renal failure is a creatinine > 2.0. Thus, patients with an elevated creatinine, especially diabetics, should have their serum creatinine checked after cardiac catheterization. If the creatinine is increased, it should be rechecked and surgery deferred, if possible, until renal function has returned to baseline. Studies have shown that a creatinine clearance (C_{CL}) less than 55 mL/min, calculated by the equation $C_{CL} = [(140 - \text{age}) \times \text{weight in kg}]/[72 \times \text{serum Cr}]$ ($\times 0.85$ for females) has a better predictive power for operative mortality than the serum creatinine level.[100] N-acetylcysteine (Mucomyst) is commonly used for cardiac catheterization to minimize renal toxicity.[101] It is given in a dose of 600 mg bid PO prior to and after catheterization or can be given intravenously as 150 mg/kg in 500 mL normal saline (NS) over 30 minutes prior to contrast exposure followed by a 50 mg/kg dose in 500 mL NS given over the subsequent 4 hours. Fenoldopam 0.1 μg/kg/min has also be used to preserve renal function during catheterization (as well as surgery).[102] Measures should be taken to optimize renal function before surgery, paying particular attention to hydration and optimizing hemodynamic status (see also Chapter 12).

C. **Liver function tests** (bilirubin, alkaline phosphatase, alanine aminotransferase, aspartate aminotransferase, albumin). Abnormalities suggestive of hepatitis or cirrhosis may warrant further evaluation. Those associated with chronic passive congestion may not improve until after surgery has been performed. Occasionally, emergency surgery is indicated in patients with cardiogenic shock with an acute hepatic insult and markedly increased liver enzymes. In this situation, there is a significant risk of severe hepatic dysfunction after surgery, which is associated with a high mortality rate.

D. **Urinalysis.** If an initial urinalysis suggests contamination, a "clean-catch" specimen with proper cleansing should be obtained. If there is the suggestion of a urinary tract infection, a culture should be obtained. The appropriate antibiotic should be given for several days prior to elective surgery. If the patient requires urgent surgery, one or two doses of an antibiotic providing gram-negative coverage should suffice prior to bypass surgery, although a few days of treatment might be considered before performing valve surgery.

E. **Chest x-ray (PA and lateral).** The x-ray is essential to rule out any active disease that should be treated prior to surgery. Identification of pulmonary nodules should prompt a chest CT scan preoperatively, since interpretation can be difficult once surgery is performed. A lateral film should always be obtained before reoperation through a median sternotomy incision. This gives an assessment of the proximity of the cardiac structures and the ITA pedicle clips to the posterior sternal table. It also allows for optimal planning of minimally invasive incisions. Additional significant information that can be derived from a chest x-ray is noted on page 61.

F. **Electrocardiogram.** A baseline study should be obtained for comparison with postoperative ECGs. Evidence of an interval infarction or new ischemia since the time of catheterization may warrant reevaluation of ventricular function and, on occasion, a repeat coronary angiogram. Patients being evaluated for elective surgery with active ischemia on ECG should be hospitalized and undergo urgent procedures.

1. If atrial fibrillation (AF) is present, it should be rate-controlled and its duration ascertained. The likelihood of conversion to sinus rhythm after surgery is nearly 80% for patients in AF less than 6 months, but it is unlikely if the AF has been of longer duration. Thus, the duration of AF would influence the aggressiveness of postoperative treatment and possibly influence the decision to perform a Maze procedure in addition to the planned operation.

2. The presence of a left bundle branch block raises the risk of heart block during the insertion of a Swan-Ganz catheter, and the catheter should not be advanced into the pulmonary artery in the operating room until the chest is open. The presence of a bundle branch block also makes it more difficult to detect ischemia.

G. Most test results are acceptable when performed within one month of surgery. However, it is beneficial to have a CBC, electrolytes, BUN, and creatinine within a few days of surgery.

V. Preoperative Blood Donation

A. Preoperative autologous blood donation is a feasible objective in patients with stable angina or valvular heart disease.[103] However, its limited use in the past few years can be ascribed to several factors: (1) the urgency of surgery in most cases; (2) concerns about precipitating angina in patients with severe coronary disease; (3) lessened concern about the transmission of hepatitis C and human immunodeficiency virus; (4) questions about its cost-effectiveness with the availability of other measures to reduce blood loss, such as antifibrinolytic drugs, cell-saving devices, and off-pump surgery; and (5) logistic blood bank considerations.[104] Thus, it is commonly not necessary or encouraged.

1. One unit of blood may be donated every week as long as the hematocrit exceeds 33%, allowing an additional 2–3 weeks before surgery for the hematocrit to return to normal.

2. The use of recombinant erythropoietin can induce erythropoiesis very rapidly. Doses of 600 U/kg SC 7 and 14 days before surgery with iron supplementation can improve the preoperative hematocrit in anemic patients and those who donate their own blood. This is particularly helpful in Jehovah's Witness patients.[105,106] Even one dose of 100 IU/kg of recombinant human erythropoietin given intravenously 4 days prior to surgery can rapidly produce erythropoiesis and reduce transfusion requirements.[107]

B. The percentage of patients requiring blood transfusions after coronary surgery has gradually been decreasing, and fewer than 50% of patients receive any blood products. In addition to the measures mentioned above, a lower transfusion trigger has evolved with the recognition that postoperative hematocrits as low as 22–24% are safe.[108,109]

C. Refinement in testing for hepatitis C (1/250,000 to 1.5 million units) and human immunodeficiency virus (1/750,000 units) has lowered their risks to extremely low levels and allayed the morbid fear of many patients of receiving transfusions.[110,111] Nonetheless, blood transfusions may still cause febrile, allergic, or transfusion reactions and may adversely affect respiratory and hemodynamic function when given in massive amounts. It has been well documented that the use of perioperative transfusions raises the risk of infection, renal dysfunction, respiratory complications, and overall mortality.

VI. Preoperative Medications

A. All antianginal medications should be continued up to and including the morning of surgery to prevent recurrence of ischemia and to provide for a more stable anesthetic course. The substitution of a shorter acting β-blocker or calcium channel blocker for a longer acting one (metoprolol for nadolol; diltiazem for Cardizem CD) should be considered. The use of preoperative β-blockers has been shown to lower the mortality rate of coronary bypass surgery.[112,113]

B. Antihypertensive medications should also be given the morning of surgery to prevent rebound hypertension and provide for a more stable anesthetic course. However, patients taking ACE inhibitors tend to have a lower systemic resistance on bypass and in the immediate postoperative period, and it is often beneficial to withhold this medication on the morning of surgery.

C. Digoxin should be given the morning of surgery if used for rate control.

D. Diuretics are continued up to the morning of surgery. Hypokalemia from diuretics is usually not a problem intraoperatively because of the high doses of potassium present in the cardioplegia solutions used for myocardial protection.

E. Anticoagulants and antiplatelet agents (see section II.B)

    1. Warfarin should be stopped four days before surgery to allow for normalization of the INR. Rapid reversal may be accomplished with 5 mg of vitamin K given intravenously, but fresh frozen plasma may be used as well.

    2. Intravenous heparin is generally continued up to the time of surgery.

    3. LMWH should be stopped more than 12 hours preoperatively.

    4. Short-acting IIb/IIIa inhibitors should be stopped 4 hours preoperatively.

    5. Aspirin should be stopped 3–7 days prior to surgery.

    6. Clopidogrel should be stopped 5–7 days prior to surgery.

    7. Surgery should be delayed 12–24 hours in patients receiving abciximab or thrombolytic therapy.

    8. If the patient requires truly urgent or emergency surgery, platelets and clotting factors must be available to combat the lingering antihemostatic effects of any of the above drugs.

F. Diabetic patients should refrain from taking their oral hypoglycemic medications or insulin on the morning of surgery. Blood sugar should be checked in the operating room and insulin given as necessary.

G. Antiarrhythmic therapy should be continued until the time of surgery. Long-term use of amiodarone may be associated with postoperative respiratory failure, and it should be stopped as soon as surgery is being contemplated if there is evidence of any pulmonary problems. Otherwise, there is little benefit in stopping it for a short period of time to reduce perioperative risks because it has a very long half-life.

H. Preoperative prophylactic antibiotics must be administered before surgical incision. A first-generation cephalosporin, such as cefazolin, is commonly chosen because of its effectiveness against gram-positive organisms. There is some evidence that over-all infection rates may be lower with use of second-generation cephalosporins, such as cefamandole or cefuroxime.[114] Vancomycin is used if there is a severe allergy to penicillin or the cephalosporins. It is more expensive than the cephalosporins, but because of its increased efficacy against gram-positive organisms, it should probably be selected for all patients undergoing valvular surgery.[115] However, it should not be used indiscriminately to minimize the emergence of strains of vancomycin-resistant enterococci, a growing concern in ICUs.

Box 3.2 • Typical Preoperative Order Sheet

1. Admit to: _____
2. Surgery date: _____
3. Planned procedure: _____
4. Laboratory tests:
   - ☐ CBC with differential
   - ☐ PT/INR   ☐ PTT
   - ☐ Electrolytes, BUN, creatinine, blood sugar
   - ☐ Bilirubin, AST, ALT, alkaline phosphatase, albumin
   - ☐ Urinalysis
   - ☐ Electrocardiogram
   - ☐ Chest x-ray PA and lateral
   - ☐ Antibody screen   ☐ Crossmatch: ___ units PRBC
   - ☐ Other:
5. Treatments/Assessments
   Admission vital signs
   Obtain room air O_2 by pulse oximetry; ABG if < 90%
   Measure height and weight
   NPO after midnight except sips of water with meds
   Shave/Hibiclens scrub to chest and legs
   Incentive spirometry teaching
6. Medications
   - ☐ Peridex gargle on-call to OR
   - ☐ Cefazolin 1 gm IV to OR with patient
   - ☐ Vancomycin 15 mg/kg = _____ g IV to OR with patient
   - ☐ Discontinue aspirin, clopidogrel, NSAIDs immediately
   - ☐ Stop heparin at _____
   - ☐ Continue heparin drip into OR
   - ☐ Discontinue low-molecular-weight heparin after AM dose on _____
   - ☐ Stop IIb/IIIa inhibitors at _____
   - ☐ Other:

I. Preoperative medications are ordered by the anesthesia service. These include sedation with narcotics (morphine), benzodiazepines (lorazepam or midazolam), scopolamine, and H_2 blockers (cimetidine or ranitidine) to decrease gastric acidity. The selection of preoperative medications usually depends on the nature of the patient's cardiac disease, as discussed in Chapter 4.

VII. Preoperative Checklist

Once the patient has been accepted for surgery, orders should be written to address general and patient-specific concerns (tests, medications) before surgery. Preprinted order sheets are helpful to avoid overlooking any details (Box 3.2). The evening before surgery, the covering physician/physician assistant/nurse practitioner should write a brief preoperative note summarizing essential information that should be reviewed before proceeding with the operation. Writing this note prevents important details from being overlooked (Box 3.3). For patients undergoing elective surgery, the surgical team must take the responsibility of confirming that all of the requisite information is present in the patient's office chart the night before admission and is available to the operating room when the patient arrives in the morning. The following should be noted:

A. The planned operative procedure

B. Indication for surgery

C. Brief summary of the cardiac catheterization data

D. Results of the laboratory data listed above

E. Surgical note and consent in chart

F. Anesthesia note and consent in chart

G. Confirmation of blood bank cross-match and blood setup

    1. The major determinants of the need for transfusion are the patient's blood volume (which correlates with body size and usually with gender) and the

---

Box 3.3 • Preoperative Checklist

1. Planned operation: _____
2. Indication for surgery: _____
3. Brief summary of cardiac catheterization results
4. Lab results
   a. Electrolytes, BUN, creatinine, blood sugar
   b. PT, PTT, platelet count, CBC
   c. Urinalysis
   d. Chest x-ray
   e. Electrocardiogram
5. Surgical note and consent in chart
6. Anesthesia note and consent in chart
7. Confirmation of blood bank setup
8. Preoperative orders written

Table 3.3 • Blood Setup Guidelines for Open-Heart Surgery

Procedure	PRBC Setup
Minimally invasive CABG without pump	Type and screen
Weight > 70 kg and hematocrit > 35%	One unit
Weight < 70 kg or hematocrit < 35%	Two units
Reoperations	Three units
Ascending aortic surgery	Three units
Descending aortic surgery	Six units

PRBC = packed red blood cells

preoperative hemoglobin level. Other risk factors for transfusion include older age, urgent or emergent operations, poor ventricular function, reoperations, more complex operations with longer duration of CPB, higher volumes of crystalloid used during surgery (>2500 mL), elevated INR preoperatively, and the presence of comorbidities, including insulin-dependent diabetes, PVD, elevated creatinine, and an albumin <4 g/dL consistent with poor nutrition.[116–119]

2. Guidelines for blood setup are shown in Table 3.3.

H. Preoperative orders are written:

1. Antibiotics: (always check for allergy)

   a. Cefazolin 1 g IV to be given in the operating room (some recommend that an appropriate dose should be either 1 g prior to induction and 1 g before going on pump, or 2 g initially to maintain an adequate serum level throughout surgery)[120,121]

   or

   b. Vancomycin 15 mg/kg. This should be available when the patient is taken into the operating room so that it may be infused over at least 30 minutes to avoid hypotension and the "red-neck syndrome" and can be completed by the time of skin incision.[122]

2. Specific orders to stop medications listed in section VI above.

3. Antiseptic scrub (chlorhexidine) with which to shower the night before surgery. Preferably this should be applied several times rather than during a single shower.[123]

4. Mupirocin (Bactroban) nasal ointment can reduce nasal carriage of staphylococcal organisms to reduce incidence of surgical site infections with methicillin-resistant *Staphylococcus aureus*.[124]

5. Peridex mouthwash (oral chlorhexidine)

6. **Skin preparation.** This is best performed the morning of surgery as it has been well documented that the closer the prep to the time of surgery, the lower the wound infection rate.[125] Use of clippers is preferable to shaving with a razor, which increases the risk of infection.

7. NPO after midnight

8. Preoperative medications per anesthesia service

VIII. Risk Assessment and Informed Consent

A. General comments

1. An important element of the preoperative preparation for cardiac surgery is an assessment of the patient's surgical risk. Risk stratification can afford patients and their families insight into the **real** risk of complications and mortality. It can also increase the awareness of the health care team to the high-risk patient for whom more aggressive therapy in the pre-, intra-, or postoperative period may be beneficial. Documentation in the chart of an informed consent discussion is **mandatory** prior to any cardiac surgical procedures. This note should quantify in some fashion the estimated mortality risk, should list some of the more common complications of the operation being performed, and should address risks that may be unique to the individual patient.

2. Although mortality rates are widely scrutinized, overall mortality for cardiac surgical procedures is quite low, being less than 3% for CABGs in the 2004 STS database. However, the overall incidence of complications after cardiac surgery is quite high, approximating 40–50%. The ability to predict and hopefully prevent postoperative morbidity has a significant impact on the patient's recovery and quality of life after surgery and in reducing hospital length of stay and costs.

B. **Risk stratification** is based on an assessment of four important interrelated categories of risk factors (see Table 3.1).

1. **Patient demographics**. These refer to patient-related factors, independent of disease, such as age, gender, and race.

2. **Comorbidities**. These refer to coexisting diseases that are not necessarily directly related to the cardiac disease but can have significant impact on the patient's ability to recover from surgery. In the vast majority of patients, mortality and complications are related to preexisting comorbidities, such as renal dysfunction, cerebrovascular disease, and COPD. These render the patient more susceptible to the insults of CPB or to complications from a low cardiac output state.

3. **Cardiac disease**. The nature and extent of cardiac disease and the degree of ventricular dysfunction are important considerations in determining the operative risk. For the vast majority of patients at low to moderate risk, they generally do not raise the operative risk significantly. However, for uncommon surgical situations, such as a very recent MI (within 24 hours), profound left ventricular dysfunction (EF < 20%), or mechanical complications of infarction, such as a ventricular septal defect (VSD) or acute mitral regurgitation, they are powerful risk factors. Postcardiotomy ventricular dysfunction associated with poor ventricular function can exacerbate preexisting comorbidities that may contribute to operative mortality, such as renal dysfunction.

4. **Preoperative status.** The immediate risk of death is greatest in patients who come to surgery on an urgent or emergent basis. Such patients may have unstable cardiac disease with ongoing ischemia or hemodynamic compromise that requires inotropes, IABP support, or even ongoing cardiopulmonary resuscitation.

C. **Types of risk models**

1. **Univariate analysis** assesses the association of an individual risk factor with a specific outcome, such as mortality. Odds ratios are calculated that compare the outcome with and without the risk factor being present. However, calculation of operative risk is difficult using univariate data. Although each individual risk factor increases the risk of surgery, it is difficult to assess the overall risk when multiple factors are present, since many are interdependent. Although some factors are discrete or dichotomous, such as gender or reoperation, others are continuous, such as patient age or ventricular function. Further subdividing continuous variables into multiple categories (e.g., age > 65, age > 75) makes risk assessment very complex when numerous risk factors are being considered.

2. **Multivariate regression models** are designed to assess the independent association of variables with a specific outcome. The inherent shortcomings of univariate models mandate the use of multivariate analysis to evaluate the independent association of factors found to be significant by univariate analysis with morbidity or mortality. Logistic (or nonlinear) regression is used for dichotomous outcomes, such as death, whereas linear regression analysis is used for continuous outcomes, such as length of stay or hospital costs.

D. **Preoperative predictors of operative mortality**

1. Numerous large surgical databases have analyzed risk factors for mortality after coronary bypass surgery (Table 3.4).[126–137] Most of these risk factors cannot be modified and the expected mortality rates have been validated in clinical studies. The surgeon can use these models to objectively provide the patient with an individualized predicted mortality rate no matter now optimal the perioperative care. The most common risk factors noted in these studies include, in approximate decreasing order of significance:

   a. Emergency surgery, which includes some of the powerful but fairly uncommon risk factors (cardiogenic shock, VSD, ongoing cardiopulmonary resuscitation)
   b. Renal dysfunction, especially if dialysis-dependent
   c. Reoperations
   d. Older age (> 75–80)
   e. Poor ventricular function (EF < 30%)
   f. Female gender
   g. Left main disease
   h. Other comorbidities, such as COPD, PVD, diabetes, and cerebrovascular disease

Table 3.4 • Predictors of Operative Mortality in Major Studies (Multivariate Analyses)

Parsonnet[127]	Cleveland Clinic[129]	STS[130]	NNE[128]	VA System[133]	New York State[131]	Toronto[134]	Israel[135]
Second reoperation	Emergency	Emergency (salvage)	Age > 75	Emergency	Disasters (VSD, cardiogenic shock)	EF < 25%	Emergency
Renal failure on dialysis	Creat > 1.9	Reoperation	Emergency	Reoperation	Second reoperation	EF < 35%	Left main disease
Cirrhosis	Severe LV dysfunction	Dialysis-dependent renal failure	Reoperation	CHF	EF < 20%	Emergency	Creatinine > 1.4
Cardiogenic shock or VSD	Reoperation	Cardiogenic shock	Age > 65	Preoperative IABP	Dialysis-dependent renal failure	Reoperation	Severe CHF
Age > 80	MR	Emergency (nonsalvage)	BSA < 1.6	IV nitroglycerin	First reoperation	Age > 75	Age > 75
First reoperation	Age > 75	Creat > 2.0	Comorbidity score > 1	Older age	CHF	Female	Diabetes mellitus
EF < 30%	Previous vascular surgery	H/o stroke	Urgent operation	Urgent indication	Diabetes	Age 65–74	Female
Age > 75	COPD	Female	LVEDP > 22	NYHA classification	Unstable angina	Three-vessel disease	Ejection fraction < 40%
EF < 50%	Anemia	Preop IABP	Age 60–64	Cerebrovascular disease	Valve operation		Urgent operation
Severe COPD	Diabetes	Peripheral vascular disease		Peripheral vascular disease	Left main disease		

VA = Veterans Affairs; MR = mitral regurgitation; LVEDP = left ventricular end-diastolic pressure; BSA = body surface area.

Table 3.5A • Preoperative Risk-Estimation Worksheet (Parsonnet)[127]

Risk Factor		Scoring	Value
Female gender		6	
Age	70–75	2.5	
	76–79	7	
	80+	11	
Congestive heart failure		2.5	
COPD (severe)		6	
Diabetes		3	
Ejection fraction	30–49%	6.5	
	< 30%	8	
Hypertension	> 140/90	3	
Left main disease	> 50%	2.5	
Morbid obesity	> 1.5 ideal body weight	1	
Preoperative IABP		4	
Reoperation	First	10	
	Second or subsequent	20	
Aortic valve replacement		0	
Mitral valve replacement		4.5	
CABG-valve		6	
Special situations			
		TOTAL	

Table 3.5B • Risk Values for Special Conditions (Parsonnet)[127]

Cardiac		Hepatorenal	
Cardiogenic shock	12	Cirrhosis	12.5
Endocarditis, active	6.5	Dialysis dependency	13.5
Endocarditis, treated	0	Renal failure, acute or chronic	3.5
LV aneurysm resection	1.5		
Tricuspid valve	5	**Vascular**	
Pacemaker dependency	0	Abdominal aortic aneurysm, asymptomatic	0.5
Transmural acute MI < 48 h	4	Carotid disease (bilateral or 100% unilateral occlusion)	2
Ventricular septal defect, acute	12	Peripheral vascular disease, severe fibrillation, aborted sudden death	2.5
Ventricular tachycardia	1		
Ventricular fibrillation, aborted sudden death			
Pulmonary		**Miscellaneous**	
Asthma	1	Blood products refused	11
Preoperative endotracheal tube	4	Severe neurologic disorder (healed CVA, paraplegia)	5
Idiopathic thrombocytopenic purpura	12	PTCA or catheterization failure	5.5
Pulmonary hypertension (mean PAP > 30)	11	Substance abuse	4.5

LV = left ventricular; CVA = cerebrovascular accident; PTCA = percutaneous transluminal coronary angioplasty; PAP = pulmonary arterial pressure.

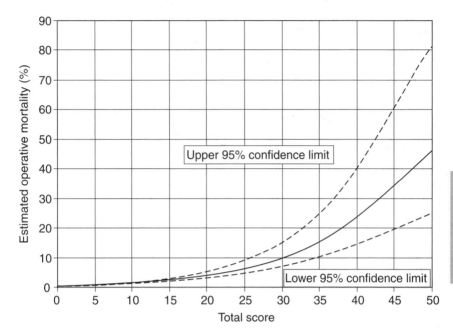

Figure 3.1 • The estimated mortality risk for patients using the preoperative risk-estimation worksheet on the previous page.[127] *Modified with permission from Bernstein AD, Parsonnet V. Bedside estimation of risk as an aid for decision-making in cardiac surgery. Ann Thorac Surg 2000;69:823–8.*

2. The calculation of operative risk can be performed with "bedside" or computerized models. The most common of the bedside models are the Parsonnet,[127] Northern New England (NNE),[128] and the Cleveland Clinic[129] risk stratification systems (Tables 3.5A, 3.5B, 3.6 and Figure 3.1). These assign weights or points to each factor based on their odds ratio, which reflects the relative contribution of each factor to mortality in a validated model. The score derived from the weight of various factors can then be used to provide an "expected" mortality. The sophisticated computer software packages compatible with the STS database require extensive data entry that can provide a precise expected mortality rate. Although the number of parameters assessed in these models differs, they all provide comparable risk assessment.

E. **Preoperative predictors of postoperative morbidity**

1. Numerous studies have also analyzed the risk factors that are predictive of overall postoperative morbidity (Table 3.7).[137–145] It is noteworthy that the overall incidence of complications for standard cardiac surgical procedures is quite high, approximating 40–50% in the STS database. The more common complications, such as AF, are fairly benign but are associated with increased length of stay and cost.[146] In contrast, the less common complications are associated with significant mortality (Table 3.8).

Table 3.6 • *Preoperative Estimation of Risk of Mortality, Cerebrovascular Accident, and Mediastinitis for Patients Undergoing Coronary Artery Bypass Surgery (Northern New England Cardiovascular Disease Study Group 1999)[128,136]*

Patient Characteristic	Mortality Score	CVA Score	Mediastinitis Score
Age 60–69	2	3.5	
Age 70–79	3	5	
Age ≥ 80	5	6	
Female sex	1.5		
EF < 40%	1.5	1.5	2
Urgent surgery	2	1.5	1.5
Emergent surgery	5	2	3.5
Prior CABG	5	1.5	
PVD	2	2	
Diabetes			1.5
Dialysis or creatinine > 2	4	2	2.5
COPD	1.5		3.5
Obesity (BMI 31–36)			2.5
Severe obesity (BMI ≥ 37)			3.5

Perioperative Risk

Total Score	Mortality	CVA	Mediastinitis
0	0.4	0.3	0.4
1	0.5	0.4	0.5
2	0.7	0.7	0.6
3	0.9	0.9	0.7
4	1.3	1.1	1.1
5	1.7	1.5	1.5
6	2.2	1.9	1.9
7	3.3	2.8	3.0
8	3.9	3.5	3.5
9	6.1	4.5	5.8
10	7.7	≥ 6.5	≥ 6.5
11	10.6		
12	13.7		
13	17.7		
14	> 28.3		

CVA = cerebrovascular accident; BMI = body mass index.

Table 3.7 • Preoperative Predictors of Postoperative Morbidity or Increased Length of Stay

Boston Univ[138]	Veterans Affairs[139]	Helsinki[140]	Pres-St. Luke's[141]	Albany[142]	Ontario[143]	Boston Univ[144]
Morbidity and Mortality	*Morbidity*	*Morbidity*	*Morbidity*	*Length of Stay*	*Length of Stay*	*Length of Stay*
Reoperation	Reoperation	Emergency	Emergency	Renal dysfunction	Emergency	Reoperation
Emergency	Emergency	Diabetes	Age ≥75	Previous stroke	Age ≥75	Valve-CABG
COPD	Peripheral vascular disease	ST changes or nonsinus rhythm	MI within 3 mo	Peripheral vascular disease	Complex operation	CHF
Pneumonia	Urgency	Low EF	CABG-valve	CHF	EF < 20% diabetes mellitus	Insulin-dependent
ST >110	Diabetes	Age >70	Renal dysfunction	Age/RBC vol	Age 65–74	Creatinine ≥ 1.5
Age >65	COPD	Creatinine >1.2	Cerebrovascular disease	Hypertension	EF 20–34%	Transfer to OR from CCU
BUN >30	NYHA class	Diabetes	Reoperation	COPD	Reoperation	
Acute MI	CHF	COPD	Female		Urgent surgery	
Remote MI	Creatinine level	Cerebrovascular disease	Pulmonary hypertension			
	Age	Body mass index >28 (kg/height in meters)				

CCU = coronary care unit; ST = sinus tachycardia; OR = operating room.

2. The preoperative predictors of postoperative morbidity are, for the most part, similar to those associated with mortality. In approximate order of significance, they include:
    a. Reoperations
    b. Emergent procedure
    c. Preoperative usage of an IABP
    d. Congestive heart failure (elevated BNP levels seen in patients with CHF have been shown to correlate with adverse clinical outcomes).[147]
    e. CABG-valve surgery
    f. Older age
    g. Comorbidities: renal dysfunction, COPD, diabetes, and cerebrovascular disease

3. In addition to predicting mortality, several studies have also elucidated the risks of specific complications based on preoperative factors. Specifically, the NNE database can provide an estimate of the risk of stroke and mediastinitis (see Table 3.6) and the STS database provides an estimated risk for stroke, reexploration for bleeding, mediastinitis, renal dysfunction, and prolonged ventilation based on preoperative parameters.[1] Awareness of these risk factors can direct attention to specific modifiable factors that might influence the occurrence of various complications.

F. **Measures to modify risk factors for morbidity and mortality**

1. The significance of identifying risk factors for postoperative events and death is evident when the mortality associated with the development of complications is analyzed (see Table 3.8).

2. Renal failure that requires dialysis carries a mortality rate greater than 40%. Optimizing renal function before, during, and after surgery is critical in patients with preexisting renal dysfunction. In fact, the odds ratio for mortality with a preoperative creatinine in excess of 2 mg/dL is greater than 3.

3. Patients requiring mechanical ventilation for more than 5 days have an operative mortality greater than 20%. Preoperative treatment (use of antibiotics for pulmonary infiltrates or bronchitis, bronchodilators) and aggressive postoperative management (intraoperative fluid restriction and use of diuretics, use of bronchodilators and steroids, early mobilization, and chest physical therapy) may minimize the duration of mechanical ventilation.

4. Older age is associated with many costly or morbid complications, including atrial arrhythmias, stroke, mediastinal bleeding, and renal dysfunction. A permanent perioperative stroke carries a greater than 25% mortality rate. Addressing carotid disease preoperatively, using epiaortic imaging in the operating room to identify ascending aortic or arch atherosclerosis, using cerebral oximetry, and maintaining a higher blood pressure on pump are a few examples of measures that should be considered in elderly patients to improve surgical results. Meticulous attention to hemostasis in elderly patients with fragile tissues can reduce the risk of bleeding, transfusions, cardiac tamponade, low cardiac output states, and subsequent respiratory and renal failure.

Table 3.8 • Postoperative Complications of Coronary Bypass Surgery and Their Mortality Risks (STS Database)*

Risk Variable	Incidence for First Operations	Risk Ratio	Mortality (%)
Multisystem failure	0.6	28.52	74.4
Cardiac arrest	1.3	29.63	64.1
Renal failure (dialysis)	0.8	17.61	47.6
Septicemia	0.9	13.92	38.6
Renal failure (no dialysis: creat > 2.0)	2.8	13.53	30.6
Ventilated > 5 days	5.5	10.73	21
Permanent stroke	1.5	10.35	28
Tamponade	0.3	8.25	25
Anticoagulation-related	0.4	8.23	24.7
Perioperative MI	1.2	6.64	19
GI complication	2.0	6.02	17
Reexploration for bleeding	2.1	4.53	13
Deep sternal infection	0.6	3.74	11

*Data obtained from STS database website in mid-1990s; data no longer available.

5. Reoperation for bleeding and the occurrence of tamponade carry significant mortality rates (13% and 25%, respectively). Reoperations, urgent surgery, older age, and renal dysfunction predispose to bleeding. Use of antifibrinolytic drugs (aprotinin) and extra vigilance in the operating room are essential. Intraoperative blood product transfusions significantly raise operative mortality. To some extent, this is because of the clinical conditions that necessitate their use.

6. The mortality rate associated with all types of anticoagulation-related complications is approximately 25% in the STS database. Heparin may be used for AF, following embolic strokes, or for valve prostheses. Tamponade, GI or retroperitoneal bleeding, or intracranial bleeding into infarcted areas may ensue. Strict criteria for usage of heparin, careful regulation of PTT and INRs, and vigilance for the insidious onset of delayed cardiac tamponade are critical in any patient receiving anticoagulation after surgery.

References

1. Shroyer ALW, Coombs LP, Peterson ED, et al. The Society of Thoracic Surgeons: 30-day mortality and morbidity risk models. Ann Thorac Surg 2003;75:1856–64.

2. Kallis P, Tooze JA, Talbot S, et al. Preoperative aspirin decreases platelet aggregation and increases postoperative blood loss: a prospective, randomized, placebo-controlled, double-blind clinical trial in 100 patients with chronic stable angina. Eur J Cardiothorac Surg 1994;8:404–9.

3. Tuman KJ, McCarthy RJ, O'Connor CJ, McCarthy WE, Ivankovich AD. Aspirin does not increase allogeneic blood transfusions in reoperative coronary artery surgery. Anesth Analg 1996;83:1178–84.

4. Reich DL, Patel GC, Vela-Cantos F, Bodian C, Lansman S. Aspirin does not increase homologous blood requirements in elective coronary bypass surgery. Anesth Analg 1994;79:4–8.

5. Furukawa K, Ohteki H. Changes in platelet aggregation after suspension of aspirin therapy. J Thorac Cardiovasc Surg 2004;127:1814–5.

6. Gibbs NM, Weightman WM, Thackray NM, Michalopoulos N, Weidmann C. The effects of recent aspirin ingestion on platelet function in cardiac surgical patients. J Cardiothorac Vasc Anesth 2001;15:55–9.

7. Weightman WM, Gibbs NM, Weidmann CR, et al. The effect of preoperative aspirin-free interval on red blood cell transfusion requirements in cardiac surgical patients. J Cardiothorac Vasc Anesth 2002;16:54–8.

8. Dacey LJ, Munoz JJ, Johnson ER, et al. Effects of preoperative aspirin use on mortality in coronary artery bypass grafting patients. Ann Thorac Surg 2000;70:1986–90.

9. Mangano DT for the Multicenter Study of Perioperative Ischemia Research Group. Aspirin and mortality from coronary bypass surgery. N Engl J Med 2002;347:1309–17.

10. Gum PA, Kottke-Marchant K, Poggio ED, et al. Profile and prevalence of aspirin resistance in patients with cardiovascular disease. Am J Cardiol 2001;88:230–5.

11. Bidstrup BP, Hunt BJ, Sheikh S, Parratt RN, Bidstrup JM, Sapsford RN. Amelioration of the bleeding tendency of preoperative aspirin after aortocoronary bypass grafting. Ann Thorac Surg 2000;69:541–7.

12. Murkin JM, Lux J, Shannon NA, et al. Aprotinin significantly decreases bleeding and transfusion-requirements in patients receiving aspirin and undergoing cardiac operations. J Thorac Cardiovasc Surg 1994;107:554–61.

13. The Clopidogrel in Unstable Angina to Prevent Recurrent Events Trial investigators. Effects of clopidogrel in addition to aspirin in patients with acute coronary syndromes without ST segment elevation. N Engl J Med 2001;345:494–502.

14. Kam PCA, Nethery CM. The thienopyridine derivatives (platelet adenosine diphosphate receptor antagonists), pharmacology, and clinical developments. Anaesthesia 2003;58:28–35.

15. Karabulut H, Toraman F, Evrenkaya S, Goksel O, Tarcan S, Alhan C. Clopidogrel does not increase bleeding and allogenic blood transfusion in coronary artery surgery. Eur J Cardiothorac Surg 2004;25:419–23.

16. Hongo RH, Ley J, Dick SE, Yee RR. The effect of clopidogrel in combination with aspirin when given before coronary artery bypass grafting. J Am Coll Cardiol 2002;40:231–7.

17. Englberger L, Faeh B, Berdat PA, Eberli F, Meier B, Carrel T. Impact of clopidogrel in coronary artery bypass grafting. Eur J Cardiothorac Surg 2004;26:96–101.

18. Genoni M, Tavakoli R, Bertel O, Turina M. Clopidogrel before urgent coronary artery bypass graft. J Thorac Cardiovasc Surg 2003;126:288–9.

19. Warkentin TE, Greinacher A. Heparin-induced thrombocytopenia and cardiac surgery. Ann Thorac Surg 2003;76:2121–31.

20. Cohen M, Demers C, Gurfinkel EP, et al. A comparison of low-molecular weight heparin with unfractionated heparin for unstable coronary artery disease. N Engl J Med 1997;337:447–52.

21. Kincaid EH, Monroe ML, Saliba D, Kon ND, Byerly WG, Reichert MG. Effects of preoperative enoxaparin versus unfractionated heparin on bleeding indices in patients undergoing coronary artery bypass grafting. Ann Thorac Surg 2003;76:124–8.

22. Jones HU, Muhlestein JB, Jones KW, et al. Preoperative use of enoxaparin compared with unfractionated heparin increases the incidence of re-exploration for postoperative bleeding after open-heart surgery in patients who present with an acute coronary syndrome. Clinical investigation and reports. Circulation 2002;106(suppl I):19–22.

23. Clark SC, Vitale N, Zacharias J, Forty J. Effect of low molecular weight heparin (Fragmin) on bleeding after cardiac surgery. Ann Thorac Surg 2000;69:762–5.

24. Hirsh J, Fuster V, Ansell J, Halperin JL. American Heart Association/American College of Cardiology Foundation guide to warfarin therapy. Circulation 2003;41:1633–52.

25. Kearon C, Hirsh J. Management of anticoagulation before and after elective surgery. N Engl J Med 1997;336:1506–11.

26. Tavel ME, Stein PD. Management of anticoagulants in a patient requiring major surgery. Chest 1998;114:1756–8.

27. Shetty HG, Backhouse G, Bentley DP, Routledge PA. Effective reversal of warfarin-induced excessive anticoagulation with low dose vitamin K$_1$. Thromb Haemost 1992;67:13–5.

28. Wentzien TH, O'Reilly RA, Kearns PJ. Prospective evaluation of anticoagulant reversal with oral vitamin K$_1$ while continuing warfarin therapy unchanged. Chest 1998;114:1546–50.

29. Roe MT, Staman KL, Pollack C, Teaff R, French PA, Peterson ED. A practical guide to understanding the 2002 ACC/AHA guidelines for the management of patients with non-ST segment elevation acute coronary syndromes. Crit Path Card 2002;1:129–49.

30. Chun R, Orser BA, Madan M. Platelet glycoprotein IIb/IIIa inhibitors: overview and implications for the anesthesiologist. Anesth Analg 2002;95:879–88.

31. Silvestry SC. Smith PK. Current status of cardiac surgery in the abciximab-treated patient. Ann Thorac Surg 2000;70:S12–9.

32. Poullis M, Manning R, Haskard D, Taylor K. ReoPro removal during cardiopulmonary bypass using a hemoconcentrator. J Thorac Cardiovasc Surg 1999;117:1032–4.

33. Bizzari F, Scolletta S, Tucci E, et al. Perioperative use of tirofiban hydrochloride (Aggrastat) does not increase surgical bleeding after emergency or urgent coronary artery bypass grafting. J Thorac Cardiovasc Surg 2001;122:1181–5.

34. Dyke CM, Bhatia D, Lorenz TJ, et al. Immediate coronary artery bypass surgery after platelet inhibition with eptifibatide: results from PURSUIT. Ann Thorac Surg 2000;70:866–72.

35. Genoni M, Zeller D, Bertel O, Maloigne M, Turina M. Tirofiban therapy does not increase risk of hemorrhage after emergency coronary surgery. J Thorac Cardiovasc Surg 2001;122:630–2.

36. Celestini A, Pulcinelli FM, Pignatelli P, et al. Vitamin E potentiates the antiplatelet activity of aspirin in collagen-stimulation platelets. Haematologica 2002;87:420–6.

37. Cupp MJ. Herbal remedies: adverse effects and drug interactions. Am Fam Physician 1999;59:1239–45.

38. Antiplatelet effects of herbal products. Dermatol Nurs 2002;14:207.

39. Freedman JE, Parker C III, Li L, et al. Select flavonoids and whole juice from purple grapes inhibit platelet function and enhance nitric oxide release. Circulation 2001;103:2792–8.

40. Hogan WJ, McBane RD, Santrach PJ, et al. Antiphospholipid syndrome and perioperative hemostatic management of cardiac valvular surgery. Mayo Clin Proc 2000;75:971–6.

41. Williams MR, D'Ambra AB, Beck JR, et al. A randomized trial of antithrombin concentrates for treatment of heparin resistance. Ann Thorac Surg 2000;70:873–7.

42. Lemmer JR JH, Despotis GJ. Antithrombin III concentrate to treat heparin resistance in patients undergoing cardiac surgery. J Thorac Cardiovasc Surg 2002;123:213–7.

43. Sabbagh AH, Chung GK, Shuttleworth P, Applegate BJ, Gabrhel W. Fresh frozen plasma: a solution to heparin resistance during cardiopulmonary bypass. Ann Thorac Surg 1984;37:466–8.

44. Cohen A, Katz M, Katz R, Hauptman E, Schachner A. Chronic obstructive pulmonary disease in patients undergoing coronary artery bypass grafting. J Thorac Cardiovasc Surg 1995;109:574–81.

45. Michalopoulos A, Geroulanos S, Papadimitriou L, et al. Mild or moderate chronic obstructive pulmonary disease risk in elective coronary artery bypass grafting surgery. World J Surg 2001;25:1507–11.

46. Samuels LE, Kaufman MS, Morris RJ, Promisloff R, Brockman SK. Coronary artery bypass grafting in patients with COPD. Chest 1998;113:878–82.

47. Hulzebos EH, Van Meeteren NL, De Bie RA, Dagnelie PC, Helders PJ. Prediction of postoperative pulmonary complications on the basis of preoperative risk factors in patients who had undergone coronary artery bypass graft surgery. Phys Ther 2003;83:8–16.

48. Zickmann B, Sablotzki A, Fussle R, Gorlach G, Hempelmann G. Perioperative microbiologic monitoring of tracheal aspirates as a predictor of pulmonary complications after cardiac operations. J Thorac Cardiovasc Surg 1996;111:1213–8.

49. Branca P, McGaw P, Light RW and Cardiovascular Surgery Associates, P.C. Factors associated with prolonged mechanical ventilation following coronary artery bypass surgery. Chest 2001;119:537–46.

50. Bevelaqua F, Garritan S, Hass F, Salazar-Schicchi J, Axen K, Reggiani JL. Complications after cardiac operations in patients with severe pulmonary impairment. Ann Thorac Surg 1990;50:602–6.

51. Cain HD, Stevens PM, Adaniya R. Preoperative pulmonary function and complications after cardiovascular surgery. Chest 1979;76:130–5.

52. Bluman LG, Mosca L, Newman N, Simon DG. Preoperative smoking habits and postoperative pulmonary complications. Chest 1998;113:883–9.

53. Warner MA, Offord KP, Warner ME, Lennon RL, Conover MA, Jansson-Schumacher U. Role of preoperative cessation of smoking and other factors in postoperative pulmonary complications: a blinded prospective study of coronary artery bypass patients. Mayo Clin Proc 1989;64:609–16.

54. Nakagawa M, Tanaka H, Tsukuma H, Kishi Y. Relationship between the duration of the preoperative smoke-free period and the incidence of postoperative pulmonary complications after pulmonary surgery. Chest 2001;120:705–10.

55. Arabaci U, Akdur H, Yigit Z. Effects of smoking on pulmonary functions and arterial blood gases following coronary artery surgery in Turkish patients. Jpn Heart J 2003;44:61–72.

56. Rajendran AJ, Pandurangi UM, Murali R, Gomathi S, Vijayan VK, Cherian KM. Preoperative short-term pulmonary rehabilitation for patients of chronic obstructive pulmonary disease undergoing coronary artery bypass graft surgery. Indian Heart J 1998;50:531–4.

57. Jacob B, Amoateng-Adjepong Y, Rasakulasuriar S, Manthous CA, Haddad R. Preoperative pulmonary function tests do not predict outcome after coronary artery bypass. Conn Med 1997; 61:327–32.

58. de Denus S, Pharand C, Williamson DR. Brain natriuretic peptide in the management of heart failure. The versatile neurohormone. Chest 2004;125:652–68.

59. Mueller C, Scholer A, Laule-Kilian K, et al. Use of B-type natriuretic peptide in the evaluation and management of acute dyspnea. N Engl J Med 2004;350:647–54.

60. Mickleborough LL, Maruyama H, Mohamed S, et al. Are patients receiving amiodarone at increased risk for cardiac operations? Ann Thorac Surg 1994;58:622–9.

61. Greenspon AJ, Kidwell GA, Hurley W, Mannion J. Amiodarone-related postoperative adult respiratory distress syndrome. Circulation 1991;84(suppl III):407–15.

62. Nalos PC, Kass RM, Gang ES, Fishbein MC, Mandel WJ, Peter T. Life-threatening postoperative pulmonary complications in patients with previous amiodarone pulmonary toxicity undergoing cardiothoracic operations. J Thorac Cardiovasc Surg 1987;93:904–12.

63. Kaushik S, Hussain A, Clarke P, Lazar HL. Acute pulmonary toxicity after low-dose amiodarone therapy. Ann Thorac Surg 2001;72:1760–1.

64. Ninomiya M, Takamoto S, Kotsuka Y, Ohtsuka T. Indication and perioperative management for cardiac surgery in patients with liver cirrhosis. Our experience with 3 patients. Jpn J Thorac Cardiovasc Surg 2001;49:391–4.

65. Klemperer JD, Ko W, Krieger KH, et al. Cardiac operations in patients with cirrhosis. Ann Thorac Surg 1998;65:85–7.

66. Bizouarn P, Ausseur A, Desseigne P, et al. Early and late outcome after elective cardiac surgery in patients with cirrhosis. Ann Thorac Surg 1999;67:1334–8.

67. Kaplan M, Cimen S, Kut MS, Demirtas MM. Cardiac operations for patients with chronic liver disease. Heart Surg Forum 2002;5:60–5.

68. Hayashida N, Shoujima T, Teshima H, et al. Clinical outcome after cardiac operations in patients with cirrhosis. Ann Thorac Surg 2004;77:500–5.

69. Yamamoto T, Takazawa K, Hariya A, Ishikawa N, Dohi S, Matsushita S. Off-pump coronary artery bypass grafting in a patient with liver cirrhosis. Jpn J Cardiovasc Surg 2002;50:526–9.

70. Thourani VH, Weintraub WS, Stein B, et al. Influence of diabetes mellitus on early and late outcome after coronary artery bypass grafting. Ann Thorac Surg 1999;67:1045–52.

71. Luciani N, Nasso G, Gaudino M, et al. Coronary artery bypass grafting in type II diabetic patients: a comparison between insulin-dependent and non-insulin-dependent patients at short- and mid-term follow-up. Ann Thorac Surg 2003;76:1149–54.

72. Hirotani T, Nakamichi T, Munakata M, Takeuchi S. Risks and benefits of bilateral internal thoracic artery grafting in diabetic patients. Ann Thorac Surg 2003;76:2017–22.

73. Lev-Ran, O, Mohr R, Pevni D, et al. Bilateral internal thoracic artery grafting in diabetic patients: short-term and long-term results of a 515 patient series. J Thorac Cardiovasc Surg 2004;127: 1145–50.

74. Matsa M, Paz Y, Gurevitch J, et al. Bilateral skeletonized internal thoracic artery grafts in patients with diabetes mellitus. J Thorac Cardiovasc Surg 2001;121:668–74.

75. Yamazaki K, Kato H, Tsujimoto S, Kitamura R. Diabetes mellitus, internal thoracic artery grafting, and the risk of an elevated hemidiaphragm after coronary artery bypass surgery. J Cardiothorac Vasc Anesth 1994;8:437–40.

76. Clement R, Rousou JA, Engleman RM, Breyer RH. Perioperative morbidity in diabetics requiring coronary artery bypass surgery. Ann Thorac Surg 1988;46:321–3.

77. Weiler JM, Gellhaus MA, Carter JG, et al. A prospective study of the risk of an immediate adverse reaction to protamine sulfate during cardiopulmonary bypass surgery. J Allergy Clin Immunol 1990;85:713–9.

78. Redmond JM, Green PS, Goldsborough MA, et al. Neurologic injury in cardiac surgical patients with a history of stroke. Ann Thorac Surg 1996;61:42–7.

79. Kallikazaros IE, Tsioufis CP, Stefanadis CI, Pitsavos CE, Toutouzas PK. Closed relation between carotid and ascending aortic atherosclerosis in cardiac patients. Circulation 2000;102(suppl III): 263–8.

80. Gott JP, Thourani VH, Wright CE, et al. Risk neutralization in cardiac operations: detection and treatment of associated carotid disease. Ann Thorac Surg 1999;68:850–7.

81. Denton TA, Trento L, Cohen M, et al. Radial artery harvesting for coronary bypass operations: neurologic complications and their potential mechanisms. J Thorac Cardiovasc Surg 2001;121: 951–6.

82. Tryba M. Sucralfate versus antacids or H_2-antagonists for stress ulcer prophylaxis: a meta-analysis on efficacy and pneumonia rate. Crit Care Med 1991;19:942–9.

83. Steinberg KP. Stress-related mucosal disease in the critically ill patient: risk factors and strategies to prevent stress-related bleeding in the intensive care unit. Crit Care Med 2002;30:S362–4.

84. Terezhalmy GT, Safadi TJ, Longworth DL, Muehrcke DD. Oral disease burden in patients undergoing prosthetic heart valve implantation. Ann Thorac Surg 1997;63:402–4.

85. Fukuda I, Gomi S, Watanabe K, Seita J. Carotid and aortic screening for coronary artery bypass grafting. Ann Thorac Surg 2000;70:2034–9.

86. D'Agostino RS, Svensson LG, Neumann DJ, Balkhy HH, Williamson WA, Shahian DM. Screening carotid ultrasonography and risk factors for stroke in coronary artery surgery patients. Ann Thorac Surg 1996;62:1714–23.

87. Hertzer NR, Loop FD, Beven EG, O'Hara PJ, Krajewski LP. Surgical staging for simultaneous coronary and carotid disease: a study including prospective randomization. J Vasc Surg 1989;9: 455–63.

88. Khaitan L, Sutter FP, Goldman SM, et al. Simultaneous carotid endarterectomy and coronary revascularization. Ann Thorac Surg 2000;69:421–4.

89. Bilfinger TV, Reda H, Giron F, Seifert FC, Ricotta JJ. Coronary and carotid operations under prospective standardized conditions: incidence and outcome. Ann Thorac Surg 2000;69:1792–8.

90. Borger MA, Fremes SE, Weisel RD, et al. Coronary bypass and carotid endarterectomy: does a combined approach increase risk? A meta-analysis. Ann Thorac Surg 1999;68:14–21.

91. Hirotani T, Kameda T, Kumamoto T, Shirota S, Yamano M. Stroke after coronary artery bypass grafting in patients with cerebrovascular disease. Ann Thorac Surg 2000;70:1571–6.

92. Sinclair MC, Singer RL, Manley NJ, Montesano RM. Cannulation of the axillary artery for cardiopulmonary bypass: safeguards and pitfalls. Ann Thorac Surg 2003;75:931–4.

93. Bitondo JM, Daggett WM, Torchiana DF, et al. Endoscopic versus open saphenous vein harvest: a comparison of postoperative wound infections. Ann Thorac Surg 2002;73:523–8.

94. Dacey LJ, DeSimone J, Braxton JH, et al. Preoperative white blood cell count and mortality and morbidity after coronary artery bypass grafting. Ann Thorac Surg 2003;76:760–4.

95. Ereth MH, Nuttall GA, Orszulak TA, Santrach PJ, Cooney WP IV, Oliver WC Jr. Blood loss from coronary angiography increases transfusion requirements for coronary artery bypass graft surgery. J Cardiothorac Vasc Anesth 2000;14:177–81.

96. Burns ER, Billett HH, Frater RW, Sisto DA. The preoperative bleeding time as a predictor of postoperative hemorrhage after cardiopulmonary bypass. J Thorac Cardiovasc Surg 1986;92:310–2.

97. Lind SE. The bleeding time does not predict surgical bleeding. Blood 1991;77:2747–52.

98. Chertow GM, Lazarus JM, Christiansen CL, et al. Preoperative renal risk stratification. Circulation 1997;95:878–84.

99. Weerasinghe A, Nornick P, Smith P, Taylor K, Ratnatunga C. Coronary artery bypass grafting in non-dialysis-dependent mild-to-moderate renal dysfunction. J Thorac Cardiovasc Surg 2001;121:1083–9.

100. Walter J, Mortasawi A, Arnrich B, et al. Creatinine clearance versus serum creatinine as a risk factor for cardiac surgery. BMC Surg 2003;17:4.

101. Kay J, Chow WH, Chan TM, et al. Acetylcysteine for prevention of acute deterioration of renal function following elective coronary angiography and intervention. A randomized controlled trial. JAMA 2003;289:553–8.

102. Kini AA, Sharma SK. Managing the high-risk patient: experience with fenoldopam, a selective dopamine receptor agonist, in prevention of radiocontrast nephropathy during percutaneous coronary intervention. Rev Cardiovasc Med 2001;2(suppl 1):S19–25.

103. Karkouti K, McCluskey S. Pro: preoperative autologous blood donation has a role in cardiac surgery. J Cardiothorac Vasc Anesth 2003;17:121–5.

104. Muirhead B. Con: preoperative autologous donation has no role in cardiac surgery. J Cardiothorac Vasc Anesth 2003;17:126–8.

105. Kiyama H, Ohshima N, Imazeki T, Yamada T. Autologous blood donation with recombinant human erythropoietin in anemic patients. Ann Thorac Surg 1999;l68:1652–6.

106. Watanabe Y, Fuse K, Naruse Y, et al. Subcutaneous use of erythropoietin in heart surgery. Ann Thorac Surg 1992;54:479–84.

107. Yazicioglu L, Eryilmaz S, Sirlak M, et al. Recombinant human erythropoietin administration in cardiac surgery. J Thorac Cardiovasc Surg 2001;122:741–5.

108. Johnson RG, Thurer RL, Kruskall MS, et al. Comparison of two transfusion strategies after elective operations for myocardial revascularization. J Thorac Cardiovasc Surg 1992;104:307–14.

109. Doak GJ, Hall RI. Does hemoglobin concentration affect perioperative myocardial lactate flux in patients undergoing coronary artery bypass surgery? Anesth Analg 1995;80:910–6.

110. Chamberland ME. Emerging infectious agents: do they pose a risk to the safety of transfused blood and blood products? Clin Infect Dis 2002;34:797–805.

111. Goodnough LT, Brecher ME, Kanter MH, AuBuchon JP. Transfusion medicine. First of two parts. Blood transfusion. N Engl J Med 1999;340:438–47.

112. ten Broecke PW, De Hert SG, Mertens E, Adriaensen HF. Effect of preoperative beta-blockade on perioperative mortality in coronary surgery. Br J Anaesth 2003;90:27–31.

113. Ferguson TB, Coombs LP, Peterson ED. Preoperative beta-blocker use and mortality and morbidity following CABG surgery in North America. JAMA 2002;287:2221–7.

114. Kreter B, Woods M. Antibiotic prophylaxis for cardiothoracic operations. Metaanalysis of thirty years of clinical trials. J Thorac Cardiovasc Surg 1992;104:590–9.

115. Maki DG, Bohn MJ, Stolz SM, Kroncke GM, Acher CW, Myerowitz PD. Comparative study of cefazolin, cefamandole, and vancomycin for surgical prophylaxis in cardiac and vascular operations. J Thorac Cardiovasc Surg 1992;104:1423–34.

116. Litmathe J, Boeken U, Feindt P, Gams E. Predictors of homologous blood transfusion for patients undergoing open heart surgery. Thorac Cardiovasc Surg 2003;51:17–21.

117. Moskowitz DM, Klein JJ, Shander A, et al. Predictors of transfusion requirements for cardiac surgical procedures at a blood conservation center. Ann Thorac Surg 2004;77:626–34.

118. Parr KG, Patel MA, Dekker R, et al. Multivariate predictors of blood product use in cardiac surgery. J Cardiothorac Vasc Anesth 2003;17:176–81.

119. Scott BH, Seifert FC, Glass PS, Grimson R. Blood use in patients undergoing coronary artery bypass surgery: impact of cardiopulmonary bypass pump, hematocrit, gender, age, and body weight. Anesth Analg 2003;97:958–63.

120. Fellinger EK, Leavitt BJ, Hebert JC. Serum levels of prophylactic cefazolin during cardiopulmonary bypass surgery. Ann Thorac Surg 2002;74:1187–90.

121. Saginur R, Croteau D, Bergeron MG, the ESPRIT group. Comparative efficacy of teicoplanin and cefazolin for cardiac operation prophylaxis in 3027 patients. J Thorac Cardiovasc Surg 2000;120:1120–30.

122. Farber BF, Karchmer AW, Buckley MJ, Moellering RC Jr. Vancomycin prophylaxis in cardiac operations: determination of the optimal dosage regimen. J Thorac Cardiovasc Surg 1983;85:933–5.

123. Kaiser AB, Kernodle DS, Barg NL, Petracek MR. Influence of preoperative showers on staphylococcal skin colonization: a comparative trial of antiseptic skin cleansers. Ann Thorac Surg 1988;45:35–8.

124. Cimochowski GE, Harostock MD, Brown R, Bernardi M, Alonzo N, Coyle K. Intranasal mupirocin reduces sternal wound infection after open heart surgery in diabetics and nondiabetics. Ann Thorac Surg 2001;71:1572–9.

125. Ko W, Lazenby WD, Zelano JA, Isom OW, Krieger KH. Effects of shaving methods and intraoperative irrigation on suppurative mediastinitis after bypass operations. Ann Thorac Surg 1992;53: 301–5.

126. Grunkemeier GL, Zerr KJ, Jin R. Cardiac surgery report cards: making the grade. Ann Thorac Surg 2001;72:1845–8.

127. Bernstein AD, Parsonnet V. Bedside estimation of risk as an aid for decision-making in cardiac surgery. Ann Thorac Surg 2000;69:823–8.

128. O'Connor GT, Plume SK, Olmstead EM, et al. Multivariate prediction of in-hospital mortality associated with coronary artery bypass graft surgery. Northern New England Cardiovascular Disease Study Group. Circulation 1992;85:2110–8.

129. Higgins TL, Estafanous FG, Loop FD, et al. ICU admission score for predicting morbidity and mortality risks after coronary artery bypass grafting. Ann Thorac Surg 1997;64:1050–8.

130. Edwards FH, Grover FL, Shroyer ALW, Schwartz M, Bero J. The Society of Thoracic Surgeons national cardiac surgery database: current risk assessment. Ann Thorac Surg 1997;63:903–8.

131. Hannan EL, Kilburn H Jr, Racz M, Shields E, Chassin MR. Improving the outcomes of coronary artery bypass surgery in New York State. JAMA 1994;27:761–6.

132. Ghali WA, Ash AS, Hall RE, Moskowitz MA, Statewide quality improvement initiatives and mortality after cardiac surgery. JAMA 1997;277:379–82.

133. Grover FL, Johnson RR, Marshall G, Hammermeister KE. Factors predictive of operative mortality among bypass subsets. Ann Thorac Surg 1993;56:1296–306.

134. Ivanov J, Tu JV, Naylor CD. Ready-made, recalibrated, or remodeled? Issues in the use of risk indexes for assessing mortality after coronary artery bypass graft surgery. Circulation 1999;99:2098–104.

135. Mozes B, Olmer L, Galai N, Simchen E, for the ISCAB Consortium. A national study of postoperative mortality associated with coronary artery bypass grafting in Israel. Ann Thorac Surg 1998;66:1254–63.

136. Eagle KA, Guyton RA, Davidoff R, et al. ACC/AHA guidelines for coronary artery bypass graft surgery. A report of the American College of Cardiology/American Heart Association Task Force on Practice Guidelines (Committee to Revise the 1991 Guidelines for Coronary Artery Bypass Graft Surgery). J Am Coll Cardiol 1999;34:1262–347.

137. Reich DL, Bodian CA, Krol M, Kuroda M, Osinski T, Thys DM. Intraoperative hemodynamic predictors of mortality, stroke, and myocardial infarction after coronary artery bypass surgery. Anesth Analg 1999;89:814–22.

138. Geraci JM, Rosen AK, Ash AS, McNiff KJ, Moskowitz MA. Predicting the occurrence of adverse events after coronary artery bypass surgery. Ann Intern Med 1993;118:18–24.

139. Grover FL, Shroyer ALW, Hammermeister KE. Calculating risk and outcome: the Veterans Affairs database. Ann Thorac Surg 1996;62:S6–11.

140. Kurki TSO, Kataja M. Preoperative prediction of postoperative morbidity in coronary artery bypass grafting. Ann Thorac Surg 1996;61:1740–5.

141. Tuman KJ, McCarthy RJ, March RJ, Najafi H, Ivankovich AD. Morbidity and duration of ICU stay after cardiac surgery. A model for preoperative risk assessment. Chest 1992;102:36–44.

142. Ferraris VA, Ferraris SP. Risk factors for postoperative morbidity. J Thorac Cardiovasc Surg 1996;111:731–41.

143. Tu JV, Jaglal SB, Naylor CD, and the Steering Committee of the Provincial Adult Cardiac Care Network of Ontario. Multicenter validation of a risk index for mortality, intensive care unit stay, and overall hospital length of stay after cardiac surgery. Circulation 1995;91:677–84.

144. Lazar HL, Fitzgerald C, Gross S, Heeren T, Aldea GS, Shemin RJ. Determinants of length of stay after coronary artery bypass graft surgery. Circulation 1995;92(suppl I):II-20–4.

145. Magovern JA, Sakert T, Magovern GJ Jr, et al. A model that predicts morbidity and mortality after coronary artery bypass graft surgery. J Am Coll Cardiol 1996;28:1147–53.

146. Aranki SF, Shaw DP, Adams DH, et al. Predictors of atrial fibrillation after coronary artery surgery. Current trends and impact on hospital resources. Circulation 1996;94:390–7.

147. Hutfless R, Kazanegra R, Madani M, et al. Utility of B-type natriuretic peptide in predicting postoperative complications and outcomes in patients undergoing heart surgery. J Am Coll Cardiol 2004;43:1873–9.

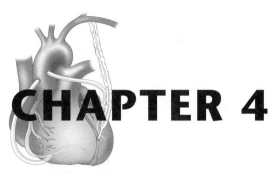

CHAPTER 4

Cardiac Anesthesia

4 Cardiac Anesthesia

Although excellence in pre- and postoperative care can often make the difference between an uneventful and a complicated recovery, the care provided in the operating room usually has the most significant impact on patient outcome. Performing a technically proficient, complete, and expeditious operation is only one component of this phase. Refinements in anesthetic techniques and monitoring, cardiopulmonary bypass (CPB), and myocardial protection have enabled surgeons to operate successfully on extremely ill patients with far advanced cardiac disease and multiple comorbidities. Use of off-pump modalities to avoid CPB is particularly useful in patients at high risk because of associated morbidities. Many patients, previously considered inoperable, will now survive the operative period to provide a challenge to postoperative care. This chapter will describe anesthesia considerations in cardiac surgery, including monitoring, transesophageal echocardiography (TEE), use of anesthetic agents, and bleeding and anticoagulation-related issues. The next two chapters will discuss issues related to CPB and myocardial protection.

I. Preoperative Visit

A. A preoperative visit by the cardiac anesthesiologist is essential before all operations. This provides an opportunity to review the patient's history, perform a relevant examination, and explain the techniques of monitoring and postoperative ventilatory support. This evaluation should identify any potential problems that might require further workup or could influence intraoperative management.

   1. History: cardiac symptoms, significant comorbidities, previous anesthetic experiences, surgical procedures, allergies, medications, recent use of steroids

   2. Examination: heart, lungs, intubation concerns (loose teeth, ability to open mouth, laxity of jaw)

B. The anesthesiologist should instruct the patient on which medications to continue up to the time of surgery and which ones to stop or have doses modified. Specifically, the anesthesiologist should tell the patient to:

   1. Continue all antihypertensive and antianginal medications up to and including the morning of surgery. One exception may be the angiotensin-converting enzyme (ACE) inhibitors, which can be withheld to reduce the risk of low systemic resistance in the perioperative period.

   2. Withhold the morning dose of insulin or oral hypoglycemic medications on the day of surgery. Blood sugars should be obtained on arrival in the operating room and frequently during surgery with coverage provided by intravenous insulin.

   3. Confirm that the patient will be off anticoagulant and antiplatelet agents prior to elective surgery (clopidogrel for 1 week, aspirin for at least 3 days)[1,2] if possible, unless the surgeon has specified otherwise (check with the surgeon if not sure). For patients awaiting surgery in hospital, the anesthesiologist should communicate with the surgical team as to the timing of cessation of various anticoagulant

medications. These include unfractionated heparin, low-molecular-weight heparin (which should be stopped at least 12 hours preoperatively)[3], and IIb/IIIa inhibitors (which should be stopped at least 4 hours preoperatively).[4,5]

C. Obtain consent from the patient for the insertion of monitoring lines with a discussion of potential complications.

D. Order appropriate preoperative medications.

II. Preoperative Medications

These should be administered 30–60 minutes before the patient is brought to the operating room. They are given to reduce the patient's anxiety and produce amnesia to allow for the safe insertion of monitoring lines without producing hemodynamic stress. Commonly used medications include lorazepam 1–2 mg PO with morphine 0.1 mg/kg IM, often with scopolamine 0.2–0.4 mg IM in younger patients. Lighter doses of preoperative medications are usually required for patients with critical valve disease or markedly depressed ventricular function. Additional sedation with midazolam is commonly given during the insertion of central lines. Prophylactic antibiotics may be given on call to the operating room, but preferentially should be administered by the anesthesiologist at the time of line insertion to make sure that the antibiotic infusion has been completed by the time of skin incision.

III. Intraoperative Monitoring and Transesophageal Echocardiography

A. Patients undergoing cardiac surgical procedures are extensively monitored. Hemodynamic alterations and myocardial ischemia that occur during the induction of anesthesia, the prebypass period, during CPB, and following resumption of cardiac activity can have significant adverse effects on myocardial function and recovery. It should be noted that even though both hypertension and tachycardia can increase myocardial oxygen demand, an increase in heart rate (HR) results in more myocardial ischemia at an equivalent increase in oxygen demand.[6]

B. Standard monitoring equipment in the operating room consists of a five-lead ECG system, a noninvasive blood pressure cuff, a radial (and occasionally femoral) arterial line, a pulse oximeter, an end-tidal CO_2 measurement, a Swan-Ganz pulmonary artery catheter to monitor filling pressures and cardiac outputs and assess for ischemia,[7] and a urinary Foley catheter to measure urine output and core body temperature. In uncomplicated coronary artery bypass surgery patients with normal or mildly depressed ventricular function, use of a central venous pressure (CVP) monitoring line instead of a pulmonary artery catheter can provide an adequate assessment of filling pressures.[8,9] TEE has become fairly routine in most centers and is cost-effective in providing useful information.[10–14] There should be provisions to perform epiaortic scanning to assess for ascending aortic atherosclerosis.[15,16]

C. **Swan-Ganz pulmonary artery catheters** are usually placed before the induction of anesthesia, especially if left ventricular (LV) dysfunction is present. These catheters are used to measure right (CVP) and left-sided filling pressures (pulmonary artery diastolic [PAD] pressure or pulmonary capillary wedge [PCW] pressure) and obtain thermodilution cardiac outputs. Despite the nearly universal use of these catheters to carefully monitor patients and provide objective data on cardiac performance, studies have not conclusively demonstrated that they influence the outcome of cardiac surgery.[9,17–19]

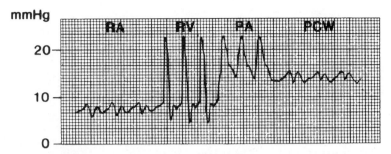

Figure 4.1 • Swan-Ganz catheter pressures. Intracardiac pressures are recorded from the distal (PA) port as the catheter is passed through the right atrium (RA), right ventricle (RV), and pulmonary artery (PA), into the pulmonary capillary wedge (PCW) position.

1. The catheter is usually inserted through an 8.5F introducer placed into the internal jugular vein or, less commonly, the subclavian vein.[20] The introducer sheath contains one side port that provides central venous access for the infusion of vasoactive medications and potassium. Multilumen introducers, such as the 8.5F and 9F high-flow advanced venous access (AVA) devices (Edwards Lifesciences and Arrow), can be used to provide additional venous access in patients with poor arm veins and limited peripheral access. A manifold with multiple stopcocks is attached to either the side port of the introducer or to one of the additional ports of the AVA through which all medications are administered.

2. The catheter is passed into the right atrium and the balloon at the catheter tip is inflated. The catheter is advanced through the right ventricle and pulmonary artery into the pulmonary capillary wedge position as confirmed by pressure tracings (Figure 4.1). The pulmonary artery tracing should reappear when the balloon is deflated. **Note:** Caution is essential when passing the catheter through the right ventricle in patients with a left bundle branch block in whom heart block might occur. In this situation, it is best to wait until the chest is open before advancing the catheter so that the surgeon can directly pace the heart if necessary.[21] External defibrillator or pacing patches may be useful.

3. The proximal port of the Swan-Ganz catheter (30 cm from the tip) is used for CVP measurements from the right atrium and for fluid injections to determine the cardiac output. Care must be exercised when injecting sterile fluid for cardiac outputs to prevent bolusing of vasoactive medications that might be running through the CVP port. **Note:** One must *never* infuse anything through this port if the catheter has been pulled back so that the tip lies in the right atrium and the CVP port lies outside the patient! This may not be noticed because the catheter is usually placed through a sterile sheath that allows for advancement or withdrawal of the catheter.

4. The distal port should always be transduced and displayed on a monitor to allow for detection of catheter advancement into the permanent wedge position, which could result in pulmonary artery injury. Balloon inflation ("wedging" of the catheter) is rarely necessary during surgery. Medications should never be given through the distal pulmonary artery port.

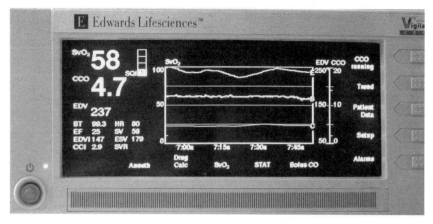

Figure 4.2 • Continuous cardiac output and mixed venous oxygen saturation obtained from a Swan-Ganz catheter commonly used during off-pump surgery. (*Image courtesy of Edwards Lifesciences, Inc.*)

5. A variety of Swan-Ganz catheters are available that provide additional functions.

   a. Some catheters contain additional ports for volume infusion or for the placement of right atrial and ventricular pacing wires. The latter is helpful during minimally invasive surgery when access to the heart is limited.

   b. Other catheters have been modified for assessment of continuous cardiac outputs and mixed venous O_2 saturations by fiberoptic oximetry (Figure 4.2). These catheters are invaluable during off-pump surgery to evaluate the patient's hemodynamic status and may contribute to a therapeutic maneuver in many patients.[22] Oximetric catheters are also helpful in patients with tricuspid regurgitation in whom thermodilution technology tends to underestimate the cardiac output.[23]

   c. Volumetric Swan-Ganz catheters use thermodilution to determine the right ventricular (RV) end-diastolic and end-systolic volumes, allowing for calculation of an RV ejection fraction.[24] This is particularly valuable in patients with pulmonary hypertension and compromised RV function.

6. The primary concerns during insertion of a pulmonary artery catheter are arterial puncture, arrhythmias during passage through the right ventricle, and potential heart block in patients with preexisting bifascicular block. Other complications of Swan-Ganz catheters are noted in Chapter 7.

7. **Pulmonary artery perforation** is a very serious complication.[25-28] It may occur during insertion of the catheter or during the surgical procedure when hypothermia causes the catheter to become rigid. Since the cold, stiff catheter may advance into the lung when the heart is manipulated, it is advisable to pull it back during CPB and readvance it after CPB. Migration of the catheter into the wedge position may be evident by loss of pulse pressure in the pulmonary artery waveform before or after bypass or by a very high pulmonary arterial

pressure measurement on bypass when the heart is decompressed. The catheter should be pulled back a short distance to prevent perforation.

    a. If perforation occurs, blood will appear in the endotracheal tube. The goals of management are to maintain gas exchange and then arrest the hemorrhage. Positive end-expiratory pressure (PEEP) should be applied to the ventilator circuit. If the degree of hemoptysis is not severe, it may abate once CPB is terminated and protamine is administered.

    b. If the airway is compromised by bleeding, CPB should be resumed with venting of the pulmonary artery. Bronchoscopy is then performed with placement of a bronchial blocker or a double-lumen endotracheal tube that can provide differential lung ventilation. The pleural space should be entered to evaluate the problem. Occluding the hilar vessels and application of PEEP may resolve the bleeding, but if it is not controlled, pulmonary resection may be required. Use of femoral artery–femoral venous extracorporeal membrane oxygenation may control bleeding by lowering the pulmonary arterial pressures. Due to the risk of recurrence, pulmonary angiography and embolization may be considered once the bleeding is controlled.

D. **Intraoperative TEE** has become routine in most cardiac surgical centers.[10–14,29–33] The probe is placed after the patient is anesthetized and before heparinization. TEE provides an analysis of regional and global right and left ventricular function, is very sensitive in detecting the presence of ischemia,[34] and identifies the presence of valvular pathology (Table 4.1). Color flow Doppler is used to analyze valvular function or suspected shunts. Although TEE may image the aorta for atheromatous disease, epiaortic imaging provides better visualization of the ascending aorta and arch when there are significant concerns about atheromatous disease.[15,16] After

---

Table 4.1 • *Specific Uses of Intraoperative Echocardiography*

All patients	Epiaortic imaging for aortic atherosclerosis Evaluation of cardiac performance (regional/global dysfunction) Evaluation of iatrogenic aortic dissections
Coronary disease	Regional dysfunction (incomplete/inadequate revascularization)
Valve surgery	Prebypass identification of valvular pathology Valve regurgitation from paravalvular leak or inadequate repair Outflow tract obstruction after mitral valve repair Valve obstruction Residual stenosis after commissurotomy Presence of intracardiac air
IABP	Location of device relative to the aortic arch
VSD closure	Residual VSD

bypass, TEE can be used to assess ventricular function, the presence of intracardiac air,[35] and the efficacy of valve repairs and replacements. An individual trained in performing and reading TEE, whether a cardiac anesthesiologist or a cardiologist, is essential to optimize its usefulness. Before the probe is placed, consideration must be given to contraindications to TEE that could produce catastrophic complications, such as esophageal perforation. These include previous esophageal surgery,

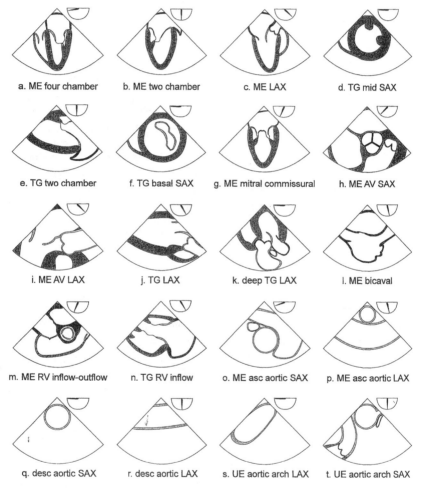

a. ME four chamber   b. ME two chamber   c. ME LAX   d. TG mid SAX

e. TG two chamber   f. TG basal SAX   g. ME mitral commissural   h. ME AV SAX

i. ME AV LAX   j. TG LAX   k. deep TG LAX   l. ME bicaval

m. ME RV inflow-outflow   n. TG RV inflow   o. ME asc aortic SAX   p. ME asc aortic LAX

q. desc aortic SAX   r. desc aortic LAX   s. UE aortic arch LAX   t. UE aortic arch SAX

Figure 4.3 • Recommended views for intraoperative transesophageal echocardiography. *(Reproduced with permission from Shanewise JS, Cheung AT, Aronson S, et al. ASE/SCA guidelines for performing a comprehensive intraoperative multiplane transesophageal echocardiography examination: Recommendations of the American Society of Echocardiography Council for Intraoperative Echocardiography and the Society of Cardiovascular Anesthesiologists Task Force for certification in perioperative transesophageal echocardiography. Anesth Analg 1999;89:870–84.)*

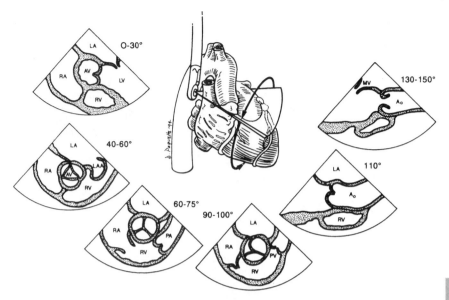

Figure 4.4 • Upper-midesophageal echocardiographic imaging of the aortic valve. Rotation of the probe allows for visualization of the aortic valve and proximal ascending aorta in short- and long-axis views. *(Reproduced with permission from Roelandt J, Pandian NG, eds. Multiplane Transesophageal Echocardiography. New York: Churchill Livingstone, 1996:33–58.)*

and known esophageal pathology, such as strictures, Schatzki's ring, or esophageal varices.[36,37]

1. Multiplane TEE has become standard and allows for rotation of the probe through 180 degrees, thus affording excellent images of the heart in multiple views. The probe is advanced up and down the esophagus and then into the stomach for transgastric views. The tip of the probe can be flexed in four different directions, and the shaft of the probe can also be rotated. The American Society of Echocardiography and the Society of Cardiovascular Anesthesiologists have defined 20 standard views for a routine examination (Figure 4.3).[31] Some of the best views during cardiac surgery include the following.

2. In the mid-upper esophagus, rotation of the probe allows for visualization of the aortic valve and proximal ascending aorta in short- and long-axis views (Figure 4.4).

3. In the mid-lower esophagus, the standard views can be obtained by rotating the probe through 135 degrees. With progressive rotation, these views include a four-chamber view (0 degrees), long-axis two-chamber view (90 degrees), and a long-axis view of the LV outflow tract (130–150 degrees) (Figure 4.5).

4. With the probe anteflexed in the transgastric views, the three standard views are the short axis of the right ventricle and left ventricle (0 degrees), longitudinal two-chamber LV view (70–90 degrees), and the LV outflow tract (110–135 degrees) (Figure 4.6).[29–31]

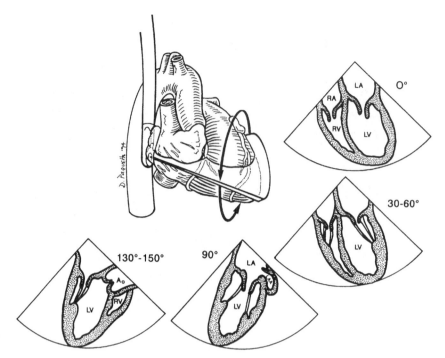

Figure 4.5 • Mid-lower esophageal echocardiographic imaging. Standard views can be obtained by rotating the probe through 135 degrees. With progressive rotation, these views include a four-chamber view (0 degrees), long-axis two-chamber view (90 degrees), and long-axis view of the LV outflow tract (130–150 degrees). *(Reproduced with permission from Roelandt J, Pandian NG, eds. Multiplane Transesophageal Echocardiography. New York: Churchill Livingstone, 1996:33–58.)*

5. During on-pump coronary artery surgery, prebypass TEE will provide a baseline analysis of regional and global ventricular function. The midpapillary long- and short-axis views are best to assess most regions of the left ventricle. The ability of the heart muscle to thicken is consistent with viability, whereas areas of thinned-out muscle represent infarcted areas. Following bypass, slight improvement in previously ischemic zones may be noted, especially with inotropic stimulation. These areas of hypokinesis may represent stunned or hibernating myocardium that have contractile reserve and may gradually recover function after revascularization. The new onset of hypokinesis raises the specter of hypoperfusion from an anastomotic or graft problem, incomplete revascularization, or inadequate myocardial protection. The new onset of mitral regurgitation (MR) may reflect loading conditions but could indicate ischemia.

6. During off-pump surgery, the midesophageal windows are best for assessing RV and LV function and the presence of MR. Baseline views are obtained. During vessel occlusion, TEE should assess for the acute development of regional LV dysfunction or acute MR during construction of left-sided grafts and for RV dysfunction during right coronary grafting. The transgastric views

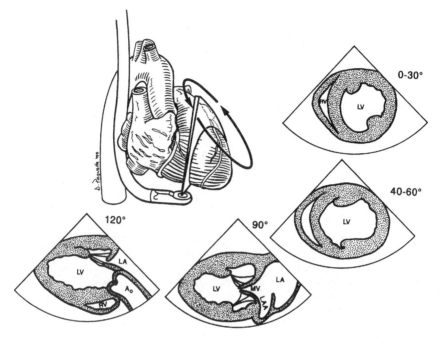

Figure 4.6 • Transgastric views. With the probe anteflexed in the transgastric views, the standard views are the short axis of the right ventricle and left ventricle (0 degrees), longitudinal two-chamber LV view (90 degrees), and the LV outflow tract (120 degrees). *(Reproduced with permission from Roelandt J, Pandian NG, eds. Multiplane Transesophageal Echocardiography. New York: Churchill Livingstone, 1996:33–58.)*

are not helpful when the heart is elevated out of the chest.[33] The development and persistence of a new regional wall motion abnormality after a graft is completed suggests a flow problem, usually at the anastomosis. However, the latter may occur even in the absence of a regional wall motion abnormality.

7. In minimally invasive procedures (usually aortic or mitral valve surgery), TEE can confirm the location of the retrograde coronary sinus catheter since it cannot be palpated by the surgeon.

8. In aortic valve operations, the best views are obtained from the mid- to upper esophagus (see Figure 4.4). TEE can quantify the degree of aortic stenosis by planimetry and pressure gradients, quantify the degree of aortic regurgitation by color flow analysis that can influence delivery of cardioplegia, and assess the degree of LV hypertrophy and its nature (concentric, septal). Annular size can be assessed. The presence of severe diastolic rather than systolic dysfunction may influence pharmacologic management. After bypass, valve opening and closing can be assessed and paravalvular leaks may be identified. Competence of homografts and autografts (Ross procedure) can be confirmed. Rarely, an unusual finding may be demonstrated, such as an aorto–left atrial fistula or ventricular septal defect (VSD).

9. The best visualization of the mitral valve is from the lower and middle esophagus. Prebypass assessment should confirm the valvular pathology and identify the mechanism of MR (e.g., a flail leaflet and the direction of the regurgitant jet). However, in some patients with MR, it is not uncommon to note a discrepancy between preoperative and intraoperative TEE due to alteration in loading conditions. Left atrial clot should be sought. During weaning from bypass, TEE is helpful in identifying intracardiac air.[35] After termination of bypass it should be used to assess the competence of valve repairs, identify paravalvular leaks after valve replacement, and assess LV and RV function. Occasionally, the TEE will reveal an unsuspected finding, such as systolic anterior motion of the anterior mitral valve leaflet obstructing the LV outflow tract, evidence of valve dysfunction with a trapped or obstructed leaflet, or aortic insufficiency after a difficult mitral valve operation (due to suture entrapment of an aortic valve cusp or distortion of the aortic annulus from placement of too small a mitral valve).

10. The diagnosis of an aortic dissection can be confirmed by TEE once the patient is anesthetized. It not only identifies the intimal flap, but can also determine whether aortic insufficiency is present, mandating aortic valve resuspension or replacement. If a large pericardial effusion is present, groin cannulation may be necessary for the emergency institution of CPB before opening the pericardium. TEE can also identify flaps in cases of iatrogenic dissections at cannulation or clamp sites.

11. In thoracic aortic surgery, TEE is useful in assessing cardiac performance and intracardiac volume status during the period of clamping and after unclamping, when pulmonary arterial pressures tend to be elevated out of proportion to preload. This may influence fluid and pharmacologic management.[38]

IV. Anesthetic Considerations for Various Types of Heart Surgery

A. Anesthetic management must be individualized, taking into consideration the patient's age, comorbidities, the nature and extent of coronary or valvular disease, and the degree of LV dysfunction. These factors will determine which medications should be selected to avoid myocardial depression, tachycardia, or bradycardia, or counteract changes in vasomotor tone. Generally, narcotic-based anesthesia is used for all open-heart surgery to minimize myocardial depression. Specific anesthetic concerns for various disease processes are presented in this section.

B. Coronary bypass surgery

1. Factors that increase myocardial oxygen demand, such as tachycardia and hypertension, must be prevented in the prebypass period, especially during the induction of anesthesia. Hypotension, often resulting from the use of narcotics and anxiolytics, such as midazolam, should be counteracted with fluids and α-agents since hypotension is more likely to produce ischemia than hypertension.

2. Detection and treatment of ischemia is critical in the prebypass period. TEE is the most sensitive means of detecting ischemic regional wall motion abnormalities but is not always used in "routine" cases.[34] Ischemia may also be manifested by an elevation in the pulmonary arterial pressures or by ST-segment elevation in the ECG leads. Aggressive management with nitroglycerin, β-blockers

(esmolol), and narcotics can usually control prebypass ischemia. If not, prompt institution of CPB may be necessary.

3. Narcotic/sedative regimens are the standard for coronary surgery, especially in patients with LV dysfunction. Use of low-dose fentanyl or sufentanil, inhalational anesthetics, midazolam, and propofol allows for early postoperative extubation.

4. Anesthetic techniques for **off-pump surgery** commonly involve use of a continuous cardiac output Swan-Ganz catheter with on-line mixed venous oxygen saturation monitoring. Tilting of the operating room table (Trendelenburg position and to the right) to augment cardiac filling, judicious fluid administration, antiarrhythmic therapy (lidocaine/magnesium), α-agents (phenylephrine) and inotropes (epinephrine/milrinone), and, on occasion, insertion of an intraaortic balloon pump (IABP) may be used. The essential elements to a successful off-pump operation include a patient surgeon who uses good judgment in deciding when off-pump surgery is feasible and when conversion to CPB or right-heart assist is necessary, an anesthesiologist who is experienced and comfortable with off-pump surgery, and a qualified, actively involved first assistant (see section IX on page 163 for a more detailed discussion of anesthesia for off-pump surgery).

C. **Left ventricular aneurysms.** Anesthetic drugs that cause myocardial depression must be avoided because of the association of LV aneurysms with significant LV dysfunction. Swan-Ganz monitoring is important in optimizing preload and contractility before and after bypass. TEE is the most sensitive means of detecting the presence of LV thrombus.

D. **Ventricular septal defects** are usually operated upon on an emergent basis when the patient is in cardiogenic shock, usually on inotropic support and often with an IABP. Thus, myocardial depression must be avoided. Systemic hypertension may increase the shunt and should be prevented.

E. **Aortic stenosis.** The induction of anesthesia is a critical period for patients with aortic stenosis. Narcotic-based anesthesia is used to minimize hemodynamic alterations such as myocardial depression, vasodilation, tachycardia, or dysrhythmias, all of which can lower cardiac output precipitously. An α-agent, such as phenylephrine or norepinephrine, is particularly valuable in supporting systemic resistance. The best TEE views of the aortic valve are obtained in the midesophageal short- and long-axis views.

F. **Aortic insufficiency.** The hemodynamic goals in the prebypass period are to maintain satisfactory preload and avoid bradycardia and hypertension. Vasodilation may be beneficial, but hypotension may reduce the diastolic perfusion pressure and precipitate ischemia. The transgastric long-axis view with color Doppler is best for assessing aortic insufficiency.

G. **Hypertrophic obstructive cardiomyopathy.** Measures that produce hypovolemia or vasodilatation must be avoided because they increase the outflow tract gradient. Volume infusions should be used to maintain preload with the use of α-agents to maintain systemic resistance. Use of β-blockers and calcium channel blockers to reduce heart rate and contractility are beneficial in the immediate preoperative and prebypass periods. Inotropic drugs with predominantly β-adrenergic effects should be avoided.

H. Mitral stenosis. Attention should be paid to maintaining preload, reducing heart rate, and preventing an increase in pulmonary vascular resistance (PVR).

1. Preload must be adjusted judiciously to ensure adequate LV filling across the stenotic valve while simultaneously avoiding excessive fluid administration that could lead to pulmonary edema. A volumetric (RV ejection fraction) Swan-Ganz catheter is valuable in the assessment of RV volumes and ejection fractions. The PA diastolic pressure may overestimate the left atrial pressure and may require placement of a left atrial line for monitoring after bypass. Balloon inflation (wedging) of a pulmonary artery catheter should be avoided or performed with a minimal amount of balloon inflation in patients with pulmonary hypertension because of the increased risk of pulmonary artery rupture.

2. The heart rate should be reduced to prolong the diastolic filling period. For patients in atrial fibrillation (AF), small doses of esmolol can be used to control a rapid ventricular response. Atropine should be avoided as a premedication. Nonetheless, cardiac output is usually marginal in patients with mitral stenosis and can be further compromised if the ventricular rate is excessively slow.

3. Factors that can increase PVR must be avoided. Preoperative sedation should be light to prevent hypercarbia. Hypoxemia, hypercarbia, acidosis, and nitrous (not nitric) oxide should be avoided in the operating room. The PVR can be reduced with pulmonary vasodilators before bypass (usually nitroglycerin), and with inotropic agents after bypass that can produce pulmonary vasodilatation (inamrinone, milrinone, or isoproterenol). Nesiritide, prostaglandin E_1 (PGE_1), nitric oxide, or Iloprost can be used to reduce PVR if there is evidence of severe RV failure (see pages 254 and 356).

I. Mitral insufficiency

1. Measures that can increase pulmonary arterial pressure, such as hypoxemia, hypercarbia, acidosis, and nitrous oxide, should be avoided. Preoperative sedation should be light.

2. In the prebypass period, adequate preload must be maintained to ensure forward output. Systemic hypertension should be avoided because it tends to increase the amount of regurgitation. If the patient has ischemic MR or a borderline cardiac output, use of systemic vasodilators or intraaortic balloon pumping will improve forward flow.

3. TEE is invaluable in identifying the precise anatomic cause for MR and in evaluating the surgical result. This is performed once the patient is anesthetized. Occasionally, there is a discrepancy between preoperative and intraoperative studies due to alterations in systemic resistance and loading conditions. Elevating the blood pressure with α-agents may increase the amount of regurgitation in patients with moderate ischemic MR and aid in the decision to repair the valve during bypass surgery. Midesophageal and transgastric long-axis views with rotation of the probe can evaluate the mitral valve quite precisely.

J. Tricuspid valve disease

1. Maintenance of an elevated CVP is essential to achieve satisfactory forward flow. A Swan-Ganz pulmonary artery catheter can be placed for monitoring of left-sided pressures in patients with tricuspid regurgitation, although cardiac

output determinations are of little value. A Swan-Ganz catheter can be used after valve repair or tissue valve replacement, but not after mechanical valve replacement. Alternatively, a left atrial line and pulmonary artery thermistor can be placed for cardiac output determinations. Other means of assessing cardiac output (esophageal Doppler or bioimpedance) can also be used.

2. A normal sinus mechanism provides better hemodynamics than AF, although the latter is frequently present. Slower HRs are preferable for tricuspid stenosis and faster HRs for tricuspid regurgitation.

3. Measures that avoid myocardial depression and lower the PVR may be helpful in improving RV function.

4. In patients with hepatic congestion, a coagulopathy may develop after CPB. Aprotinin should be considered in these patients and fresh frozen plasma should be available due to depletion of coagulation factors normally produced by the liver.

K. Endocarditis

1. Anesthetic management is dictated by the hemodynamic derangements associated with the particular valve involved.

2. Patients with aortic valve endocarditis may have evidence of heart block from involvement of the conduction system by periannular infection. This may require preoperative placement of a transvenous pacing wire.

3. Ongoing sepsis may produce refractory hypotension on pump despite use of α-agents. Vasopressin may be necessary to maintain the blood pressure.

L. Aortic dissections

1. Maintenance of hemodynamic stability and especially avoidance of hypertension are critical to prevent aortic rupture, especially during the induction of anesthesia and line insertion. Use of a Swan-Ganz catheter is important to optimize perioperative hemodynamics. Its insertion can be delayed until after intubation to minimize the stress response.

2. Most patients require emergency surgery and should be considered to have a full stomach. A modified rapid sequence induction should be performed to minimize the risk of aspiration while ensuring hemodynamic stability.

3. TEE is invaluable in localizing the site and often the extent of the dissection, the degree of aortic insufficiency, and the presence of hemopericardium. This must be performed **very cautiously** in the awake patient with a suspected dissection for fear of precipitating hypertension, rupture, and then tamponade. If the diagnosis has been confirmed by other means, TEE should be performed in the anesthetized patient.

4. Repair of type A dissections is usually performed during a period of deep hypothermic circulatory arrest. The head is packed in ice, and medications are given to potentially provide additional cerebral protection (see section M.1).

5. Repair of type B dissections requires a period of descending aortic cross-clamping. Because less collateral flow is present in patients with dissections than with atherosclerotic aneurysms, the risk of paraplegia is greater. A cerebrospinal fluid (CSF) drainage catheter should be placed before the patient is anesthetized. Proximal hypertension must be controlled during application of the cross-clamp but should not be so low as to compromise spinal cord perfusion.

M. Ascending aortic and arch aneurysms

1. Aneurysms limited to the proximal and mid-ascending aorta are repaired with CPB and application of an aortic cross-clamp. If they extend more distally or the arch is extensively involved, a period of deep hypothermic circulatory arrest at 18°C is used. This should provide 45–60 minutes of safe arrest time in minimizing the risk of neurologic insult. Adjuncts to improve cerebral protection include packing the head in ice, and administration of methylprednisolone 30 mg/kg and thiopental or pentobarbital 5–10 mg/kg. Continuous retrograde perfusion of the superior vena cava (SVC) may be used to maintain cerebral hypothermia, and the CVP should be monitored and kept less than 20 mm Hg. Alternatively, antegrade perfusion of the cerebral vessels may be provided.

2. Profound hypothermia and warming are associated with a coagulopathy. Platelets, fresh frozen plasma, and cryoprecipitate are helpful in achieving hemostasis. Supplemental use of warming devices, such as the Arctic Sun device (MediVance, Inc., Louisville, CO), is helpful in warming the patient faster and preventing temperature afterdrop.

3. Aprotinin is arguably helpful in reducing intraoperative bleeding with use of deep hypothermic circulatory arrest, although there are concerns about adverse neurologic sequelae.[39] Proponents of aprotinin believe that it is safe as long as certain measures are taken. This includes ensuring an adequate activated clotting time (kaolin ACT > 750–1000 seconds), giving additional heparin (1 mg/kg just prior to period of circulatory arrest), and stopping the infusion of aprotinin during the arrest period.[40–42] Alternatively, aprotinin may be given just during the rewarming phase.

N. Descending aortic aneurysms

1. Arterial monitoring lines are inserted in the right radial and the right femoral artery to monitor proximal and distal pressures during the period of aortic cross-clamping. The femoral line is valuable when left-heart bypass techniques are used.

2. A Swan-Ganz catheter is important to monitor filling pressures during the period of cross-clamping. TEE is helpful in evaluating myocardial function and often demonstrates a hypovolemic LV chamber despite elevated pulmonary arterial pressures when the cross-clamp is removed.[38] Ensuring adequate intravascular volume will reduce the risk of "declamping shock" upon release of the aortic cross-clamp.

3. One-lung anesthesia using a double-lumen or Univent tube improves operative exposure.

4. Several medications have been used in an attempt to improve renal perfusion during the period of aortic cross-clamping. An infusion of fenoldopam 0.03–0.1 μg/kg/min appears to be promising.[43]

5. Control of proximal hypertension is essential during the cross-clamp period. A catheter for CSF drainage should be placed before the patient is positioned and anesthetized to reduce the incidence of spinal ischemia. Nitroprusside must be used cautiously because it can reduce renal and spinal cord perfusion and increase CSF pressure.[44]

O. Implantable cardioverter-defibrillator placement

1. ICD implantation is usually performed in an electrophysiology laboratory under moderate sedation with midazolam, allowing the patient to breath spontaneously.

When ventricular fibrillation is induced, deepening of the level of sedation with propofol and assisted ventilation usually suffice. This requires close nursing or anesthesia attendance and careful monitoring. Most patients have markedly depressed ventricular function. Provisions for cardiac resuscitation (personnel and equipment) should be immediately available. External defibrillator pads should be placed for rescue defibrillation.

   2. Medications that could be potentially arrhythmogenic, such as the catecholamines, must be avoided. Antiarrhythmic medications are continued unless there are plans for an electrophysiologic study, which is usually performed with the patient off medications.

P. **Surgery for atrial fibrillation**

   1. Procedures to correct AF may not be successful for several months. Therefore, medications used for rate control or for AF prophylaxis can be continued up to the time of surgery.

   2. Other considerations pertain to the specific lesion for which surgery is being performed if the arrhythmia surgery is an adjunctive procedure.

Q. **Surgery for pericardial disease**

   1. Cardiac output and blood pressure are dependent on adequate preload, increased heart rate, and increased sympathetic tone. Swan-Ganz monitoring is helpful in maintaining adequate preload and in assessing the hemodynamic response to the procedure. Agents that produce vasodilatation, bradycardia, or myocardial depression must be avoided. Volume infusions and α-agents are beneficial in maintaining hemodynamic stability. Since loss of sympathetic tone can be catastrophic in a patient with tamponade physiology, prepping and draping of the patient before the induction of anesthesia should be strongly considered.

   2. TEE is invaluable in identifying the size and hemodynamic effects of an effusion. With limited surgical approaches, such as a subxiphoid window or thoracoscopy, it can identify whether the effusion has been adequately drained.

   3. After resolution of tamponade, filling pressures generally fall, blood pressure increases, and a brisk diuresis occurs. Depending on the duration of tamponade, some patients may require transient inotropic support after the fluid is removed.

   4. After the constricted heart is decorticated, filling pressures may transiently fall, but many patients develop a low output state associated with ventricular dilatation requiring inotropic support. Inadequate decortication may be evident when a fluid challenge that restores the preoperative filling pressures fails to increase cardiac output. Pulmonary edema may develop if the surgeon decorticates the right ventricle while the left ventricle remains constricted.

V. Induction and Maintenance of Anesthesia

A. Cardiac anesthesia is provided by a combination of medications that includes induction agents, anxiolytics, amnestics, analgesics, muscle relaxants, and inhalational anesthetics.

B. Induction agents include thiopental, propofol, etomidate, ketamine, and the benzodiazepines. Most commonly, anesthesia is induced with a combination of thiopental, narcotics, and neuromuscular blockers to provide muscle relaxation and prevent chest wall rigidity that is associated with high-dose narcotic inductions. Ketamine given

Table 4.2 • Hemodynamic Effects of Commonly Used Anesthetic Agents

Agent	HR	Contractility	SVR	Net Effect on BP
Induction Agents				
Thiopental	↑	↓	↓	↓
Propofol	↓	↓	↓↓	↓↓
Etomidate	↔	↔	↔	↔
Anxiolytics				
Midazolam	↑	↔	↓	↓
Propofol	↓	↓	↓↓	↓↓
Lorazepam	↔	↔	↓	↓
Narcotics				
Fentanyl	↓	↔	↓	↓
Sufentanil	↓↓	↔	↓	↓
Alfentanil	↓	↔	↓	↓
Remifentanil	↓	↔	↓	↓
Muscle Relaxants				
Pancuronium	↑	↔	↔	↑
Vecuronium	↔	↔	↔	↔
Doxacurium	↔	↔	↔	↔
Atracurium	↔	↔	↓	↓
Rocuronium	↔	↔	↔	↔
Succinylcholine	↑↓	↓	↔	↑↓

with a benzodiazepine is very useful in patients with compromised hemodynamics or tamponade. Ketamine does not produce myocardial depression, and its dissociative effects and sympathetic stimulant properties that produce hypertension and tachycardia are attenuated by use of a benzodiazepine.[45]

C. Subsequently, anesthesia is maintained by additional dosing of narcotics and muscle relaxants in combination with an anxiolytic (midazolam or propofol) and an inhalational agent (Tables 4.2 and 4.3). Bispectral (BIS) electroencephalographic monitoring can be used to titrate and minimize the amount of medication required to maintain adequate anesthesia (a level around 55–60) while preventing awareness.[46,47] This is useful during bypass when hemodilution increases the effective volume of distribution and may necessitate redosing of anesthetic medications. The dose and selection of anesthetic agents must provide adequate anesthesia and analgesia during surgery, but may be modified to allow for extubation in the operating room or, more commonly, several hours after arrival in the ICU.

Table 4.3 • Dosages and Metabolism of Commonly Used Anesthetic Agents

Agent	Usual Dosage	Duration of Action
Induction Agents		
Thiopental	3–5 mg/kg	5–10 min
Propofol	1–3 mg/kg →	2–8 min
	10–100 µg/kg/min	
Etomidate	0.2–0.4 mg/kg →	3–8 min
	5–10 µg/kg/min	
Anxiolytics		
Propofol	25–75 µg/kg/min	Up to 20 min
Midazolam	2.5–5 mg IV q2h or	Up to 10 h
	1–4 mg/h	
Lorazepam	1–4 mg q4h or	4–6 h
	0.02–0.05 mg/kg	
Narcotics		
Fentanyl	5–10 µg/kg → 1–5 µg/kg/h	1–4 h
Sufentanil	0.5–1 µg/kg →	1–4 h
	0.25–0.75 µg/kg/h	
Alfentanil	50–75 µg/kg →	1–1.6 h
	0.5–3 µg/kg/min	
Remifentanil	1 µg/kg →	10 min
	0.05–2 µg/kg/min	
Muscle Relaxants		
Pancuronium	0.1 mg/kg →	180–240 min[a]/0–60 min[b]
	0.01 mg/kg q1h	
Vecuronium	0.1 mg/kg →	45–90 min[a]/25–40 min[b]
	0.01 mg/kg q30–45 min	
Doxacurium	0.06 mg/kg →	180–240 min[a]/45–60 min[b]
	0.005 mg/kg q30 min	
Atracurium	0.4–0.5 mg/kg →	30–45 min[a]/15–30 min[b]
	0.3–0.6 mg/kg/h	
Rocuronium	0.6–1.2 mg/kg IV	30–60 min
Succinylcholine	1 mg/kg	5–10 min

[a]After initial intubating dose.
[b]After repeat dose.

D. Traditional regimens that included high-dose fentanyl have been supplanted by protocols using low-dose fentanyl, sufentanil, or alfentanil.[48–50] The least expensive regimen combines low-dose fentanyl with an inhalational anesthetic to facilitate early extubation. Sufentanil has a half-life of about 20–40 minutes and allows patients to awaken within hours of completion of the operation. Remifentanil is a very short-acting narcotic with a context-sensitive half-life of 3–5 minutes that may be beneficial in shorter operations and in elderly patients.[51–54] Although more expensive, it allows for a reduction in the dose of propofol and is usually selected for patients who can be extubated promptly after surgery. Thus, it has not been shown to increase overall hospital costs.[54]

E. Midazolam has been shown to have an elimination half-life of more than 10 hours in patients undergoing cardiac surgery.[55] Although early extubation can be achieved in patients receiving midazolam throughout surgery, most groups limit its use to the prebypass period and then initiate a propofol infusion at the termination of bypass and continue it in the ICU. Propofol can be used to control post-bypass hypertension because of its strong vasodilator properties. When the patient is stable, the propofol is turned off and the patient is allowed to awaken.[56]

F. Inhalational agents provide muscle relaxation and unconsciousness, with variable effects on myocardial depression.[57] Agents commonly used include isoflurane, enflurane, desflurane, and sevoflurane. They are generally given during CPB to maintain anesthesia and reduce blood pressure, and allow for usage of lower doses of intravenous medications, although they provide no analgesia. Desflurane and sevoflurane have less lipid solubility with a rapid onset of action and are quickly reversible, allowing for early extubation. Nitrous oxide is contraindicated in that it reduces the amount of oxygen that can be delivered and may also increase pulmonary arterial pressures.

G. Muscle relaxants are given throughout the operation to minimize patient movement and suppress shivering during hypothermia. Adequate muscle relaxation might reduce some of the paraspinal muscle soreness often noted after surgery due to sternal retraction.

   1. Pancuronium is the most commonly used neuromuscular blocker. It increases both heart rate and blood pressure and mitigates narcotic-induced bradycardia and hypotension. In contrast, vecuronium and doxacurium have very few hemodynamic effects. Rocuronium is a short-acting neuromuscular blocker with a rapid onset of action and vagolytic properties. It is especially helpful for the induction of anesthesia. Atracurium does not undergo renal elimination and is the best agent to use in patients with renal insufficiency (see Tables 4.2 and 4.3).[58–60]

   2. Although some centers reverse muscle relaxants at the end of the operation, this can be detrimental if the patient becomes agitated and develops hemodynamic alterations. A conservative approach is to observe the patient in the ICU for several hours during which time most of the neuromuscular blockade dissipates and extubation can then be achieved. **Adequate sedation must be maintained in the ICU while a patient remains pharmacologically paralyzed.**

H. Dexmedetomidine is an α_2-adrenergic agonist with numerous properties, including sedation, analgesia, anxiolysis, and sympatholysis. During surgery, it can be used to reduce the dosage of other medications, allowing for early, comfortable extubation. It may also reduce shivering and myocardial ischemia.[61,62] Its role in perioperative management is still being defined.[63] It is given as a loading dose of 1 µg/kg over 10 minutes followed by a continuous infusion of 0.2–0.7 mg/kg/h.

VI. Prebypass Considerations

A. Avoidance of ischemia prior to initiating bypass is critical for all types of heart surgery. Identification of ischemic electrocardiographic changes, elevation in filling pressures, or regional wall motion abnormalities on TEE requires prompt attention. Manipulation of the heart by the surgeon for cannula placement, blood loss during redo dissections, ongoing blood loss from leg incisions, and AF during atrial cannulation are a few of the potential insults that must be addressed. Judicious use of fluids and α-agents to counteract vasodilatation and hypotension, β-blockers or additional anesthetic agents for hypertension or tachycardia, and nitroglycerin for ischemia must be selected appropriately to maintain stable hemodynamics. In the prebypass period, fluids are usually administered in the form of crystalloid.

B. **TEE** should be performed at this time to provide a baseline assessment of regional wall motion abnormalities and identify known or overlooked valvular pathology.[29–32]

C. **Autologous blood withdrawal** before the institution of bypass protects platelets from the damaging effects of CPB. The quality of this blood is excellent, with only slight activation of platelets, and it has been demonstrated to preserve red cell mass and reduce transfusion requirements.[64] It should be considered in patients for whom the calculated hematocrit on pump will remain adequate after withdrawal of 1–2 units of blood with nonheme fluid replacement.

D. Pharmacologic intervention may be considered to reduce the systemic inflammatory response to bypass. This may include use of aprotinin (see below) or steroids. Although use of preoperative methylprednisolone or dexamethasone may reduce the inflammatory response, little clinical benefit other than an improvement in emetic symptoms or appetite has been demonstrated.[65–68]

E. **Antifibrinolytic drugs** have been demonstrated unequivocally to reduce perioperative blood loss in cardiac operations. They should be used for all on-pump cardiac surgical procedures and may be of benefit in off-pump cases as well.[69–72] Most protocols include giving the first dose at the time of skin incision or before heparinization, giving a dose in the pump prime, and administering a constant infusion during the operation (Box 4.1).

1. **Aprotinin** is a serine protease inhibitor that has been demonstrated in numerous studies to be extremely effective in reducing perioperative bleeding and also in producing an antiinflammatory effect.[73]

   a. Mechanisms of action of aprotinin include:

   i. Preservation of platelet function by blocking the platelet glycoprotein Ib receptor.

   ii. Inhibition of fibrinolysis by inhibiting circulating plasmin directly and by blocking kallikrein-induced conversion of plasminogen to plasmin.

   iii. Inhibition of kallikrein-induced kinin formation, minimizing its vasoactive effects that contribute to increased vascular permeability.

   iv. Inhibition of neutrophil activation and degranulation.

   v. Decrease in complement activation.

   b. Because aprotinin is so effective in reducing perioperative bleeding, there have been concerns about its prothrombotic tendencies, especially in patients with small coronary arteries.[74] However, it has been shown that aprotinin selectively blocks the proteolytically activated thrombin receptor (PAR1) on platelets, thus inhibiting platelet aggregation induced by thrombin

---

Box 4.1 • Doses of Antifibrinolytic Drugs

Aprotinin	(1) High dose:	2 million KIU prior to heparinization
		2 million KIU in pump prime
		0.5 million KIU/h
	(2) Low dose:	half of above
	(3) Weight adjusted:	3.5 mg/kg IV bolus
		70 mg pump prime load
		3.5 mg/kg/h for 1 hour
		1 mg/kg/h continuous infusion[83]
ε-aminocaproic acid	5 g prior to heparinization	
	5 g in pump prime	
	1 g/h during surgery	
Tranexamic acid	(1) 10 mg/kg over 20 minutes followed by a 1 mg/kg/h infusion[99,103]	
	(2) 1-g bolus followed by an infusion of 400 mg/h with 500 mg in the pump prime[93]	
	(3) 100 mg/kg given before CPB[104]	
	(4) 5.4 mg/kg load, 50 mg in the pump prime (for a 2.5-L circuit), and a 5 mg/kg/h continuous infusion[98]	

(antithrombotic effect). At the same time, it does not inhibit platelet aggregation induced by collagen or adenosine diphosphate (ADP), thus allowing for normal hemostatic activity in surgical wounds.[75] Most studies have not demonstrated adverse effects of aprotinin on graft patency.[76] Additionally, use of high-dose, but not low-dose, aprotinin reduces the risk of stroke.[77]

   c. Because of its expense, aprotinin should generally be reserved for complex operations, reoperations, and other situations where the bleeding risk is increased (hepatic dysfunction, thrombocytopenia, uremia, use of aspirin and possibly clopidogrel).[78,79]

   d. Traditionally, aprotinin protocols have been subdivided into high-dose, low-dose, and ultra-low-dose as follows:

   i. High-dose aprotinin: 2 million kallikrein inactivation units (KIU) (280 mg) after the induction of anesthesia over 30 minutes, 2 million KIU (280 mg) in the pump prime, and a maintenance infusion of 0.5 million KIU/h (70 mg/h) until the completion of the operation.

   ii. Half-dose aprotinin: 1 million KIU (140 mg) after induction, 1 million KIU (140 mg) in the pump prime, and a continuous infusion of 250,000 KIU/h (35 mg/h).

   iii. "Minimal dose" and "ultra-low-dose" protocols include giving 0.5 million KIU (70 mg) before incision with additional 0.5 million KIU (70 mg) on pump or giving 1–2 million KIU (140–280 mg) in the pump prime alone.

e. The antifibrinolytic effects of aprotinin are noted at plasma concentrations of 125 KIU/L, which is sufficient to inhibit 90% of plasmin activity. This may be seen with lower dosing regimens and is effective in reducing bleeding. However, the antiinflammatory effects require a plasma level of 200 KIU/mL, which is required to inhibit kallikrein by approximately 50%.[80-82] This usually requires the higher dosing regimen.

f. Due to the expense of using aprotinin, weight-based protocols to maintain a serum level of 200 KIU/mL have been devised.[83,84] The recommendation of the Mayo clinic group is as follows:

   i. 3.5 mg/kg IV bolus

   ii. 70-mg pump prime load

   iii. 3.5 mg/kg/h for 1 hour, then 1 mg/kg/h continuous infusion

g. Aprotinin is useful in minimizing uremic bleeding due to platelet dysfunction in patients with dialysis-dependent renal failure. However, in patients with moderate renal dysfunction, it must be used cautiously because it may worsen renal function. Approximately 20% of patients will develop an increase in serum creatinine >0.5 mg/dL and 4% will have more than a 2 mg/dL increase, both of which are greater than in patients not receiving aprotinin.[85] Aprotinin is actively absorbed by the renal tubular system where it remains for 5–6 days and produces reversible overload of tubular reabsorption mechanisms. Patients with normal preoperative renal function usually compensate for this abnormality with little increase in creatinine, but those with altered tubular function may sustain additional tubular injury. Although guidelines for dosing in patients with moderate renal dysfunction are not available, lower doses should probably be used because of the increased half-life in patients with renal dysfunction.[86-88] Note that aprotinin is removed by intraoperative hemofiltration; this must be taken into consideration when hemofiltration is used during surgery to remove fluid.

h. Aprotinin raises the ACT and can lead to underheparinization. Aprotinin is absorbed by kaolin, so a kaolin ACT >480 seconds is adequate. It is not absorbed by celite, so a celite ACT must exceed 750 seconds.[89] If readily available, heparin levels should be measured and maintained >2.7 IU/mL.

i. There has been a reported association of neurologic deficits and renal dysfunction in patients undergoing deep hypothermic circulatory arrest with the use of aprotinin.[39] Safe use of aprotinin involves administering additional heparin before the period of circulatory arrest to achieve a higher ACT (at least >600 seconds and perhaps >1000 seconds), maintaining a heparin level >2.7 U/kg, recirculating the pump during the period of circulatory arrest, and avoiding infusion of aprotinin during the arrest period. Alternatively, the aprotinin infusion can be initiated during the rewarming phase.

j. Despite its antigenic properties (50% of patients will have detectable IgG immunoglobulins within 3 months of exposure), allergic reactions upon reexposure to aprotinin are relatively uncommon (about 3%).[90] Nonetheless, reexposure is best avoided for 6 months. A small test dose of 1 mL is optional before an initial dose of aprotinin because a severe anaphylactic reaction has been reported upon primary exposure.[91]

2. **ε-aminocaproic acid** (Amicar) is an inexpensive medication that can be used to reduce blood loss in first-time and uncomplicated reoperations. It has antifibrinolytic properties and may also preserve platelet function by inhibiting the

conversion of plasminogen to plasmin. It has no effect on the ACT. Although a meta-analysis concluded that it was as effective as aprotinin in reducing bleeding after cardiac surgery,[92] many studies have not demonstrated this, consistent with most surgeons' experiences.[93]

a. One common regimen is to give 5 g after the induction of anesthesia, 5 g on pump, and 1 g/h during the procedure. Twice this dose is commonly used in patients weighing more than 100 kg. Giving a 5–10-g dose only at the time of heparinization for bypass also reduces blood loss.

b. A pharmacokinetic study showed that the clearance of ε-aminocaproic acid decreases and the volume of distribution increases during CPB. To maintain a plasma level of 260 μg/mL, a recommended dosing regimen of a 50 mg/kg load over 20 minutes followed by a maintenance infusion of 25 mg/kg/h has been recommended.[94]

c. Few adverse clinical effects have been noted with use of ε-aminocaproic acid. There is no increased risk of stroke.[95] Although a subtle degree of renal tubular dysfunction may occur, as demonstrated by an increase in urine β_2-microglobulin levels, a 10 g dose was not shown to alter creatinine clearance.[96,97]

d. ε-Aminocaproic acid is primarily effective when given prophylactically, but might be of benefit in reducing blood loss if given only after bypass by inhibiting fibrinolysis. If extensive bleeding is encountered after its prophylactic use, aprotinin may be considered to control bleeding. However, the combination of these two medications might theoretically promote a prothrombotic state, and this must be taken into consideration if one takes this approach.

3. **Tranexamic acid** (Cyclokapron) has similar properties to ε-aminocaproic acid, inhibiting fibrinolysis at a serum concentration of 10 μg/mL, and reducing plasmin-induced platelet activation at a level of 16 μg/mL.[98] It has been shown to reduce perioperative blood loss in on- and off-pump surgery[71,99] and in several studies was found to be as effective as aprotinin.[100,101] It does not affect the ACT.[102]

a. The appropriate dosing of tranexamic acid is not well defined. One common recommendation is 10 mg/kg over 20 minutes followed by a 1 mg/kg/h infusion; another is a 1 g bolus followed by an infusion of 400 mg/h with 500 mg in the pump prime.[93,99–101,103] Another study showed that one dose of 100 mg/kg given before CPB was very effective in reducing bleeding.[104]

b. A weight-based protocol to achieve a plasma level >20 μg/mL entails a 5.4 mg/kg load, 50 mg in the pump prime (for a 2.5-L circuit), and a 5 mg/kg/h continuous infusion, to be modified by the serum creatinine.[98]

c. Topical use of tranexamic acid in the pericardial space has been shown to significantly reduce perioperative bleeding.[105]

d. Tranexamic acid is substantially less expensive than aprotinin, but more expensive than ε-aminocaproic acid.

F. **Anticoagulation for cardiopulmonary bypass**

1. Anticoagulation is essential during CPB to prevent the production of thrombin and fibrin monomers caused by interaction of blood with a synthetic interface. Advances in the design of extracorporeal circuits, such as heparin-bonded systems (Carmeda, Duraflo), have reduced, but not completely eliminated, the necessity for anticoagulation (see Chapter 5).[106,107]

2. **Heparin dosing.** Heparin inhibits the coagulation system by binding to antithrombin III. It also contributes to platelet dysfunction and induces a fibrinolytic state.[108,109] A baseline ACT should be drawn after the operation has commenced and before systemic heparinization. A small dose of heparin (5000 units) is given before division of the internal thoracic artery or radial artery, but a total dose of approximately 3–4 mg/kg of heparin must be given prior to cannulation for CPB. Porcine heparin may be associated with a lower risk of heparin antibody formation than bovine heparin and is therefore preferentially recommended.[110]

3. **Heparin** monitoring is performed using a number of systems that measure the ACT. This widely used test qualitatively assesses the anticoagulant effect of heparin. Although a standard dose of heparin is usually given, there is great variability in patient response to heparin. An individualized dose-response curve that relates the heparin dose to its effect on the ACT can be performed to determine the requisite amount of heparin. The ACT is influenced by many factors besides heparin, including hypothermia, hemodilution, and, to a lesser degree, thrombocytopenia. Furthermore, the ACT does not measure or necessarily correlate with heparin concentrations. Achieving higher patient-specific heparin levels more effectively suppresses hemostatic system activation than standard dosing based on ACT alone.[111] Nonetheless, due to its simplicity and overall safety, achieving a satisfactory ACT level is acceptable and universally utilized. The ACT should be monitored every 20–30 minutes during bypass (or prior to bypass if there is a significant delay after initial heparinization) and additional heparin administered as necessary.

   a. The ACT should be maintained over 480 seconds throughout the pump run. Lower ACTs are acceptable with the use of heparin-coated circuits during routine coronary bypass surgery, but probably are not acceptable during complex open heart operations.[106,107]

   b. With the use of aprotinin, which itself raises the ACT level, kaolin ACTs must be maintained longer than 480 seconds, whereas celite ACTs must exceed 750 seconds to avoid underheparinization.

   c. During off-pump surgery, the optimal ACT is not known. Using 2.5 mg/kg of heparin with a target ACT over 300 seconds is satisfactory and is not associated with any increased risk of thrombotic complications.[112]

   d. Because of individual patient variability in response to heparin and the effects of hypothermia and hemodilution on the ACT, anticoagulation can also be assessed by calculating dose-response curves and measuring circulating levels of heparin (desired level is > 2.7 U/mL) using the Medtronic Hepcon system. This directly measures circulating heparin levels and also allows for determination of a neutralizing dose of protamine to return the ACT to baseline.[113]

   e. An alternative means of assessing anticoagulation is the high-dose thrombin time. This correlates better with heparin concentration and is not affected by temperature, hemodilution, or aprotinin.[114]

4. **Heparin resistance** is present when a heparin dose of 5 mg/kg fails to raise the ACT to an adequate level (> 400 seconds). This is an unpredictable occurrence but is more commonly noted in patients on preoperative heparin, IV nitroglycerin, an IABP, and in patients with infective endocarditis.[115] It is usually related to antithrombin III deficiency. If additional heparin does not elevate the ACT,

antithrombin III must be given, either in fresh frozen plasma or in a commercially available pooled product (Thrombate III), which provides 500 units per vial.[116–118]

5. **Heparin-induced thrombocytopenia** documented by positive serologic tests (enzyme-linked immunosorbent assay) or platelet aggregation testing (heparin-platelet factor 4 or serotonin release assay) poses a dilemma for the patient requiring cardiac surgery.[119] Ideally, surgery should be delayed for about 3 months, at which time antibodies have usually disappeared. At that time, a heparin challenge is considered to be safe and is usually not associated with the reappearance of antibodies. However, when surgery is necessary on a more urgent basis and HIT is confirmed (i.e., *both* antibodies and thrombocytopenia are present), the readministration of heparin can produce profound thrombocytopenia and widespread thrombosis. Not infrequently, a heparin antibody is present in patients receiving preoperative heparin (up to 35% in one study),[120] but in the absence of thrombocytopenia its presence is not a contraindication to use of heparin during surgery. However, when HIT is present, an alternative means of achieving satisfactory anticoagulation during CPB and for off-pump surgery must be employed. Several regimens have been investigated (Table 4.4).

   a. Standard doses of heparin can be used in association with the three following options:

      i. Preoperative **aspirin and dipyridamole** as platelet pretreatment (a somewhat risky approach).[121]

      ii. Platelet inhibition with the short-acting **glycoprotein IIb/IIIa inhibitors** (tirofiban or eptifibatide). One recommended dosing regimen for tirofiban is 10 μg/kg 10 minutes prior to administration of standard-dose heparin, followed by a continuous infusion of 0.15 μg/kg/min that should be stopped 1 hour before the anticipated cessation of CPB. The effects of tirofiban on platelet function cannot be reversed, but 80% of their effect dissipates within 4 hours. Thus, bleeding may persist for a period of time after CPB has terminated.[122]

      iii. **Prostaglandin analogs** (PGE$_1$, epoprostenol [prostacyclin], or iloprost) can be used to inhibit platelet function during heparinization.
         • PGE$_1$ is given in a dose of 0.5–1.0 μg/min.
         • Epoprostenol is given in a dose of 5 ng/kg/min and increased by 5 ng/kg increments every 5 minutes (to observe for systemic hypotension) up to 25–30 ng/kg/min, following which a heparin bolus is given. After protamine administration, the dose is weaned in 5 ng/kg decrements.[123]
         • Iloprost can be given starting at a dose of 3 ng/kg/min with a doubling of dose every 5 minutes to a dose determined by preoperative in vitro testing. The usual dose required is 6–24 ng/kg/min.[124]

   b. **Bivalirudin** is a synthetic hirudin analog that is a direct thrombin inhibitor. It has a rapid onset of action and a half-life of 25 minutes. It is primarily metabolized by proteolytic cleavage by thrombin in the bloodstream. There is some renal elimination, so modification is necessary in patients with renal dysfunction. The effects of bivalirudin cannot be reversed, but it can be eliminated by hemofiltration and plasmapheresis.[125] After discontinuation, it is not associated with a hypercoagulable state (cf. argatroban).

Table 4.4 • Alternative Drugs for Anticoagulation During Cardiopulmonary Bypass in Patients with Heparin-Induced Thrombocytopenia

Drug	Half-life	Reversal	Metabolism	Monitoring	Dosing Regimen
Bivalirudin	25 min	None	Metabolic > renal	ACT, ECT	1.5 mg/kg bolus, 50 mg in pump, then 2.5 mg/kg/h infusion
Lepirudin	80 min	None	Renal	PTT, ECT	0.25 mg/kg, 2 mg/kg in pump prime, 0.5 mg/min infusion
Argatroban	30 min	None	Hepatic > renal	PTT, ACT	0.1 μg/kg bolus, then 5–10 μg/kg/min
Danaparoid	20 h	None	Renal	Factor Xa levels	125 U/kg, 3 U/kg in pump prime, 7 U/kg/h

    i. For off-pump surgery, bivalirudin has been given as a loading dose of 0.75 mg/kg followed by an infusion of 1.75 mg/kg/h to obtain an ACT of 300–350 seconds.[126]

    ii. For on-pump surgery, the recommended dose is a 1.5 mg/kg initial bolus, followed by a continuous infusion of 2.5 mg/kg/h infusion with 50 mg placed in the pump.[119] The infusion rate is then modified depending on the ecarin clotting time (ECT) as noted below. Other studies have used a 50-mg bolus followed by an infusion of 1.5–1.75 mg/kg/h.[127,128]

    iii. Adequacy of anticoagulation can be monitored with an ACT or an ECT drawn every 30 minutes. Studies have suggested that plasma bivalirudin levels of 10–15 µg/mL should be achieved. The correlation of the ECT with plasma levels is as follows: >500 seconds (> 15 µg/mL), 400–500 seconds (10–15 µg/mL), and <400 seconds (<10 µg/mL).[119,129]

c. R-hirudin (lepirudin) is a recombinant hirudin analog that is a direct thrombin inhibitor. It has a slow onset of action and a long half-life, estimated at around 80 minutes in a patient with normal renal function. Since it is primarily excreted by the kidneys, any impairment in renal function contraindicates its use. Its effects cannot be reversed, although it can be eliminated by hemofiltration.[130] Significant bleeding has been reported in most cases in which lepirudin has been used.

    i. The recommended dosing regimen is 0.25 mg/kg before CPB, 0.2 mg/kg in pump prime, and a continuous infusion of 0.5 mg/min. It should be discontinued 15–30 minutes before the anticipated end of CPB.[131,132]

    ii. The ACT is unreliable in assessing anticoagulation with hirudin at levels required for CPB. Thus, anticoagulation must be monitored by the ECT, attempting to achieve a level of 400–450 seconds. This corresponds to a hirudin level greater than 4 µg/mL.[119]

d. Argatroban is a direct thrombin inhibitor that takes about 1–3 hours to reach a steady-state level and has a half-life of about 30 minutes. It is primarily metabolized by the liver with about 25% excretion by the kidneys. Thus it is preferable to lepirudin in patients with renal impairment. It is monitored by the ACT, aiming for a level of 300–400 seconds. For off-pump surgery, one recommended dose is 2.5 µg/kg/min to achieve an ACT of twice baseline.[133] For on-pump surgery, the recommended dose is 0.1 mg/kg followed by a continuous infusion of 5–10 µg/kg/min.[134]

e. Danaparoid sodium is a heparinoid that inhibits factor Xa, resulting in inhibition of thrombin generation. It has low cross-reactivity with antiheparin antibodies (about 10%). Although it has been used during cardiac surgery, its disadvantages are that it has a half-life of 20 hours, undergoes renal metabolism, and its effects are not reversible.[135,136] Thus, it is invariably associated with significant bleeding after CPB.

    i. The recommended dosing protocol is 125 antifactor Xa U/kg IV bolus, 3 U/kg in the pump prime, and a continuous infusion of 7 U/kg/h that should be stopped 45 minutes before the anticipated end of CPB.

    ii. Appropriate monitoring requires measurement of factor Xa levels, trying to maintain a plasma concentration of 0.7–1.3 U/mL. Since such testing is not feasible during CPB, this medication is very risky and has been associated with thrombotic events on bypass. Although useful in postoperative patients with HIT, it is best avoided during CPB. It is no longer available in the United States.

G. Although one dose of antibiotics administered prior to skin incision usually suffices to provide adequate tissue levels, an additional 1-g dose of cefazolin may be beneficial just before going on bypass.

VII. Considerations During Cardiopulmonary Bypass

A. Virtually all valve surgery and most coronary bypass surgery is performed using CPB. The essential components of the CPB circuit are discussed in the next chapter. Basically, the blood drains by gravity from the right atrium into a reservoir, is oxygenated, cooled or warmed, and then returned to the patient through an arterial cannula usually placed in the ascending aorta. Desired hemodynamic and laboratory values during bypass are noted in Table 5.2.

B. The lungs are not ventilated during bypass since oxygenation occurs within the oxygenator and carbon dioxide is eliminated by the gas flow into the oxygenator (the sweep rate). Although studies have suggested that the efficacy of gas exchange postpump is improved in patients whose lungs remain inflated during CPB, this is not a common practice.[137] Arterial blood gases are measured to ensure that the oxygenator is providing adequate oxygenation and that CO_2 extraction is sufficient. Venous oxygen saturation is measured to determine if the systemic flow rate is adequate. If on-line monitoring is not available, studies should be repeated every 15–20 minutes.

C. The optimal mean blood pressure during CPB is controversial.[138,139] Although there is some evidence that a higher mean blood pressure (around 80 mm Hg) may reduce some of the neurocognitive changes seen after bypass, the standard management is to maintain a mean blood pressure around 65 mm Hg using vasodilators (narcotics or inhalational anesthetics) or vasopressors (phenylephrine, norepinephrine, or vasopressin). Perfusion pressure is determined by a number of variables.

    1. Hypotension may be related to hemodilution; use of preoperative vasodilators, including ACE inhibitors, calcium channel blockers, and amiodarone; vasodilatation during rewarming; and autonomic dysfunction. It may also occur due to inadequate systemic flow rates, impairment of venous drainage, aortic insufficiency, administration of cardioplegia, and during return of large amounts of cardiotomy-suctioned blood into the circulation.

    2. Hypertension may be related to vasoconstriction, the level of anesthesia and analgesia, elevation in endogenous catecholamine levels, and alterations in acid-base balance and blood gas exchange.

D. A venous oxygen saturation exceeding 65% indicates that the systemic flow rate is satisfactory, although there may be differences in regional flow (i.e., less to the kidneys and splanchnic circulation). It tends to be higher during systemic hypothermia due to lessened oxygen extraction, and may decrease significantly during rewarming, necessitating an increased flow rate.

E. Studies have suggested that cerebral blood flow is more dependent on blood pressure than on flow rate.[140,141] If flow rate is adequate, α-agents must be utilized to maintain a blood pressure of at least 40 mm Hg and probably higher. Cerebral blood flow is maintained by autoregulation until the pressure falls below 40 mm Hg, but this response is inadequate in diabetic and hypertensive patients, in whom a higher pressure must be maintained. Measurement of cerebral oxygenation by cerebral oximetry using bifrontal sensors with near-infrared spectroscopy

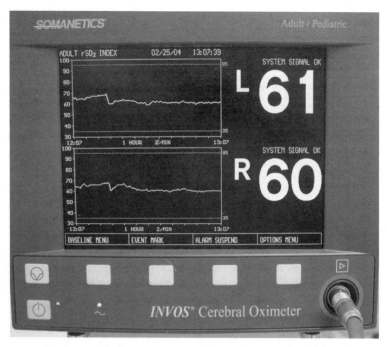

Figure 4.1 • The Somanetics INVOS Cerebral Oximeter. This device uses near infrared spectroscopy to measure the regional oxygen saturation of predominantly venous blood directly in the brain through optical sensors placed on the right and left side of the forehead. *(Image courtesy of Somanetics Corporation)*

(Somanetics INVOS Cerebral Oximeter) can be used to assess the adequacy of cerebral perfusion (ScO_2) during on-pump and off-pump surgery (Figure 4.7)[142–144] There is increasing evidence that modifications in anesthetic and perfusion management by changes in flow rate, blood pressure, PCO_2, and/or hematocrit in response to a fall in ScO_2 below 40 mm Hg reduces neurological complications.[145]

F. Blood sugar tends to be elevated due to the hormonal stress response to surgery and CPB with insulin resistance. The infusion of insulin to control blood sugar has not been shown to reduce inotropic requirements or the occurrence of arrhythmias but may reduce the incidence of neurocognitive dysfunction.[146,147]

G. Measures to optimize renal function should be considered in patients with preoperative renal dysfunction (creatinine > 1.5 mg/dL), especially in diabetic, hypertensive patients. The primary considerations should be maintaining a higher mean perfusion pressure (around 80 mm Hg) and keeping the pump run as short as possible (or avoiding it entirely with off-pump techniques). Pharmacologic means to optimize renal perfusion may include fenoldopam (0.03–0.1 µg/kg/min) or nesiritide, although the potential renoprotective role of nesiritide has not yet been defined.[148–150] Although both renal-dose dopamine (3 µg/kg/min) and furosemide may increase urine output during CPB, neither has been found to be renoprotective.[151–153] In fact, furosemide has been shown to increase the incidence of postoperative renal dysfunction.[151] However, the major cause of postoperative renal dysfunction is a low output state, so maintenance of satisfactory hemodynamics at the termination of CPB is essential so that any intraoperative renal insults are transient.

H. When the cross-clamp is removed, lidocaine and magnesium may be given to reduce the incidence of atrial and ventricular arrhythmias.[154] Ventricular fibrillation tends to occur when the heart was maintained at a cold temperature during the period of cardioplegic arrest and usually requires defibrillation, although spontaneous conversion to a sinus mechanism may occur.

VIII. Termination of Bypass and Reversal of Anticoagulation

A. Once the cardiac portion of the operation has been completed, the lungs are ventilated and pacing is initiated, if necessary. Just prior to weaning bypass, 1 g of calcium chloride may be given to increase systemic vascular resistance (SVR) and provide some initial inotropic support.

B. Inotropic medications can be started prior to terminating bypass if it is anticipated that the heart may require some support. This should be considered in patients with preexisting LV dysfunction, prebypass ischemia, recent infarction, suboptimal or incomplete revascularization, LV hypertrophy, and long cross-clamp periods. If α-agents (phenylephrine, norepinephrine) were necessary on pump to support systemic pressure, they are usually necessary for a brief period of time after CPB is terminated.

C. Bypass is weaned by gradually reducing the venous return, increasing intravascular volume in the patient, and reducing the arterial flow rate.

D. **Arterial blood pressure** monitoring is often inconsistent due to the presence of peripheral vasoconstriction. Measurement of the central aortic pressure using a stopcock on the aortic line is very helpful in sorting out discrepancies. If this problem persists for more than 10–15 minutes, it is helpful to insert a femoral arterial monitoring line.[155,156]

E. TEE is utilized as the patient is being weaned from bypass to (see Table 4.1):

1. Identify intracardiac air. This is essential in valvular heart procedures or any procedure in which the left side of the heart has been entered (including venting). It is particularly valuable during minimally invasive procedures in which exposure to the heart for deairing is limited.

2. Assess regional and global ventricular function and loading conditions. TEE is the only means of assessing intravascular volume directly (other than by direct visualization) since the volume-pressure relationship is altered by decreased ventricular compliance. Thus, it is helpful in determining whether hypotension should be treated by volume infusions, inotropic medications, or α-agents.

3. Detect paravalvular leaks or the competence of a valve repair

F. If hemodynamic performance is not ideal, the anesthesiologist must work in concert with the surgeon in assessing myocardial function and the need for inotropes.[157] When myocardial performance is adequate, fluid administration to optimize preload is sufficient to obtain adequate hemodynamics. Initially this can be achieved by transfusing volume from the pump. After protamine administration, the blood remaining in the pump is processed through the cell-saving device and returned to the patient. If this is not immediately available, a colloid is often chosen to maintain intravascular volume. Albumin is preferable to hetastarch, which has been shown to increase bleeding and transfusion requirements.[158]

1. Once the patient is off bypass, visual inspection of the heart, assessment of serial cardiac outputs and filling pressures with a Swan-Ganz catheter, and TEE can be used to assess ventricular function and identify potential problems. For example, a new regional wall motion abnormality may suggest a technical problem with graft flow that can be remedied. If intracardiac air is identified, it is not uncommon for it to pass into the right coronary artery, causing RV dysfunction and dilatation. An additional short course on bypass with deairing of the aorta and any bypass grafts usually suffices. This is not an uncommon phenomenon in mitral valve surgery.

2. Fluid loading with concomitant TEE assessment and cardiac output measurements is helpful is determining the optimal filling pressures for subsequent management, although it is anticipated that filling pressures will eventually fall with improvement in cardiac performance. It should be remembered that the heart is less compliant after a period of ischemic arrest, and higher filling pressures will be necessary to achieve adequate intravascular volume.

3. If necessary, inotropic support is usually initiated with a catecholamine, such as epinephrine (1–2 µg/min) or dobutamine (5–10 µg/kg/min). If cardiac performance remains unsatisfactory, use of either inamrinone or milrinone is extremely helpful in unloading the heart and providing inotropic support. Their preemptive use just prior to terminating bypass has been suggested as a means of ameliorating postoperative deterioration in cardiac performance and oxygen transport, and reducing the need for catecholamine support.[159]

4. If cardiac performance is still suboptimal, reinstitution of CPB to reperfuse the heart at a low workload will frequently result in improved ventricular function. If the heart still does not function well, insertion of an IABP is usually necessary. When all of the above fail, consideration must be given to use of a circulatory assist device.

G. Protamine is a polycationic peptide administered to counteract the effects of heparin and is usually given in a 1:1 mg/mg ratio to return the ACT to baseline. Despite complete neutralization of heparin, the ACT may remain elevated in patients with significant thrombocytopenia or coagulopathies. Although moderate thrombocytopenia has not been shown to increase the ACT in patients with normally functioning platelets, it does seem to increase it when associated with platelet dysfunction after bypass.[160] Thus, although additional protamine can be administered for a slightly elevated ACT, it will not necessarily return the ACT to baseline.

1. The Medtronic Hepcon system provides a heparin-protamine titration test that can be utilized to measure heparin levels in the bloodstream and determine the appropriate dose of protamine necessary to neutralize the remaining heparin. Use of this system usually results in less protamine being administered than empiric dosing based on the heparin dose. Thus it can avoid the unnecessary use of protamine to correct an abnormal ACT that is not attributable to excessive heparin. Use of lower doses of protamine has been shown to restore platelet responsiveness to thrombin and attenuate platelet α-granule secretion.[161]

2. Residual heparin effect may account for an elevated ACT. Thus it is not inappropriate to give small additional doses of protamine to try to reduce the ACT

to baseline. Infusion of blood that is spun down in the cell-saving devices does contain some heparin (up to 10% of the heparin is retained), and additional protamine (about 50 mg) may be useful to counteract its effects.

3. "Heparin rebound" may occur when heparin reappears in the bloodstream after protamine neutralization. This is more likely to occur in patients who have received large doses of heparin during bypass and is more common in obese patients.[162] This may occur because the half-life of protamine is only about 5 minutes.[163] An elevated ACT or PTT commonly reflects this phenomenon and can be reversed with additional doses of protamine.

4. Empiric use of large amounts of additional protamine should be discouraged because protamine itself is an anticoagulant and may contribute to mediastinal bleeding. Although a dose exceeding that of heparin by 3:1 is usually necessary to produce this effect, studies have demonstrated that an elevated PT from protamine can occur when the ratio exceeds 1.5:1.[164]

5. Hemodynamic studies have shown that intravenous administration of protamine may cause histamine release from the lungs, contributing to a decrease in systemic resistance and blood pressure, an effect not seen with intraarterial injection.[165] Nonetheless, other studies have shown no hemodynamic benefit to intraarterial as opposed to intravenous administration of protamine.[166]

H. **Protamine reactions** are unusual and are often unpredictable, although they have been noted with greater frequency in patients taking NPH insulin (risk may be increased 30- to 50-fold), those with fish or medication allergies, those with previous protamine exposure, and those who have had vasectomies.[167–169] Awareness of the possibility of their development and a prompt response if a reaction is noted are essential because protamine reactions are associated with increased perioperative mortality.[170,171]

1. **Type I.** Systemic hypotension from rapid administration (entire neutralizing dose after CPB given within 3 minutes). This is caused by a histamine-related reduction in systemic and pulmonary vascular resistance. It can be avoided by infusing the protamine over a 10–15 minute period and should be reversible with α-agent support.

2. **Type II.** Anaphylactic or anaphylactoid reaction resulting in hypotension, tachycardia, bronchospasm, flushing, and pulmonary edema.

   a. IIA. Idiosyncratic IgE- or IgG-mediated anaphylactic reaction. Release of histamine, leukotrienes, and kinins produces a systemic capillary leak causing hypotension and pulmonary edema. This tends to occur within the first 10 minutes of administration.

   b. IIB. Immediate nonimmunologic anaphylactoid reaction.

   c. IIC. Delayed reactions, usually occurring 20 minutes or more after the protamine infusion has been started, probably related to complement activation and leukotriene release, producing wheezing, hypovolemia, and noncardiogenic pulmonary edema from a pulmonary capillary leak.

3. **Type III.** Catastrophic pulmonary vasoconstriction manifested by elevated pulmonary arterial pressures, systemic hypotension from peripheral vasodilation, decreased left atrial pressures, RV dilatation, and myocardial depression. This reaction tends to occur about 10–20 minutes after the protamine infusion has started. One proposed mechanism involves activation of complement

by the heparin-protamine complex that triggers leukocyte aggregation and release of liposomal enzymes that damage pulmonary tissue leading to pulmonary edema. Activation of the arachidonic acid pathway produces thromboxane, which constricts the pulmonary vessels. Pulmonary vasoconstriction usually abates after about 10 minutes.

4. Prevention of protamine reactions is usually not possible. Skin testing has not proved of any value. In patients considered at high risk, type II reactions might be attenuated by the prophylactic use of histamine blockers (cimetidine 300 mg IV, diphenhydramine 50 mg IV) and steroids (hydrocortisone 100 mg IV). This common practice has not been shown clinically to be of much benefit.

5. Treatment of protamine reactions involves correction of hemodynamic abnormalities that are identified. They must be differentiated from other conditions that can cause hemodynamic deterioration, such as hypoperfusion, air embolism, poor myocardial protection, or valve dysfunction. Measures must be taken to support systemic blood pressure while reversing pulmonary vasoconstriction if it is also present. Preparations to reinstitute CPB are frequently necessary. The following options may be effective:

a. Calcium chloride 500 mg IV to support systemic resistance and provide some inotropic support.

b. α-agents (phenylephrine, norepinephrine) to support systemic resistance.

c. β-agents for inotropic support that can also reduce pulmonary resistance (low-dose epinephrine, dobutamine, inamrinone, milrinone).

d. Drugs to reduce preload and pulmonary pressures (nitroglycerin, PGE_1, nitric oxide).[172]

e. Aminophylline for wheezing.

f. Readministration of heparin has been used to reverse the protamine reaction.[173,174]

I. **Alternatives to reverse anticoagulation.** Although simply not reversing heparin and administering clotting factors may suffice in ameliorating the bleeding tendency of heparinization,[175] other measures have been evaluated to arrest bleeding without use of protamine.

1. **Heparinase-I** is a heparin-degrading enzyme that reverses the ACT in a dose-dependent fashion without causing hemodynamic changes. It is given as a bolus injection of 7–10 mg/kg. Although it returns the ACT to normal, it neutralizes only 70% of antifactor Xa (protamine neutralizes 100%) and returns antifactor IIA activity to zero. This is a promising alternative to use of protamine.[176]

2. **Recombinant platelet factor 4** neutralizes heparin by a polycationic-polyanionic interaction. It reverses heparin when given in a ratio of 3:1 to the dose of heparin.[177]

3. A **heparin removal device** has been developed and used clinically in a few patients with protamine sensitivity. This system uses a double-lumen cannula placed in the right atrium and a venovenous circuit. This contains a pheresis chamber in which heparin binds to poly-L-lysine and is removed from the blood.[178,179]

4. **Hexadimethrine** has been used on a compassionate basis in a few patients with protamine allergies but is not clinically available in the United States.[180]

5. A low-molecular-weight protamine preparation has been investigated in canine models and has been shown to be effective in neutralizing heparin without demonstrating any adverse hemodynamic responses caused by nonimmunologic mechanisms.[181]

J. **Treatment of coagulopathy.** A meticulous operation and routine use of antifibrinolytic drugs in a patient with no preexisting coagulation problem should result in minimal postoperative bleeding. However, a coagulopathy is present in all patients to varying degrees after CPB. Generally, the longer the duration of CPB and the greater the number of blood transfusions required on pump, the greater the coagulopathy. Furthermore, preoperative medications, especially the ubiquitous antiplatelet agents, have adverse effects on hemostasis.

1. Most groups treat coagulopathies in the operating room by the "shotgun approach." This entails the empiric administration of additional protamine and transfusion of platelets, fresh frozen plasma, and, occasionally, cryoprecipitate. However, it is best to prioritize these products based on suspicion of the hemostatic defect. For example, platelet transfusions should be given first to patients on aspirin or clopidogrel or with uremia; fresh frozen plasma should be considered first for patients on preoperative warfarin, with hepatic dysfunction, or when multiple transfusions are given on pump; and uremic patients might benefit from desmopressin (see Chapter 9).

2. Although these approaches will usually stem the "coagulopathic tide," it is more scientific and cost-effective to use point-of-care testing to assess the specific hemostatic defect and direct care accordingly. Systems are available to measure the PT, PTT, and platelet count, and several are capable of measuring platelet function as well.[114,182,183] Other tests, such as the thromboelastogram, can provide an assessment of the exact hemostatic defect, but this test is time-consuming and rarely used.

3. Further comments on the treatment of bleeding and specific coagulation defects associated with aspirin, clopidogrel, and the IIb/IIIa inhibitors are presented on pages 95–98.

IX. Anesthetic Considerations During Off-Pump Surgery (Box 4.2)[184]

A. Monitoring considerations

1. In contrast to on-pump surgery, off-pump surgery via a median sternotomy requires that the heart provide adequate systemic perfusion at all times. Hemodynamics may be compromised by positioning of the heart, myocardial ischemia, ventricular arrhythmias, bleeding, and valvular regurgitation.

2. To ideally monitor a patient for myocardial ischemia and dysfunction when the heart is positioned at unorthodox angles, more intense monitoring is required than for on-pump surgery. Swan-Ganz catheters that provide on-line continuous cardiac output and mixed venous oxygen saturation are essential. These will dictate whether volume infusion or pharmacologic management is indicated. Simply maintaining an adequate blood pressure and heart rate pharmacologically may not suffice and often will provide no premonitory indication that the heart is becoming ischemic and subject to precipitous deterioration into ventricular fibrillation.

Box 4.2 • Key Elements of Anesthetic Management for Off-Pump Surgery

1. Continuous cardiac output and mixed venous oxygen monitoring
2. Transesophageal echocardiography
3. Antifibrinolytic drugs (probably of benefit)
4. Low-level heparinization with ACT of 300 seconds
5. Short-acting anesthetic agents
6. Maintenance of systemic normothermia
7. Arrhythmia prophylaxis with lidocaine and magnesium
8. Availability of pacing capability
9. Maintenance of hemodynamics with fluid, α-agents, and inotropes
10. Patience and emotional support for the surgeon!

---

3. TEE is helpful in assessing for the development of regional wall motion abnormalities during construction of an anastomosis. The anesthesiologist should be well trained in TEE and must immediately communicate any problem to the surgeon. Steps can then be taken to resolve the problem, often with the placement of a shunt to improve flow. During vessel occlusion, TEE should assess for the acute development of regional LV dysfunction or acute MR during construction of left-sided grafts and for RV or inferior wall dysfunction during right-sided grafting. If regional wall motion abnormalities persist after the graft is completed, a technical problem with the anastomosis should be suspected. The midesophageal windows are best for assessing RV and LV function. The transgastric views are not helpful when the heart is elevated out of the chest.[33]

B. **Anesthetic agents** are similar to those used for on-pump surgery, although shorter-acting medications may be selected depending on plans for extubation. Although patients can be extubated in the operating room, a more common practice is to use propofol for sedation at the end of surgery and for several hours in the ICU before considering extubation.

C. **Heparinization** is essential during off-pump surgery because coagulation is still activated by release of tissue factor and activation of the extrinsic pathway. The requisite amounts of heparin and minimally acceptable ACT levels have not been delineated. Usually 2.5 mg/kg of heparin suffices to raise the ACT to a level of 300 seconds. There have been concerns about the prothrombotic tendency noted after off-pump coronary artery bypass (OPCAB), since the hemodilution, platelet dysfunction, and fibrinolysis associated with CPB may not be seen. This prothrombotic tendency may be related to procoagulant activity of platelets or the activation of fibrinogen and other acute-phase reactants that result from the surgery itself.[185–189] However, clinical evidence of these problems, primarily graft closure, has not been confirmed at ACTs greater than 300 seconds.[112]

D. **Antifibrinolytic therapy** has not been studied extensively for off-pump surgery, although limited studies of aprotinin and tranexamic acid have shown benefits in reducing bleeding.[71,72] Although the blood is not subject to contact activation in an extracorporeal circuit, heparinization does induce fibrinolysis, and thus use of any of the antifibrinolytic agents may be beneficial. ε-aminocaproic acid has been used routinely for OPCABs at many centers.

E. **Patient temperature** tends to drift during open-chest procedures but should be maintained as close to normothermia as possible to prevent arrhythmias, bleeding, and subsequent shivering in the ICU. The ambient room temperature must be raised into the mid-70sºF and some form of warming blanket should be used. These include a sterile Bair Hugger and heat-emitting devices, such as the Arctic Sun temperature-controlling system.[190] All fluids must be warmed and a heated humidifier placed in the ventilatory circuit

F. **Maintenance of hemodynamics.** During cardiac positioning, the patient is placed in Trendelenburg position and the operating room table is rotated to the right. Deep pericardial sutures are placed to aid with retraction. Apical suction devices can also be used to rotate the heart cephalad and to the right. Central venous and pulmonary arterial pressures increase in the head-down position, and care must be taken not to administer too much fluid and increase these pressures even more. Transducer location may need to be adjusted to ensure accuracy. The possibility of producing cerebral edema should be kept in mind.

   1. Magnesium and lidocaine should be given to increase the arrhythmic threshold.

   2. Blood pressure should be maintained in the 120–140 mm Hg systolic range to optimize coronary perfusion, especially collateral flow. This can be done with some fluid administration but usually with liberal administration of α-agents.

   3. Atrial pacing wires may be placed if there is a concern about bradycardia developing with heart positioning. Transesophageal pacing may be utilized. Induced bradycardia is not essential with the latest generation of stabilizing devices. However, tachycardia should be controlled. Ventricular pacing cables should be immediately available in case heart block develops.

   4. Detection of ischemia can be difficult, since the monitor ECG and TEE images can be difficult to interpret in the translocated heart. A reduction in the SvO_2 is one of the first signs of the struggling heart. Intracoronary shunting or aortocoronary shunting during construction of an anastomosis ameliorates distal ischemia. This is more likely to be required during bypass of the distal right coronary artery, which compromises flow to the atrioventricular node and produces heart block. Upon the first suspicion of ventricular dysfunction, the surgeon should be informed immediately so that a shunt may be placed, if not done so prophylactically, to try to minimize ischemia.

   5. If inotropic support is required, low-dose epinephrine is given first, followed by inamrinone or milrinone if more support is needed. In high-risk cases, such as severe left main disease, a prophylactic IABP may be helpful.[191] Unless there is a strong indication for OPCAB, such as severe comorbidities, immediate conversion to an on-pump procedure may be a wise decision if instability persists.

G. **Blood loss** can be insidious during OPCAB. Blood should be scavenged into a cell saver and retransfused to the patient. Not infrequently, about 1 L of blood is lost and scavenged during these operations.

H. **Proximal anastomoses** are usually performed last. The blood pressure should be lowered to about 80–90 mm Hg systolic for application of the side clamp to minimize the risk of aortic injury and atheroembolization. Induced hypotension may increase the risk of renal dysfunction. Distal perfusion is compromised after a graft is sewn to the aorta until the clamp is removed, and the patient can become unstable at this time.

I. Protamine is given in a 1:1 ratio to heparin. Bleeding should be minimal if the anastomoses are hemostatic. Pacing wires should be placed on the atrium and ventricle, chest tubes are placed, and the chest is closed.

J. The patient may be extubated in the operating room but more commonly is maintained on a propofol drip for several hours in the ICU. When the patient is normothermic, hemodynamically stable, and not bleeding, the propofol is gradually weaned off, and standard criteria for respiratory weaning and extubation are followed. Most patients are extubated within a few hours.

References

1. Gibbs NM, Weightman WM, Thrackray NM, Michalopoulos N, Weidmann C. The effects of recent aspirin ingestion on platelet function in cardiac surgical patients. J Cardiothorac Vasc Anesth 2001;15:55–9.

2. Weightman WM, Gibbs NM, Weidmann CR, et al. The effect of preoperative aspirin-free interval on red blood cell transfusion requirements in cardiac surgical patients. J Cardiothorac Vasc Anesth 2002;16:54–68.

3. Kincaid EH, Monroe ML, Saliba D, Kon N, Byerly WG, Reichert MG. Effects of preoperative enoxaparin versus unfractionated heparin on bleeding indices in patients undergoing coronary artery bypass grafting. Ann Thorac Surg 2003;76:124–8.

4. Chun R, Orser BA, Madan M. Platelet glycoprotein IIb IIIa inhibitors: overview and implications for the anesthesiologist. Anesth Analg 2002;95:879–88.

5. Sreeram GM, Sharma AD, Slaughter TF. Platelet glycoprotein IIb/IIIa antagonists: perioperative implications. J Cardiothorac Vasc Anesth 2001;15:237–40.

6. Loeb HS, Saudye A, Croke RP, et al. Effects of pharmacologically-induced hypertension on myocardial ischemia and coronary hemodynamics in patients with fixed coronary obstruction. Circulation 1978;57:41–6.

7. Sanchez R, Wee M. Perioperative myocardial ischemia: early diagnosis using the pulmonary artery catheter. J Cardiothorac Vasc Anesth 1991;5:604–7.

8. Stewart RD, Psyhojos T, Lahey SJ, Levitsky S, Campos CT. Central venous catheter use in low-risk coronary artery bypass grafting. Ann Thorac Surg 1998;66:1306–11.

9. Schwann TA, Zacharias A, Riordan CJ, Durham SJ, Engoren M, Habib RH. Safe, highly selective use of pulmonary artery catheters in coronary artery bypass grafting: an objective patient selection method. Ann Thorac Surg 2002;73:1394–1402.

10. Forrest AP, Lovelock ND, Hu JM, Fletcher SN. The impact of intraoperative echocardiography on an unselected cardiac surgical population: a review of 2343 cases. Anaesth Crit Care 2002;30:734–41.

11. Michel-Cherqui M, Ceddaha A, Liu N, et al. Assessment of the systematic use of intraoperative transesophageal echocardiography during cardiac surgery in adults: a prospective study of 203 patients. J Cardiothorac Vasc Anesth 2000;14:45–50.

12. Mishra M, Chauhan R, Sharma KK, et al. Real-time intraoperative transesophageal echocardiography: how useful? Experience of 5,016 cases. J Cardiothorac Vasc Anesth 1998;12:625–32.

13. Fanshawe M, Ellis C, Habib S, Konstadt SN, Reich DL. A retrospective analysis of the costs and benefits in cardiac surgery from routine intraoperative transesophageal echocardiography. Anesth Analg 2002;95:824–7.

14. Al-Tabbaa A, Gonzalez RM, Lee D. The role of state-of-the-art echocardiography in the assessment of myocardial injury during and following cardiac surgery. Ann Thorac Surg 2001; 72:S2214–9.

15. Grigore AM, Grocott HP. Pro Epiaortic scanning is routinely necessary for cardiac surgery. J Cardiothorac Vasc Anesth 2002;14:87–90.

16. Wilson MJ, Boyd SY, Lisagor PG, Rubal BJ, Cohen DJ. Ascending aortic atheroma assessed intraoperatively by epiaortic and transesophageal echocardiography. Ann Thorac Surg 2000;70:25–30.

17. Ramsey SD, Saint S, Sullivan SD, Dey L, Kelley K, Bowdle A. Clinical and economic effects of pulmonary artery catheterization in nonemergent coronary artery bypass graft surgery. J Cardiothorac Vasc Anesth 2000;14:113–8.

18. Tuman KJ, McCarthy RJ, Spiess BD, et al. Effect of pulmonary artery catheterization on outcome in patients undergoing coronary artery surgery. Anesthesiology 1989;70:199–206.

19. Spackman TN. A theoretical evaluation of cost-effectiveness of pulmonary artery catheters in patients undergoing coronary artery surgery. J Cardiothorac Vasc Anesth 1994;8:570–6.

20. Ruesch S, Walder B, Tramer MR. Complications of central venous catheters: internal jugular versus subclavian access: a systematic review. Crit Care Med 2002;30:454–60.

21. Wadsworth R, Littler C. Cardiac standstill, pulmonary artery catheterisation and left bundle branch block. Anaesthesia 1996;51:97.

22. Vedrinne C, Bastien O, De Varax R, et al. Predictive factors for usefulness of fiberoptic pulmonary artery catheter for continuous oxygen saturation in mixed venous blood monitoring in cardiac surgery. Anesth Analg 1997;85:2–10.

23. Balik K, Pachil J, Hendl J, Martin B, Jan P, Han H. Effect of the degree of tricuspid regurgitation on cardiac output measurements by thermodilution. Intensive Care Med 2002;28:1117–21.

24. Perings SM, Perings C, Kelm M, Strauer BE. Comparative evaluation of thermodilution and gated blood pool method for determination of right ventricular ejection fraction at rest and during exercise. Cardiology 2001;95:161–3.

25. Smythe WR, Gorman RC, DeCampli WM, Spray TL, Kaiser LR, Acker MA. Management of exsanguinating hemoptysis during cardiopulmonary bypass. Ann Thorac Surg 1999;67:1288–91.

26. Urschel JD, Myerowitz PD. Catheter-induced pulmonary artery rupture in the setting of cardiopulmonary bypass. Ann Thorac Surg 1993;56:585–9.

27. Mullerworth MH, Angelopoulos P, Couyant MA, et al. Recognition and management of catheter-induced pulmonary artery rupture. Ann Thorac Surg 1998;66:1242–5.

28. Sirivella S, Gielchinsky I, Parsonnet V. Management of catheter-induced pulmonary artery perforation: a rare complication in cardiovascular operations. Ann Thorac Surg 2001;72:2056–9.

29. Seward JB, Khandheria BK, Freeman WK, et al. Multiplane transesophageal echocardiography: image orientation, examination technique, anatomic correlations, and clinical applications. Mayo Clin Proc 1993;68:523–51.

30. Schneider AT, Hsu TL, Schwartz SL, Pandian NG. Single, biplane, multiplane, and three-dimensional transesophageal echocardiography. Echocardiographic-anatomic correlations. Cardiol Clin 1993;11:361–87.

31. Shanewise JS, Cheung AT, Aronson S, et al. ASE/SCA guidelines for performing a comprehensive intraoperative multiplane transesophageal echocardiography examination: Recommendations of the American Society of Echocardiography Council for Intraoperative Echocardiography and the Society of Cardiovascular Anesthesiologists Task Force for certification in perioperative transesophageal echocardiography. Anesth Analg 1999;89:870–84.

32. Oh JK, Seward JB, Tajik AJ. The Echo Manual, 2nd ed. Philadelphia: Lippincott Williams & Wilkins, 1999.

33. Shanewise JS, Zaffer R, Martin RP. Intraoperative echocardiography and minimally invasive cardiac surgery. Echocardiography 2002;19:579–82.

34. Koide Y, Keehn L, Nomura T, Long T, Oka Y. Relationship of regional wall motion abnormalities detected by biplane transesophageal echocardiography and electrocardiographic changes in patients undergoing coronary artery bypass graft surgery. J Cardiothorac Vasc Anesth 1996;10:719–27.

35. Tingleff J, Joyce FS, Pettersson G. Intraoperative echocardiographic study of air embolism during cardiac operations. Ann Thorac Surg 1995;60:673–7.

36. Brinkman WT, Shanewise JS, Clements SD, Mansour KA. Transesophageal echocardiography: not an innocuous procedure. Ann Thorac Surg 2001;72:1725–6.

37. Kallmeyer I, Morse CS, Body SC, Collard CD. Transesophageal echocardiography: associated gastrointestinal trauma. J Cardiothorac Vasc Anesth 2000;14:212–6.

38. Iafrati MD, Gordon G, Staples MH, et al. Transesophageal echocardiography for hemodynamic management of thoracoabdominal aneurysm repair. Am J Surg 1993;166:179–85.

39. Gravlee GP. Con: aprotinin should not be used in patients undergoing hypothermic circulatory arrest. J Cardiovasc Vasc Anesth 2001;15:126–8.

40. Mora Mangano CT, Neville NJ, Hsu PH, Mignea I, King J, Miller DC. Aprotinin, blood loss, and renal dysfunction in deep hypothermic circulatory arrest. Circulation 2001;104:1276–81.

41. Smith CR, Spanier TB. Aprotinin in deep hypothermic circulatory arrest. Ann Thorac Surg 1999;68:278–86.

42. Royston D. Pro: aprotinin should be used in patients undergoing circulatory arrest. J Cardiothorac Vasc Anesth 2001;15:121–5.

43. Sheinbaum R, Ignacio C, Safi HJ, Estrera A. Contemporary strategies to preserve renal function during cardiac and vascular surgery. Rev Cardiovasc Med 2003;4(suppl 1):S21–8.

44. Marini CP, Levison J, Caliendo F, Nathan IM, Cohen JR. Control of proximal hypertension during aortic cross-clamping: its effect on cerebrospinal fluid dynamics and spinal cord perfusion pressures. Semin Thorac Cardiovasc Surg 1998;10:51–6.

45. Dhadphale PR, Jackson AP, Alseri S. Comparison of anesthesia with diazepam and ketamine vs. morphine in patients undergoing heart-valve replacement. Anesthesiology 1979;51:200–3.

46. Mourisse J, Booij L. Bispectral index detects period of cerebral hypoperfusion during cardiopulmonary bypass. J Cardiothorac Vasc Anesth 2003;17:76–8.

47. Sebel PS. Central nervous system monitoring during open heart surgery: an update. J Cardiothorac Vasc Anesth 1998;12:3–8.

48. Thomson IR, Harding G, Hudson RJ. A comparison of fentanyl and sufentanil in patients undergoing coronary artery bypass graft surgery. J Cardiothorac Vasc Anesth 2002;14:652–6.

49. Tritapepe L, Voci P, Di Giovanni C, et al. Alfentanil and sufentanil in fast-track anesthesia for coronary artery bypass graft surgery. J Cardiothorac Vasc Anesth 2002;16:157–62.

50. Howie MB, Cheng D, Newman MF, et al. A randomized double-blinded multicenter comparison of remifentanil versus fentanyl when combined with isoflurane/propofol for early extubation in coronary artery bypass graft surgery. Anesth Analg 2001;92:1084–93.

51. Guarracino F, Penzo D, De Cosmo D, Vardanega A, De Stefani R. Pharmacokinetic-based total intravenous anesthesia using remifentanil and propofol for surgical myocardial revascularization. Eur J Anaesthesiol 2003;20:385–90.

52. Howie MB, Michelson LG, Hug CC Jr, et al. Comparison of three remifentanil dose-finding regimens for coronary artery surgery. J Cardiothorac Vasc Anesth 2003;17:51–9.

53. Geisler FE, de Lange S, Royston D, et al. Efficacy and safety of remifentanil in coronary artery bypass graft surgery: a randomized, double-blind dose comparison study. J Cardiothorac Vasc Anesth 2003;17:60–8.

54. Myles PS, Hunt JO, Fletcher H, et al. Remifentanil, fentanyl, and cardiac surgery: a double-blinded, randomized controlled trial of costs and outcomes. Anesth Analg 2002;95:805–12.

55. Maitre PO, Funk B, Crevoisier C, Ha HR. Pharmacokinetics of midazolam in patients recovering from cardiac surgery. Eur J Clin Pharmacol 1989;37:161–6.

56. Engoren MC, Kraras C, Garzia F. Propofol-based versus fentanyl-isoflurane-based anesthesia for cardiac surgery. J Cardiothorac Vasc Anesth 1998;12:177–81.

57. De Hert S, ten Broecke PW, Mertens E, et al. Sevoflurane but not propofol preserves myocardial function in coronary surgery patients. Anesthesiology 2002;97:42–9.

58. Searle NR, Sahab P, Blain R, et al. Hemodynamic and pharmacodynamic comparison of doxacurium and high-dose vecuronium during coronary artery bypass surgery: a cost–benefit study. J Cardiothorac Vasc Anesth 1994;8:490–4.

59. Smith CE, Botero C, Holbook C, Pinchak AC, Hagen JF. Rocuronium versus vecuronium during fentanyl induction in patients undergoing coronary artery surgery. J Cardiothorac Vasc Anesth 1999;13:567–73.

60. Berntman L, Rosberg B, Shweikh I, Yousef H. Atracurium and pancuronium in renal insufficiency. Acta Anaesthesiol Scand 1989;33:48–52.

61. Kamibayashi T, Maze M. Clinical uses of alpha-2 adrenergic agonists. Anesthesiology 2000;93:1345–49.

62. Doufas AG, Lin CM, Suleman MI, et al. Dexmedetomidine and meperidine additively reduce shivering threshold in humans. Stroke 2003;34:1218–23.

63. Herr DL, Sum-Ping ST, England M. ICU sedation after coronary artery bypass graft surgery: dexmedetomidine-based versus propofol-based sedation regiments. J Cardiothorac Vasc Anesth 2003;17:576–84.

64. Flom-Halvorsen HI, Ovrum E, Oystese R, Brosstad F. Quality of intraoperative autologous blood withdrawal for retransfusion after cardiopulmonary bypass. Ann Thorac Surg 2003;76:744–8.

65. Laffey JG, Boylan JF, Cheng DCH. The systemic inflammatory response to cardiac surgery. implications for the anesthesiologist. Anesthesiology 2002;97:215–52.

66. Fillinger MP, Rassias AJ, Guyre PM, et al. Glucocorticoid effects on the inflammatory and clinical responses to cardiac surgery. J Cardiothorac Vasc Anesth 2002;16:163–9.

67. Halvorsen P, Raeder J, White PF, et al. The effect of dexamethasone on side effects after coronary revascularization procedures. Anesth Analg 2003;96:1578–83.

68. Tassani P, Richter JA, Barankay A, et al. Does high-dose methylprednisolone in aprotinin-treated patients attenuate the systemic inflammatory response during coronary artery bypass grafting? J Cardiothorac Vasc Anesth 1999;13:165–72.

69. Levi M, Cromheecke ME, de Jonge E, et al. Pharmacological strategies to decrease excessive blood loss in cardiac surgery: a meta-analysis of clinically relevant endpoints. Lancet 1999;354:1940–7.

70. Laupacis A, Fergusson D. Drugs to minimize perioperative blood loss in cardiac surgery: meta-analyses using perioperative blood transfusions as the outcome. The International Study of Perioperative Transfusions (ISPOT) Investigators. Anesth Analg 1997;85:258–67.

71. Casati V, Valle PD, Benussi S, et al. Effects of tranexamic acid on postoperative bleeding and related histochemical variables in coronary surgery: comparison between on-pump and off-pump techniques. J Thorac Cardiovasc Surg 2004;128:83–91.

72. Englberger L, Markart P, Eckstein FS, Immer FF, Berdat PA, Carrel TP. Aprotinin reduces blood loss in off-pump coronary artery (OPCAB) surgery. Eur J Cardiothorac Surg 2002;22:545–51.

73. Rich JB. The efficacy and safety of aprotinin use in cardiac surgery. Ann Thorac Surg 1998;66:S6–11.

74. Alderman EL, Levy JH, Rich JB, et al. Analyses of coronary graft patency after aprotinin use: results from the International Multicenter Aprotinin Graft Patency Experience (IMAGE) trial. J Thorac Cardiovasc Surg 1998;116:716–30.

75. Landis RC, Asimakopoulos G, Poullis M, Haskard DO, Taylor KM. The antithrombotic and anti-inflammatory mechanisms of action of aprotinin. Ann Thorac Surg 2001;72:2169–75.

76. Westaby S, Katsumata T. Editorial: aprotinin and vein graft occlusion: the controversy continues. J Thorac Cardiovasc Surg 1998;116:731–3.

77. Frumento RJ, O'Malley CMN, Bennett-Guerrero E. Stroke after cardiac surgery: a retrospective analysis of the effects of aprotinin dosing regimens. Ann Thorac Surg 2003;75:479–83.

78. Murkin JM, Lux J, Shannon NA, et al. Aprotinin significantly decreases bleeding and transfusion requirements in patients receiving aspirin and undergoing cardiac operations. J Thorac Cardiovasc Surg 1994;107:554–61.

79. Bidstrup BP, Hunt BJ, Sheikh S, Parratt RN, Bidstrup M, Sapsford RN. Amelioration of the bleeding tendency of preoperative aspirin after aortocoronary bypass grafting. Ann Thorac Surg 2000;69:541–7.

80. Dignan RJ, Law DW, Seah PW, et al. Ultra-low dose aprotinin decreases transfusion requirements and is cost effective in coronary operations. Ann Thorac Surg 2001;71:158–64.

81. Englberger L, Kipfer B, Berdat PA, Nydegger UE, Carrel TP. Aprotinin in coronary operation with cardiopulmonary bypass: does "low-dose" aprotinin inhibit the inflammatory response? Ann Thorac Surg 2002;73:1897–904.

82. Royston D, Cardigan R, Gippner-Steppert C, Jochum M. Is perioperative plasma aprotinin concentration more predictable and constant after a weight-related dose regimen? Anesth Analg 2001;92:830–6.

83. Nuttall GA, Fass DN, Oyen LJ, Oliver WC Jr, Ereth MH. A study of weight-adjusted aprotinin dosing schedule during cardiac surgery. Anesth Analg 2002;94:283–9.

84. Beath SM, Nuttall G, Fass N, Oliver OC Jr, Ereth MH, Oyen LJ. Plasma aprotinin concentrations during cardiac surgery: full- versus half-dose regimens. Anesth Analg 2000;92:257–64.

85. Smith PK. Overview of aprotinin. Innovative strategies to improve open-heart surgery outcomes. Symposium, Washington DC May 2002.

86. Schweizer A, Hohn L, Morel MR, Kalangos A, Licker M. Aprotinin does not impair renal haemodynamics and function after cardiac surgery. Br J Anaesth 2000;84:16–22.

87. Feindt PR, Walcher S, Volkmer I, et al. Effects of high-dose aprotinin on renal function in aortocoronary bypass grafting. Ann Thorac Surg 1995;60:1076–80.

88. O'Connor CJ, Brown DV, Avramov M, Barnes S, O'Connor HN, Tuman KJ. The impact of renal dysfunction on aprotinin. Pharmacokinetics during cardiopulmonary bypass. Anesth Analg 1999;89:1101–7.

89. Dietrich W, Jochum M. Effect of celite and kaolin on activated clotting time in the presence of aprotinin: activated clotting time is reduced by binding of aprotinin to kaolin (Letter). J Thorac Cardiovasc Surg 1995;1090:177–8.

90. Dietrich W, Spath P, Ebell A, Richter JA. Prevalence of anaphylactic reactions to aprotinin: analysis of two hundred forty-two reexposures to aprotinin in heart operations. J Thorac Cardiovasc Surg 1997;113:194–201.

91. Cohen DM, Norberto J, Cartabuke R, Ryu G. Severe anaphylactic reaction after primary exposure to aprotinin. Ann Thorac Surg 1999;67:837–8.

92. Munoz JJ, Birkmeyer NJO, Birkmeyer JD, O'Connor GT, Dacey LJ. Is ε-aminocaproic acid as effective as aprotinin in reducing bleeding with cardiac surgery? A meta-analysis. Circulation 1999;99:81–9.

93. Casati V, Guzzon D, Oppizzi M, et al. Hemostatic effects of aprotinin, tranexamic acid and epsilon-aminocaproic acid in primary cardiac surgery. Ann Thorac Surg 1999;68:2252–7.

94. Butterworth J, James RL, Lin Y, Prielipp RC, Hudspeth AS. Pharmacokinetics of epsilon-aminocaproic acid in patients undergoing aortocoronary bypass surgery. Anesthesiology 1999;90:1624–35.

95. Bennett-Guerrero E, Spillane WF, White WD, et al. ε-aminocaproic acid administration and stroke following coronary artery bypass surgery. Ann Thorac Surg 1999;67:1283–7.

96. Garwood S, Mathew J, Barash PG, Hines R. Reduced blood loss at the expense of renal function: is epsilon-aminocaproic acid a blow to the kidney? Presented at the American Society of Anesthesiologists 1997 Annual meeting. San Diego, CA. October 1997.

97. Stafford-Smith M, Phillips-Bute B, Reddan DN, Black J, Newman MF. The association of epsilon-aminocaproic acid with postoperative decrease in creatinine clearance in 1502 coronary bypass patients. Anesth Analg 2000;91:1085–90.

98. Fiechter BK, Nuttall GA, Johnson ME, et al. Plasma tranexamic acid concentrations during cardiopulmonary bypass. Anesth Analg 2001;92:1131–6.

99. Zabeeda D, Medalion B, Sverdlow M, et al. Tranexamic acid reduces bleeding and the need for blood transfusion in primary myocardial revascularization. Ann Thorac Surg 2002;74:733–8.

100. Casati V, Guzzon D, Oppizzi M, et al. Tranexamic acid compared with high-dose aprotinin in primary elective heart operations: effects on perioperative bleeding and allogeneic transfusions. J Thorac Cardiovasc Surg 2000;120:520–7.

101. Wong BI, McLean RF, Fremes SE, et al. Aprotinin and tranexamic acid for high transfusion risk cardiac surgery. Ann Thorac Surg 2000;69:808–16.

102. Bechtel JFM, Prosch J, Sievers HH, Bartels C. Is the kaolin or celite activated clotting time affected by tranexamic acid? Ann Thorac Surg 2002;74:390–3.

103. Horrow JC, Van Riper DF, Strong MD, Grunewald KE, Parmet JL. Is the dose-response relationship of tranexamic acid. Anesthesiology 1995;82:383–92.

104. Karski JM, Dowd NP, Joiner R, et al. The effect of three different doses of tranexamic acid on blood loss after cardiac surgery with mild systemic hypothermia (32°C). J Cardiothorac Vasc Anesth 1998;12:642–6.

105. De Bonis M, Cavaliere F, Alessandrini F, et al. Topical use of tranexamic acid in coronary artery bypass operations: a double-blind, prospective, randomized, placebo-controlled trial. J Thorac Cardiovasc Surg 2000;119:575–80.

106. Kuitunen AH, Heikkila LJ, Salmenpera MT. Cardiopulmonary bypass with heparin-coated circuits and reduced systemic anticoagulation. Ann Thorac Surg 1997;63:438–44.

107. Aldea GS, Doursounian M, O'Gara P, et al. Heparin-bonded circuits with a reduced anticoagulation protocol in primary CABG: a prospective, randomized study. Ann Thorac Surg 1996;62:410–8.

108. Jobes DR, Safety issues in heparin and protamine administration for extracorporeal circulation. J Cardiothorac Vasc Anesth 1998;12:17–20.

109. Upchurch GR, Valeri CR. Khuri SF, et al. Effect of heparin on fibrinolytic activity and platelet function in vivo. Am J Physiol 1996;27:H528–34.

110. Warkentin TE. Pork or beef? Ann Thorac Surg 2003;75:15–6.

111. Despotis GJ, Joist JH, Hogue CW Jr, et al. More effective suppression of hemostatic system activation in patients undergoing cardiac surgery by heparin dosing based on heparin blood concentrations rather than ACT. Thromb Haemost 1996;76:902–8.

112. Cartier R, Robitaille D. Thrombotic complications in beating heart operations. J Thorac Cardiovasc Surg 2001;121:920–2.

113. Despotis GJ, Joist JH. Anticoagulation and anticoagulation reversal with cardiac surgery involving cardiopulmonary bypass: an update. J Cardiothorac Vasc Anesth 1999;13(4Suppl I):18–29.

114. Shore-Lesserson L. Point-of-care coagulation monitoring for cardiovascular patients: past and present. J Cardiothorac Vasc Anesth 2002;16:99–106.

115. Dietrich W, Spannagl M, Schramm W, Vogt W, Barankay A, Richter JA. The influence of preoperative anticoagulation on heparin response during cardiopulmonary bypass. J Thorac Cardiovasc Surg 1991;102:505–14.

116. Williams MR, D'Ambra AB, Beck JR, et al. A randomized trial of antithrombin concentrates for treatment of heparin resistance. Ann Thorac Surg 2000;70:873–7.

117. Lemmer JR JH, Despotis GJ. Antithrombin III concentrate to treat heparin resistance in patients undergoing cardiac surgery. J Thorac Cardiovasc Surg 2002;123:213–7.

118. Sabbagh AH, Chung GK, Shuttleworth P, Applegate BJ, Gabrhel W. Fresh frozen plasma: a solution to heparin resistance during cardiopulmonary bypass. Ann Thorac Surg 1984;37:466–8.

119. Warkentin TE, Greinacher A. Heparin-induced thrombocytopenia and cardiac surgery. Ann Thorac Surg 2003;76:2121–31.

120. Bauer TL, Arepally G, Konkle BA, et al. Prevalence of heparin-associated antibodies without thrombosis in patients undergoing cardiopulmonary bypass surgery. Circulation 1997;95:1242–6.

121. Makoul RG, McCann RL, Austin EH, Greenberg CS, Lowe JE. Management of patients with heparin-associated thrombocytopenia and thrombosis requiring cardiac surgery. Ann Thorac Surg 1987;43:617–21.

122. Koster A, Meyer O, Fischer T, et al. One-year experience with the platelet glycoprotein IIb/IIIa antagonist tirofiban and heparin during cardiopulmonary bypass in patients with heparin-induced thrombocytopenia type II. J Thorac Cardiovasc Surg 2001;122:1254–5.

123. Mertzlufft F, Kuppe H, Koster A. Management of urgent high-risk cardiopulmonary bypass with heparin-induced thrombocytopenia type II and coexisting disorders of renal function: use of heparin and epoprostenol combined with on-line monitoring of platelet function. J Cardiothorac Vasc Anesth 2000;14:304–8.

124. Palatianos GM, Foroulis CN, Vassili MI, et al. Preoperative detection and management of immune heparin-induced thrombocytopenia in patients undergoing heart surgery with Iloprost. J Thorac Cardiovasc Surg 2003;127:548–54.

125. Koster A, Chew D, Grundel M, et al. An assessment of different filter systems for extracorporeal elimination of bivalirudin: an in vitro study. Anesth Analg 2003;96:1316–9.

126. Merry AF, Raudkivi PJ, Middleton NG, et al. Bivalirudin versus heparin and protamine in off-pump coronary artery bypass surgery. Ann Thorac Surg 2004;77:925–31.

127. Davis Z, Anderson R, Short D, Garber D, Valgiusti A. Favorable outcome with bivalirudin anticoagulation during cardiopulmonary bypass. Ann Thorac Surg 2003;75:264–5.

128. Vasquez JC, Vichiendilokkul A, Mahmood S, Baciewicz FA Jr. Anticoagulation with bivalirudin during cardiopulmonary bypass in cardiac surgery. Ann Thorac Surg 2003;74:2177–9.

129. Koster A, Chew D, Grundel M, Bauer M, Kuppe H, Speiss BD. Bivalirudin monitored with the ecarin clotting time for anticoagulation during cardiopulmonary bypass. Anesth Analg 2003;96:383–6.

130. Koster A, Merkle F, Hansen R, et al. Elimination of recombinant hirudin by modified ultrafiltration during simulated cardiopulmonary bypass: assessment of different filter systems. Anesth Analg 2000;91:265–9.

131. Nuttall GA, Oliver WC Jr, Santrach PJ, et al. Patients with a history of type II heparin-induced thrombocytopenia with thrombosis requiring cardiac surgery with cardiopulmonary bypass: a prospective observational case series. Anesth Analg 2003;96:344–50.

132. Koster A, Hansen R, Kuppe H, Hetzer R, Crystal GJ, Mertzlufft F. Recombinant hirudin as an alternative for anticoagulation during cardiopulmonary bypass in patients with heparin-induced thrombocytopenia type II: a 1-year experience in 57 patients. J Cardiothorac Vasc Anesth 2000;14:243–8.

133. Kieta DR, McGammon AT, Holman WL, Nielson VG. Hemostatic analysis of a patient undergoing off-pump coronary artery bypass surgery with argatroban anticoagulation. Anesth Analg 2003;96:956–8.

134. Furukawa K, Ohteki J, Hirahara K, Narita Y, Koga S. The use of argatroban as an anticoagulant for cardiopulmonary bypass in cardiac operations. J Thorac Cardiovasc Surg 2001;122:1255–6.

135. Olin DA, Urdaneta F, Lobato EB. Use of danaparoid during cardiopulmonary bypass in patients with heparin-induced thrombocytopenia. J Cardiothorac Vasc Anesth 2000;14:707–9.

136. Ariano RE, Bhattacharya SK, Moon M, Brownwell LG. Failure of danaparoid anticoagulation for cardiopulmonary bypass. J Thorac Cardiovasc Surg 2000;119:167–8.

137. Loeckinger A, Kleinsasser A, Lindner KH, Margreiter J, Keller C, Hoermann C. Continuous positive airway pressure at 10 cm H_2O during cardiopulmonary bypass improves postoperative gas exchange. Anesth Analg 2000;91:522–7.

138. DiNardo JA, Wegner JA. Pro: low-flow cardiopulmonary bypass is the preferred technique for patients undergoing cardiac surgical procedures. J Cardiothorac Vasc Anesth 2001;15:649–51.

139. Cook DJ. Con: low-flow cardiopulmonary bypass is not the preferred technique for patients undergoing cardiac surgical procedures. J Cardiothorac Vasc Anesth 2001;15:652–4.

140. Schwartz AE, Sandhu AA, Kaplon RJ, et al. Cerebral blood flow is determined by arterial pressure and not cardiopulmonary bypass flow rate. Ann Thorac Surg 1995;60:165–70.

141. Schwartz AE. Regulation of cerebral blood flow during hypothermic cardiopulmonary bypass. Review of experimental results and recommendations for clinical practice. CVE 1997;2:133–7.

142. Reents W, Muellges W, Franke D, Babin-Ebell J, Elert O. Cerebral oxygen saturation assessed by near-infrared spectroscopy during coronary artery bypass grafting and early postoperative cognitive dysfunction. Ann Thorac Surg 2002;74:109–14.

143. Edmonds Jr HL. Cerebral oximetry provides early warning of oxygen delivery failure during cardiopulmonary bypass. J Cardiothorac Vasc Anesth 2002;16:204–6.

144. Talpahewa SP, Ascione R, Angelini GD, Lovell AT. Cerebral cortical oxygenation changes during OPCAB surgery. Ann Thorac Surg 2003;Nov;76(5):1516–22.

145. Yao FSF, Tseng CC, Woo D, Huang SW, Levin SK. Maintaining cerebral oxygen saturation during cardiac surgery decreased neurological complications. Anesthesiology 2001;95:A–152.

146. Lanier WL. Glucose management during cardiopulmonary bypass: cardiovascular and neurologic implications. Anesth Analg 1991;72:423–7.

147. Groban L, Butterworth J, Legault C, Rogers AT, Kon ND, Hammon JW. Intraoperative insulin therapy does not reduce the need for inotropic or antiarrhythmic therapy after cardiopulmonary bypass. J Cardiothorac Vasc Anesth 2002;16:405–12.

148. Garwood S, Swamidoss CP, Davis EA, Samson L, Hines RL. A case series of low-dose fenoldopam in seventy cardiac surgical patients at increased risk of renal dysfunction. J Cardiothorac Vasc Anesth 2003;17:17–21.

149. Caimmi PP, Pagani L, Micalizzi E, et al. Fenoldopam for renal protection in patients undergoing cardiopulmonary bypass. J Cardiothorac Vasc Anesth 2003;17:491–4.

150. Ranucci M, Soro G, Barzaghi N, et al. Fenoldopam prophylaxis of postoperative acute renal failure in high-risk cardiac surgery patients. Ann Thorac Surg 2004;78:1332–8.

151. Lassnigg A, Donner E, Grubhoger G, Presterl E, Druml W, Hiesmayr M. Lack of renoprotective effects of dopamine and furosemide during cardiac surgery. J Am Soc Nephrol 2000;11:97–104.

152. Woo EB, Tang AT, el-Gamel A, et al. Dopamine therapy for patients at risk for renal dysfunction following cardiac surgery: science or fiction? Eur J Cardiothorac Surg 2002;22:106–11.

153. Aronson S, Blumenthal R. Perioperative renal dysfunction and cardiovascular anesthesia: concerns and controversies. J Cardiothorac Vasc Anesth 1998;12:567–86.

154. Wilkes NJ, Mallett SV, Peachey T, Di Salvo C, Walesby R. Correction of ionized magnesium during cardiopulmonary bypass reduces the risk of postoperative cardiac arrhythmia. Anesth Analg 2002;95:828–34.

155. Mohr R, Lavee J, Goor DA. Inaccuracy of radial artery pressure measurement after cardiac operations. J Thorac Cardiovasc Surg 1987;94:286–90.

156. Gravlee GP, Wong AB, Adkins TG, Case LD, Pauca AL. A comparison of radial, brachial, and aortic pressures after cardiopulmonary bypass. J Cardiothorac Anesth 1989;3:20–6.

157. Griffin MJ, Hines RL. Management of perioperative ventricular dysfunction. J Cardiothorac Vasc Anesth 2001;15:90–106.

158. Knutson JE, Deering JA, Hall FW, et al. Does intraoperative hetastarch administration increase blood loss and transfusion requirements after cardiac surgery? Anesth Analg 2000;80:801–7.

159. Kikura M, Sato S. The efficacy of preemptive milrinone or amrinone in patients undergoing coronary artery bypass grafting. Anesth Analg 2002;94:22–30.

160. Ammar T, Fisher CF, Sarier K, Coller BS. The effects of thrombocytopenia on the activated coagulation time. Anesth Analg 1996;83:1185–8.

161. Shigeta O, Kojima H, Hiramatsu Y, et al. Low-dose protamine based on heparin-protamine titration method reduces platelet dysfunction after cardiopulmonary bypass. J Thorac Cardiovasc Surg 1999;118:354–60.

162. Gravlee GP, Rogers AT, Dudas DM, et al. Heparin management protocol for cardiopulmonary bypass influences postoperative heparin rebound but not bleeding. Anesthesiology 1992;76: 393–401.

163. Butterworth J, Lin YA, Prielipp RC, Bennett J, Hammon JW, James RL. Rapid disappearance of protamine in adults undergoing cardiac operation with cardiopulmonary bypass. Ann Thorac Surg 2002;74:1589–95.

164. Vertrees RA, Engelman RM, Breyer RH, Johnson J III, Auvil J, Rousou JA. Protamine-induced anticoagulation following coronary bypass. Proc Am Acad Cardiovasc Perfusion 1986;7:94–7.

165. Frater RW, Oka Y, Hong Y, Tsubo T, Loubser PG, Masone R. Protamine-induced circulatory changes. J Thorac Cardiovasc Surg 1984;87:687–92.

166. Milne B, Rogers K, Cervenko F, Salerno T. The haemodynamic effects of intraaortic versus intravenous administration of protamine for reversal of heparin in man. Can Anaesth Soc J 1983; 30:347–51.

167. Kimmel SE, Sekeres MA, Berlin JA, et al. Risk factors for clinically important adverse events after protamine administration following cardiopulmonary bypass. J Am Coll Cardiol 1998;32: 1916–22.

168. Comunale ME, Maslow A, Robertson LK, Haering JM, Mashikian JS, Lowenstein E. Effect of site of venous protamine administration, previously alleged risk factors, and preoperative use of aspirin on acute protamine-induced pulmonary vasoconstriction. J Cardiothorac Vasc Anesth 2003;17:309–13.

169. Weiler JM, Gellhaus MA, Carter JG, et al. A prospective study of the risk of an immediate adverse reaction to protamine sulfate during cardiopulmonary bypass surgery. J Allergy Clin Immunol 1990;85:713–9.

170. Kimmel SE, Sekeres M, Berlin JA, Ellison N. Mortality and adverse events after protamine administration in patients undergoing cardiopulmonary bypass. Anesth Analg 2002;94:1402–8.

171. Horrow JC. Protamine allergy. J Cardiothorac Anesth 1988;2:225–42.

172. Abe K, Sakakibara T, Miyamoto Y, Ohnishi K. Effect of prostaglandin E1 on pulmonary hypertension after protamine injection during cardiac surgery. Eur J Clin Pharmacol 1998;54:21–5.

173. Lock R, Hessell EA II. Probable reversal of protamine reactions by heparin administration. J Cardiothorac Anesthesia 1990;4:604–8.

174. Horrow JC. Heparin reversal of protamine toxicity: have we come full circle? J Cardiothorac Anesth 1990;4:539–42.

175. Mukadam ME, Pritchard P, Riddington D, et al. Management during cardiopulmonary bypass of patients with presumed fish allergy. J Cardiothorac Vasc Anesth 2001;15:512–9.

176. Heres EK, Horrow JC, Gravlee GP, et al. A dose-determining trial of heparinase-I (Neutralase TM) for heparin neutralization in coronary artery surgery. Anesth Analg 2001;93:1446–52.

177. Levy JH, Cormack JG, Morales A. Heparin neutralization by recombinant platelet factor 4 and protamine. Anesth Analg 1995;81:35–7.

178. Zwishchenberger JB, Vertrees RA, Brunston RL Jr, Tao W, Alpard SK, Brown PS Jr. Application of a heparin removal device in patients with known protamine hypersensitivity. J Thorac Cardiovasc Surg 1998;115:729–31.

179. Zwischenberger JB, Tao W, Deyo DJ, Vertrees RA, Alpard SK, Shulman G. Safety and efficacy of a heparin removal device: a prospective randomized preclinical outcomes study. Ann Thorac Surg 2001;71:270–7.

180. Cooney A, Mann TJ. Recent experiences with hexadimethrine for neutralizing heparin after cardiopulmonary bypass. Anaesth Intensive Care 1999;27:298–300.

181. Lee LM, Chang LC, Wrobleski S, Wakefield TW, Yang VC. Low molecular weight protamine as nontoxic heparin/low molecular weight heparin antidote (III): preliminary in vivo evaluation of efficacy and toxicity using a canine model. AAPS PharmSci 2001;3:article 19.

182. Despotis GJ, Santoro SA, Spitznagel E, et al Prospective evaluation and clinical utility of on-site monitoring of coagulation in patients undergoing cardiac operation. J Thorac Cardiovasc Surg 1994;107:271–9.

183. Johi RR, Cross MH, Hansbro SD. Near-patient testing for coagulopathy after cardiac surgery. Br J Anaesth 2003;90:499–501.

184. Michelsen LG, Horswell S. Anesthesia for off-pump coronary artery bypass grafting. Semin Thorac Cardiovasc Surg 2003;15:71–82.

185. Mariani AM, Gu J, Boonstra PW, et al. Procoagulant activity after off-pump coronary operation: is the current anticoagulation adequate? Ann Thorac Surg 1999;68:1370–5.

186. Casati V, Gerli C, Franco A, et al. Activation of coagulation and fibrinolysis during coronary surgery: on-pump versus off-pump techniques. Anesthesiology 2001;95:1103–9.

187. Moller CH, Steinbruchel DA. Platelet function after coronary artery bypass surgery: is there pro-coagulant activity after off-pump compared with on-pump surgery? Scand Cardiovasc J 2003;37:149–53.

188. Kurlansky PA. Is there a hypercoagulable state after off-pump bypass surgery? What do we know and what can we do? J Thorac Cardiovasc Surg 2003;126:7–10.

189. Englberger L, Immer FF, Eckstein FS, Perdat PA, Haeberli A, Carrel TP. Off-pump coronary artery bypass operation does not increase procoagulant and fibrinolytic activity: preliminary results. Ann Thorac Surg 2004;77:1560–6.

190. Grocott HP, Mathew JP, Carver EH, et al. A randomized controlled trial of the Arctic Sun Temperature Management System versus conventional methods for preventing hypothermia during off-pump cardiac surgery. Anesth Analg 2004;98:298–302.

191. Babatasi G, Massetti M, Bruno PG, et al. Pre-operative balloon counterpulsation and off-pump coronary surgery for high-risk patients. Cardiovasc Surg 2003;11:145–8.

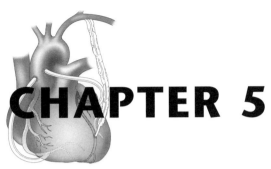

CHAPTER 5

Cardiopulmonary Bypass

Cardiopulmonary Bypass

Over the past 50 years, extracorporeal circulation has evolved into a remarkably safe means of providing systemic perfusion during open-heart surgery. A greater understanding has been gained of its effects at the molecular and biochemical level that can adversely affect organ system function and a patient's recovery from surgery. Although cardiopulmonary bypass (CPB) remains essential for virtually all valvular operations, concerns about some of its adverse effects, especially those on neurocognitive function, have encouraged the development of off-pump techniques for coronary bypass surgery (see Chapter 1).[1] Nonetheless, the vast majority of coronary bypass surgery is still performed with CPB, and many surgeons are reverting back to this traditional approach as questions about the completeness of revascularization and the true benefits of off-pump surgery surface. This section will provide the reader with the essential elements of extracorporeal circulation and its uses during open-heart surgery.[2,3]

I. General Comments

A. CPB involves an extracorporeal circuit that provides oxygenated systemic blood flow when the heart and lungs are not functional. CPB is accompanied by normovolemic hemodilution and nonpulsatile flow.

B. The contact of blood with the extracorporeal circuit results in the activation of numerous cascades, including the kallikrein, coagulation, and complement systems.[4-7] Among the consequences of this contact are the release of proinflammatory cytokines and a systemic inflammatory response. Neutrophil-endothelial cell adhesion contributes to endothelial activation and dysfunction that have been implicated in myocardial reperfusion damage, pulmonary and renal dysfunction, neurocognitive changes, and a generalized capillary leak. Fortunately, adverse effects of this inflammatory response are not clinically significant in most patients. However, in patients requiring long pump runs or in those with significant hemodynamic compromise after surgery, this systemic inflammatory response may persist for days, leading to multiple organ system compromise.

C. Use of membrane oxygenators, heparin-coated circuits, centrifugal pumps, intraoperative steroids, leukocyte filters, or mannitol may reduce the extent of some of these derangements.[8-14] Aprotinin is a serine protease inhibitor that, when given in high doses, may ameliorate the consequences of the inflammatory cascade in addition to reducing blood loss.[15,16]

D. Despite adequate heparinization, the bypass circuit is a potent activator of the coagulation system with generation of factor Xa and thrombin that contribute to the inflammatory response. A coagulopathy may develop from activation of platelets and the fibrinolytic system, as well as from dilution of clotting factors and platelets during bypass.

II. The Cardiopulmonary Bypass Circuit

A. The extracorporeal circuit consists of polyvinylchloride tubing and polycarbonate connectors. Circuits coated with heparin (Duraflo II, Carmeda Bioactive Surface) or poly(2-methoxyethylacrylate) (PMEA) have been shown to improve biocompatibility; reduce complement, neutrophil, and platelet activation; and minimize the release of proinflammatory mediators.[11-14] Some studies have demonstrated clinical benefits with use of these circuits, including a reduction in platelet activation and bleeding, less pulmonary and renal dysfunction in high-risk patients, and fewer neurocognitive changes. However, other studies have not demonstrated any clinical benefits in low-risk patients.[15-23] Less heparin seems to be necessary with Duraflo II than Carmeda circuits,[22] but some degree of heparinization still remains essential for safe conduct of bypass with these circuits.[23-25] Some have recommended that giving enough heparin to achieve an activated clotting time (ACT) greater than 250 seconds is satisfactory in low-risk coronary cases, but an ACT greater than 400 seconds remains essential for high-risk cases, including reoperations and valvular surgery.[26]

B. The pump is primed with a balanced electrolyte solution. The average priming volume is 1500–2000 mL. A colloid, usually albumin, is commonly added to the pump prime to increase oncotic pressure, reduce fluid requirements, and decrease the time to extubation. It may also ameliorate bleeding by delaying fibrinogen absorption and reducing platelet activation.[27] Albumin is preferable to hetastarch, which has been associated with increased perioperative bleeding.[28]

C. Venous blood drains by gravity from the right atrium or vena cavae into a cardiotomy reservoir, passes through an oxygenator/heat exchanger attached to a heater/cooler unit, and returns to the arterial system through a filter using either a roller or a centrifugal pump (Figure 5.1). Active drainage using a centrifugal pump or vacuum-assisted venous drainage can be used to augment venous drainage and is valuable during minimally invasive procedures and when small venous catheters are utilized. The possibility of venous air entrainment in the bypass circuit and undetected air microembolism must always be entertained when this technique is utilized.[29]

D. Systemic flow is provided by either a roller pump or a centrifugal pump, but is nonpulsatile with both systems unless additional technology is utilized to provide pulsatile flow. Roller pumps are pressure insensitive and can pressurize the arterial line in the face of outflow obstruction. Centrifugal pumps are afterload sensitive, such that they will reduce flow if outflow is obstructed. Studies have indicated that centrifugal pumps might cause less blood trauma, but the inflammatory response and effects on perioperative bleeding are fairly similar with both types of pumps.[30,31]

E. Suction lines return extravasated blood to the cardiotomy reservoir to conserve blood and blood elements and to maintain pump volume. Despite the universal use of these suction lines, studies have shown that blood that is aspirated from the surgical field is replete with fat and procoagulant and proinflammatory mediators.[32,33] These cytokines may contribute to adverse clinical outcomes, including increased perioperative bleeding and neurologic sequelae. Notably, return of this blood to the circuit usually causes systemic hypotension. Aspiration of blood contaminated by tissue contact is a significant activator of coagulation with increased thrombin generation, promoting inflammation, and also contributes to hemolysis.[34] Elimination

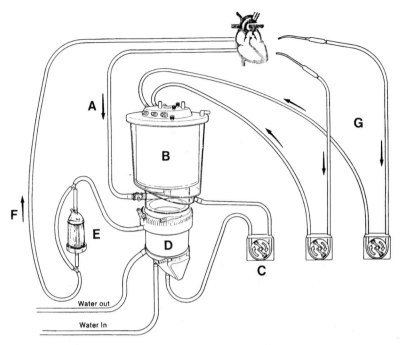

Figure 5.1 • The basics of an extracorporeal circuit. Blood drains by gravity through the venous lines (A) into a cardiotomy reservoir (B), is pumped using a roller head (C) or centrifugal pump through the oxygenator/heat exchanger (D) and arterial line filter (E) back into the arterial circuit (F). Additional suction lines (G) can be used for intracardiac venting and scavenging of blood from the operative field.

of cardiotomy suction has been demonstrated to reduce thrombin generation, platelet activation, and the systemic inflammatory response.[35, 36] Use of cell-saving devices to aspirate and wash shed blood generally can eliminate many of these factors and eliminate fat from the blood while preserving red cells, although coagulation factors and platelets are eliminated during centrifugation.[37,38]

F. An additional suction line can be connected to an intracardiac vent, draining blood from the left ventricle or other cardiac chamber into the reservoir by active suctioning by a roller pump head. These lines are useful in providing ventricular decompression and/or improving surgical exposure.

G. Oxygen and compressed air pass into the oxygenator through a blender, which regulates oxygen concentration by adjusting the F_{IO_2} and also determines the gas flow by adjusting a "sweep rate." The sweep rate is generally maintained slightly less than the systemic flow rate to eliminate CO_2 from the blood to achieve a desired value (generally around 40 mm Hg). To minimize blood activation, the oxygenator may be coated with heparin or silicone to improve biocompatibility.[39]

H. The bypass setup includes a separate heat exchanger for cardioplegia delivery. Tubes of differing diameters are passed through the same roller pump head delivering a preselected ratio of pump volume to cardioplegia solution (such as 4:1). The final mixture then passes through a separate heat exchanger for delivery of cold or warm cardioplegia. Pressure monitoring of infusion pressure is essential, especially for retrograde delivery, which generally provides about 200 mL/min of flow at a pressure that should not exceed 40 mm Hg to prevent coronary sinus rupture. Very high line pressures indicate obstruction to flow, either because the line is clamped or the cardioplegia catheter is obstructed. A low line pressure generally indicates misplacement of the catheter.

I. Additional features of the CPB circuit may include the following:

1. On-line monitoring of arterial and venous blood gases, electrolytes, hematocrit, and multiple temperatures. This is useful during deep hypothermia cases.

2. A direct connection to the cell-saving device, through which excess volume can be directed during the pump run and for centrifugation of pump contents at the end of surgery.

3. An arterial line filter (usually 40 μm), which is essential to remove microemboli before returning blood to the patient. Microemboli may consist of air, blood or platelet microaggregates, or other particulate matter. Fat microemboli are found in abundance in cardiotomy suction and can be removed by 20-μm filters.[37,38]

4. Recirculation lines to allow for venting of air and to prevent stagnation of blood. This is essential with use of aprotinin during circulatory arrest cases and also when direct thrombin inhibitors are used for anticoagulation in patients with heparin-induced thrombocytopenia.

5. Hemofilters or hemoconcentrators that can be placed in the circuit to remove excessive volume in patients with preexisting fluid overload or renal dysfunction. They can be used to perform modified ultrafiltration at the end of the pump run to hemoconcentrate the pump contents for retransfusion through the venous cannula.[40,41]

J. A detailed checklist must be utilized by the perfusionists before every case to make sure that no detail is overlooked because the patient's life is dependent on the function of the heart-lung machine. Accurate record keeping during bypass is essential (Figures 5.2 and 5.3).

III. Cannulation for Bypass

A. **Arterial cannulation** is usually accomplished by placement of a cannula in the ascending aorta just proximal to the innominate artery (Figure 5.4). Cannula size is determined by the anticipated flow rate for that patient based on body surface area so as to minimize line pressure and shear forces (Table 5.1).

1. Cannula designs have been modified in a variety of ways to minimize shear forces and jet effects on the aortic wall (Figure 5.5). Some have end holes, whereas others have multiple side holes or other designs through which blood exits at lower velocity (soft flow and dispersion cannulas).[42] The latter might theoretically reduce the risk of cerebral embolization, especially to the left hemisphere.[43] A cannula with a small distal net has been designed to trap embolic material upon aortic unclamping and has been shown to reduce the risk of stroke (Embol-X, Edwards Lifesciences).[44,45] Distal arch cannulation with placement of the tip of the cannula beyond the left subclavian artery has been proposed as a means of reducing cerebral emboli in patients with severe ascending aortic atherosclerosis.[46]

Saint Vincent Hospital at Worcester Medical Center
DEPARTMENT OF SURGERY

Perfusion Record

☐ Patient chart reviewed and assessed
☐ Heart-Lung machine properly plugged in; all batteries checked and operational
☐ Centrifugal pump in correct position and properly mounted
☐ Hand cranks available
☐ All pump tubing connections correct and tightened
☐ MPS machine properly set up and primed, correct ratio, KCL, MgSO4 and temps
☐ Cardioplegia tubing placement in correct direction in pump head raceway and occlusions checked and set
☐ Adequate tubing clamps available
☐ Sweep gas line attached to oxygenator / FIO2 and gas flow selected
☐ Fluotec checked and filled with Isoflourane
☐ Scavenger line prepared
☐ Venous sat. monitor, battery checked
☐ Venous sat. probe attached and checked for proper functioning and positioning
☐ Pump cart available with adequate supply of drugs, solutions, syringes, needles, filters, etc.
☐ Centrifugal pump flow probe attched properly
☐ Oxygen analyzer calibrated and battery checked
☐ Connections to table lines properly made and checked, A-V Loop primed
☐ Heater/Cooler connected and primed and properly set
☐ Ice in room and added to appropriate heater/cooler
☐ Cardioplegia solution prepared and correct for surgeon
☐ Hepcon machine set up, with adequate supplies and patient data entered
☐ Baseline ACT performed and heparin dose calculated/reported to anesthesiologist
☐ Heparin given by anesthesiologist
☐ Adequate post-heparin ACT achieved
☐ Arterial and venous lines properly clamped
☐ Cardiotomy reservoir set up and vented
☐ Pump suction and vent line placed correctly in pump head
☐ Occlusions properly checked and set
☐ Blood gas analyzer shift Q.C. completed

Signature: _____   Date: _____

DISPOSABLES   **MANUFACTURER**   **LOT #**
Oxygenator: _____
Cardioplegia: _____
Tubing Pack: _____
Cell Saver: _____
Hemoconcentrator: _____

Figure 5.2 • Prebypass checklist.

2. Although most surgeons palpate the ascending aorta to assess for the presence of atherosclerotic plaque and calcification, this is a very insensitive means of detecting plaque. Transesophageal echocardiography (TEE) may identify protruding atheromas, but epiaortic imaging is the gold standard for identifying plaque.[47,48]

3. If ascending aortic cannulation is not feasible, an alternative cannulation site must be sought. Traditionally, the femoral artery has been accessed if there is

Saint Vincent Hospital at Worcester Medical Center
DEPARTMENT OF SURGERY
Perfusion Record

				Date	OR #	Case #	
				Preop Diagnosis		Procedure	
Surgeon		Anesthesiologist		Perfusionist		Assistant	
BSA	Ht.	Wt.	☐ M ☐ F	Age	Bld. Type	Preop Heparin: ☐ Yes ☐ No	
Labs	BUN/Creat	K	Glucose	WBC	HGB	Hct	Plts
PMH and Meds			On Pump	Xclamp On	IABP ☐ Preop ☐ Intraop	Art. Can.	Prime
			Off Pump	Xclamp Off	Inotropes ☐ Yes ☐ No	Ven. Can.	Blood ID #
			ECP Total	Xclamp Time	Defibx	Retro. Can	Cell Saver Vol.

Map X Flows *			Grafts	Flows
	Time			
	MAP/(L) Flows			
	100	5		
	90			
	80	4		
	70			
	60	3		
	50			
	40	2		
	30			
	20	1		
	10			

In-Line	SVO_2%		Comments:
Temp			
Gas	FiO_2%		
	Flow L/m		
Labs	pH	A	
Prebypass	pCO_2	A	
	pO_2	A	
	HCO3	A	
	BE		
	Sat	A	
	%		
	K+		
	Hct/Hgb		
	Glucose		
	iCa/Na+		
	ACT		
Fluid	Crystalloid		
	Colloid		Cardioplegia: ☐ MPS ☐ 4:1
ccs	Blood		Time / Temp / Ant cc / Ret cc
	FFP		
	Urine		
	Hemoconc		
Drugs	HCO3		
	Heparin		
	Mannitol		
	Forane		
	CaCl		
	Lidocaine		
	Pressor (NEO)		
	Dilator (TNG)		
			Total Blood:
			Cryst:

FORM #11132 (Rev. 11/00)

Figure 5.3 • Typical perfusion record.

minimal aortoiliac atherosclerosis, but it always runs the risk of a retrograde dissection. Cannulas can be placed percutaneously or via cutdown. Femoral artery disease is frequently encountered and often requires elaborate repair after decannulation. TEE is helpful in identifying descending aortic atherosclerosis that could produce retrograde cerebral atheroembolism and contraindicates femoral cannulation. In this situation, cannulation of the distal subclavian/

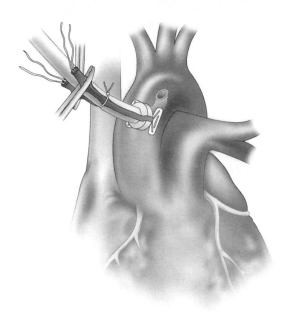

Figure 5.4 • Arterial cannulation. The arterial cannula is placed amidst two pursestrings in the ascending aorta just proximal to the innominate artery.

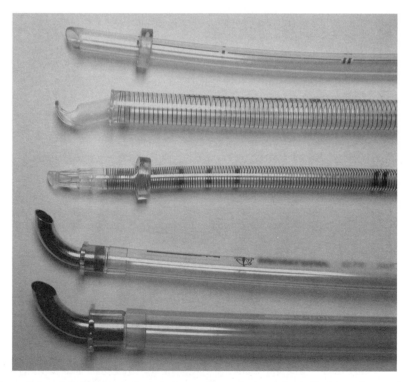

Figure 5.5 • Arterial cannulas include (top to bottom): a straight tip flexible arch cannula, the Edwards dispersion cannula, the soft-flow cannula with multiple side holes, and Medtronic DLP 20F and Sarns 8-mm curved metal tip cannulas.

axillary is an excellent alternative. This may be performed directly through an arteriotomy or through a side-arm graft anastomosed to the vessel, which provides distal arm circulation during bypass.[49]

B. **Venous drainage** for most open-heart surgery is accomplished with a single double-staged cavoatrial cannula (Figure 5.6). This is placed through the right atrial appendage or right atrial free wall with the distal end situated in the inferior vena cava (IVC) (Figure 5.7A). Blood drains from the IVC through several apertures near the end and from the right atrium through side holes about 9–10 cm from the tip. This catheter is used for most procedures that do not require opening of the right side of the heart.

1. Bicaval cannulation is used for mitral valve surgery if a biatrial transseptal approach is planned, although many surgeons use it routinely for this operation. Tricuspid valve surgery always requires bicaval cannulation with placement of caval snares around the cannulas to prevent entry of air into the venous lines. A cannula may be placed directly into the superior vena cava (SVC) or passed through an atriotomy in the right atrial appendage into the SVC. The IVC cannula is placed through a pursestring low in the right atrial free wall (Figure 5.7B).

2. Femoral venous cannulation may be necessary when it is essential to initiate CPB prior to or soon after sternal entry. This may include ruptured ascending aortic aneurysms (usually a type A dissection) or reoperative surgery when there is concern about potential cardiac, aortic, or graft damage during sternotomy. A 50-cm long venous line is passed through the femoral vein to lie within the right atrium to ensure adequate venous drainage. Shorter venous catheters can be used, if necessary.

3. Femoral arterial and venous cannulation have been used to systemically warm patients presenting with profound accidental hypothermia.

C. Figure 5.8 provides an illustration of cannulation and clamping for a routine on-pump coronary bypass operation.

IV. Initiation and Conduct of Cardiopulmonary Bypass (Table 5.2)

A. **Heparin management**. Anticoagulation is essential to minimize thrombin formation within the extracorporeal circuit. Heparin is administered in a dose of 3–4 mg/kg with monitoring of its anticoagulant effect by the ACT. A blood sample is drawn 3–5 minutes after heparin administration and should achieve an ACT greater than 480 seconds. Since aprotinin can elevate the ACT, it is imperative to achieve an adequate ACT if it is utilized. Most groups use kaolin tubes, which absorb the aprotinin, so an ACT greater than 480 seconds is sufficient. If celite ACTs are utilized, the ACT must exceed 750 seconds. ACTs should be rechecked every 15 minutes on pump. Because of patient variability in response to heparin and the effects of hypothermia and hemodilution on the ACT, an individual dose-response curve can be generated using the Medtronic Hepcon system that calculates the precise amount of heparin necessary to achieve a specified ACT.[50] Also, the high-dose thrombin time correlates better with heparin concentration and is not affected by temperature, hemodilution, or aprotinin.[51]

Table 5.1 • Flow Rates and Desired Cannula Sizes

BSA	Venous		Arterial		Flow (L/min)
	Double	2-Stage	French	Metric (mm)	
1.3	26 × 28				3.1
1.4		37/29	18		3.4
1.5	28 × 30				3.6
1.6					3.8
1.7	30 × 32			6.5	4.1
1.8					4.3
1.9		40/32	20		4.6
2.0	32 × 34				4.8
2.1					5.0
2.2					5.3
2.3					5.5
2.4	34 × 36	46/34	24	8.0	5.8
2.5					6.0
2.6					6.2

B. In a patient with documented **heparin-induced thrombocytopenia,** an alternative means of anticoagulation must be sought. This may entail pretreatment with or simultaneous use of antiplatelet medications (ASA, glycoprotein IIb/IIIa inhibitors, prostaglandin analogs) to permit safe heparinization. Alternatively, direct thrombin inhibitors, such as lepirudin, bivalirudin, or argatroban, can be used to avoid heparin entirely. This issue is discussed in more detail on pages 154–156.

C. **Retrograde autologous priming** can be used to reduce the hemodilutional effects of the priming solution and maintain a higher hematocrit on pump. The crystalloid

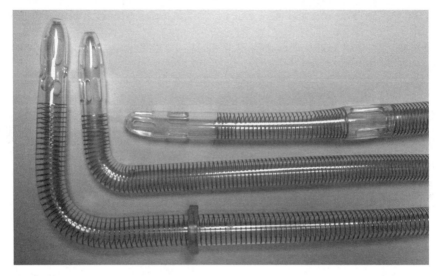

Figure 5.6 • Venous cannulas include (top to bottom): a 40/32 cavoatrial cannula, and short and long right-angle cannulas.

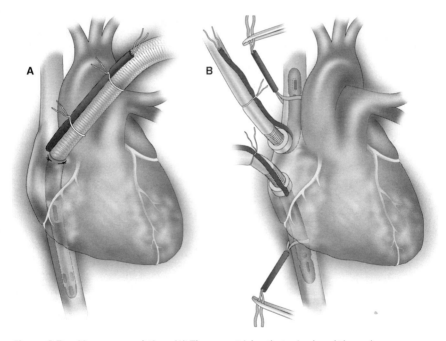

Figure 5.7 • Venous cannulation. (A) The cavoatrial catheter is placed through a purse-string in the right atrial appendage. The tip consists of multiple side holes and is placed into the inferior vena cava. The "basket" lies in the midatrium, and drains flow from the superior vena cava and coronary sinus through multiple holes 9 cm back from the tip. (B) Bicaval cannulation. The superior vena cava (SVC) cannula may be placed directly into the SVC or via the right atrial appendage. The inferior vena cava (IVC) cannula is placed through a purse-string low on the right atrial free wall.

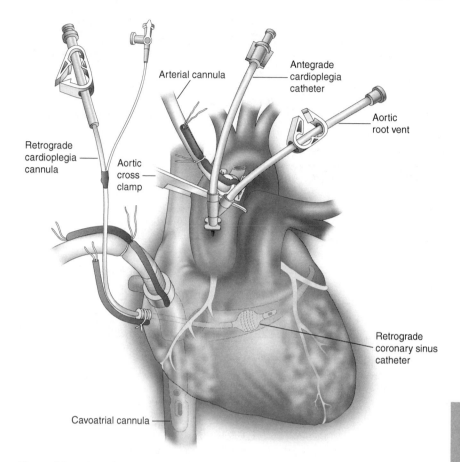

Figure 5.8 • Cannulation and clamping during a routine on-pump coronary bypass operation. Note aortic and venous cannulation, antegrade and retrograde cardioplegia catheters, and the aortic cross-clamp.

prime is back drained from the venous line to the bypass circuit and aspirated into the cell saver before initiating bypass. Simultaneously, an α-agent is given to maintain systemic pressure. Often an infusion of albumin is necessary to minimize the reduction in circulating volume, although, to some degree, this may offset the benefits of a reduced priming volume on maintaining a higher hematocrit. Retrograde autologous priming does maintain a higher oncotic pressure during the pump run and has been shown to minimize the accumulation of extravascular lung water. It is probably most beneficial in small patients with low blood volumes and low hematocrits.[52-54]

D. Systemic pressures and flows. When the pump is turned on, the patient's pulsatile perfusion is replaced by nonpulsatile flow. The blood pressure initially decreases from hemodilution and a reduction in blood viscosity. It should then be maintained between 50–70 mm Hg during the pump run. It may transiently

Table 5.2 • Desired Values on Pump

1. ACT	>480 seconds (less if heparin coated circuit)
2. Systemic flow rates	2–2.5 L/min/m² at 37°C 1.7–2.0 (low flow) or 2.0–2.5 L/min/m² (high flow) at 30°C
3. Systemic blood pressure	50–70 mm Hg

4. Arterial blood gases	Po_2 >250 mm Hg, Pco_2 35–45 mm Hg with pH 7.40
	Deep hypothermia:
	    α stat pH 7.40 measured at 37°C
	    pH stat pH 7.40 at systemic temperature

5. Svo_2	>65%
6. Hematocrit	>20%
7. Blood glucose	100–180 mg/dL

decrease during cardioplegia delivery (probably from potassium delivery into the systemic circulation), from return of large volumes of cardiotomy suction, and during rewarming. Blood pressure may rise due to vasoconstriction from hypothermia and from dilution of narcotics by the pump prime.

1. The systemic flow rate is calculated based on the patient's body surface area and is modified by the degree of hypothermia and the venous oxygen saturation (Svo_2). It should also take into account the degree of anemia that can influence whole-body oxygen delivery. The flow rate should exceed 2 L/min/m² at normothermia and can be reduced to 1.5–1.7 L/min/m² at 30°C with "low flow" bypass. Flow needs to be increased during rewarming, when increased metabolism usually decreases the Svo_2. Low flow bypass during moderate hypothermia has been shown to improve myocardial protection, reduce collateral flow improving exposure, reduce hemolysis, and reduce fluid requirements without any compromise in tissue perfusion.[55]

2. As long as the venous oxygen saturation exceeds 65%, the flow rate is considered to be adequate, although this may not reflect regional flow.[56, 57] For example, at normothermia, the brain and kidney autoregulate to maintain perfusion as the flow rate is reduced at the expense of skeletal muscle and splanchnic flow. However, renal blood flow is determined primarily by the systemic flow rate and can be adversely affected during hypothermia when renal autoregulation is impaired.[58,59] Due to concerns that the combination of hemodilution and a lower flow rate may reduce the mean arterial pressure below the autoregulatory threshold and compromise organ system function, there are proponents of using "high flow bypass" (2–2.4 L/min/m²) rather than "low flow" during hypothermia.[60]

3. One of the primary concerns with CPB is maintenance of adequate cerebral oxygenation, which is determined by both blood pressure and systemic flow rate. Cerebral autoregulation allows for maintenance of cerebral blood flow down to mean arterial pressures as low as 40–50 mm, but autoregulation is considered to be inadequate in hypertensive, diabetic patients in whom it may be desirable to maintain a higher pressure. In fact, some studies have shown that cerebral oxygenation is impaired at this level even if the flow rate is satisfactory, so the blood pressure must be maintained at an adequate level regardless of the flow rate, usually using vasopressors, such as phenylephrine, norepinephrine, or vasopressin.[61,62] This may improve cerebral oxygenation but reduce flow to other regions, specifically the kidneys and splanchnic viscera.

4. Several techniques have been used to assess the adequacy of cerebral oxygenation during CPB.[63-68] Both fiberoptic jugular bulb oximetry and cerebral oximetry using bifrontal sensors with near-infrared spectroscopy (Somanetics INVOS cerebral oximeter) (see Figure 4.7) can be used to detect cerebral oxygenation (Sco_2). The Sco_2 tends to fall during initiation of bypass and during rewarming, even with an increase in systemic flow.[64] In fact, it may even be reduced when the mixed venous oxygen saturation is normal.[66] Several studies have demonstrated benefits of this technology in reducing the incidence of neurocognitive changes. One study showed that desaturation was more common in elderly patients and did correlate with short-term cognitive impairment.[67] Another showed that modification of flow rate, blood pressure, increase in Pco_2 (a potent cerebral vasodilator), and/or increase in hematocrit in response to a fall in Sco_2 below 40 mm Hg reduced neurologic complications.[68]

E. Both the **hematocrit** on pump and the systemic flow rate determine the amount of oxygen delivery to the body. Hemodilution from the pump prime commonly reduces oxygen delivery by 25% as estimated from the following equation:[2]

$$\text{Predicted HCT on pump} = \frac{(70 \times \text{kg} \times \text{preop HCT}/100)}{(70 \times \text{kg}) + \text{prime volume} + \text{IV fluids pre-CPB}}$$

where $70 \times$ kg equals the blood volume and $70 \times$ kg $\times$ preop HCT is the RBC volume

Hemodilution reduces blood viscosity and improves microcirculatory flow, but at the extremes of hemodilution, there is a substantial reduction in oncotic pressure that increases fluid requirements. This can exacerbate the systemic inflammatory response and capillary leak, causing substantial tissue edema. This may contribute to cerebral edema, papilledema and ischemic optic neuropathy, and respiratory compromise, among other adverse effects.[69] Generally, the lower limit of hematocrit on pump has been considered to be 18%, although one study reported that a hematocrit less than 22% was associated with greater mortality and an increased risk of multisystem organ dysfunction. This occurred presumably on the basis of inadequate oxygen delivery, causing ischemic or inflammatory organ system injury.[70] Considering the increasing age and increased severity of illness of the current patient population, maintaining a hematocrit at this level seems prudent.

F. **Temperature management.** The systemic temperature may be maintained at normothermia or at varying degrees of hypothermia depending on the surgeon's preference and the operative procedure. Most surgeons use moderate hypothermia to provide some organ system protection during nonpulsatile perfusion and also in the event that a temporary problem arises with surgery (need to reduce flow to place sutures) or with perfusion (impaired drainage, low blood pressure, air embolism, pump head failure, oxygenator failure, etc.). Although the rate of rewarming may affect neurocognitive outcome, no conclusive benefit of either temperature management scheme has been established in terms of inflammatory activation, perioperative hemostasis, or neurocognitive outcome.[71-75]

G. Gas exchange. Oxygenation and elimination of carbon dioxide are determined by the sweep rate, which is adjusted on the blender. Most oxygenators currently available are not stressed until the flow rate exceeds 7 L/min, which should be adequate for even a 175-kg patient. The PO_2 should be maintained above 250 mm Hg in the event of a temporary reduction in flow or pump malfunction, and can be monitored on-line or by intermittent blood gases every 30 minutes. Inhalational anesthetics, such as sevoflurane, desflurane, or isoflurane, are administered through the blender and must be scavenged via the oxygenator.

H. pH management. With progressive hypothermia, CO_2 production decreases and pH normally rises. With mild or moderate hypothermia, pH is generally maintained between 7.40 and 7.50 by adjusting the sweep rate and maintaining the Pco_2 around 40 mm Hg. Evidence of metabolic acidosis on pump may be a sign of inadequate tissue oxygenation despite normal blood gases. Regional hypoperfusion, especially of the splanchnic bed, may contribute to this problem. In fact, lactate release with levels greater than 4 mmol/L during reperfusion is predictive of an increased risk of complications and death.[76] During deep hypothermia, two pH management strategies can be used. With pH stat, the pH is temperature-corrected and maintained at 7.40 by adding a mixture of O_2 and CO_2 to the circuit. With this strategy, there is an increase in cerebral blood flow and a potentially increased risk of cerebral microembolism. In contrast, with α stat, the pH is maintained at 7.40 measured at 37°C (i.e., not temperature-corrected). Cerebral blood flow is autoregulated and coupled to cerebral oxygen demand. The latter strategy is preferred during deep hypothermic circulatory arrest (DHCA) cases.[77]

I. Medications to maintain anesthesia or control blood pressure are given into a sampling manifold that flows into the venous reservoir. Other medications that may be given by the perfusionist into the circuit during bypass include mannitol, furosemide, insulin, sodium bicarbonate, antibiotics, vasopressors, and inotropes.

J. Intermittent measurements of serum potassium, glucose, and hematocrit should be performed in addition to arterial and venous blood gases and ACTs. An elevated potassium may necessitate a change in the composition or frequency of cardioplegia delivery and may require administration of diuretics or insulin for control. An elevated glucose may be related to increased levels of endogenous epinephrine and insulin resistance and may be associated with an increased risk of neurologic injury.[78] Blood sugar should generally be maintained at a level below 180 mg/dL.

V. Terminating Bypass

A. Before terminating bypass, the patient should be warmed toward normothermia. Overwarming the patient with inflow temperatures greater than 38°C should be avoided to minimize protein denaturation and potential cerebral damage. If significant hypothermia is used, the gradient between the arterial and venous return temperature should be less than 10–12°C to minimize the formation of gaseous emboli. The rate of rewarming may affect neurocognitive outcome.[72]

B. The lungs are ventilated and pacing is initiated, if necessary. Calcium chloride 1 g may be given prior to coming off bypass to provide an increase in systemic vascular resistance and some inotropic support. The heart is filled by restricting venous return as bypass flow is reduced and turned off. Inotropic support should be considered for marginal cardiac performance (see Chapter 11). Low systemic resistance is common, and α-agents may be necessary to improve the blood pressure. On rare occasions, the patient may manifest "vasoplegia," a condition of profound peripheral vasodilatation despite adequate cardiac output. It is more frequently seen in patients on preoperative angiotensin-converting enzyme inhibitors as well as those on amiodarone, which may be associated with α- and β-receptor blockade. Vasopressin is usually successful in reversing the low systemic vascular resistance in these patients.[79,80]

C. When the patient is stable, protamine is administered to reverse heparin effect and should return the ACT to normal. The dosage is commonly based on a 1:1 mg/mg ratio to the administered heparin, although with use of the Hepcon system, which measures heparin levels, a more precise amount of protamine to reverse heparin can be calculated. Protamine reactions are uncommon, but can be life-threatening (see page 161). They require immediate attention, occasionally requiring reinstitution of bypass after additional administration of heparin.

D. The heart is decannulated and the cannulation sites are secured. Hemostasis is then achieved and the chest is closed.

VI. Potential Problems Encountered During Cardiopulmonary Bypass (Box 5.1)

A. **Inadequate ACT** from standard doses of heparin usually results from antithrombin III (ATIII) deficiency. This has been noted most frequently in patients maintained preoperatively on heparin therapy or IV nitroglycerin. Additional administration of 1–2 mg/kg of heparin will usually achieve an adequate ACT. If not, ATIII must be given in the form of fresh frozen plasma or, if available, a commercial ATIII product (Thrombate III™), which provides 500 units per vial.[81-83]

B. **Inadequate venous drainage** will be detected by the surgeon as a distended right heart and by the perfusionist as a drop in blood level in the venous reservoir (which should trigger a low volume alarm) and an inability to maintain systemic flow rates. It may result from an airlock in the venous line, kinking of the line on the field or close to the reservoir, inadvertent clamping of the venous line, retraction of the heart impeding flow into the venous cannula, or malposition of the venous cannula (either being too far in or not far in enough). Inadequate venous drainage not only warms the heart during systemic hypothermia, potentially compromising myocardial protection, but it may adversely affect the organs that are not drained well. A high CVP may indicate impaired SVC drainage and can produce cerebral edema (usually only noted with bicaval cannulation). More commonly, drainage from the IVC is impaired and can result in hepatic or splanchnic congestion with significant fluid sequestration in the bowel and in renal impairment. In this situation, the surgeon may note that the right atrium is well drained but the perfusionist notes a distinct reduction in venous return.

Box 5.1 • Potential Problems on Pump

1. Inadequate heparinization (low ACT)
2. Inadequate venous drainage
3. Air entry into venous lines
4. High arterial line pressure
5. Ventricular distention
6. Inadequate systemic pressures
7. Inadequate retrograde cardioplegia delivery pressure
8. Systemic or coronary air embolism
9. Inadequate systemic oxygenation
10. Red cell agglutination in the bypass circuit

C. **Air entry into the venous lines** usually arises from the venous cannulation site or the retrograde cardioplegia site and can be controlled by an additional suture around the catheter. Rarely, it may result from inadvertent damage to the IVC or from an atrial septal defect.

D. **High arterial line pressure** measured by the perfusionist is a potentially alarming situation. With pressurized roller pumps, this could result in a catastrophic line disconnection. With centrifugal pumps, which are afterload sensitive, high line pressures cannot occur because the pump head automatically reduces flow. A high line pressure caused by a high flow rate through a small cannula should not occur if the appropriately sized cannula is selected. For example, a 20F or 7-mm aortic cannula should be able to flow up to 6 L/min but may be inadequate for higher flows. Malposition of the tip of the aortic cannula or an aortic dissection can account for a high line pressure. When a dissection occurs, the high line pressure is accompanied by very low systemic pressures, and mandates immediate cessation of pump flow and relocation of the arterial inflow cannula.

E. **Distention of the heart** on bypass is indicative of poor venous drainage, aortic insufficiency, or tremendous collateral flow. It may stretch the ventricular fibers producing myocardial injury, increase pulmonary arterial pressures producing pulmonary barotrauma, or increase ventricular warming impairing myocardial protection. The cause of distention should be remedied, either by readjusting the venous line or placing a vent in the left ventricle or in the pulmonary artery.

F. **Inadequate systemic pressures** have been incriminated as causes of multiorgan system dysfunction, including neurocognitive changes, renal failure, and splanchnic hypoperfusion. Whether low-flow or high-flow CPB is optimal for organ system protection is controversial, but a minimum pressure of 50–60 mm Hg should be maintained unless it is desired to intentionally maintain a higher pressure (e.g., the patient with significant uncorrected carotid disease or the hypertensive, diabetic patient with preexisting renal dysfunction). Phenylephrine or norepinephrine is commonly used on pump to maintain systemic pressures, accepting the transient dips that occur with cardioplegia infusion or reinfusion of shed blood aspirated through the cardiotomy suckers. However, adequate flow rates must be maintained because use of α-agents will shunt blood away from the muscles and splanchnic circulation. Occasionally, in the patient on numerous anti-hypertensive medications, including angiotensin-converting enzyme inhibitors, amiodarone, and/or calcium channel blockers, a state of refractory hypotension exists. This state of autonomic dysfunction, or vasoplegia, may require the infusion of vasopressin to maintain blood pressure.[79,80] On rare occasions, methylene blue 1–2 mg/kg has been used to maintain blood pressure.[84]

G. **Inadequate retrograde cardioplegia delivery** may produce inadequate myocardial protection. Low retrograde cardioplegia line pressures may be associated with rupture of the coronary sinus, a left SVC, or catheter displacement back into the right atrium.[85] Catheter placement too far into the sinus may reduce flow to the right ventricle and impair its protection. Filling of the posterior descending vein suggests that the right ventricle is being adequately protected, but this may not always be the case.

H. **Systemic air embolism** noted during bypass is a catastrophic problem usually related to inattention to the venous reservoir level with delivery of air through a roller pump head. It requires cessation of bypass with immediate venting of air from the aorta with a needle or through a stopcock on the aortic line and then removal of air from the bypass circuit. Ventilation with 100% oxygen, steep Trendelenburg position, and retrograde SVC perfusion should be used in an effort to eliminate air from the cerebral circulation. Steroids, barbiturates, and reinstitution of bypass with deep hypothermia may also reduce the degree of cerebral injury.[86] Air embolism may also occur on bypass when air is trapped in the left side of the heart and the pressure generated by the left ventricle exceeds that in the aorta. Careful attention to deairing, either by needle aspiration of the left ventricle or constant venting of the aortic root, is important when there has been cardiac entry or active intracardiac or root venting. Flooding the field with carbon dioxide may be helpful as the cardiac chambers are being closed.[87] TEE monitoring is the best means of identifying retained air. The most common site for systemic air embolism during valve surgery is the right coronary artery, frequently resulting in transient right ventricular dysfunction. This generally resolves after a brief return to CPB and additional deairing.

I. **Inadequate oxygenation** may result from failure of the oxygenator, the oxygen blender, or disconnection from an oxygen source. Evidence of cerebral oxygen desaturation may precede a reduction in systemic venous oxygen saturation. This problem should be immediately recognizable by a change in the color of the arterial blood return line. Mild systemic hypothermia can provide some element of organ system protection during the period of poor oxygenation as emergency steps are being taken by the perfusionist to correct the problem. On rare occasions, when the patient is no longer on pump, this may result from the anesthesiologist failing to provide ventilation to the patient (usually after the surgeon has asked that the lungs not be ventilated to improve exposure).

J. **Cold-reactive autoimmune diseases** are rarely detected preoperatively but may result in red cell agglutination and hemolysis on bypass at cold temperatures. This may be noted in the bypass or cardioplegia circuit.[88-90]

1. Cold hemagglutinin disease is caused by an IgM autoimmune antibody that causes red cell agglutination and hemolysis at cold temperatures. This may cause microvascular thrombosis that may contribute to myocardial infarction, renal failure, or other organ system failure. Since less than 1% of patients have cold agglutinins, screening is not routinely performed, and it rarely poses a

problem during bypass because hemodilution lowers antibody titers. However, should antibody titers be measured and be in high concentration (>1:1000), agglutination will occur at warmer temperatures.

    a. If high-titer agglutinins are present, systemic hypothermia and cold blood cardioplegia must be avoided. Either warm cardioplegia or cold crystalloid cardioplegia after an initial normothermic flush can be used. Even better would be performance of off-pump coronary bypass surgery or on-pump beating or fibrillating heart surgery.[91]

    b. De novo discovery of cold agglutinins may occur on pump by detecting agglutination and sedimentation in the blood cardioplegia heat exchanger or any stagnant line containing blood. It has also been identified when the retrograde cardioplegia line develops high pressure due to obstruction from agglutination.[89] In these circumstances, the patient should be warmed back to normothermia and crystalloid cardioplegia used to flush out the coronary arteries.

  2. Paroxysmal cold hemoglobinuria is an autoimmune disease in which a nonagglutinating IgG antibody binds to red cells in the cold causing hemolysis. It should be managed in a similar fashion.[92]

VII. Special Types of Extracorporeal Circulation

  A. **Deep hypothermic circulatory arrest** is used primarily in situations when the aorta cannot be clamped safely to perform an aortic anastomosis.

    1. Indications for DHCA include:

      a. Severe aortic atherosclerosis or calcification (porcelain aorta for aortic valve replacement, proximal venous anastomoses in coronary surgery).

      b. Desire to avoid aortic wall damage to improve the quality of an anastomosis (type A dissections).

      c. Clamp placement is too close to the suture line: ascending aortic or hemiarch repairs, descending thoracic aneurysms involving the arch.

      d. Complex thoracic aortic surgery to improve anastomotic exposure while providing neuroprotection for the brain and/or spinal cord.

      e. Resection of IVC tumors.

    2. The patient is cooled systemically to 18°C to achieve electroencephalographic (EEG) silence. The temperature is measured at multiple sites, including the tympanic, nasopharyngeal, bladder, and/or rectal temperatures, with the presumption that this will ensure uniform cooling of the cerebral cortex. Since an EEG is usually not performed, surgeons rely on clinical studies that have shown 45–60 minutes of DHCA at 18°C is safe in minimizing cerebral damage.[93]

    3. The head is packed in ice and medications are given to minimize cerebral injury. These include methylprednisolone 20 mg/kg and thiopental 10 mg/kg. The arterial line is clamped and blood is drained from the circulation, taking care not to allow air entry in the lines. Measures that may extend the acceptable period of DHCA include antegrade cerebral perfusion (providing flow into the arch vessels during the period of circulatory arrest) and retrograde cerebral perfusion (providing oxygenated, cold blood into the SVC at a flow rate up to 500 mL/min at a pressure of up to 20 mm Hg).[94-96] The former is technically more demanding but probably more effective in providing nutrients to the brain; the latter is probably beneficial because it maintains cerebral hypothermia. It is also beneficial in flushing air and debris out of the cerebral vessels.

4. Extensive cooling and rewarming are often associated with a coagulopathy. Use of aprotinin is controversial during DHCA cases, but adherence to a strict protocol that ensures adequate ACTs during the period of circulatory arrest has been shown to minimize the risk of neurologic complications (see page 151).[97,98]

5. When bypass flow is reinstituted, care must be taken to eliminate air or atherosclerotic debris from the arterial tree. Warming generally takes twice as long as cooling, and the gradient between the arterial inflow and the patient's temperature must be maintained at less than 10°C to prevent generation of gaseous emboli.

B. Left heart bypass for thoracic aortic surgery

1. Impairment of blood supply to the lower body is inherent to any aortic procedure involving descending aortic cross-clamping. The greatest risks are those of paraplegia and renal dysfunction. Left heart bypass entails draining of oxygenated blood from the left side of the heart and returning it more distally in the arterial tree (Figure 5.9).[99,100]

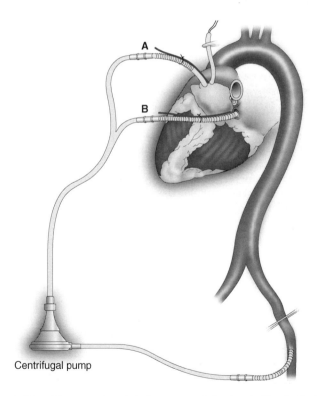

A

B

Centrifugal pump

Figure 5.9 • Left heart bypass setup. A drainage cannula is placed either in the left atrial appendage (A) or the left inferior pulmonary vein (B). Blood is then returned by a centrifugal pump to the femoral artery or to the distal aorta in cases of limited disease, such as traumatic tears of the aorta.

2. Inflow to a centrifugal pump may come from the left atrium or preferentially from the inferior pulmonary vein, which may be associated with fewer complications.[101] The blood is returned to either the femoral artery or to the distal aorta below the lowest clamp in patients with limited disease, such as traumatic tears or Crawford type I aneurysms (see page 37). The blood does not pass through an oxygenator, although one can be placed in the circuit to improve oxygenation during one-lung anesthesia.[102]

3. Minimal heparinization is necessary for this setup (about 5000 units to achieve an ACT of 250 seconds) and is beneficial in trauma cases or cases requiring extensive dissection. Flow rates of up to 3 L/min can be used, with monitoring of lower extremity mean pressures in the femoral artery that should approximate 50 mm Hg. Drainage should not be so excessive as to compromise antegrade flow from the heart to the brain.

C. **Assisted right heart bypass for off-pump surgery.** During manipulation of the heart for off-pump surgery, especially with enlarged hearts, there may be compromise of right ventricular filling. Several devices have been designed that provide right heart assist by draining blood from the right atrium and pumping it into the pulmonary artery during these procedures.[103]

D. **Perfusion-assisted direct coronary artery bypass (PADCAB).** During off-pump surgery, there is compromise of distal flow during temporary vessel occlusion required for construction of an anastomosis. This may lead to subtle or severe degrees of ischemia and potential myocardial necrosis. Intracoronary or aortocoronary shunts can be used to provide distal perfusion during the anastomosis, either routinely or if there is evidence of ischemia.[104] PADCAB provides perfusion-assisted flow at a designated pressure (usually 120 mm Hg) that is independent of the systemic blood pressure. Additionally, medications, such as nitroglycerin, can be administered in the perfusate to provide coronary vasodilatation. Placing a small catheter directly into the coronary artery allows for distal perfusion as the anastomosis is being constructed. Subsequently, flow can be directed through 2–3 mm cannulas placed into the conduits until the proximal anastomoses are performed.[105,106] A comparative study of no shunting, passive shunting, and active perfusion showed that myocardial protection (measured by troponin levels) and performance were superior with active perfusion.[107]

References

1. Kilo J, Czerny M, Gorlitzer M, et al. Cardiopulmonary bypass affects cognitive brain function after coronary artery bypass grafting. Ann Thorac Surg 2001;72:1926–32.
2. Gravlee GP, Davis RF, Kurusz M, Utley JR. Cardiopulmonary bypass: principles and practice. 2nd ed. Philadelphia: Lippincott Williams & Wilkins, 2000.
3. Lich BV, Brown DM. The Mannual of clinical perfusion. 2nd ed updated. Fort Meyers, FL: Perfusion.com, Inc.
4. Levy JH, Tanaka KA. Inflammatory response to cardiopulmonary bypass. Ann Thorac Surg 2003;75:S715–20.
5. Laffey JG, Boylan JF, Cheng DCH. The systemic inflammatory response to cardiac surgery. Implications for the anesthesiologist. Anesthesiology 2002;97:215–52.
6. Asimakopoulos G, Taylor KM. Effects of cardiopulmonary bypass on leukocyte and endothelial adhesion molecules. Ann Thorac Surg 1998;66:2135–44.
7. Boyle EM Jr, Pohlman TH, Johnson MC, Verrier ED. The systemic inflammatory response. Ann Thorac Surg 1997;64:S31–7.
8. Gott JP, Cooper WA, Schmidt FE Jr, et al. Modifying risk for extracorporeal circulation: trial of four antiinflammatory strategies. Ann Thorac Surg 1998;66:747–54.
9. Gu YJ, de Vries AJ, Vos P, Boonstra PW, van Oeveren W. Leukocyte depletion during cardiac operation: a new approach through the venous bypass circuit. Ann Thorac Surg 1999;67:604–9.
10. Chen YF, Tsai WC, Lin CC, et al. Leukocyte depletion attenuates expression of neutrophil adhesion molecules during cardiopulmonary bypass in human beings. J Thorac Cardiovasc Surg 2002;123:218–24.
11. Videm V, Mollnes TE, Fosse E, et al. Heparin-coated cardiopulmonary bypass equipment. I. Biocompatibility markers and development of complications in a high-risk population. J Thorac Cardiovasc Surg 1999;117:794–802.
12. Moen O, Fosse E, Dregelid E, et al. Centrifugal pump and heparin coating improves cardiopulmonary bypass biocompatibility. Ann Thorac Surg 1996;62:1134–40.
13. Weerwind PW, Maessen JG, van Tits LJH, et al. Influence of Duraflo II heparin-treated extracorporeal circuits on the systemic inflammatory response in patients having coronary bypass. J Thorac Cardiovasc Surg 1995;110:1633–41.
14. Ikuta T, Fujii H, Shibata T, et al. A new poly-2-methoxyethylacrylate-coated cardiopulmonary bypass circuit possesses superior platelet preservation and inflammatory suppression efficacy. Ann Thorac Surg 2004;77:1678–83.
15. Murkin JM. Cardiopulmonary bypass and the inflammatory response: a role for serine protease inhibitors? J Cardiothorac Vasc Anesth 1997;11:19–23.
16. Hill GE, Alonso A, Spurzem JR, Stammers AH, Robbins RA. Aprotinin and methylprednisolone equally blunt cardiopulmonary bypass–induced inflammation in humans. J Thorac Cardiovasc Surg 1995;110:1658–62.
17. Defraigne JO, Pincemail J, Dekoster G, et al. SMA circuits reduce platelet consumption and platelet factor release during cardiac surgery. Ann Thorac Surg 2000;70:2075–81.
18. McCarthy PM, Yared JPP, Foster RC, Ogella DA, Borsh JA, Cosgrove DM III. A prospective randomized trial of Duraflo II heparin-coated circuits in cardiac reoperations. Ann Thorac Surg 1999;67:1268–73.
19. Gunaydin S, Farsak B, Kocakulak M, Sari T, Yorcangioglu C, Zorlutana Y. Clinical performance and biocompatibility of poly(2-methoxyethylacrylate)-coated extracorporeal circuits. Ann Thorac Surg 2002;74:819–24.
20. Ranucci M, Mazzucco A, Pessotto R, et al. Heparin-coated circuits for high-risk patients: a multicenter, prospective, randomized trial. Ann Thorac Surg 1999;67:994–1000.
21. Heyer EJ, Lee KS, Manspeizer HE, et al. Heparin-bonded cardiopulmonary bypass circuits reduce cognitive dysfunction. J Cardiothorac Vasc Anesth 2002;16:37–42.
22. Ovrum E, Tangen G, Oystese R, Ringdal MAL, Istad R. Comparison of two heparin-coated extracorporeal circuits with reduced systemic anticoagulation in routine coronary artery bypass operations. J Thorac Cardiovasc Surg 2001;121:324–30.

23. Kumano H, Suehiro S, Hattori K, et al. Coagulofibrinolysis during heparin-coated cardiopulmonary bypass with reduced heparinization. Ann Thorac Surg 1999;68:1252–6.

24. Ovrum E, Tangen G, Tollofsrud S, Ringdal MAL. Heparin-coated circuits and reduced systemic anticoagulation applied to 2500 consecutive first-time coronary artery bypass grafting procedures. Ann Thorac Surg 2003;76:1144–8.

25. von Segesser LK, Weiss BM, Garcia E, von Felten A, Turina MI. Reduction and elimination of systemic heparinization during cardiopulmonary bypass. J Thorac Cardiovasc Surg 1992;103:790–9.

26. Weiss BM, von Segesser LK. Pro and con of heparin-bonded circuits for cardiopulmonary bypass. J Cardiothorac Vasc Anesth 1999;13:646–58.

27. Kaplan M, Cimen S, Demirtas MM. Effects of different pump prime solutions on postoperative fluid balance and hemostasis. Chest 2001;120:172S.

28. Wilkes MM, Navickis RJ, Sibbald WJ. Albumin versus hydroxyethyl starch in cardiopulmonary bypass surgery: a meta-analysis of postoperative bleeding. Ann Thorac Surg 2001;72:527–33.

29. Willcox TW, Mitchell SJ, Gorman DF. Venous air in the bypass circuit: a source of arterial line emboli exacerbated by vacuum-assisted drainage. Ann Thorac Surg 1999;68:1285–9.

30. Baufreton C, Intrator L, Jansen PGM, et al. Inflammatory response to cardiopulmonary bypass using roller or centrifugal pumps. Ann Thorac Surg 1999;67:972–7.

31. Scott DA, Silbert BS, Blyth C, O'Brien J, Santamaria J. Blood loss in elective coronary artery surgery: a comparison of centrifugal versus roller pump heads during cardiopulmonary bypass. J Cardiothorac Vasc Anesth 2001;15:322–5.

32. Chung JH, Gikakis N, Rao AK, Drake TA, Colman RW, Edmunds LH Jr. Pericardial blood activates the extrinsic coagulation pathway during clinical cardiopulmonary bypass. Circulation 1996;93:2014–8.

33. Tabuchi N, de Hann J, Boonstra PWW, van Oeveren W. Activation of fibrinolysis in the pericardial cavity during cardiopulmonary bypass surgery. J Thorac Cardiovasc Surg 1993;106: 828–33.

34. De Somer F, Van Belleghem Y, Caes F, et al. Tissue factor as the main activator of the coagulation system during cardiopulmonary bypass. J Thorac Cardiovasc Surg 2002;123:951–8.

35. Aldea GS, Soltow LO, Chandler WL, et al. Limitation of thrombin generation, platelet activation, and inflammation by elimination of cardiotomy suction in patients undergoing coronary artery bypass grafting treated with heparin-coated circuits. J Thorac Cardiovasc Surg 2002;123:742–55.

36. Westerberg M, Bengtsson A, Jeppsson A. Coronary surgery without cardiotomy suction and autotransfusion reduces the postoperative systemic inflammatory response. Ann Thorac Surg 2004;78:54–9.

37. Kaza AK, Cope JT, Fiser SM, et al. Elimination of fat microemboli during cardiopulmonary bypass. Ann Thorac Surg 2003;75:555–9.

38. Jewell AE, Akowuah EF, Suvarna SK, Braidley P, Hopkinson D, Cooper G. A prospective randomized comparison of cardiotomy suction and cell saver for recycling shed blood during cardiac surgery. Eur J Cardiothorac Surg 2003;23:633–6.

39. Shimamoto A, Kanemitsu S, Fujinaga K, et al. Biocompatibility of silicone-coated oxygenator in cardiopulmonary bypass. Ann Thorac Surg 2000;69:115–20.

40. Lee LW, Gabbott S. High-volume ultrafiltration with extracellular fluid replacement for the management of dialysis patients during cardiopulmonary bypass. J Cardiothorac Vasc Anesth 2002; 16:70–2.

41. Boga M, Islamoglu F, Badak I, et al. The effects of modified hemofiltration on inflammatory mediators and cardiac performance in coronary artery bypass grafting. Perfusion 2000;15:143–50.

42. Grooters RK, Ver Steeg DA, Stewart MJ, Thieman KC, Schneider RF. Echocardiographic comparison of the standard end-hole cannula, the soft-flow cannula, and the dispersion cannula during perfusion into the aortic arch. Ann Thorac Surg 2003;75:1919–23.

43. Weinstein GS. Left hemispheric strokes in coronary surgery: implications for end-hole aortic cannulas. Ann Thorac Surg 2001;71:128–32.

44. Banbury MK, Kouchoukos NT, Allen KB, et al. Emboli capture using the Embol-X intraaortic filter in cardiac surgery: a multicenter randomized trial of 1,289 patients. Ann Thorac Surg 2003;76:508–15.

45. Wimmer-Greinecker G. Reduction of neurologic complications by intra-aortic filtration in patients undergoing combined intracardiac and CABG procedures. Eur J Cardiothorac Surg 2003;23:159–64.

46. Borger MA, Taylor RL, Weisel RD, et al. Decreased cerebral emboli during distal aortic arch cannulation: a randomized clinical trial. J Thorac Cardiovasc Surg 1999;118:740–5.

47. Wilson MJ, Boyd SY, Lisagor PG, Rubal BJ, Cohen DJ. Ascending aortic atheroma assessed intraoperatively by epiaortic and transesophageal echocardiography. Ann Thorac Surg 2000;70:25–30.

48. Ura M, Sakata R, Nakayama Y, Miyamoto TA, Goto T. Extracorporeal circulation before and after ultrasonographic evaluation of the ascending aorta. Ann Thorac Surg 1999;67:478–83.

49. Sinclair MC, Singer RL, Manley NJ, Montesano RM. Cannulation of the axillary artery for cardiopulmonary bypass: safeguards and pitfalls. Ann Thorac Surg 2003;75:931–4.

50. Despotis GJ, Joist JH. Anticoagulation and anticoagulation reversal with cardiac surgery involving cardiopulmonary bypass: an update. J Cardiothorac Vasc Anesth 1999;13(4 suppl I):18–29.

51. Shore-Lesserson L. Point-of-care coagulation monitoring for cardiovascular patients: past and present. J Cardiothorac Vasc Anesth 2002;16:99–106.

52. Rosengart TK, DeBois W, O'Hara M, et al. Retrograde autologous priming for cardiopulmonary bypass. A safe and effective means of decreasing hemodilution and transfusion requirements. J Thorac Cardiovasc Surg 1998;115:426–39.

53. Balachandran S, Cross MH, Karthikeyan S, Mulpur A, Hansbro SD, Hobson P. Retrograde autologous priming of the cardiopulmonary bypass circuit reduces blood transfusion after coronary artery surgery. Ann Thorac Surg 2002;73:1912–8.

54. Eising GP, Pfauder M, Niemeyer M, et al. Retrograde autologous priming: is it useful in elective on-pump coronary artery bypass surgery? Ann Thorac Surg 2003;75:23–7.

55. DiNardo JA, Wegner JA. Pro: low-flow cardiopulmonary bypass is the preferred technique for patients undergoing cardiac surgical procedures. J Cardiothorac Vasc Anesth 2001;15:649–51.

56. Boston US, Slater JM, Orszulak TA, Cook DJ. Hierarchy of regional oxygen delivery during cardiopulmonary bypass. Ann Thorac Surg 2001;71:260–4.

57. Johnston WE, Zwischenberger JB. Improving splanchnic perfusion during cardiopulmonary bypass. Anesthesiology 2000;92:305–7.

58. Andersson LG, Bratteby LE, Ekroth R, et al. Renal function during cardiopulmonary bypass: influence of pump flow and systemic blood pressure. Eur J Cardiothorac Surg 1994;8:597–602.

59. Slogoff S, Reul GJ, Keats AS, et al. Role of perfusion pressure and flow in major organ dysfunction after cardiopulmonary bypass. Ann Thorac Surg 1990;50:911–8.

60. Cook DJ. Con: low-flow cardiopulmonary bypass is not the preferred technique for patients undergoing cardiac surgical procedures. J Cardiothorac Vasc Anesth 2001;15:652–4.

61. Sungurtekin H, Boston US, Cook DJ. Bypass flow, mean arterial pressure, and cerebral perfusion during cardiopulmonary bypass in dogs. J Cardiothorac Vasc Anesth 2000;14:25–8.

62. Schwartz AE, Sandhu AA, Kaplon RJ, et al. Cerebral blood flow is determined by arterial pressure and not cardiopulmonary bypass flow rate. Ann Thorac Surg 1995;60:165–70.

63. Anastasiou E, Gerolioliou K, Karakoulas K, Peftoulidou M, Giala M. Reliability of continuous jugular venous bulb hemoglobin oxygen saturation during cardiac surgery. J Cardiothorac Vasc Anesth 1999;13:276–9.

64. von Knobelsdorff G, Hanel F, Werner C, Schulte am Esch J. Jugular bulb oxygen saturation and middle cerebral blood flow velocity during cardiopulmonary bypass. J Neurosurg Anesthesiol 1997;9:128–33.

65. Reents W, Muellges W, Franke D, Babin-Ebell J, Elert O. Cerebral oxygen saturation assessed by near-infrared spectroscopy during coronary artery bypass grafting and early postoperative cognitive dysfunction. Ann Thorac Surg 2002;74:109–14.

66. Prabhune A, Sehic A, Spence PA, Church T, Edmonds HL Jr. Cerebral oximetry provides early warning of oxygen delivery failure during cardiopulmonary bypass. J Cardiothorac Vasc Anesth 2002;16:204–6.

67. Kadoi Y, Saito S, Goto F, Fujita N. Decrease in jugular venous oxygen saturation during normothermic cardiopulmonary bypass predicts short-term postoperative neurologic dysfunction in elderly patients. J Am Coll Cardiol 2001;38:1450–5.

68. Yao FSF, Tseng CC, Woo D, Huang SW, Levin SK. Maintaining cerebral oxygen saturation during cardiac surgery decreased neurological complications. Anesthesiology 2001;95:A-152.

69. Shapira OM, Kimmel WA, Lindsey PS, Shahian DM. Anterior ischemic optic neuropathy after open heart operations. Ann Thorac Surg 1996;61:660–6.

70. Habib RH, Zacharias A, Schwann TA, Riordan CJ, Durham SJ, Shah A. Adverse effects of low hematocrit during cardiopulmonary bypass in the adult: should current practice be changed? J Thorac Cardiovasc Surg 2003;125:1438–50.

71. Bert AA, Stearns GT, Feng W, Singh AK. Normothermic cardiopulmonary bypass. J Cardiothorac Vasc Anesth 1997;11:91–9.

72. Grigore AM, Grocott HP, Mathew JP, et al. The rewarming rate and increased peak temperature alter neurocognitive outcome after cardiac surgery. Anesth Analg 2002;94:4–10.

73. Stensrud PE, Nuttall GA, de Castro MA, et al. A prospective, randomized study of cardiopulmonary bypass temperature and blood transfusion. Ann Thorac Surg 1999;67:711–5.

74. Engelman RM, Pleet AB, Rousou JA, et al. Influence of cardiopulmonary bypass perfusion temperature on neurologic and hematologic function after coronary artery bypass grafting. Ann Thorac Surg 1999;67:1547–56.

75. Gaudino N, Zamparelli R, Andreotti F, et al. Normothermia does not improve postoperative hemostasis nor does it reduce inflammatory activation in patients undergoing primary isolated coronary artery bypass. J Thorac Cardiovasc Surg 2002;123:1092–100.

76. Demers P, Elkouri S, Martineau R, Couturier A, Cartier R. Outcome with high blood lactate levels during cardiopulmonary bypass in adult cardiac operation. Ann Thorac Surg 2000;70:2082–6.

77. Patel RL, Turtle MR, Chambers DJ, James DN, Newman S, Venn GE. Alpha-stat acid-base regulation during cardiopulmonary bypass improves neuropsychological outcome in patients undergoing coronary artery bypass grafting. J Thorac Cardiovasc Surg 1996;111:1267–79.

78. Lanier WL. Glucose management during cardiopulmonary bypass: cardiovascular and neurologic implications. Anesth Analg 1991;72:423–7.

79. Mekontso-Dessap A, Houel R, Soustelle C, Kirsch M, Thebert D, Loisance DY. Risk factors for post-cardiopulmonary bypass vasoplegia in patients with preserved left ventricular function. Ann Thorac Surg 2001;71:1428–32.

80. Mets B, Michler RE, Delphin ED, Oz MC, Landry DW. Refractory vasodilation after cardiopulmonary bypass for heart transplantation in recipients on combined amiodarone and angiotensin-converting enzyme inhibitor therapy: a role for vasopressin administration. J Cardiothorac Vasc Anesth 1998;12:326–9.

81. Sabbagh AH, Chung GK, Shuttleworth P, Applegate BJ, Gabrhel W. Fresh frozen plasma: a solution to heparin resistance during cardiopulmonary bypass. Ann Thorac Surg 1984;37:466–8.

82. Lemmer JR JH, Despotis GJ. Antithrombin III concentrate to treat heparin resistance in patients undergoing cardiac surgery. J Thorac Cardiovasc Surg 2002;123:213.

83. Williams MR, D'Ambra AB, Beck JR, et al. A randomized trial of antithrombin concentrates for treatment of heparin resistance. Ann Thorac Surg 2000;70:873–7.

84. Leyh RG, Kofidis T, Struder M, et al. Methylene blue: the drug of choice for catecholamine-refractory vasoplegia after cardiopulmonary bypass? J Thorac Cardiovasc Surg 2003;125:1426–31.

85. Langenberg CJM, Pietersen HG, Geskes G, et al. Coronary sinus catheter placement. Assessment of placement criteria and cardiac complications. Chest 2003;124:1259–65.

86. Mills NL, Ochsner JL. Massive air embolism during cardiopulmonary bypass. J Thorac Cardiovasc Surg 1980;80:708–17.

87. Webb WR, Harrison LH Jr, Helmcke FR, Aharon A. Carbon dioxide field flooding minimizes residual intracardiac air after open heart operations. Ann Thorac Surg 1997;64:1489–91.

88. Agarwal SK, Ghosh PK, Gupta D. Cardiac surgery and cold-reactive proteins. Ann Thorac Surg 1995;60:1143–50.

89. Fisher GD, Claypoole V, Collard CD. Increased pressures in the retrograde blood cardioplegia line: an unusual presentation of cold agglutinins during cardiopulmonary bypass. Anesth Analg 1997;84:454–6.

90. Dake SB, Johnston MF, Brueggeman P, Barner HB. Detection of cold hemagglutination in a blood cardioplegia unit before systemic cooling of a patient with unsuspected cold agglutinin disease. Ann Thorac Surg 1989;47:914–5.

91. Gokhale AGK, Suhasini T, Saraswati V, Chandrasekhar N, Rajagopal P. Cold agglutinins and warm heart surgery. J Thorac Cardiovasc Surg 1993;105:557.

92. Kuypson AP, Warner JJ, Telen MJ, Milano CA. Paroxysmal cold hemoglobinuria and cardiopulmonary bypass. Ann Thorac Surg 2003;75:579–81.

93. Kirklin JW, Barratt-Boyes MG. Cardiac Surgery. New York: John Wiley & Sons, 1986:42–3.

94. Griepp RB. Cerebral protection during aortic arch surgery. J Thorac Cardiovasc Surg 2001; 121:425–7.

95. Kazui T, Yamashita K, Washiyama N, et al. Usefulness of antegrade selective cerebral perfusion during aortic arch operations. Ann Thorac Surg 2002;74:S1806–9.

96. Reich DL, Uysal S, Ergin MA, Griepp RB. Retrograde cerebral perfusion as a method of neuroprotection during thoracic aortic surgery. Ann Thorac Surg 2001;72:1774–82.

97. Royston D. Pro: aprotinin should be used in patients undergoing hypothermic circulatory arrest. J Cardiothorac Vasc Anesth 2001;15:121–5.

98. Smith CR, Spanier TB. Aprotinin in deep hypothermic circulatory arrest. Ann Thorac Surg 1999;68:278–86.

99. Coselli JS, LeMaire SA. Left heart bypass reduces paraplegia rates after thoracoabdominal aortic aneurysm repair. Ann Thorac Surg 1999;67:1931–4.

100. Szwerc MF, Benckhart DH, Lin JC, et al. Recent clinical experience with left heart bypass using a centrifugal pump for repair of traumatic aortic transection. Ann Surg 1999;230:484–90.

101. Karmy-Jones R, Carter Y, Meissner M, Mulligan MS. Choice of venous cannulation for bypass during repair of traumatic rupture of the aorta. Ann Thorac Surg 2001;71:39–41.

102. Leach WR, Sundt TM III, Moon MR. Oxygenator support for partial left-heart bypass. Ann Thorac Surg 2001;72:1770–1.

103. Mathison M, Buffolo E, Jatene AD, et al. Right heart circulatory support facilitates coronary artery bypass without cardiopulmonary bypass. Ann Thorac Surg 2000;70:1083–5.

104. Yeatman M, Caputo M, Narayan P, et al. Intracoronary shunts reduce transient intraoperative myocardial dysfunction during off-pump coronary operations. Ann Thorac Surg 2002;73:1411–7.

105. Cooper WA, Corvera JS, Thourani VH, et al. Perfusion-assisted direct coronary artery bypass provides early reperfusion of ischemic myocardium and facilitates complete revascularization. Ann Thorac Surg 2003;75:1132–9.

106. Muraki S, Tsukamoto M, Komatsu K, et al. Minimally ischemic off-pump coronary artery bypass grafting: active perfusion assist with nitroglycerin-supplemented blood. Ann Thorac Surg 2003;76:298–300.

107. Vassiliades TA Jr, Nielsen JL, Lonquist JL. Coronary perfusion methods during off-pump coronary artery bypass: results of a randomized clinical trial. Ann Thorac Surg 2002;74:S1383–9.

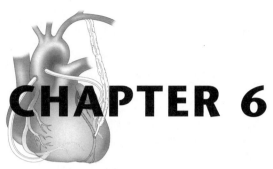

CHAPTER 6

Myocardial Protection

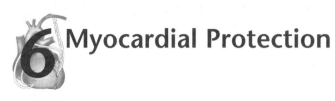Myocardial Protection

Obtaining an optimal surgical result depends on performing a technically proficient operation while protecting the heart from potential damage. With the use of extracorporeal circulation, surgeons can take advantage of a period of aortic cross-clamping and ischemic cardiac arrest to produce a quiet, bloodless field that allows for precise surgical techniques. The development of cardioplegia solutions almost 30 years ago was one of the major advances in cardiac surgery that allowed surgeons to extend this period of ischemic arrest to well over 3 hours to perform complex surgical procedures without adversely affecting myocardial function. Conscientious application of well-developed principles is essential to minimize ischemia/reperfusion injury that contributes to postischemic myocardial dysfunction, thus optimizing both the short- and long-term results of surgery.[1]

I. Types of Myocardial Protection (Box 6.1)

A. **Cardioplegia** is used to arrest the heart after application of an aortic cross-clamp that interrupts the coronary circulation. Cross-clamping of the aorta without the use of cardioplegia results in anaerobic metabolism and depletion of myocardial energy stores. Thus, without a reduction in myocardial metabolism, either by hypothermia or chemical cardiac arrest, cross-clamping to induce ischemic arrest for more than 15–20 minutes would result in severe myocardial dysfunction.

B. **Off-pump coronary artery bypass surgery** (OPCAB) is performed without cardiopulmonary bypass and thus on a beating heart. The need to provide myocardial protection is limited because, in the absence of ongoing ischemia, only the region subtended by the artery being bypassed should be in ischemic jeopardy. If ischemia develops, as evidenced by electrocardiographic changes or ventricular dysfunction, intracoronary shunting or aortocoronary shunting can be used to provide distal flow until the anastomosis is completed.[2] Perfusion-assisted shunting may provide the best myocardial protection during OPCAB.[3,4]

C. Ischemic preconditioning refers to a phenomenon by which a transient reduction in blood flow to the myocardial tissue enables it to tolerate a subsequent longer period of ischemia.[5] The ideal application of this concept is in off-pump surgery because, in the absence of collateral flow, there is obligatory transient ischemia with occlusion of a target vessel that might be lessened by ischemic preconditioning.[6]

D. On-pump surgery can be performed without aortic cross-clamping, thus obviating the need to provide myocardial protection (so-called **on-pump beating-heart surgery**). With the availability of stabilizing platforms used for OPCAB, this technique allows for construction of distal anastomoses on a beating heart while the pump provides systemic flow. This should be considered when safe aortic clamping cannot be performed and when the risk of arresting the heart is considered very high due to severe ventricular dysfunction. Due to the lower oxygen demand of the empty, beating heart, ischemia should be better tolerated than standard OPCAB, but shunting techniques can still be used to optimize protection. The on-pump beating-heart technique

---

Box 6.1 • Options for Myocardial Protection

1. Off-pump surgery
   a. Aortocoronary shunting
   b. Perfusion-assisted shunting
   c. Ischemic preconditioning
2. On-pump surgery
   a. On-pump beating heart
   b. Cardioplegic arrest
   c. Hypothermic fibrillatory arrest
   d. Intermittent ischemic arrest

---

can also be used for intracardiac operations, such as resection of a left ventricular aneurysm or repair of an atrial septal defect.

E. **Intermittent ischemic arrest** involves multiple short periods of cross-clamping with mild systemic hypothermia to perform each distal anastomosis. Conceptually, this is a violation of the principle of preserving the heart by inducing diastolic arrest during the period of aortic cross-clamping. However, the heart can tolerate these brief periods without adverse sequelae.[7] With the technique of **hypothermic fibrillatory arrest,** the aorta remains unclamped and distal anastomoses are performed with the heart cold and fibrillating at high perfusion pressures. This technique is useful when safe clamping of the aorta is not feasible due to extensive calcification or atherosclerosis.[8] However, this technique provides less than ideal protection, especially in the hypertrophied heart. With the availability of stabilizing platforms, surgery that must be performed without clamping is best performed on a beating heart, either at normothermia or mild hypothermia.

II. Principles of Cardioplegia[9–13] (Table 6.1)

A. Prompt **diastolic arrest** of the heart is achieved using a delivery solution containing about 20–25 mEq/L of potassium chloride (KCl). The potassium may be added to a crystalloid solution that is administered undiluted ("crystalloid cardioplegia") or it may be concentrated in a smaller bag of crystalloid solution and administered in a mixture with blood in varying ratios (most commonly 4:1 blood) ("blood cardioplegia"). Systems are available that add the potassium directly to blood to minimize hemodilution ("miniplegia").

1. **Crystalloid cardioplegia** provides little substrate and no oxygen to the heart during the period of ischemic arrest. It functions primarily by arresting the heart at cold temperatures. It can be oxygenated by bubbling oxygen through the solution, but this is not a common practice.

2. **Blood cardioplegia** solutions provide oxygen, natural buffering agents, antioxidants, and free-radical scavengers. Standard supplemental additives to these solutions include other buffers to achieve an alkaline pH (THAM), citrate-phosphate-dextrose (CPD) to lower the level of calcium, and occasionally drugs to maintain slight hyperosmolarity (mannitol). The cardioplegia mixture passes

Table 6.1 • Principles and Composition of Cardioplegia

Principle	Composition
1. Prompt diastolic arrest	KCl 20–25 mEq/L
2. Buffering	THAM, bicarbonate
3. Reduction of calcium levels	CPD
4. Adequate delivery	Antegrade ± retrograde administration
5. Temperature	Cold vs. tepid vs. warm
6. Substrate additives to optimize myocardial metabolism or prevent cell damage	Aspartate-glutamate Na^+-H^+ exchange inhibitors Insulin Magnesium Procainamide L-arginine Calcium channel blockers

THAM = tris(hydroxymethyl)aminomethane; CPD = citrate-phosphate-dextrose.

through a separate heater/cooler system in the extracorporeal circuit with the infusion rate and pressure controlled by the perfusionist.

3. The oxygen demand of the heart is reduced by nearly 90% by simply arresting the heart at normothermia, so maintenance of arrest during the cross-clamp period is essential (Figure 6.1). This is accomplished by readministering the solution every 15–20 minutes to deliver potassium and wash out metabolic byproducts. A low potassium solution (12–15 mEq/L) is then used to maintain the arrest while avoiding an excess potassium load; the high-potassium solution should be used if the heart resumes any activity. Cold blood alone can be given retrograde into the coronary sinus as an alternative to subsequent doses of cardioplegia to optimize tissue oxygenation and metabolism while minimizing the potassium load. This is adequate as long as the heart remains arrested.

4. Clinical studies have not demonstrated the superiority of one type of cardioplegia over the other in routine cases,[14] but they do suggest that patients with more advanced left ventricular dysfunction may fare better with blood cardioplegia, especially if given both antegrade and retrograde.[15]

5. Polarized arrest, using a potassium-channel opener (nicorandil, pinacidil, aprikalim), is being investigated as an alternative to the depolarized arrest induced by potassium. This has been shown to attenuate the elevation of intracellular calcium, and may improve contractile function compared with standard potassium arrest.[16–18]

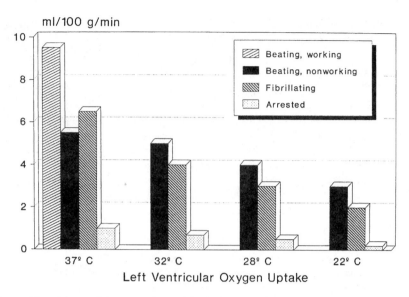

ml/100 g/min

Figure 6.1 • Myocardial oxygen demand (mvO$_2$). Notice that the most significant decrease in mvO$_2$ occurs with the induction of the arrested state and secondarily by the production of hypothermia. *(Modified with permission from Buckberg GD, Brazier JR, Nelson RL, Goldstein SM, McConnell DH, Cooper N. Studies of the effects of hypothermia on regional myocardial blood flow and metabolism during cardiopulmonary bypass. I. The adequately perfused beating, fibrillating, and arrested heart. J Thorac Cardiovasc Surg 1977;73:87–94.)*

B. Temperature. Before the development of cardioplegia solutions, myocardial protection was provided entirely by systemic and topical hypothermia. It seemed logical that administering cardioplegia at a cold temperature would be a significant factor in decreasing myocardial metabolism. However, the reduction in myocardial metabolism attributable to hypothermia is actually quite insignificant compared with that achieved by diastolic arrest (Figure 6.1). Nonetheless, systemic hypothermia supplemented by use of topical cold (not iced) saline and topical cooling devices that surround the left ventricle and protect the phrenic nerve from cold injury are routinely used in patients receiving cold cardioplegia.

1. Some surgeons monitor myocardial temperatures with the presumption that adequate hypothermia (< 15°C) of the myocardium is providing satisfactory myocardial protection. However, in clinical practice, only one site is usually selected for monitoring, and there is commonly a significant discrepancy between the temperatures of different areas of the left ventricle and especially between the left and right ventricles. It should be understood that temperature monitoring provides only a relative assessment of the degree of myocardial protection.[19] A more scientific means of assessing the degree of myocardial protection is use of a pH probe. The development of significant acidosis caused by a derangement in myocardial metabolism is indicative of poor protection.[20]

2. Since enzymatic and cellular reparative processes function better at normothermia, some surgeons use "warm cardioplegia" for myocardial protection with excellent results.[21,22] However, because of the tendency for the heart to resume electrical activity at normothermia, this must be given continuously or with only

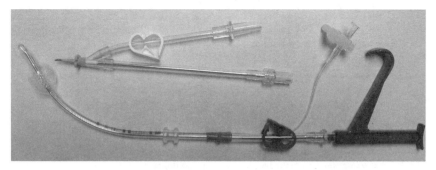

Figure 6.2 • (Top) Antegrade cardioplegia catheter with a side port for venting. (Bottom) A 14F retrograde catheter with self-inflating balloon for measuring coronary sinus pressures.

brief interruptions to protect the heart. When given continuously, it can obscure the operative field. To minimize hemodilution from excessive cardioplegia administration, the "miniplegia" system that simply adds potassium or other substances (magnesium) to the blood is useful.

3. Use of intermittent "tepid" blood cardioplegia (whether at 32°C or 20°C) has been shown to provide better metabolic and functional recovery than cold cardioplegia in several studies, and may also be associated with improved long-term results.[23–26]

4. Warm cardioplegia can be used as an adjunct to cold cardioplegia when given at the beginning and the end of the period of aortic cross-clamping.

   a. **Warm induction** involves administering 500 mL of warm cardioplegia immediately after aortic cross-clamping. Studies suggest that this may be beneficial in actively ischemic hearts with energy depletion by providing a brief period of time during which oxygen can be used to repair cell damage and replace energy stores. This may be further beneficial if the solution is enriched with glutamate and aspartate.[9,11,27]

   b. Terminal warm blood cardioplegia (**"hot shot"**) is commonly given just before removal of the aortic cross-clamp because it has been shown to improve myocardial metabolism.[28] The heart tends to remain asystolic for several minutes after removal of the aortic cross-clamp, during which time the heart is able to "repair" cellular processes or replenish energy stores while the oxygen demand is low.

C. **Route of delivery.** Cardioplegia is initially administered antegrade into the aortic root and then may be given retrograde through a catheter placed in the coronary sinus (Figure 6.2).

   1. The efficacy of antegrade cardioplegia (ACP) delivery may be compromised by severe coronary artery stenosis and is often dependent on collateral flow.[29] In addition, sufficient root distention may not be achieved in patients with more than mild aortic insufficiency. ACP can also be cumbersome to readminister during aortic and mitral valve operations. If root venting is utilized, care must be taken to eliminate air from the aortic root when the cardioplegia is readministered.

   2. Retrograde cardioplegia (RCP) is easy to administer, either intermittently or continuously, and does not interrupt the flow of an operation. It is helpful in reducing the risk of atheroembolism from patent yet diseased saphenous vein

grafts at reoperation. It provides excellent myocardial protection, although there is always concern about maldistribution of this solution, especially to the right ventricle. Some studies have shown excellent and others poor protection of the right ventricle with this approach.[30-32] Careful monitoring of coronary sinus pressure during the administration of retrograde cardioplegia is essential: if it is too high (>50 mm Hg), coronary sinus rupture can occur; if it is too low (< 20 mm Hg), there is usually a problem with catheter malposition.[33]

3. Studies that have analyzed the distribution of cardioplegia solutions suggest that the routes of delivery should be complementary, not exclusive. Contrast echocardiography studies have shown that perfusion of the left ventricle is better with warm antegrade delivery than retrograde delivery. They have also shown that delivery to the right ventricle is poor with either approach, especially if there is right coronary artery occlusion.[13,29,34] Although warm RCP should ideally be run as continuously as possible, most surgeons who administer cold RCP do so intermittently. However, one study demonstrated that cold RCP given continuously improved ventricular performance with reduced myocardial ischemia compared with intermittent administration.[35]

D. **Cardioplegia additives.** A variety of medications that might potentially be cardioprotective when given in the cardioplegia solution have been studied. Those showing the greatest promise include the Na^+-H^+ exchange inhibitors (such as cariporide), adenosine, and L-arginine.[36-41] Aspartate and glutamate are Krebs' cycle intermediates that have been used to improve myocardial energy metabolism with variable success.[9,27] Other drugs include procainamide, magnesium (which has been shown to reduce arrhythmias),[42] and free-radical scavengers. The insulin cardioplegia trial involved use of tepid cardioplegia enriched with glucose and insulin. This demonstrated metabolic and functional benefits to patients undergoing elective but not urgent surgery.[43-45]

E. **Modified reperfusion.** Just prior to removal of the cross-clamp, the administration of a modified cardioplegia solution given under specific conditions has been shown to improve myocardial function.[9,11] Such controlled reperfusion with or without substrate enhancement, such as aspartate and glutamate, should provide a low potassium load (8 to 10 mEq/L), include CPD to limit calcium influx, should be hyperosmolar, and should be given at low pressures (< 50 mm Hg) over several minutes. Benefits of such a regimen may only be beneficial in high-risk cases if these principles are adhered to.[46,47] Neutrophil depletion by leukocyte filtration in cardiac reperfusate solutions may also reduce ischemia/reperfusion injury.[48]

III. Cardioplegia Strategy

Numerous studies have been done to elucidate the best cardioplegia strategy. Comparisons have been based on myocardial contrast echocardiography or assessments of perfusion, clinical results (hemodynamic performance, use of inotropes, rates of infarction, mortality), or enzyme elevation (troponin, a very sensitive marker of myocardial injury). For example, one study showed that troponin levels were more elevated in patients receiving antegrade rather than retrograde crystalloid cardioplegia, but this had no clinical relevance.[49] The extent of coronary disease and especially of collateral flow can significantly impact the efficacy of both antegrade and retrograde flow and confound the analysis.[29] There are so many variations in cardioplegia strategies and solutions that it is often difficult to ascertain which specific element provides the true benefit.

A. Most studies suggest that in low-risk cases, multidose cold crystalloid, or cold or warm blood cardioplegia, whether given antegrade and/or retrograde, produce relatively comparable clinical results. In general, protection of the right ventricle is suboptimal with all strategies, especially in patients with right coronary artery disease. In high-risk cases, combined ACP/RCP cold or tepid blood cardioplegia seems best.

B. A proposal for blood cardioplegia strategy is as follows:

1. Use warm induction for severely ischemic hearts only.

2. Induce cardioplegic arrest with about 500 mL of antegrade infusion (cold or tepid); then complete the initial dose by administering cardioplegia retrograde. This is especially important in patients with severe coronary artery disease. If temperature monitoring is used for cold cardioplegia, it should be maintained at less than 20°C.

3. For valve surgery, use either continuous warm retrograde cardioplegia or intermittent cold retrograde blood cardioplegia with a low-potassium solution every 20 minutes.

4. For coronary surgery, perform the right coronary graft first and administer low-potassium cardioplegia down that graft simultaneously with retrograde cardioplegia for all subsequent administrations.

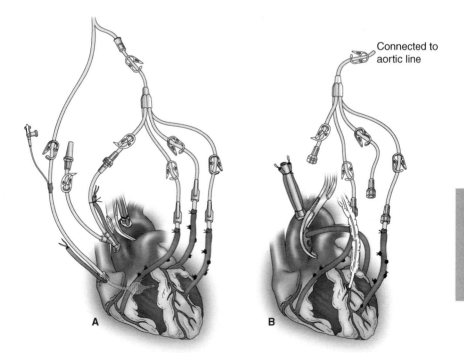

Connected to
aortic line

A   B

Figure 6.3 • (A) Technique of administering cardioplegia simultaneously down the completed vein grafts and the retrograde cannula. (B) Blood can be delivered off the aortic line during construction of the proximal anastomoses.

5. If warm retrograde cardioplegia is used, it should be run as continuously as possible as long as it does not interfere with exposure. A high-potassium solution should be used if there is a return of cardiac activity.

6. Administer cardioplegia down each bypass graft as it is completed along with additional retrograde cardioplegia. Concomitant administration down all completed grafts might be helpful but has not been studied (Figure 6.3).

7. Administer 500 mL of hot shot retrograde just prior to removal of the cross-clamp. If retrograde is not used, give this into the aortic root at a pressure not exceeding 50–80 mm Hg.

C. Careful adherence to the basic principles of cardioplegia (maintaining arrest and multidosing, in particular) should allow surgeons to patiently yet expeditiously perform even the most complex, time-consuming surgery without worrying about poor myocardial protection.

References

1. Nicolini F, Beghi C, Muscari C, et al. Myocardial protection in adult cardiac surgery: current options and future challenges. Eur J Cardiothorac Surg 2003;24:986–93.

2. Yeatman M, Caputo M, Narayan P, et al. Intracoronary shunts reduce transient intraoperative myocardial dysfunction during off-pump coronary operations. Ann Thorac Surg 2002;73: 1411–7.

3. Cooper WA, Corvera JS, Thourani VH, et al. Perfusion-assisted direct coronary artery bypass provides early reperfusion of ischemic myocardium and facilitates complete revascularization. Ann Thorac Surg 2003;75:1132–9.

4. Vassiliades TA Jr, Nielsen JL, Lonquist JL. Coronary perfusion methods during off-pump coronary artery bypass: results of a randomized clinical trial. Ann Thorac Surg 2002;74:S1383–9.

5. Teoh LK, Grant R, Hulf JA, Pugsley WB, Yellon DM. A comparison of ischemic preconditioning, intermittent cross-clamp fibrillation and cold crystalloid cardioplegia for myocardial protection during coronary artery bypass graft surgery. Cardiovasc Surg 2002;10:251–5.

6. Laurikka J, Wu ZK, Iisalo P, et al. Regional ischemic preconditioning enhances myocardial performance in off-pump coronary artery bypass grafting. Chest 2002;121:1183–9.

7. Raco L, Mills E, Millner RJW. Isolated myocardial revascularization with intermittent aortic cross-clamping: experience with 800 cases. Ann Thorac Surg 2002;73:1436–40.

8. Akins CW. Noncardioplegic myocardial preservation for coronary revascularization. J Thorac Cardiovasc Surg 1984;88:174–81.

9. Buckberg GD, Beyersdorf F, Allen BS, Robertson JM. Integrated myocardial management: background and initial application. J Card Surg 1995;10:68–89.

10. Buckberg GD. Update on current techniques of myocardial protection. Ann Thorac Surg 1995; 60:805–14.

11. Beyersdorf F, Buckberg GD. Myocardial protection with blood cardioplegia during valve operations. J Heart Valve Dis 1994;3:388–403.

12. Buckberg GD. Antegrade/retrograde cardioplegia to ensure cardioplegic distribution: operative techniques and objectives. J Card Surg 1989;4:216–38.

13. Cohen G, Borger MA, Weisel RD, Rao V. Intraoperative myocardial protection: current trends and future perspectives. Ann Thorac Surg 1999;68:1995–2001.

14. Hendriks M, Jiang H, Gutermann H, et al. Release of cardiac troponin I in antegrade crystalloid versus cold blood cardioplegia. J Thorac Cardiovasc Surg 1999;118:452–9.

15. Flack JE III, Cook JR, May SJ, et al. Does cardioplegia type affect outcome and survival in patients with advanced left ventricular dysfunction? Results from the CABG patch trial. Circulation 2000;102(suppl III):84–9.

16. Chambers DJ. Mechanisms and alternative methods of achieving cardiac arrest. Ann Thorac Surg 2003;75:S661–6.

17. Ducko CT, Stephenson ER Jr, Jayawant AM, Vigilance DW, Damiano RJ Jr. Potassium channel openers: are they effective as pretreatment or additives to cardioplegia? Ann Thorac Surg 2000;69:1363–8.

18. Li HY, Wu S, He GW, Wong TM. Aprikalim reduces the Na^+-Ca^{2+} exchange outward current enhanced by hyperkalemia in rat ventricular myocytes. Ann Thorac Surg 2002;73:1253–60.

19. Dearani JA, Axford TC, Patel MA, Healey NA, Lavin PT, Khuri SF. Role of myocardial temperature measurement in monitoring the adequacy of myocardial protection during cardiac surgery. Ann Thorac Surg 2001;72:S235–44.

20. Khabbaz KR, Zankoul F, Warner KG. Intraoperative metabolic monitoring of the heart: II. Online measurement of myocardial tissue pH. Ann Thorac Surg 2001;72:S2227–33.

21. Franke UFW, Korsch S, Wittwer T, et al. Intermittent antegrade warm myocardial protection compared to intermittent cold blood cardioplegia in elective coronary surgery: do we have to change? Eur J Cardiothorac Surg 2003;23:341–6.

22. Salerno TA, Houck JP, Barrozo CA, et al. Retrograde continuous warm blood cardioplegia: a new concept in myocardial protection. Ann Thorac Surg 1991;51:245–7.

23. Chocron S, Kaili D, Yan Y, et al. Intermittent lukewarm (20°C) antegrade intermittent blood cardioplegia compared with cold and warm blood cardioplegia. J Thorac Cardiovasc Surg 2000;119:610–6.

24. Hayashida N, Isomura T, Sato T, et al. Minimally diluted tepid blood cardioplegia. Ann Thorac Surg 1998;65:615–21.

25. Elwatidy AMF, Fadalah MA, Bukhari EA, et al. Antegrade crystalloid cardioplegia vs. antegrade/retrograde cold and tepid blood cardioplegia in CABG. Ann Thorac Surg 1999;68:447–53.

26. Mallidi HR, Sever J, Tamariz M, et al. The short-term and long-term effects of warm or tepid cardioplegia. J Thorac Cardiovasc Surg 2003;125:711–20.

27. Wallace AW, Ratcliffe MB, Nosé PS, et al. Effect of induction and reperfusion with warm substrate–enriched cardioplegia on ventricular function. Ann Thorac Surg 2000;70:1301–7.

28. Teoh KH, Christakis GT, Weisel RD, et al. Accelerated myocardial metabolic recovery with terminal warm blood cardioplegia. J Thorac Cardiovasc Surg 1986;91:888–95.

29. Aronson S, Jacobsohn E, Savage R, Albertucci M. The influence of collateral flow on the antegrade and retrograde distribution of cardioplegia in patients with an occluded right coronary artery. Anesthesiology 1998;89:1099–1107.

30. Ruengsakulrach P, Buxton BF. Anatomic and hemodynamic considerations influencing the efficiency of retrograde cardioplegia. Ann Thorac Surg 2001;71:1389–95.

31. Kulshrestha P, Rousou JA, Engelman RM, et al. Does warm blood retrograde cardioplegia preserve right ventricular function? Ann Thorac Surg 2001;72:1572–5.

32. Allen BS, Winkelmann JW, Hanafy JH, et al. Retrograde cardioplegia does not adequately perfuse the right ventricle. J Thorac Cardiovasc Surg 1995;109:1116–26.

33. Langenberg CJM, Pietersen JG, Geskes G, et al. Coronary sinus catheter placement. Assessment of placement criteria and cardiac complications. Chest 2003;124:1259–65.

34. Borger MA, Wei KS, Weisel RD, et al. Myocardial perfusion during warm antegrade and retrograde cardioplegia: a contrast echo study. Ann Thorac Surg 1999;68:955–61.

35. Louagie YAG, Jamart J, Gonzalez M, et al. Continuous cold blood cardioplegia improves myocardial protection: a prospective randomized study. Ann Thorac Surg 2004;77:664–71.

36. Boyce SW, Bartels C, Bolli R, et al. Impact of sodium-hydrogen exchange inhibition by cariporide on death or myocardial infarction in high-risk CABG surgery patients: results of the CABG surgery cohort of the GUARDIAN study. J Thorac Cardiovasc Surg 2003;126:420–7.

37. Cox CS Jr, Allen SJ, Sauer H, Laine GA. Improved myocardial function using a Na^+/H^+ exchanger during cardioplegic arrest and cardiopulmonary bypass. Chest 2003;123:187–94.

38. Mentzer RM Jr, Lasley RD, Jessel A, Karmazyn M. Intracellular sodium hydrogen exchange inhibition and clinical myocardial protection. Ann Thorac Surg 2003;75:S700–8.

39. Chauhan S, Wasir HS, Bhan A, Rao BH, Saxena N, Venugopal P. Adenosine for cardioplegia induction: a comparison with St. Thomas' solution. J Cardiothorac Vasc Anesth 2000;14:21–4.

40. Vinten-Johansen J, Zhao ZQ, Corvera JS, et al. Adenosine in myocardial protection in on-pump and off-pump cardiac surgery. Ann Thorac Surg 2003;75:S691–9.

41. Carrier M, Pellerin M, Perrault LP, et al. Cardioplegic arrest with L-arginine improves myocardial protection: results of a prospective randomized clinical trial. Ann Thorac Surg 2002;73:837–42.

42. Yeatman M, Caputo M, Narayan P, et al. Magnesium-supplemented warm blood cardioplegia in patients undergoing coronary artery revascularization. Ann Thorac Surg 2002;73:112–8.

43. Rao V, Christakis GT, Weisel RD, et al. The Insulin Cardioplegia Trial: myocardial protection for urgent coronary artery bypass grafting. J Thorac Cardiovasc Surg 2002;123:928–35.

44. Rao V, Borger MA, Weisel RD, et al. Insulin cardioplegia for elective coronary bypass surgery. J Thorac Cardiovasc Surg 2000;119:1176–84.

45. Doenst T, Bothe W, Beyersdorf F. Therapy with insulin in cardiac surgery: controversies and possible solutions. Ann Thorac Surg 2003;75:S721–8.

46. Edwards R, Treasure T, Hossein-Nia M, Murday A, Kantidakis GH, Holt DW. A controlled trial of substrate-enhanced, warm reperfusion ("hot shot") versus simple reperfusion. Ann Thorac Surg 2000;69:551–5.

47. Buckberg GD. Substrate enriched warm blood cardioplegia reperfusion: an alternate view. Ann Thorac Surg 2000;69:334–5.

48. Palatianos GM, Balentine G, Papadakis EG, et al. Neutrophil depletion reduces myocardial reperfusion morbidity. Ann Thorac Surg 2004;77:956–61.

49. Franke U, Wahlers T, Cohnert TU, et al. Retrograde versus antegrade crystalloid cardioplegia in coronary surgery: value of troponin-I measurement. Ann Thorac Surg 2001;71:249–53.

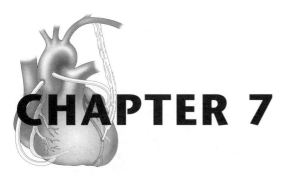

CHAPTER 7

Admission to the ICU
and Monitoring Techniques

Admission to the ICU and Monitoring Techniques

I. Admission to the ICU

A. The first critical phase of postoperative care starts at the completion of the surgical procedure. During transfer from the operating room table to an intensive care unit (ICU) bed, from one monitoring system to another, and from the operating room to the ICU, the potential exists for airway and ventilation problems, sudden hypotension or hypertension, arrhythmias, inadvertent medication changes, and unidentified problems with invasive catheters, monitoring, and bleeding. The electrocardiogram (ECG) and pressure tracings (arterial, central venous, and/or pulmonary arterial) are transferred one at a time from the operating room monitor to the transport module to ensure that the patient is monitored at all times. Ventilation is provided by a manual resuscitator bag (Ambu®) connected to a portable oxygen tank. Drug infusions should be placed on battery-powered infusion pumps to ensure accurate infusion rates. A selection of cardiac medications should always be available in the event of an emergency during transport.

B. Upon arrival in the ICU, the endotracheal tube is connected to a mechanical ventilator, and the ECG and pressure lines are transduced on the bedside monitors. A pulse oximeter is attached to one of the patient's fingertips. Medication drip rates are confirmed or readjusted on controlled-infusion pumps, preferably using the same pumps that were used in the operating room to avoid temporary disconnection from the patient. The thoracic drainage system is connected to suction.

C. During this transition phase, much attention is directed to getting the patient connected to the monitors and attached to the ventilator. To ensure that the patient remains stable while getting settled in, it is critical that the accompanying anesthesia and/or surgical personnel as well as the accepting nurses and respiratory therapists make sure that:

1. The patient is being well-ventilated by observing chest movement and auscultating bilateral breath sounds.

2. The ECG demonstrates satisfactory rate and rhythm on the transport and then on the bedside monitor.

3. The blood pressure is adequate on the portable monitor and remains so after the arterial line is transduced and calibrated on the bedside monitor.

D. Immediate assessment and response to any abnormalities suspected to be present at the time of admission to the ICU, whether real or spurious, is imperative. The two most common problems encountered are low blood pressure and an indecipherable ECG.

E. **Low blood pressure** (systolic pressure < 90 mm Hg or mean pressure < 60 mm Hg) is caused most commonly by hypovolemia or sudden termination of a drug infusion.

However, the possibility of more critical problems, such as myocardial ischemia, severe myocardial dysfunction, arrhythmias, or ventilatory problems, should always be kept in mind. Low blood pressure may also result from inadequate zeroing of the transducer, or kinking or transient occlusion of the line, producing a dampened tracing. If the transduced blood pressure is low, do the following:

1. Resume manual ventilation and listen for bilateral breath sounds.
2. Palpate the brachial or femoral artery to confirm a pulse and a satisfactory blood pressure. Attach the blood pressure cuff above the radial arterial line site and take an auscultatory or occlusion blood pressure. This is done by inflating the cuff until the arterial tracing is obliterated; when the pressure tracing reappears, the systolic pressure can be read from the sphygmomanometer. **Never assume that a low blood pressure recording is caused by dampening of the arterial line unless a higher pressure can be confirmed by another method.** Insertion of an additional arterial monitoring line (usually in the femoral artery) may be indicated.
3. Make sure that all medication bottles are appropriately labeled and are connected to the patient and infusing at the designated rate through patent intravenous lines. **Note:** If hypotension is present, quickly ascertain whether the patient is receiving nitroglycerin or nitroprusside (in the silver wrapper) because they can lower the blood pressure precipitously. Unless you know how to change the drip rate on the particular drug infusion pump, let someone else who is familiar with it take care of it!
4. Quickly examine the chest tubes for massive mediastinal bleeding. Exsanguinating hemorrhage may require emergency sternotomy.
5. The initial **treatment** for hypotension should include volume infusion and, if there is no immediate response, administration of calcium chloride 500 mg IV. Vasoactive medications may be started or the rate of medications already being used can be adjusted. **If there is no response to these measures and the ECG is abnormal, assume the worst and prepare to treat the patient as an imminent cardiac arrest until the problem is sorted out. If the patient cannot be immediately resuscitated, call for help and prepare for an emergency sternotomy.**

F. An indeterminate or undecipherable **ECG** is usually caused by artifact with jostling or detachment of the ECG leads. If the arterial waveform is normal or the pulse oximeter sounds normal, this is usually the case. However, if the arterial pressure is low or not transduced, the pulse is irregular or slow, or the monitor is difficult to interpret, palpate for a pulse and take the steps mentioned above. **If the blood pressure is undetectable and ECG reading is not available, assume the worst and treat the patient as a cardiac arrest.** Readjust the ECG leads on the patient and monitor. If interpretation remains difficult, attach a standard ECG machine to limb leads to ascertain the rhythm.

1. If ventricular fibrillation or tachycardia is present, immediate defibrillation and a cardiac arrest protocol are indicated (see page 400)
2. If a pacemaker is being used, examine the connections and settings and confirm capture on an ECG.
3. Attach a pacemaker and initiate pacing if bradycardia or heart block is present. Always try to pace the atrium (AOO) or initiate atrioventricular pacing (DDD or DVI) if atrial pacing wires are present and heart block is present. If there is no response, initiate ventricular pacing (VVI). If the patient has a rhythm but the ventricle fails to pace, consider placing a skin wire as a ground, in case one of the wires has been dislodged from the heart.

Box 7.1 • Initial Evaluation of the Patient in the Intensive Care Unit

1. The patient should be examined thoroughly (heart, lungs, peripheral perfusion).
2. Hemodynamic measurements (central venous, pulmonary artery diastolic, pulmonary capillary wedge, and/or left atrial pressures) should be obtained, cardiac output measured, and systemic vascular resistance calculated (see Table 11.1).
3. A portable supine chest x-ray should be obtained. Specific attention should be paid to the position of the endotracheal tube and Swan-Ganz catheter, the width of the mediastinum, and the presence of a pneumothorax, fluid overload, atelectasis, or pleural effusion.
4. A 12-lead ECG should be reviewed for ischemic changes or arrhythmias.
5. Laboratory tests should be drawn (see Box 7.2 for sample admission order sheet).

---

4. Look for the undetected development of atrial fibrillation that can develop during atrioventricular pacing. This may account for a fall in cardiac output and blood pressure despite an adequate ventricular pacing rate.

5. Look for evidence of ischemia or other arrhythmias that may require management.

G. Once the patient's heart rate, rhythm, and blood pressure are found to be satisfactory and adequate ventilation from the ventilator is confirmed, a full report should be given to the ICU staff by the accompanying anesthesiologist and/or surgical house staff. This should include the patient's cardiac disease, comorbidities, operative procedure, intraoperative course, medications being administered, and special instructions for postoperative care. Further assessment as delineated in Box 7.1 can then be carried out to address the subtleties of patient care. A standardized set of preprinted orders that can be adapted to each patient is invaluable for ensuring that no essential elements in early postoperative care are overlooked (Box 7.2).

H. It is very important to review the immediate postoperative chest x-ray to assess the position of the endotracheal tube and make sure that a pneumothorax is not overlooked. In addition, review of an ECG obtained soon after the patient's arrival in the ICU is essential to identify any ischemic changes that might prompt urgent attention.

II. Monitoring in the ICU: Techniques and Problems

Careful monitoring is required in the early postoperative period to optimize clinical management and outcome.[1,2] A continuous display of the ECG is provided and pressures derived from invasive catheters, including arterial and Swan-Ganz catheters placed in the operating room, are transduced on bedside monitors (Figure 7.1). The endotracheal tube is securely connected to the mechanical ventilator and appropriate ventilator settings are selected. A continuous readout of the arterial oxygen saturation (Sao_2) determined by pulse oximetry should be displayed. The drainage outputs of chest tubes and the Foley catheter are measured and recorded. A comprehensive flowsheet, whether handwritten or entered into a computerized system, is essential (Appendix 4).

Box 7.2 • Typical Orders for Admission to the ICU

1. Admit to ICU
2. Procedure: _____
3. Condition: _____
4. Vital signs q15 min until stable, then q30 min
5. Continuous ECG, arterial, PA tracings, Sao_2 on bedside monitor
6. Cardiac output q15 min × 1h, then q1h × 4 h, then q2–4h when stable
7. Chest tubes to chest drainage system with 20 cm H_2O suction; record hourly
8. Urinary catheter to gravity drainage and record hourly
9. Elevate head of bed to 30 degrees
10. Hourly I&O
11. Daily weights
12. Advance activity after extubation (dangle, out of bed to chair)
13. GI/nutrition: □ NPO while intubated
                      □ Nasogastric tube to low suction
                      □ Clear liquids as tolerated 1h after extubation and removal of NG tube
14. Ventilator settings
    Fio_2: _____ in SIMV mode
    IMV rate: _____ breaths/min
    Tidal volume: _____ mL
    PEEP: _____cm H_2O
    Pressure support: ____ cm H_2O
15. Respiratory care
    □ Endotracheal suction q4h, then prn
    □ Wean ventilator to extubate per protocol
    □ O_2 via face mask with Fio_2 0.6–1.0 per protocol
    □ O_2 via nasal prongs @ 2–6 liters/min to keep Sao_2 > 95%
    □ Incentive spirometer q1h when awake
16. Laboratory tests
    □ STAT ABGs, CBC, electrolytes, glucose
    □ STAT PT, PTT, platelet count if chest tube output > 100/h
    □ STAT chest x-ray
    □ STAT ECG
    □ ABGs 4 h after arrival, prior to weaning and prior to extubation
    □ HCT, K^+ every 4–6 h and prn
    □ In morning of POD #1: ECG, CXR, electrolytes, BUN, creatinine, CBC

(*Continued*)

Box 7.2 • (Continued)

17. Pacemaker settings: Mode: □ Atrial □ VVI □ DVI □ DDD
    Atrial output: ___ mA Ventricular output ____ mA
    Rate ___ /min AV interval: ___ /msecs
    □ Pacer attached but off

18. Notify MD/PA for:

    a. Systolic blood pressure <90 or >140 mm Hg
    b. Cardiac index <1.8 liters/min/m²
    c. Urine output <30 mL/h × 2 h
    d. Chest tube drainage >100 mL/h
    e. Temperature >38.5°C

19. Medications

Allergies _____

    a. IV drips
       □ Dextrose 5% in 0.45 NS 250 mL via Cordis/triple lumen at KVO
       □ Arterial line and distal Swan-Ganz port: heparin 250 U/250 mL NS at 3 mL/h
       □ Epinephrine 1 mg/250 mL D5W: _____ µg/min to maintain cardiac index >2.0
       □ Milrinone 20 mg/100 mL NS: _____ µg/kg/min
       □ Norepinephrine 8 mg/250 mL D5W: _____ µg/min to keep systolic BP >100
       □ Phenylephrine 40 mg/250 mL D5W: _____ µg/min to keep systolic BP >100
       □ Nitroprusside 50 mg/250 mL D5W: _____ µg/kg/min to keep systolic BP <130
       □ Nitroglycerin 100 mg/250 mL D5W: _____ µg/kg/min
       □ Lidocaine 2 g/250 mL D5W: _____ mg/min IV; wean off at 06:00 POD #1
       □ Diltiazem: 100 mg/100 mL D5W: _____ mg/h
       □ Other: _____
       □ Other: _____

    b. Antibiotics
       □ Cefazolin 1 g IV q8h for 6 doses
       □ Vancomycin 1 g IV q12h for 4 doses

    c. Sedatives/analgesics
       □ Propofol infusion 10 mg/mL: 25–50 µg/kg/min per protocol
       □ Midazolam 2 mg IV q2h prn agitation; stop after extubation
       □ Morphine sulfate 25 mg/100 mL D5W: 0.01–0.02 mg/kg continuous IV infusion; supplement with 2–5 mg IV q1–2h prn for breakthrough pain; discontinue in AM POD #1
       □ Meperidine 25 mg IV prn shivering
       □ Ketorolac 15–30 mg IV q6h prn for breakthrough pain; d/c after 72 h

(Continued)

Box 7.2 • (Continued)

d. Other medications

☐ Metoprolol 25 mg PO/per NG tube starting 8 h after arrival, then q12h; hold for HR <60 or SBP <100

☐ Digoxin 0.25 mg IV q6h × 2 doses starting 8 h after arrival; then 0.25 mg PO q6h × 2 doses, then 0.25 mg PO qd; hold for HR <60

☐ Magnesium sulfate 2 g IV on POD #1 in AM

☐ Sucralfate 1 g per NG tube q6h until NG tube removed

☐ Pantoprazole (Protonix) 40 mg PO qd

☐ Aspirin ☐ 325 mg ☐ 81 mg PO qd (starting 6 hours after arrival); hold for platelet count <75,000 or chest tube drainage > 50 mL/h

☐ Warfarin _____ mg starting _____ ; check with HO for daily dose

e. PRN medications

☐ Acetaminophen 650 mg PO/PR q4h prn temp > 38.5°C

☐ Droperidol 0.625–1.25 mg IV q6h prn nausea

☐ Ondansetron 4 mg IV prn nausea

☐ KCl 80mEq/250 mL D5W via central line to keep K^+ > 4.5 mEq/liter:

    K^+ 4.0–4.5 KCl 10 mEq over 30 min

    K^+ 3.5–3.9 KCl 20 mEq over 60 min

    K^+ < 3.5   KCl 40 mEq over 90 min

☐ Initiate hyperglycemia protocol if BS > 240 mg/dL on admission or >180 mg/dL 8 h after admission

☐ Other

Each invasive technique is used to provide an essential function or obtain special information about the patient's postoperative course, but each has potential complications. Each should be used only as long as necessary to maximize benefit while minimizing morbidity.

A. **Electrocardiographic display** on a bedside monitor is critical to allow for rapid interpretation of rhythm changes. The use of cartridge modules allows for the simultaneous display and recording of standard limb leads and atrial electrograms for the analysis of complex rhythms (see Chapter 11). Most bedside monitors have a memory, and abnormal rhythms will activate a printout. This is helpful in detecting the mechanism of arrhythmia development (such as an R-on-T phenomenon leading to ventricular tachycardia or fibrillation). ST-segment analysis is provided by most monitoring systems, but abnormalities often must be more thoroughly analyzed from a 12-lead ECG.

B. Mechanical ventilation via an endotracheal tube is used for all patients except those who are extubated in the operating room. The initial settings are determined by the

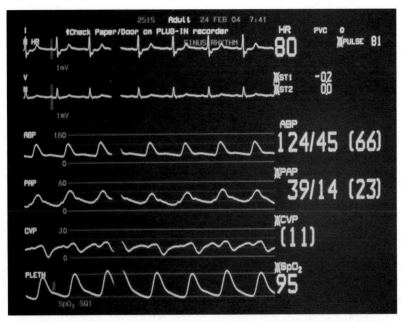

Figure 7.1 • Monitoring in the ICU. From top to bottom: ECG leads, arterial blood pressure (ABP), pulmonary artery systolic/diastolic waveform (PAP), central venous pressure (CVP), and pulse oximetry (SpO_2).

anesthesiologist and respiratory therapist and generally provide a tidal volume of 8–10 mL/kg at a rate of 8–10/min with the initial FIO_2 set at 1.0. Confirmation of bilateral breath sounds and chest movement, intermittent rechecking of ventilator settings, and assessment of the adequacy of gas exchange are essential.

1. **Pulse oximetry** is routinely used to continuously assess the status of peripheral perfusion and arterial oxygen saturation. It can draw attention to major problems with oxygenation during the period of intubation and following extubation.[3] If the patient is severely vasoconstricted, the recordings from the patient's fingers may be inadequate and a better signal may be derived from the earlobe. Use of pulse oximetry obviates the need to draw arterial blood gases more than a few times during the period of intubation. Nonetheless, it should be kept in mind that pulse oximetry provides only the Sao_2 and does not provide the same information as an arterial blood gas (ABG). In addition to a Pao_2, the ABG provides an assessment of Pco_2 and pH that can be important in determining the patient's respiratory drive during the weaning process. Furthermore, an ABG can identify whether the patient has a metabolic or respiratory acidosis/alkalosis. This is particularly valuable in determining when a patient with borderline hemodynamic function has a metabolic acidosis that requires further pharmacologic intervention.

2. Suctioning should be performed gently every few hours or as necessary to maintain a tube free of secretions but not so frequently as to induce endobronchial trauma or bronchospasm.[4] The endotracheal tube bypasses the protective mechanism of

the upper airway and predisposes the patient to pulmonary infection. It should be removed as soon as the patient is maintaining satisfactory ventilation and oxygenation and is able to protect his or her airway. This is generally accomplished within 12 hours of surgery. A standard protocol for weaning and extubation is essential in any cardiac surgical ICU (see Tables 10.4 to 10.6).

C. **Arterial lines** are placed in either the radial or femoral artery and are transduced on the bedside monitor. Accurate pressure recording depends on proper calibration and elimination of air from the transducer. Radial arterial pressure measurements may not reflect the central aortic pressure immediately after bypass, but this problem usually abates by the time the patient reaches the ICU. If a discrepancy persists, placement of a femoral arterial line in the ICU might be necessary. Femoral lines tend to demonstrate comparable mean pressures to radial lines, although they frequently demonstrate systolic overshoot, which can be eliminated by resonance overshoot filters present on most monitors.[5,6]

1. There is often a discrepancy between the auscultatory or occlusion blood pressure and that recorded digitally on the bedside monitor. This may be ascribed to the dynamic response characteristics of catheter-transducer systems.[7] The overdampening of signals usually results from gas bubbles within the fluid-filled system. Underdampening of signals is related to excessive compliance, length, or diameter of the tubing connecting the arterial line to the transducer. If the intraarterial pressure appears to be dampened or exhibits overshoot, the analog display of the mean pressure is most reliable. The occlusion pressure is probably the most accurate measurement of the systolic pressure.

2. Arterial lines should be connected to continuous heparin flushes to improve patency rates and minimize thrombus formation. Maintaining a radial arterial line for more than 3 days is associated with an increased risk of vessel thrombosis and line sepsis.[8] Arterial lines are invaluable for sampling ABGs and obtaining blood for other laboratory tests, but they are often retained when invasive pressure monitoring is no longer essential but intravenous access for blood sampling is limited. Arterial lines should generally be removed when there is no longer a requirement for pharmacologic support and when satisfactory postextubation ABGs have been achieved. A room air blood gas before removal may give a baseline assessment of the patient's oxygenation. If the patient requires continuous arterial pressure monitoring in the ICU, the line should be changed every 4 days. **Note:** If a patient has suggestive evidence of heparin-induced thrombocytopenia but still requires arterial line monitoring, it is important to use saline flushes and eliminate any heparin from the flush lines.

3. Attention must always be directed to perfusion of the hand when a radial arterial line is present. Removal is indicated urgently if hand ischemia develops. Fortunately, the incidence of serious complications associated with radial artery catheterization is extremely low.

D. **Central venous pressure (CVP)** monitoring may provide adequate information about filling pressures in patients with preserved ventricular function.[9,10] Because of the potential complications associated with Swan-Ganz catheters and the failure of multiple studies to document a beneficial impact on surgical outcome,[10–12] monitoring of the CVP can be considered safe and sufficient in managing patients undergoing uneventful, low-risk surgery. Generally, the CVP and the pulmonary artery diastolic

(PAD) pressure correlate fairly well in these patients and can guide fluid management appropriately. However, the decision to use inotropes has to be based on an integration of CVP, blood pressure response to volume, urine output, and clinical exam. One study found little correlation between the physician's or nurse's estimate of cardiac output and the actual output, suggesting that use of α-agents or inotropes may at times be inappropriate, although it may not influence outcome.[13]

E. **Swan-Ganz pulmonary artery catheters** are commonly placed in patients undergoing open-heart surgery to assist with intraoperative and postoperative hemodynamic management. They are valuable in guiding evidence-based, scientific decisions about fluid, inotropic, or vasopressor support, although their impact on clinical outcome may only be evident in high-risk patients. They are generally placed before the induction of anesthesia, but may have to be placed in the ICU when a patient exhibits hemodynamic instability or clinical deterioration. These catheters measure the CVP, PA, and pulmonary capillary wedge pressures indicative of left-sided filling, and allow for the determination of a thermodilution cardiac output. Sampling blood from the PA port allows for measurement of a mixed venous oxygen saturation (Svo_2). Although the correlation of Svo_2 and cardiac output is subject to many variables, the Svo_2 is helpful when the thermodilution output seems inconsistent with the patient's clinical course.[14,15] It is helpful in patients with tricuspid regurgitation in whom the thermodilution cardiac output is inaccurate.[16]

1. Some Swan-Ganz catheters have the capability of providing continuous cardiac output measurements and on-line Svo_2. They are particularly useful in patients undergoing off-pump surgery. Other catheters calculate right ventricular volumes and ejection fraction, while others have additional ports for volume infusions or pacing wires.

2. The proximal port of the Swan-Ganz catheter (30 cm from the tip) is used for CVP measurements from the right atrium and for fluid injections to determine the cardiac output. Care must be exercised when injecting sterile fluid for cardiac outputs to prevent bolusing of vasoactive medications that might be running through the CVP port. **Note:** One must **never** infuse anything through this port if the catheter has been pulled back so that the tip lies in the right atrium!

3. The distal port should always be transduced and displayed on the bedside monitor to allow detection of catheter advancement into the permanent wedge position, which could result in pulmonary artery injury. This will be detected by loss of the phasic PA trace on the monitor and is also suggested by the position of the catheter on a chest x-ray. Balloon inflation ("wedging" of the catheter) need not be performed more than once every few hours and the balloon should not be inflated for more than two respiratory cycles to prevent PA injury. Balloon inflation should be performed cautiously with minimal inflation volume or should be avoided entirely in patients with pulmonary hypertension. Medications should never be given through the distal PA port.

4. Although there is a significant incidence of minor complications associated with the insertion and use of the Swan-Ganz catheter, serious life-threatening complications are very uncommon.[17] The catheter is more commonly placed through the internal jugular vein than the subclavian vein for cardiac surgery. The former is more likely to be associated with arterial puncture, but less likely to result in catheter malposition.[18,19]

   a. Complications associated with insertion include:
   - Arrhythmias and heart block (especially in patients with bifascicular block)
   - Arterial puncture
   - Pneumothorax
   - Air embolism
   - Catheter knotting
   b. Complications of indwelling PA catheters include:
   - Arrhythmias and heart block
   - Heparin-induced thrombocytopenia (from heparin-coated catheters)
   - Infection
   - Pulmonary artery rupture and hemorrhage
   - Endocardial and valvular damage
   - Pulmonary infarction
   - Pulmonary infiltrates
   - Venous thrombosis

5. **Pulmonary artery perforation** is a very serious complication.[20] It may occur during insertion of the catheter, during surgery, or at any time in the ICU. The position of the catheter should always be inspected on an immediate postoperative or any postinsertion chest x-ray. Migration of the catheter into wedge position should be noted on the bedside monitor and the catheter should be pulled back immediately. Perforation may lead to hemoptysis, bleeding into the endotracheal tube, or intrapleural hemorrhage. The chest x-ray may demonstrate a hematoma surrounding the tip of the catheter. If perforation is suspected, the catheter should be withdrawn and positive end-expiratory pressure added to the ventilator circuit. If bleeding persists, bronchoscopy can be performed with placement of a bronchial blocker to isolate the lung. Use of a double-lumen endotracheal tube or even a thoracotomy with pulmonary resection may be indicated for ongoing pulmonary hemorrhage. Rarely, a false aneurysm of the pulmonary artery branches may develop. This can be managed by transcatheter embolization.[21]

6. The PA catheter should be removed when the patient no longer requires vasoactive drug support. If the catheter is removed but the introducer sheath is left in place for fluid or medication administration, the port must be covered with a small adhesive drape to minimize the risk of infection. A one-way valve present on most introducer sheaths eliminates the possibility of air embolism. The introducer should be removed as soon as possible because of its size and the attendant risk of infection and venous thrombosis (let alone patient discomfort). If less intensive central venous monitoring is required or venous access is limited, a smaller double- or triple-lumen catheter should replace the large-bore introducer.

7. **Alternative means of assessing cardiac output** (see also page 342). Although the Swan-Ganz catheter is the gold standard for measurement of cardiac output, it is an invasive catheter associated with a number of potential complications. Alternative less invasive means of determining the cardiac output have been developed, including esophageal Doppler, thoracic bioimpedance, and pulse contour analysis, which provide comparable cardiac output measurements to thermodilution.[22-26] The esophageal Doppler provides Doppler flow velocity waveforms that include flow time and peak velocity. These waveforms allow for assessment of left ventricular contractility, filling, and systemic vascular resistance (Figure 7.2).[22-26]

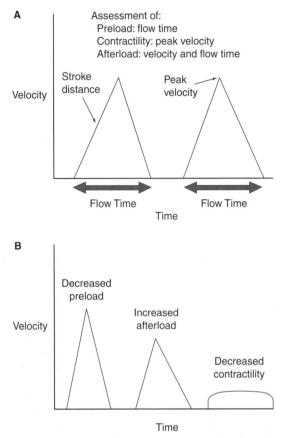

Figure 7.2 • Doppler flow waveforms obtained with the esophageal Doppler. (A) A normal waveform. Preload is estimated by the flow time, contractility by the peak velocity, and afterload (systemic resistance) by both the velocity and flow time. (B) Waveforms that are associated with decreased preload, increased afterload, or decreased contractility. These conditions can be improved by volume infusions, vasodilators, and inotropes, respectively.

F. **Left atrial (LA) lines** are used in special circumstances, such as severe left ventricular dysfunction, severe pulmonary hypertension secondary to mitral valve disease, use of circulatory assist devices, or heart transplantation. They are placed through the right superior pulmonary vein and passed into the left atrium during surgery. These lines are helpful in providing important hemodynamic information in these patients and are associated with infrequent but potentially significant complications.[27]

1. LA lines provide the most accurate assessment of left-sided filling pressures, especially when a high transpulmonary gradient is present. This is most helpful in patients with biventricular assist devices to assess the degree of left-sided filling.

2. An LA line should always be considered dangerous because of the risk of air embolism.[28] It must always be aspirated before being flushed to make sure there is no air or thrombus present within the system. It is then connected to a constant

infusion flush line that includes an air filter to reduce the risk of systemic air embolism. The line should be removed when the chest tubes are still in place in the event that bleeding from the insertion site should occur.

G. **Chest tubes** are placed in the mediastinum and into the pleural spaces if they are entered during surgery. Drainage should be recorded hourly or more frequently if there is evidence of significant bleeding.

1. The chest tubes are connected to a drainage system to which 20 cm of H_2O suction is applied. The tubes should be gently milked or stripped to prevent blood clotting within them. There is no particular advantage of any of the common practices (milking, stripping, fanfolding, or tapping) to maintain chest tube patency.[29,30] Aggressive stripping creates a negative pressure of up to -300 cm H_2O in the mediastinum. This may actually increase bleeding and is quite painful to the patient who has regained consciousness and is not adequately sedated. Suctioning of clotted chest tubes with endotracheal suction catheters should be discouraged because of the risk of introducing infection.

2. Bloody drainage through chest tubes can be best observed if the tubes are not completely covered with tape. Plastic connectors must be tightly and securely attached to both the chest tubes and the drainage tubing to maintain sterility and prevent air leaks within the system.

3. Excessive mediastinal bleeding requires immediate attention because it often leads to hemodynamic instability, metabolic acidosis, the requirement for multiple blood products, and, potentially, cardiac tamponade (see Chapter 9).

4. A variety of collection systems are available for autotransfusion of shed mediastinal blood. Blood may be reinfused from soft plastic collection bags or directly from the plastic shell via a pump and a 20–40 µm filter. This blood has low levels of platelets, fibrinogen, and factor VIII with high levels of fibrin split products. Autotransfused blood can provide some red cell salvage and act as a volume expander in the bleeding patient, but its use is somewhat cumbersome and its benefits controversial. Studies have shown that autotransfusion is not cost-effective when less than 250 mL is transfused. Reinfusion of moderate volumes (500–1000 mL) reduces transfusion requirements without significantly altering coagulation parameters. However, reinfusion of greater amounts should be avoided since it can perpetuate a coagulopathy. Generally, if a patient bleeds more than 1000 mL within the first 3–4 hours of surgery, reexploration is indicated.[31–33]

H. The **urinary Foley catheter** is attached to gravity drainage and the urine output is recorded hourly. Urine output is an excellent measure of myocardial function although it is subject to many variables.

1. Foley catheters incorporating temperature probes are commonly used during surgery and can be used in the ICU to record the patient's core temperature.

2. The Foley catheter is usually removed on the second postoperative morning. It may be left in place if the patient is undergoing a significant diuresis or has a history of prostatic hypertrophy or urinary retention and has not been mobilized. The risk of urinary infection increases as the duration of indwelling catheter time lengthens, and early removal should be considered in patients with prosthetic valves and grafts when its use is no longer essential.

3. Suprapubic tubes should be left in place and clamped after several days to see if the patient can void per urethra.

I. **Nasogastric tubes** may be inserted in the operating room or after the patient's arrival in the ICU to aid with gastric decompression. Insertion may cause hypertension, bradycardia, tachycardia, or arrhythmias if the patient is not well sedated. Additional sedation may be required if insertion is difficult. Insertion may also cause nasopharyngeal bleeding if the patient is still heparinized (during surgery) or has a coagulopathy. Instillation of medication to reduce stress ulceration, such as sucralfate, should be considered for all patients for the first 12–24 hours. This is as efficacious as the H_2 blockers and proton pump inhibitors, both of which raise gastric pH. One could consider the supplemental use of a proton pump inhibitor if the patient is at extremely high risk for stress ulcer–related bleeding.[34–36]

J. **Pacing wires.** Most surgeons place two atrial and two ventricular temporary epicardial pacing wire electrodes at the conclusion of open-heart surgery. If the pacing wires are being used, they must be securely attached to the patient and to the cable connector, and the cable must be securely attached to the pacing box. The pacemaker box itself should be easily accessible. **Everyone caring for the patient should understand how the particular pacemaker generator works.** Pacing wires that are not being used should be placed in insulating needle caps to isolate them from stray electrical currents that could potentially trigger arrhythmias.

III. Summary of Guidelines for Removal of Lines and Tubes in the ICU

A. The Swan-Ganz catheter should be removed when inotropic support and vasodilators are no longer necessary. If central venous access is required after several days but hemodynamic monitoring is no longer essential, the Swan-Ganz catheter should be replaced by a double- or triple-lumen catheter.

B. Any central line should be removed when no longer necessary to reduce the risk of infection. The literature suggests that the catheter need only be replaced for a clinical indication, such as a fever of unknown origin or suspected bacteremia. If the catheter site is infected or bacteremia is confirmed, the catheter should be withdrawn and another inserted at a different site. If neither of these indications is present, the catheter can be changed over a guidewire to reduce the risk of mechanical complications associated with a new insertion site. The catheter tip is cultured. If this returns positive, the catheter should be changed to a new site.[18, 37,38]

C. The arterial line should be removed after a stable postextubation blood gas has been obtained. An additional ABG obtained on room air is frequently worthwhile because it provides a relative indication of the patient's baseline postoperative oxygenation. The arterial line should not be left in place for more than 3 days as a convenience for blood sampling.

D. Left atrial lines must be removed in the ICU while the chest tubes remain in place in the event that intrapericardial bleeding should occur.

E. The urinary catheter can be left in place if the patient is undergoing a vigorous diuresis or has an increased risk of urinary retention. It should otherwise be removed once the patient is mobilized out of bed, usually on the second postoperative day.

F. Chest tubes should be removed when the total drainage is less than 100 mL for 8 hours. Prolonging the duration of drainage may increase total chest tube output without any effect on the incidence of postoperative pericardial effusions.[39] One study showed that there was no difference in the incidence of pericardial effusions if tubes were withdrawn when drainage was less than 50 mL over 5 hours or when the fluid became serosanguineous (either upon visual inspection or when the drain/blood hematocrit ratio was < 0.3).[40] In contrast to the standard 32F chest tubes that are commonly used, small Silastic (Blake) drains may be placed in the mediastinum or into the pleural space and provide comparable drainage efficiency. However, they are more comfortable for the patient.[41–43] Leaving a supplemental drain in the pleural space for 3–5 days is useful in reducing the incidence of symptomatic pleural effusions.[44] Mediastinal tubes should always be removed off suction because graft avulsion might theoretically occur if suction is maintained. Chest radiography is not essential after mediastinal tube removal but should be performed after removal of pleural chest tubes to rule out a pneumothorax.

References

1. Wiedemann HP, Matthay MA, Matthay RA. Cardiovascular-pulmonary monitoring in the intensive care unit (Part 1). Chest 1984;85:537–49.

2. Wiedemann HP, Matthay MA, Matthay RA. Cardiovascular-pulmonary monitoring in the intensive care unit (Part 2). Chest 1984;85:656–68.

3. Bierman MI, Stein KL, Snyder JV. Pulse oximetry in the postoperative care of cardiac surgical patients. A randomized controlled trial. Chest 1992;102:1367–70.

4. Guglielminotti J, Desmonts JM, Dureuil B. Effects of tracheal suctioning on respiratory resistances in mechanically ventilated patients. Chest 1999;113:1135–8.

5. Gravlee GP, Wong AB, Adkins TG, Case LD, Pauca AL. A comparison of radial, brachial, and aortic pressures after cardiopulmonary bypass. J Cardiothorac Anesth 1989;3:20–6.

6. Thrush DN, Steighner ML, Rasanen J, Vijayanagar R. Blood pressure after cardiopulmonary bypass: which technique is accurate? J Cardiothorac Vasc Anesth 1994;8:269–72.

7. Gibbs NC, Gardner RM. Dynamics of invasive pressure monitoring systems: clinical and laboratory evaluation. Heart Lung 1988;17:43–51.

8. Martin C, Saux P, Papazian L, Gouin F. Long term arterial cannulation in ICU patients using the radial artery or dorsalis pedis artery. Chest 2001;119:901–6.

9. Stewart RD, Psyhojos T, Lahey SJ, Levitsky S, Campos CT. Central venous catheter use in low-risk coronary artery bypass grafting. Ann Thorac Surg 1998;66:1306–11.

10. Schwann TA, Zacharias A, Riordan CJ, Durham SJ, Engoren M, Habib RH. Safe, highly selective use of pulmonary artery catheters in coronary artery bypass grafting; an objective patient selection method. Ann Thorac Surg 2002;73:1394–1402.

11. Ramsey SD, Saint S, Sullivan SD, Dey L Kelley K, Bowdle A. Clinical and economic effects of pulmonary artery catheterization in nonemergent coronary artery bypass graft surgery. J Cardiothorac Vasc Anesth 2000;14:113–8.

12. Tuman KJ, McCarthy RJ, Spiess BD, et al. Effect of pulmonary artery catheterization on outcome in patients undergoing coronary artery surgery. Anesthesiology 1989;70:199–206.

13. Linton RAF, Linton NWF, Kelly F. Is clinical assessment of the circulation reliable in postoperative cardiac surgical patients? J Cardiothorac Vasc Anesth 2002;16:4–7.

14. Sommers MS, Stevenson JS, Hamlin RL, Ivey TD, Russell AC. Mixed venous oxygen saturation and oxygen partial pressure as predictors of cardiac index after coronary artery bypass grafting. Heart Lung 1993;22:112–20.

15. Magilligan DJ Jr, Teasdall R, Eisinminger R, Peterson E. Mixed venous oxygen saturation as a predictor of cardiac output in the postoperative cardiac surgical patient. Ann Thorac Surg 1987;44:260–2.

16. Balik K, Pachl J, Hendl J, Martin B, Jan P, Jan H. Effect of the degree of tricuspid regurgitation on cardiac output measurements by thermodilution. Intensive Care Med 2002;28:1117–21.

17. Shah KB, Rao TLK, Laughlin S, El-Etr AA. A review of pulmonary artery catheterization in 6,245 patients. Anesthesiology 1984;61:271–5.

18. McGee DC, Gould MK. Preventing complications of central venous catheterization. N Engl J Med 2003;348:1123–33.

19. Ruesch S, Walder B, Tramer MR. Complications of central venous catheters: internal jugular versus subclavian access: a systematic review. Crit Care Med 2002;30:454–60.

20. Mullerworth MH, Angelopoulos P, Couyant MA, et al. Recognition and management of catheter-induced pulmonary artery rupture. Ann Thorac Surg 1998;66:1242–5.

21. Karak P, Dimick R, Hamrick KM, Schwartzberg M, Saddekni S. Immediate transcatheter embolization of Swan-Ganz catheter–induced pulmonary artery pseudoaneurysm. Chest 1997;111:1450–2.

22. DiCorte CJ, Latham P, Greilich PE, Cooley MV, Grayburn PA, Jessen ME. Esophageal Doppler monitor determinations of cardiac output and preload during cardiac operations. Ann Thorac Surg 2000;69:1782–6.

23. Gan TJ. The esophageal Doppler as an alternative to the pulmonary artery catheter. Curr Opin Crit Care 2000;6:214–21.

24. Botero M, Lobato EB. Advances in noninvasive cardiac output monitoring: an update. J Cardiothorac Vasc Anesth 2001;15:631–40.

25. Poeze M, Ramsay G, Greve JWM, Singer M. Prediction of postoperative cardiac surgical morbidity and organ failure within 4 hours of intensive care unit admission using esophageal Doppler ultrasonography. Crit Care Med 1999;27:1288–94.

26. Bein B, Worthmann F, Tonner PH, et al. Comparison of esophageal Doppler, pulse contour analysis, and real-time pulmonary artery thermodilution for the continuous measurement of cardiac output. J Cardiothorac Vasc Anesth 2004;18:185–9.

27. Santini F, Gatti G, Borghetti V, Oppido G, Mazzucco A. Routine left atrial catheterization for the post-operative management of cardiac surgical patients: is the risk justified? Eur J Cardiothorac Surg 1999;16:218–21.

28. Feerick AE, Church JA, Zwischenberger J, Conti V, Johnston WE. Systemic gaseous microembolism during left atrial catheterization: a common occurrence? J Cardiothorac Vasc Anesth 1995;9:395–8.

29. Wallen M, Morrison A, Gillies D, O'Riordan E, Bridge C, Stoddard F. Mediastinal chest drain clearance for cardiac surgery. Cochrane Database Syst Rev 2002;2:CD003042.

30. Charnock Y, Evans D. Nursing management of chest drains: a systematic review. Aust Crit Care 2001;14:156–60.

31. Axford TC, Dearani JA, Ragno G, et al. Safety and therapeutic effectiveness of reinfused shed blood after open heart surgery. Ann Thorac Surg 1994;57:615–22.

32. Vertrees RA, Conti VR, Lick SD, Zwischenberger JB, McDaniel LB, Schulman G. Adverse effects of postoperative infusion of shed mediastinal blood. Ann Thorac Surg 1996;62:717–23.

33. Hartz RS, Smith JA, Green D. Autotransfusion after cardiac operation. Assessment of hemostatic factors. J Thorac Cardiovasc Surg 1988;96:178–82.

34. Steinberg KP. Stress-related mucosal disease in the critically ill patient: risk factors and strategies to prevent stress-related bleeding in the intensive care unit. Crit Care Med 2002;30(6 suppl):S362–4.

35. Yang YX, Lewis JD. Prevention and treatment of stress ulcers in critically ill patients. Semin Gastrointest Dis 2003;14:11–19.

36. Jung R, MacLaren R. Proton-pump inhibitors for stress ulcer prophylaxis in critically ill patients. Ann Pharmacother 2002;36:1929–37.

37. Cobb DK, High KP, Sawyer RG, et al. A controlled trial of scheduled replacement of central venous and pulmonary-artery catheters. N Engl J Med 1992;327:1062–8.

38. Hagley MT, Martin B, Gast P, Traeger SM. Infectious and mechanical complications of central venous catheters placed by percutaneous venipuncture and over guidewires. Crit Care Med 1992;20:1426–30.

39. Smulders YM, Wiepking ME, Moulijn AC, et al. How soon should drainage tubes be removed after cardiac operations? Ann Thorac Surg 1989;48:540–3.

40. Gercekoglu H, Aydin NB, Dagdeviren B, et al. Effect of timing of chest tube removal on development of pericardial effusion following cardiac surgery. J Card Surg 2003;18:217–24.

41. Obney JA, Barnes MJ, Lisagor PG, Cohen DJ. A method for mediastinal drainage after cardiac procedures using small silastic drains. Ann Thorac Surg 2000;70:1109–10.

42. Frankel TL, Hill PC, Stamou SC, et al. Silastic drains vs conventional chest tubes after coronary artery bypass. Chest 2003;124:108–13.

43. Lancey RA, Gaca C, Vander Salm TJ. The use of smaller, more flexible chest drains following open-heart surgery: an initial evaluation. Chest 2001:119:19–24.

44. Payne M, Magovern GJ Jr, Benckart DH, et al. Left pleural effusion after coronary artery bypass decreases with a supplemental pleural drain. Ann Thorac Surg 2002;73:149–52.

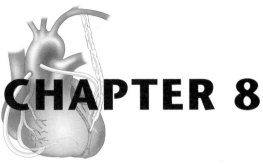

CHAPTER 8

Early Postoperative Care

Early Postoperative Care

The early postoperative course for most patients undergoing cardiac surgery with use of cardiopulmonary bypass (CPB) is characterized by a typical pattern of pathophysiologic derangements that benefits from standardized management.[1] Anesthetic techniques and early postoperative protocols should be designed to achieve early extubation and "fast-track" recovery of most patients (Table 8.1).[2] The pathophysiology noted after off-pump surgery is slightly different in that patients are not subjected to the insults of CPB and cardioplegia, two factors that contribute to a systemic inflammatory response and transient myocardial depression. This chapter will summarize the basic clinical features of the post-CPB patient and will then present scenarios commonly seen in the early postoperative period. It will then discuss aspects of postoperative care unique to various types of cardiac surgical procedures. The subsequent chapters will describe in greater detail the assessment and management of the major concerns of the postoperative period: mediastinal bleeding, respiratory, cardiovascular, renal, and metabolic problems.

I. Basic Features of the Early Postoperative Period

A. Overview

1. Patients are commonly mildly hypothermic and fully anesthetized upon arrival in the ICU, requiring full mechanical ventilation for several hours. Adequate pain control is essential at this time and during the weaning process from the ventilator, which generally should be started once standard criteria are met (see Box 10.2).

2. Inotropic support may be required to terminate CPB and is usually maintained for at least 6–8 hours to optimize cardiac output as the heart recovers from the insult imposed by ischemia and reperfusion associated with cardioplegic arrest.

3. Urine output is usually copious because of hemodilution during surgery. However, even though the patient is total body fluid overloaded, fluid administration is usually necessary to maintain intravascular volume to optimize hemodynamic status. Hypokalemia associated with excellent urine output must be monitored and managed. Renal function is a good marker of hemodynamic function, although it is subject to numerous variables.

4. Patients may have mediastinal bleeding as a result of technical problems or a coagulopathy.

5. Postoperative care requires an integration of a myriad of hemodynamic measurements and other laboratory tests to ensure a swift and uneventful recovery from surgery. Use of a comprehensive flowsheet is essential in evaluating the patient's course in the ICU (Appendix 4).

B. Warming from hypothermia to 37°C

1. CPB is usually accompanied by moderate systemic hypothermia to 32–34°C and is terminated after the patient has been rewarmed to a core body temperature of at least 36°C. Although it is common practice to warm patients to 37°C before

Table 8.1 • Options for a Fast-Track Protocol

Operating Room	
Anesthetic agents	Sufentanil 0.5 µg/kg for induction, then 0.25 µg/kg/h Fentanyl 5–10 µg/kg, then 0.3–5 µg/kg/h or inhalational agents + propofol Remifentanil 1 µg/kg for induction, then 0.05–2 µg/kg/min
Sedatives	Midazolam 2.5–5 mg before bypass Propofol 50–75 µg/kg/min (2–10 mg/kg/h) after bypass
Cardiopulmonary bypass	Withdrawal of autologous blood before starting bypass Consider retrograde autologous priming to maintain higher hematocrit Echo imaging for aortic atherosclerosis Maintain blood sugar < 180 mg/dL Consider fenoldopam if renal dysfunction Warm to 37°C before terminating bypass
Myocardial protection	Antegrade/retrograde blood cardioplegia with terminal "hot shot"
Antifibrinolytic agents	ε-aminocaproic acid 5 g at skin incision and in pump prime, and 1 g/h infusion Aprotinin 280 mg at skin incision and in pump prime, and 70 mg/h
Fluids	Minimize fluid administration
Other medications	Methylprednisolone 1 g before bypass, then dexamethasone 4 mg q6h × 4
Intensive Care Unit	
Analgesia	Morphine infusion 0.01–0.02 mg/kg/h depending on age Ketorolac 15–30 mg IV after extubation PCA pump with morphine on POD #1
Anxiolysis	Propofol 25 µg/kg/min
Shivering	Meperidine 25–50 mg IV
Hypertension	Sodium nitroprusside/esmolol (avoid sedatives)
Anemia	Tolerate hematocrit of 22% if stable
Medications	Metoprolol by POD #1 (AF prophylaxis) Magnesium sulfate 2 g on POD #1 (AF prophylaxis) Consider amiodarone for AF prophylaxis Metoclopramide 10 mg tid

POD = postoperative day

terminating bypass, this may require higher arterial inflow temperatures and may be associated with impairment in neurocognitive function.[3,4] In fact, studies have shown that the brain temperature is several degrees warmer than the nasopharyngeal temperature, suggesting that temperatures measured at other sites may underestimate the degree of cerebral hyperthermia.[5] Even the rectum or bladder, two commonly monitored sites considered to represent the core temperature, are in an "intermediate compartment" where the temperature is close but not identical to core temperature. Thus, although hypothermia has potential adverse effects, aggressive "overwarming" during CPB may also prove detrimental.

2. Despite adequate core rewarming on pump, progressive hypothermia may ensue in the postpump period when the chest is still open and hemostasis is being achieved ("afterdrop"). This results from insufficient rewarming of peripheral tissues that leaves a significant temperature gradient between core temperature and the periphery. Thus, heat is subsequently redistributed to the periphery resulting in a gradual reduction in core temperature. Heat loss is further exacerbated by continued intraoperative heat loss from exposure to cool ambient temperatures, poor peripheral perfusion, and by anesthetic-induced inhibition of normal thermoregulatory control.[6] Even with normothermic bypass, active warming is usually required to maintain patients at temperatures greater than 35°C on CPB, and even these patients may cool down several degrees. Progressive intraoperative cooling is of particular concern with off-pump surgery (see page 165). Consequently, patients usually arrive in the ICU with core temperatures around 35°C.

3. Prevention of afterdrop can be achieved by prolonging the warming phase on CPB, warming the periphery, or using pharmacologic vasodilatation. Since most heat loss during surgery occurs by convection from the anterior surface of the body, use of warm heating coils placed posteriorly has only marginal benefit in preventing heat loss. The Arctic Sun temperature-controlling system has been used during off-pump surgery to provide more circumferential coverage.[7] Intraoperative use of a cutaneous forced-air warming device, such as the Bair Hugger, is also useful in preventing afterdrop, although it does not reduce redistribution of heat.[8] Sodium nitroprusside has been successful in reducing postbypass afterdrop because it produces peripheral vasodilatation and improves peripheral perfusion. However, this benefit is usually noticed only in patients cooled to less than 32°C.[8–10]

4. Hypothermia (< 36°C) upon admission to the ICU has been associated with adverse outcome.[11] Thus, hypothermia must be treated in the ICU to avoid potential adverse effects.[12] Hypothermia may:

    a. Predispose to atrial and ventricular arrhythmias and lower the ventricular fibrillation threshold.

    b. Increase systemic vascular resistance (SVR) and cause hypertension. This may contribute to increased mediastinal bleeding; it raises afterload and myocardial oxygen demand, potentially depressing contractility and cardiac output; and it may elevate filling pressures and mask hypovolemia by producing peripheral vasoconstriction.

    c. Precipitate shivering, which increases peripheral O_2 consumption and CO_2 production.[13,14]

    d. Produce platelet dysfunction and a generalized impairment of the coagulation cascade.[15]

    e. Prolong the time to extubation.

5. In the ICU, most patients are peripherally vasoconstricted as a compensatory mechanism to provide core warming. Pharmacologic vasodilatation with medications such as nitroprusside or propofol may facilitate the redistribution of core heat to peripheral tissues and improve tissue perfusion, but at the same time, they may delay central warming because peripheral vasodilatation augments heat loss. The adjunctive use of warming blankets and radiant heating hoods is thus quite beneficial in minimizing peripheral heat loss, although they do not directly promote core warming. Generally, forced-air warming systems (such as the Bair Hugger system) or a conductive electric overblanket are more effective than "space blankets" in limiting the duration of postoperative hypothermia, thus reducing shivering and oxygen consumption and expediting early extubation.[16–18]

6. Other measures, such as heating intravenous fluids or using heated humidifiers in the ventilator circuit, are of some benefit in preventing progressive hypothermia, but generally do not contribute to warming.

7. Shivering is associated with hypothermia and increases oxygen consumption and patient discomfort. Control of shivering is important in the postoperative period and is best controlled with meperidine (25 mg), which has specific antishivering properties related to several possible mechanisms.[13] Other medications that have been shown to be of benefit in controlling shivering include dexmedetomidine,[19] clonidine 150 µg, ketanserin 10 mg, and doxapram 100 mg.[20] Propofol reduces total body oxygen consumption and may also reduce shivering. [21]

8. Occasionally a patient may rapidly rewarm to 37°C and then "overwarm" to higher temperatures due to resetting of the central thermoregulating system. Narcotics, but not propofol, tend to increase the core temperature required for sweating and may contribute to this problem.[22,23] Since warming may lead to profound peripheral vasodilatation and hypotension, gradual vasodilatation with nitroprusside and concomitant volume infusion can minimize this problem (see postoperative scenarios III.A and III.B).

C. **Control of mediastinal bleeding** (see Chapter 9)
1. Numerous factors may predispose to mediastinal bleeding following CPB.[24] These include residual heparin effect, thrombocytopenia and platelet dysfunction, clotting factor depletion, fibrinolysis, poor surgical technique, hypothermia, and postoperative hypertension.

2. Nearly all cardiac surgical services use one of the antifibrinolytic medications (aprotinin, ε-aminocaproic acid, or tranexamic acid) to reduce intraoperative bleeding.[25] These medications not only inhibit fibrinolysis but, to varying degrees, also preserve platelet function. Thus, intra- and postoperative bleeding have become relatively uncommon problems. Nonetheless, use of these medications is not a substitute for careful hemostasis in the operating room.

3. Careful monitoring of the extent of postoperative bleeding dictates the aggressiveness with which bleeding should be managed. Many patients with "nonsurgical" causes will drain about 100 mL/h for several hours before bleeding eventually tapers. A faster rate of bleeding without evidence of diminution requires systematic evaluation and treatment (often prompting reexploration) as described in Chapter 9.

4. Recognition of the early signs of cardiac tamponade and the importance of prompt mediastinal exploration for severe bleeding or tamponade are critical to improving patient outcome.

D. **Ventilatory support**, emergence from anesthesia, weaning, and extubation (see Chapter 10)

1. Although patients can be extubated in the operating room using short-acting medications, most centers use narcotic-based anesthesia for cardiac surgery that leaves the patient sedated upon arrival in the ICU, requiring mechanical ventilation for a short period. The initial inspired oxygen tension of 1.0 is gradually weaned to below 0.5 as long as the Pao_2 remains above 80 torr or the arterial oxygen saturation (Sao_2) exceeds 95%. The respiratory rate or tidal volume of the mechanical ventilator is adjusted to accommodate the increased CO_2 production that occurs with warming, awakening, and shivering.

2. Oxygenation is influenced by the patient's baseline pulmonary status, hemodynamic performance, the use and duration of CPB, and the amount of fluid administered during surgery. CPB is associated with a "capillary leak" that is produced by the various vasoactive substances released during extracorporeal circulation, and this results in increased interstitial lung water. Various measures can be used in the operating room to optimize postoperative pulmonary function. Minimizing the positive fluid balance during surgery is a major factor that improves the likelihood of successful early extubation and fosters a faster recovery from surgery.[26] Use of a centrifugal pump, membrane oxygenator, heparin-coated circuit, aprotinin, steroids, and/or leukocyte filters during CPB may reduce the systemic inflammatory response and contribute to a faster convalescence.[27]

3. Early extubation (within 8–12 hours) is feasible in most patients, but depends on the anesthetic agents used during surgery, medications given in the ICU, the patient's age and comorbid factors, the extent of the operative procedure, and the patient's hemodynamic performance.[2,28] Low-dose fentanyl or other shorter-acting narcotics (sufentanil, alfentanil, remifentanil) allow patients to awaken more readily.[29–31] Amnestic agents with long half-lives, such as midazolam, are given only in the prebypass period, and short-acting drugs, such as propofol, are commonly given after bypass and continued into the early postoperative period. Although patients can be extubated fairly promptly by pharmacologic reversal of neuromuscular blockade, most centers prefer to observe the patient for a few hours in the ICU and then consider weaning once the patient is stable. If the patient develops hypertension during awakening, antihypertensive medications, such as nitroprusside, should be used, rather than sedatives.

4. As long as certain criteria are met (see Table 10.1), there is no reason to exclude elderly patients or even those with impaired ventricular function or significant comorbidities from a protocol of early extubation. Even if it takes a few hours longer to extubate these patients than younger healthier ones, the benefits of early extubation usually translate into a quicker recovery from surgery. Generally patients are more alert at an earlier stage of recovery, capable of being mobilized by the first postoperative day, and discharged routinely by the fourth day after uneventful and sometimes complex surgery.[32]

E. **Analgesia and sedation**

1. An essential element of postoperative care is the provision of adequate analgesia and sedation.[33,34] Unless extubated in the operating room, the patient will arrive in the ICU anesthetized from the residual effects of anesthetic agents, which also provide some element of analgesia. When early extubation is anticipated, short-acting

medications should be used to provide relief from pain and anxiety while minimizing respiratory depression. Small doses of narcotics may be given along with low-dose propofol. Just before the propofol is discontinued, a nonsteroidal antiinflammatory medication, such as indomethacin 50 mg PR or diclofenac 75 mg PR, can be given to provide analgesia.[35,36]

2. Rather than administering boluses of narcotics, an alternative protocol is to provide a continuous infusion of low-dose morphine sulfate (0.02 mg/kg/h for patients under age 65 and 0.01 mg/kg/h for patients over age 65). This usually produces minimal respiratory depression and can be continued after extubation. If the patient remains overly sedated, the infusion rate can be decreased. Alternatively, an infusion of dexmedetomidine can be used to provide anxiolysis and analgesia and allow for a reduction in the dosage of other drugs. It can be continued after the patient is extubated.[37]

3. Breakthrough pain in intubated patients may be treated with small additional doses of IV morphine or IV ketorolac (15–30 mg). Following extubation, the IV morphine infusion can be continued until the patient is transferred out of the ICU. Many patients benefit from morphine delivered by a patient-controlled analgesia (PCA) pump on the first postoperative day, although use of IV ketorolac (15–30 mg q6h for a maximum of 72 hours) may be sufficient.[38] If delayed extubation is anticipated, such as when significant inotropic support or an IABP is required, a longer-acting sedative, such as midazolam, can be combined with morphine. If more prolonged ventilation is likely, an infusion of fentanyl can provide both sedation and analgesia.

F. **Hemodynamic support** during a period of transient myocardial depression (see Chapter 11)[39]

1. Myocardial function is temporarily depressed as the heart recovers from the period of ischemia and reperfusion. Hypothermia and elevated levels of catecholamines lead to an increase in SVR and systemic hypertension, which increase afterload and depress myocardial performance.

2. Serial assessments of filling pressures, cardiac output, and SVR allow for the appropriate selection of fluids, inotropes, and/or vasodilators to optimize preload, afterload, and contractility to provide hemodynamic support during this period of temporary myocardial depression. The objective is to maintain a cardiac index above 2.2 L/min/m^2 with a stable blood pressure (systolic 100–130 mm Hg or a mean pressure of 80–90 mm Hg). Adequate tissue oxygenation is the primary goal of hemodynamic management and can be assessed by measuring the mixed venous O_2 saturation (Svo_2) from the pulmonary artery port of the Swan-Ganz catheter (normal >65%).

3. Atrial or atrioventricular pacing at a rate of 90–100/min is commonly required at the conclusion of surgery to achieve optimal hemodynamics. This is especially true in patients taking β-blockers before surgery.

4. Monitoring of serial hematocrits is important to ensure the adequacy of tissue oxygen delivery. The hematocrit may be influenced by hemodilution or mediastinal bleeding and should generally be maintained at a level greater than 22–24%. In elderly or critically ill patients, transfusion to a higher level should be considered, weighing the potential benefits and risks of transfusion.

G. **Fluid administration** to maintain filling pressures in the presence of a capillary leak and vasodilatation (see Chapter 12)

1. Following CPB, the patient will be total body salt and water overloaded and should theoretically be aggressively diuresed. However, the use of CPB results in a "systemic inflammatory response" that produces a capillary leak. Furthermore, peripheral vasoconstriction masks intravascular hypovolemia despite adequate left-heart filling pressures.

2. Fluid resuscitation is therefore necessary to offset the capillary leak and the vasodilatation caused by numerous medications and warming to normothermia. Crystalloid and colloid infusions are used to maintain intravascular volume, although this usually occurs at the expense of expansion of the interstitial space.[40,41] After the capillary leak has ceased and hemodynamics have stabilized, the patient may be aggressively diuresed to eliminate the excessive salt and water administered during surgery and the early postoperative period.

H. Monitoring of serum potassium and glucose is essential in the early postoperative period. Potassium levels may be elevated from cardioplegia solutions delivered for myocardial protection, but most patients with normal renal function and preserved myocardial function will make large quantities of urine during the first few hours after CPB, often resulting in hypokalemia. To minimize the risk of developing arrhythmias, potassium levels should be checked every 4 hours and replaced as necessary.

I. Strict management of hyperglycemia has been shown to reduce the incidence of sternal wound infection and surgical mortality.[42,43] Factors that contribute to hyperglycemia are insulin resistance, endogenous catecholamine release on pump, and use of epinephrine postpump for hemodynamic support. A hyperglycemia protocol should be utilized to determine the appropriate amount of insulin to be given (usually as a continuous infusion) to maintain the blood sugar less than 180 mg/dL (see Appendix 6).

II. Management of Common Postoperative Scenarios

There are several typical hemodynamic scenarios that are noted during the early phase of recovery from open-heart surgery. An understanding of these patterns allows for therapeutic maneuvers to be undertaken in anticipation of hemodynamic changes, rather than as reactions to problems once they have occurred.

A. **Vasoconstriction from hypothermia with hypertension and borderline cardiac output.**

1. The patient arriving in the ICU with a temperature below 35–36°C will vasoconstrict in an attempt to increase core body temperature. The elevation in SVR may produce hypertension at a time when cardiac function is still somewhat depressed from surgery. These patients should be treated with a combination of fluid replacement to reach a pulmonary artery diastolic (PAD) or pulmonary capillary wedge pressure (PCWP) of 15–20 mm Hg, vasodilatation with sodium nitroprusside (SNP) to maintain a systolic pressure of 100–130 mm Hg (mean pressure 80–90 mm Hg), and inotropic support if the cardiac index remains less than 2.0 L/min/m². Warming methods noted above should also be employed. SNP is preferable to nitroglycerin (NTG), which tends to lower preload and reduce cardiac output to a greater degree while producing less systemic vasodilatation.

2. The use of SNP is beneficial in the vasoconstricted patient for several reasons:

   a. It lowers afterload, improving myocardial metabolism and left ventricular (LV) function.

b. It improves peripheral tissue perfusion and redistributes heat to the periphery.

c. It facilitates gentle and adequate fluid administration.

3. SNP is administered starting at a dose of 0.1 μg/kg/min (often less) and titrating to a maximum of 8 μg/kg/min. As the SVR and blood pressure decrease, left-sided filling pressures will fall modestly, requiring the simultaneous infusion of fluids to maintain cardiac output. The optimal left-sided filling pressures depend on the state of myocardial contractility and compliance. Preload should generally not be raised above 20 mm Hg because of the deleterious effects of elevated wall tension on myocardial metabolism and function. However, if preload is allowed to fall too low during SNP infusion, the patient may become hypovolemic and hypotensive when normothermia is achieved. The general principle is to "optimize preload → reduce afterload → optimize preload."

4. If the patient is vasoconstricted and the cardiac index (CI) is very marginal (e.g., <2.0 L/min/m^2), it is advisable to start an inotrope in addition to SNP. **Stopping an inotropic medication in a hypertensive patient without first ensuring that a satisfactory cardiac output is present can be very dangerous.** Some patients with very marginal cardiac function maintain a satisfactory blood pressure by intense vasoconstriction from enhanced sympathetic tone and hypothermia. Loss of this compensatory mechanism may result in rapid deterioration from loss of perfusion pressure.

B. Vasodilatation and hypotension during the rewarming phase

1. Vasodilatation reduces filling pressures and, in the hypovolemic patient, may produce hypotension and often a decrease in cardiac output. There are several reasons why a patient may vasodilate during the early postoperative period.

a. Medications used for analgesia and anxiolysis are vasodilators (narcotics, midazolam, propofol).

b. NTG used in the operating room or ICU to control blood pressure or minimize ischemia will lower preload and cardiac output as well as blood pressure. To counteract these problems, significant fluid administration is frequently required. Unless active ischemia is present, IV NTG is best avoided during the rewarming phase to reduce fluid requirements.

c. Resolution of hypothermia leads to peripheral vasodilatation, which is accentuated in patients who warm to higher than 37°C.

d. Improvement in cardiac output often leads to relaxation of peripheral vasoconstriction.

2. To avoid hypotension, fluids must be given to maintain filling pressures. The quandary is whether crystalloid or colloid should be selected and how much should be given. If the basic reason for hypovolemia is a capillary leak syndrome, the use of colloid could be detrimental because its oncotic elements may pass into the interstitial tissues and exacerbate tissue edema and compromise organ function. However, if vasodilatation of the peripheral and splanchnic beds is the major problem, then colloids should be preferable because they will augment the intravascular volume to a greater extent than crystalloids.[40] Generally, if the PCWP is not elevated, the amount of extravascular lung water will not be influenced significantly by whether colloid or crystalloid is infused.[41]

3. It is generally best to start with a 500 mL bolus of Ringer's lactate. If there is minimal increase in filling pressures, a colloid, such as 5% albumin or hetastarch, may be chosen. Hetastarch increases the intravascular volume more effectively than crystalloid and longer than 5% albumin. However, the total infusion volume should be limited to 1500–1750 mL (20 mL/kg) per 24 hours to minimize adverse effects on the coagulation mechanism. Hetastarch should be avoided in the patient with significant mediastinal bleeding because it may increase bleeding. If the patient's hematocrit is low, a packed red cell transfusion is best to increase intravascular volume.

4. There is often a tendency to administer a tremendous amount of fluid during the period of vasodilatation in order to maintain filling pressures and systemic blood pressure. Furthermore, most patients with satisfactory cardiac function are simultaneously producing a copious amount of urine. One should resist the temptation to "flood" the patient with fluid. Excessive fluid administration (>2 L within 6 hours) may exacerbate interstitial edema and delay extubation.[26] It also produces significant hemodilution, often necessitating blood transfusions for anemia, and reduces the levels of clotting factors, possibly increasing mediastinal bleeding and necessitating plasma or platelet administration. **Preload should be increased only as necessary to maintain satisfactory cardiac output and tissue perfusion.**

5. The response to fluid administration is not always predictable and depends on the compliance of the left atrium and ventricle, the degree of capillary leakage, and the intensity of peripheral vasoconstriction.

   a. An increase in preload with repeated fluid challenges will generally raise the cardiac output to satisfactory levels. Peripheral vasoconstriction tends to relax as the cardiac output improves and the patient warms. As this occurs, filling pressures tend to fall and some additional volume may be necessary. However, if cardiac function and filling pressures are adequate, use of an α-agent to support the blood pressure can limit the amount of fluid that needs to be given. If these drugs cannot maintain a satisfactory BP with adequate filling pressures, yet the cardiac output is satisfactory, a "vasoplegic syndrome" may be present. This generally responds to vasopressin 0.04–0.1 units/min. This syndrome may be attributable to leukocyte activation and release of proinflammatory mediators caused by the systemic inflammatory response to CPB, although it has been described after off-pump surgery as well.[44-46]

   b. Failure of filling pressures to rise with volume infusions may reflect not only vasodilatation, but also the capillary leak of fluid into the interstitial space rather than retention in the intravascular space. This is particularly common in very sick patients with a long duration of CPB. Sometimes it seems virtually impossible to maintain filling pressures and cardiac output despite a tremendous amount of fluid administration, yet, on occasion, this may be necessary. One often has to accept the adverse consequences of excessive total body water to improve hemodynamics. Use of drugs to provide inotropic support and some increase in systemic resistance may reduce the amount of fluid that is administered.

   c. If filling pressures do rise with fluid administration, but the blood pressure and cardiac output remain marginal, right and left ventricular distention may ensue, increasing myocardial oxygen demand and decreasing coronary blood flow. Further fluid administration is contraindicated, and inotropic support must be initiated.

6. The following is a general guideline to hemodynamic management during the rewarming phase.

   a. If blood pressure is marginal, push the PCWP to 18–20 mm Hg using crystalloid and then colloid. Once this level is reached, or if urine volume begins to match the infused volume, or if more than 2000 mL of fluid has been administered and filling pressures are not rising, consider the following:

      i. If CI > 2.2 L/min/m², use phenylephrine (pure α).
      ii. If CI is 1.8–2.2 L/min/m², use norepinephrine (α and β).
      iii. If CI < 1.8 L/min/m², use an inotrope, then norepinephrine PRN.

   b. Note: Use of an α-agent may not be adequate to minimize a capillary leak, but it does counteract vasodilatation. This may decrease the volume requirement and improve SVR and blood pressure with little effect on myocardial function.

C. Copious urine output and falling PCWP. Some patients will make large quantities of urine, resulting in a reduction in filling pressures, blood pressure, and cardiac output. Several factors should be considered when determining why this might be occurring.

   1. Is the patient on "renal dose" dopamine producing copious urine output out of proportion to its hemodynamic effects? If so, and the patient requires inotropic support, consider changing to another drug, such as dobutamine or epinephrine.

   2. Did the patient receive mannitol or furosemide in the operating room because of a low urine output or hyperkalemia? Urine output is no longer a direct reflection of myocardial function when a diuretic has been administered. Excessive urine output often necessitates a significant amount of fluid administration to maintain filling pressures and confounds the selection of the appropriate fluid to administer (crystalloid versus colloid).

   3. Is the patient hyperglycemic and developing an osmotic diuresis? A hyperglycemia protocol should be used routinely to maintain the blood glucose below 180 mg/dL (see Appendix 6).

   4. Does the patient have normal LV function and the kidneys are simply mobilizing excessive interstitial fluid from hemodilution on pump? This beneficial effect is often seen in healthy patients with a short CPB run, and reflects excellent cardiac output and renal function that should lead to a rapid postoperative recovery. However, copious urine output can be problematic when it lowers filling pressures, blood pressure, and cardiac output.

      a. Any contributing factors or medications to the diuresis should be addressed.

      b. Crystalloid and colloid should be administered to keep the fluid balance modestly negative during this phase of spontaneous diuresis. One should resist the temptation to administer too much colloid, which can produce hemodilution and progressive anemia despite the negative fluid balance and can dilute clotting factors, potentially contributing to mediastinal bleeding. Use of an α-agent may maintain filling pressures and decrease the volume requirement in some of these patients.

D. Normal LV function but low cardiac output (diastolic dysfunction and right ventricular failure)

1. A disturbing postoperative scenario is that of a low cardiac output syndrome associated with normal or elevated left heart filling pressures yet preserved ventricular function. This scenario is noted most commonly in small women with systemic hypertension who have small, hypertrophied left ventricles. A variant of this problem is seen in patients with aortic stenosis (AS) and hyperdynamic hearts that manifest near-cavity obliteration.[47,48]

2. This problem of severe diastolic dysfunction is characterized by reduced ventricular compliance exacerbated by myocardial edema from ischemic/reperfusion injury. Contributing factors to the low cardiac output are lack of atrioventricular (AV) synchrony with impaired ventricular filling, occasionally impaired right ventricular (RV) function, and perhaps excessive use of inotropic agents.

3. The hemodynamic data derived from the Swan-Ganz catheter typically show elevated filling pressures and a low cardiac output, consistent with LV dysfunction. Thus, a typical therapeutic response would be to ensure AV conduction, administer some volume, and initiate inotropic support. However, this may lead to little improvement in cardiac output, even higher filling pressures leading to pulmonary congestion, a reduction in renal blood flow (often exacerbated by systemic venous hypertension), and progressive oliguria. The use of inotropes may also produce a significant sinus tachycardia that is detrimental to myocardial metabolism and recovery.

4. Transesophageal echocardiography (TEE) has been invaluable in the assessment and management of this problem. TEE usually confirms a hypertrophic, stiff left ventricle with hyperdynamic function. Fluid should be administered to raise the PCWP to about 20–25 mm Hg. This will increase the left ventricular end-diastolic volume, which tends to be smaller than would be suggested by pressure measurements because of poor LV compliance. Lusitropic drugs that relax the left ventricle should be substituted for catecholamines that have β-adrenergic inotropic and chronotropic properties. Inamrinone or milrinone may be beneficial in this regard and can support RV function as well. Nesiritide, a synthetic β-type natriuretic peptide, is a pulmonary and systemic vasodilator with lusitropic properties that has been noted anecdotally to benefit patients with severe diastolic dysfunction.[49]

5. Other considerations include use of low-dose calcium channel blockers or β-blockers to improve diastolic relaxation, although it is conceptually difficult to start these when the cardiac output is compromised. Aggressive diuresis to reduce interstitial edema while providing colloid (salt-poor albumin) to maintain intravascular volume may also improve diastolic relaxation. If the patient can survive the first few days of low cardiac output syndrome without end-organ dysfunction, a gradual improvement in cardiac output generally results.

6. The problem of a marginal cardiac output and blood pressure with preserved LV function may be noted in patients with markedly impaired RV function. This may result from RV infarction or poor intraoperative protection of an enlarged right ventricle in patients with pulmonary hypertension. This problem is not uncommon in cardiac transplant recipients with preexisting pulmonary hypertension and may be noted in patients with advanced mitral valve disease. The use

of blood products also increases pulmonary vascular resistance (PVR) and can exacerbate RV dysfunction. Fluid administration, inotropic support with medications such as inamrinone or milrinone, or use of nesiritide or inhaled nitric oxide (a pure pulmonary vasodilator) may be beneficial. If not, a circulatory assist device might be necessary. The management of RV dysfunction is discussed in more detail on pages 353–358.

III. Postoperative Considerations Following Commonly Performed Procedures

A. Coronary artery bypass grafting (on-pump CABG)

1. The patient with excellent ventricular function usually requires a vasodilator (SNP or NTG) to control hypertension more often than an inotrope. With the use of propofol, immediate postbypass hypertension tends to be less common. Although patients who are β-blocked preoperatively frequently require pacing at the conclusion of bypass, tachycardia may be present in those who are not β-blocked, especially in young anxious patients. Both the hypertension and the tachycardia can be managed by β-blockers (esmolol or intermittent doses of IV metoprolol) if cardiac output is satisfactory. Patients with a **hyperdynamic left ventricle** may develop progressive tachycardia when vasodilators are used to control hypertension. This should be managed by allowing the blood pressure to drift up to 140 systolic (mean 100–110) and then using β-blockers to control both the tachycardia and the hypertension.

2. Use of NTG to control hypertension reduces preload and cardiac output because of its venodilatory effects. SNP is the preferable medication because it primarily lowers the SVR with less effect on preload and thus requires less volume infusion. However, NTG should be used if there is any evidence of ischemia. Nicardipine is another satisfactory alternative to control hypertension.

3. **Inotropic support** is usually initiated at the termination of bypass and may be required for several hours in the ICU.[39] The initial first-line drug may be epinephrine, dobutamine, or dopamine. Epinephrine is a strong inotrope, usually produces less tachycardia than the other drugs, and is the preferred medication. If there is an inadequate response to one of these catecholamines, inamrinone or milrinone is of great benefit in improving cardiac output. These two phosphodiesterase inhibitors are positive inotropes that produce systemic vasodilatation that frequently requires the addition of norepinephrine to support systemic resistance. When hemodynamic performance remains very marginal, placement of an intraaortic balloon pump (IABP) should be considered. In contrast to the catecholamines, the IABP can reduce myocardial oxygen demand and improve coronary perfusion. Support beyond 6–12 hours may be necessary if the patient has sustained a perioperative infarction or has a severely "stunned" myocardium that exhibits a prolonged period of dysfunction in the absence of infarction.

4. Lidocaine is often started in the operating room when the aortic cross-clamp is removed and is continued on a prophylactic basis until the following morning. This may decrease the incidence of **ventricular ectopy** that may be associated with hypothermia, hemodynamic instability, or the presence of the endotracheal tube or Swan-Ganz catheter. Subsequent use of antiarrhythmic therapy should be based on the presence and severity of any arrhythmias as well as the patient's

ejection fraction. The occurrence of nonsustained or sustained ventricular tachycardia after surgery in the patient with depressed LV function is an indication for an electrophysiologic study and usually the insertion of an implantable cardioverter-defibrillator (ICD). Otherwise medical therapy with β-blockers and possibly amiodarone may be indicated.

5. **Atrial fibrillation (AF)** is noted in about 25% of patients following CABG. It may be related to poor atrial preservation during surgery or to withdrawal of β-blockers. Most centers initiate β-blocker treatment by the first postoperative morning (usually metoprolol 25–50 mg bid) because of the overwhelming evidence that β-blockers reduce the incidence of AF.[50] The concomitant administration of digoxin may lower the incidence of AF even further.[51] Magnesium sulfate has been shown in some, but not all, studies to reduce the incidence of AF (and ventricular arrhythmias) as well as aid in conversion to sinus rhythm.[52,53] Amiodarone may also be considered for AF prophylaxis. A detailed discussion of the prevention and management of AF is presented on pages 427–435.

6. Close attention must be paid to the postoperative **electrocardiogram (ECG)**. Evidence of ischemia may represent incomplete revascularization, poor myocardial protection, or impaired flow due to anastomotic stenosis, acute graft occlusion, or coronary spasm. Regardless of the cause, IV NTG (starting at 0.25 μg/kg/min) is usually indicated. Calcium channel blockers (nifedipine 30 mg SL or diltiazem 0.25 mg/kg IV over 2 minutes, then 5–15 mg/h IV) are useful if coronary spasm is suspected. These medications may resolve ischemic changes or minimize infarct size if necrosis is already underway. Placement of an IABP should also be considered. If a problem with a bypass graft is suspected as the cause of the ischemia, emergency angiography followed by percutaneous coronary intervention or reexploration may be indicated.

7. For patients receiving **radial artery grafts**, a vasodilator is used to prevent graft spasm. Common options include diltiazem 10 mg/h IV or NTG 10–15 μg/min (0.1–0.2 μg/kg/min) started in the operating room and continuing for 18–24 hours postoperatively. These intravenous medications are then converted to long-acting diltiazem 120–180 mg PO qd or Imdur 20 mg PO qd and arbitrarily continued for 6 months.

8. The diagnosis of a perioperative **myocardial infarction (MI)** can be difficult to make, but is usually confirmed by persistent ECG changes and new regional wall motion abnormalities on echocardiography (see pages 404–407). Cardiac enzymes are elevated in over 90% of patients after open-heart surgery, but a level of creatine kinase MB that exceeds 10 times the upper limit of normal or a troponin level > 15–20 μg/dL is consistent with a perioperative MI.[54,55] Management consists of hemodynamic support and other standard measures. A common finding in the patient sustaining a small perioperative MI is a low SVR that necessitates use of a vasopressor for several days to support blood pressure. A more extensive MI may require pharmacologic support or an IABP for longer periods and is associated with increased operative mortality and a decrease in long-term survival.

9. **Antiplatelet therapy** inhibits platelet deposition on vein grafts and has been shown to improve graft patency. Enteric-coated aspirin 75–325 mg qd should be started 6h after surgery, or as soon as possible thereafter once mediastinal bleeding has tapered. It should be continued at this dose for 1 year and then given

indefinitely in a dose of 75–162 mg qd. Clopidogrel 75 mg qd should also be considered for 1 year if surgery was performed for a non-STEMI.[56]

B. **Minimally invasive direct coronary artery surgery (MIDCAB)** entails performance of an anastomosis of the left internal thoracic artery to the left anterior descending artery. This is performed through a left thoracotomy incision using one-lung anesthesia.

1. Patients are generally extubated in the operating room or soon after arrival in the ICU. Epidural analgesia (Duramorph) and intercostal bupivacaine (Marcaine) are helpful in reducing splinting and improving respiratory efforts in patients who might otherwise have significant chest wall pain from rib retraction, resection, or fracture.

2. No pacing wires are placed, so a heart rate in the 60–70/min range is acceptable. Ventricular pacing wires placed through the Swan-Ganz catheter can be used for bradycardia but generally do not provide optimal hemodynamics. External pacing may be used, if necessary.

3. A postoperative ECG must be obtained and carefully reviewed for any evidence of ischemia because anastomotic problems are more common when surgery is performed on a beating rather than an arrested heart.

4. Intrapericardial or intrapleural bleeding may originate from the chest wall, the anastomotic site, or side branches of the internal thoracic artery. Blood will more readily accumulate in the pleural space during spontaneous ventilation. The possibility of bleeding should be monitored by observing chest tube drainage and a postoperative chest x-ray.

C. **Off-pump coronary artery bypass (OPCAB)** is performed through a sternotomy incision and should achieve complete revascularization comparable to traditional on-pump surgery. Numerous studies have documented that OPCAB is associated with reduced blood loss, reduced transfusion requirements, less renal dysfunction, and, arguably, less AF, less neurocognitive decline, and a lower risk of stroke.[57–67] Patients are more intensively monitored during OPCAB than routine CABG, using continuous cardiac output measurements, on-line mixed venous oxygen saturations, and TEE to ensure stability during the procedure.[68,69] Aspects of this operation that can impact postoperative care include temperature regulation, the influence of intraoperative ischemia on cardiac performance, potential anastomotic problems or incomplete revascularization causing perioperative ischemia or infarction, fluid administration to maintain hemodynamics during cardiac positioning, and bleeding due to use of heparin or transfusion of scavenged blood.

1. Patient temperature tends to drift during surgery and must be maintained by having a higher temperature in the operating room, warming all intravenous fluids, using heated humidifiers in the ventilator circuit, and using a topical warming device, such as the Bair Hugger or the Arctic Sun temperature-controlling system.[7] Hypothermia can lead to a number of problems, including ventricular arrhythmias, and must be avoided. If the patient arrives in the unit hypothermic, the standard measures noted in section I.B should be taken.

2. Hemodynamic performance is generally stable after the patient's arrival in the ICU, although ischemia occurring during construction of anastomoses may lead to transient diminution in cardiac performance. Generally, the initial deterioration

in cardiac output noted in CPB patients does not occur. However, low doses of inotropes are commonly used during surgery, especially in patients with impaired ventricular function, and should be continued until a satisfactory output can be maintained.

3. The immediate postoperative ECG must be evaluated. Although intraoperative assessment of graft patency can be performed by Doppler flow analysis or epicardial echocardiography, this is not a common practice.[70,71] The likelihood of an anastomotic problem is greater during OPCAB due to suboptimal visualization from bleeding or movement. This may be evident by ECG changes or regional wall motion abnormalities on TEE. Occasionally, an abnormal ECG reflects incomplete revascularization when small coronary arteries are not bypassed. There should be a low threshold for postoperative coronary angiography if there is any question about graft flow and patency.

4. Pacing wires should be placed on all patients because patients who are treated preoperatively with β-blockers will have slower heart rates that will persist into the postoperative period. Although heart rates of 60–70/min are acceptable, cardiac output can be optimized by achieving a heart rate of at least 80/min in the early postoperative period.

5. The benefits of OPCAB in reducing the incidence of AF are controversial.[66,67] Thus, the early initiation of β-blockers remains essential. Magnesium is usually given in the operating room to lower the arrhythmia threshold during construction of anastomoses; it may also be given on the first postoperative day to reduce the risk of AF.

6. Many cardiac surgical groups extubate patients in the operating room or soon after arrival in the ICU. Standard criteria for weaning and extubation should be used. These include the achievement of normothermia, hemodynamic stability, absence of bleeding, an adequate level of alertness without significant pain, and satisfactory gas exchange. Use of short-acting anesthetic agents and propofol should allow for the safe, early extubation of most patients once these criteria are met. Although OPCAB is performed without CPB, there is little evidence that avoidance of CPB preserves respiratory function any better when evaluating postoperative pulmonary function test results, arterial blood gases, or the duration of extubation.[72,73]

7. Although the hemodilution of CPB has been avoided, there is a tendency for anesthesiologists to administer a significant amount of volume during surgery to maintain preload and offset the adverse effects of cardiac manipulation and positioning on hemodynamic performance. Thus, patients tend to be somewhat fluid overloaded and need to be diuresed once hemodynamic stability has been achieved. Although the incidence of renal dysfunction may be less with OPCAB, there is an obligatory period of relative hypotension during the construction of proximal anastomoses that can adversely affect kidney function in patients with preexisting renal dysfunction.

8. Anemia is less common after OPCAB than on-pump surgery because hemodilution and other adverse effects of CPB on the coagulation system are avoided.[60–62] Thus, significant mediastinal bleeding should be extremely uncommon in the absence of a surgical bleeding site. However, the potential for a coagulopathy may still exist.

    a. Heparinization is necessary during the procedure, and some degree of fibrinolysis is also probably present. The antifibrinolytic drugs have been shown to be beneficial in reducing bleeding in OPCAB, and thus should be utilized.[74,75]

    b. Insidious blood loss occurring during the construction of anastomoses is scavenged into a cell saver device. Centrifugation and washing eliminate clotting factors and platelets from reinfused blood.

    c. Both pleural spaces are entered during OPCAB, and failure to place a chest tube in a pleural cavity (or poor drainage through a pleural tube that is placed) may result in the undetected collection of blood spilling over from the mediastinum. Vigilance is necessary in assessing and managing any mediastinal bleeding that is noted and having a high level of suspicion that such might be occurring if the patient is hemodynamically unstable.

D. Aortic valve surgery

  1. Aortic stenosis

    a. Aortic stenosis (AS) leads to the development of a hypertrophied, noncompliant left ventricle that depends on synchronous atrial and ventricular contractions for nearly 30% of its stroke volume. Postoperatively, it is imperative that sinus rhythm be present or that atrial or AV pacing be used. There should be a low threshold for cardioversion of AF because profound hemodynamic deterioration may occur, especially during the first 24 hours after surgery.

    b. Adequate **preload** must be maintained (PCWP > 15 mm Hg) to ensure adequate LV filling. Filling pressures may rise rapidly with minimal volume infusion because of the noncompliant hypertrophied ventricle.

    c. Although LV pressures often exceed 200 mm Hg preoperatively in patients with AS, significant **systolic hypertension** is usually not seen at the conclusion of bypass despite elimination of the transvalvular gradient and satisfactory myocardial protection. However, hypertension tends to develop after several hours in the ICU and must be controlled to reduce myocardial oxygen demand and protect the aortic suture line. Use of vasodilators for a hyperdynamic heart may reduce diastolic perfusion pressure and produce a tachycardia. Use of a β-blocker, such as esmolol, is beneficial in this situation.

    d. Patients with a hyperdynamic left ventricle with midcavity obliteration and intracavitary flow acceleration have a higher risk of postoperative morbidity and mortality. [47,48] These patients have diastolic dysfunction with low stroke volumes and low cardiac output. Hypovolemia and inotropes must be avoided. A careful TEE in the operating room can define the nature of the pathophysiology because inotropic support with catecholamines for a low cardiac output state associated with a hyperdynamic ventricle is counterproductive.

  2. Aortic regurgitation

    a. Aortic regurgitation (AR) produces both volume and pressure overload of the left ventricle, resulting in a dilated and frequently hypertrophied ventricle. Maintenance of a supraventricular rhythm is important. Filling pressures often rise minimally despite large fluid challenges because of the enlarged, compliant left ventricle.

b. Despite the placement of a competent aortic valvular prosthesis, most patients with AR remain vasodilated after surgery and require the use of an α-agent, such as phenylephrine or norepinephrine, to maintain a satisfactory blood pressure. Systolic hypertension is often better controlled with β-blockers than with vasodilators.

3. **Heart block** may complicate an aortic valve replacement (AVR) because of edema, hemorrhage, suturing, or debridement near the conduction system, which lies adjacent to the base of the right coronary cusp near the commissure with the noncoronary cusp. Epicardial **AV** pacing may be necessary for several days. The presence of a bundle branch block following AVR is of adverse prognostic significance.[76] If complete heart block persists for more than a few days, during which time edema or hemorrhage should subside, placement of a permanent DDD pacemaker should be considered.

4. **Anticoagulation**

a. Tissue valves: The American College of Chest Physicians (ACCP) 2004 guidelines suggest that warfarin should be used for 3 months (target international normalized ratio [INR] 2.5, range 2.0–3.0) to reduce the incidence of thromboembolism from tissue aortic valves.[77] Since numerous studies have shown that aspirin is just as effective as warfarin, most surgeons use the alternative recommendation of aspirin 81–100 mg qd following surgery.[77–80]

b. Mechanical valves: all patients with current-generation single tilting-disk or bileaflet valves should receive warfarin indefinitely to achieve a target INR of 2.5 (range 2.0–3.0). In patients at higher risk of thromboembolism (atrial fibrillation, MI, left atrial enlargement, endocardial damage, low EF, or history of systemic embolism), aspirin 75–100 mg/day should be added and the target INR raised to 3.0. Heparin may be started around the fourth postoperative day if the INR is less than 1.8, always being cognizant of the potential for delayed tamponade in the anticoagulated postoperative patient. The patient can usually be discharged home once the INR is approaching the therapeutic range (generally > 1.8).

E. **Mitral valve surgery**

1. **Mitral stenosis (MS).** Most patients with MS have a small LV cavity with preserved function. They are prone to a low cardiac output syndrome following surgery because of small LV end-diastolic and end-systolic volumes. Maintenance of adequate filling pressures is essential to ensure a satisfactory stroke volume. The "ideal" filling pressure varies for each patient, depending on the level of preexisting pulmonary hypertension and the degree of its reversibility. Hemodynamic support is more often required for RV rather than LV dysfunction.

a. Postoperative ventilatory failure is not uncommon in patients with chronic MS as a result of pulmonary hypertension, fluid overload, and chronic cachexia with poor ventilatory reserve. Aggressive diuresis, nutritional support, and a plan for ventilatory support and weaning are essential.

b. Most patients with MS are diuretic-dependent. Despite correction of their valvular abnormality, they often require substantial doses of diuretics during the hospital stay to achieve their preoperative weight. They should be maintained on diuretics for several months after discharge.

2. **Mitral regurgitation (MR)** reduces left ventricular wall stress by systolic unloading through the regurgitant valve. When mitral valve competence has

been restored, there may be unmasking of LV dysfunction because of the greater systolic wall stress required to achieve forward ejection. This may be attenuated to some degree by a reduction in volume overload. This so-called afterload mismatch may result in LV failure and require inotropic support and systemic unloading with vasodilators.[81]

3. **Right ventricular dysfunction** is not uncommon following mitral valve surgery for either MS or MR, especially in patients with significant preexisting pulmonary hypertension. RV failure may be precipitated by poor myocardial protection or by factors that increase RV afterload. These include positive-pressure ventilation, increased extravascular lung water, blood and blood component transfusions, blood gas and acid-base abnormalities, and reversible pulmonary vascular spasm related to perfusion-related phenomena and the systemic inflammatory response.

   a. Isolated RV dysfunction is manifested by a high CVP, variable PA pressures, a hypovolemic left ventricle, and a low cardiac output. The use of volumetric Swan-Ganz catheters can better define the degree of RV dysfunction by calculating the RV ejection fraction,[82] but the presence of functional tricuspid regurgitation may render thermodilution cardiac outputs unreliable. In this situation, an alternative means of measuring cardiac output may be necessary (see pages 228 and 342).

   b. The initial management of RV dysfunction is fluid administration to optimize preload. However, if the CVP rises above 20 mm Hg without achieving a satisfactory cardiac output, further volume should not be given. This may cause further deterioration of RV function and also impair LV filling by producing a septal shift.

   c. Inotropic drugs should be given to support both RV and LV performance. Preferably, those that can also reduce the PVR, such as inamrinone or milrinone, should be chosen. Isoproterenol may lower the PVR, but its use is usually limited by a tachycardia.[83] Low dose-epinephrine or dobutamine may be helpful.

   d. Pulmonary vasodilators should then be selected and may improve RV function by lowering RV afterload. Nesiritide is a readily available vasodilator that is very effective in reducing PA pressures while concomitantly producing a strong diuretic effect. In higher doses, it does produce some degree of systemic vasodilatation. Nitroglycerin is effective in lowering preload, although it also produces systemic vasodilatation at higher doses. Selective pulmonary vasodilators that may not be as readily available include inhaled nitric oxide (20–40 PPM through the ventilator)[84] and inhaled prostacyclin (up to 50 ng/kg/min).[85] Intravenous prostaglandin E_1 may achieve pulmonary vasodilatation without producing systemic hypotension at doses up to 0.1 µg/kg/min.[86] However, higher doses usually require infusion of an α-agent directly into a left atrial line to maintain systemic blood pressure.

   e. Additional comments on the management of RV failure are noted on pages 353–358.

4. **Left ventricular dysfunction** may occur after surgery for mitral regurgitation because a newly competent mitral valve reduces low pressure unloading of the left ventricle and may unmask LV dysfunction. Deterioration of LV function is minimized by mitral valve reparative techniques or preservation of the

subchordal apparatus during mitral valve replacement. On rare occasions, it may be attributable to inadvertent circumferential entrapment of the circumflex coronary artery during suture placement. This should be evident by the identification of significant regional wall motion abnormalities on TEE and ECG changes in the distribution of the artery.

   a. To optimize the systemic output, the left ventricular volume status usually has to be maintained at fairly high levels. Administering a large quantity of fluid is frequently required because of the increased left atrial and ventricular compliance. In the presence of severe RV dysfunction, this can be problematic, because attempts to achieve adequate left-sided filling may lead to progressive RV dilatation and failure, and subsequent impairment in LV filling. Careful monitoring of CVP and RV end-diastolic volumes may indicate when fluid challenges are detrimental rather than beneficial.

   b. Assessment of LV filling can be somewhat difficult in the ICU. Although there is some decrease in PA pressure after surgery, the degree and rapidity of reversibility of pulmonary hypertension are unpredictable, and thus the PA pressures may not be indicative of the degree of LV filling. Optimal volume status can frequently be determined by observing myocardial function by echocardiography at various filling pressures at the conclusion of CPB.

   c. Aside from echocardiography, the left atrial pressure is the most accurate means of assessing LV filling. Left atrial lines are safe as long as certain precautions regarding air embolism and observation after their removal are taken.[87] They also permit the selective infusion of α-agents to counteract the systemic vasodilatation of some vasodilators (although this is rarely necessary).

   d. PAD pressures may give an inaccurate assessment of left heart filling because a significant transpulmonary gradient (PA mean pressure minus the PCWP) is commonly present in patients with mitral valve disease. Although the PCWP is more accurate, balloon inflation is usually best avoided in the patient with pulmonary hypertension to avoid the risk of pulmonary artery rupture.

5. Maintenance of **sinus rhythm** is beneficial to optimize cardiac output. When mitral valve surgery is performed through the biatrial transseptal approach, the sinus node artery is usually divided, and sinus rhythm is frequently absent.[88,89] Commonly, it is difficult to pace the atrium despite preoperative sinus rhythm. In patients with long-standing AF, it is frequently possible to AV pace the heart for several hours or days after surgery. Maintenance of sinus rhythm beyond the early postoperative period is highly unlikely, however, when AF has been present for more than a year or the left atrial dimension exceeds 50 mm. β-blockers, calcium channel blockers, and/or digoxin may be used for rate control, but medications to maintain sinus rhythm, such as procainamide or amiodarone, are generally not indicated in the patient with chronic AF.

6. The Maze procedure (see Figures 1.18 and 1.19) can be used to treat paroxysmal or chronic AF and is most commonly performed as an adjunct to mitral valve surgery. Pulmonary vein isolation can be performed in the electrophysiology lab or during surgery using various ablative technologies with a 90% success rate for paroxysmal AF. Chronic AF responds best to the "cut and sew" Cox-Maze III operation, following which about 10–15% of patients require

pacemakers. Successful conversion can be achieved in about 70% of patients with chronic AF using radiofrequency, microwave, or cryoablation. Anticoagulation with warfarin is recommended for 3 months if the patient converts to sinus rhythm (SR) or indefinitely if they do not. Amiodarone is usually given for 3 months even if there is early conversion to SR. If AF persists, an elective cardioversion is performed after 1–3 months; if successful, the amiodarone may be continued for 3 more months. If AF still persists, the amiodarone may be stopped, but commonly is continued for a few months to improve the likelihood of converting to sinus rhythm.

7. **Anticoagulation**

   a. Tissue valves and mitral rings. Warfarin should be given for 3 months to achieve a target INR of 2.5 (range 2.0–3.0) and should then be converted to aspirin 75–100 mg qd if the patient is in sinus rhythm.[77] Warfarin should be continued indefinitely in patients with AF, an enlarged left atrium (> 50 mm in diameter), or a history of thromboembolism. Some surgeons prefer not to utilize warfarin after placement of mitral valve rings. The decision to initiate heparin if the INR is not therapeutic by the fourth postoperative day must be individualized, taking into consideration the potential benefits and risks (i.e., delayed tamponade) for that patient.

   b. Mechanical valves. Warfarin is started on the first postoperative day to achieve a target INR of 3.0 (range 2.5–3.5) and is given indefinitely. The addition of aspirin 75–100 mg is safe and may further reduce the incidence of thromboembolism especially in patients at high risk (AF, enlarged left atrium). Heparin should be started around the fourth postoperative day if the INR is less than 2.0.

   c. The patient can usually be discharged from the hospital when the INR is approaching the target range. Acceptable values include an INR of 1.5 for tissue valves and rings (1.8 if in AF), and 2.0 for mechanical valves. If the patient is at increased risk of thromboembolism (e.g., large left atrium), low-molecular weight heparin (1 mg/kg SC bid) may also be prescribed (as an off-label use) until the INR has reached the target range.

8. The acute onset of exsanguinating bleeding through the chest tubes or the development of tamponade soon after MVR suggests the possibility of **LV rupture**. This may occur at the atrioventricular groove, at the base of the papillary muscles, or in between. This problem can be avoided by chordal preservation during MVR, avoiding tissue valves (which have protruding struts) in patients with a very small left ventricle (usually elderly women with MS), and using meticulous surgical technique. It may be precipitated by left ventricular distention or excessive afterload after bypass. Once identified, emergency surgical intervention on CPB is required and carries a significant mortality rate.[90]

F. Aortic dissections

1. Virtually all patients with dissections that involve the ascending aorta (type A dissection) undergo surgical repair. The reestablishment of vascular continuity involves suturing of a Dacron graft to very fragile tissues, and suture line bleeding is commonly noted. Use of an adjunct such as BioGlue™ has been helpful in reducing this problem.[91] In addition, surgical repair is predicated on stabilization of the entry site of the dissection but does not completely eliminate the distal false channel. Thus, surgery is palliative and leaves the patient predisposed to distal aneurysm formation in the future.

2. The antihypertensive regimen used in the early postoperative period should be similar to that used preoperatively in reducing systolic blood pressure and the force of cardiac contraction (dp/dt). The most common regimens are esmolol alone or esmolol combined with SNP. The patient is then converted to oral medications, such as the β-blockers (labetalol is an excellent choice), with use of additional antihypertensives, such as calcium channel blockers or ACE inhibitors as necessary.

3. The repair of a type A dissection usually involves a period of deep hypothermic circulatory arrest during which time the distal anastomosis is constructed. The extensive cooling and rewarming may be associated with a significant coagulopathy, but bleeding can usually be minimized by the use of BioGlue and aprotinin.[92] The use of aprotinin is somewhat controversial because it has been associated with neurologic problems and renal dysfunction after circulatory arrest.[93] However, adherence to strict protocols of heparinization during surgery (see page 144) should minimize this risk.[94,95] Careful preoperative and postoperative neurologic assessments are important.

4. Patients undergoing surgery for repair of type B dissections, usually for "complicated" dissections, may develop paraplegia and/or renal failure related to aortic cross-clamping. A careful preoperative and postoperative neurologic examination and measures to support renal function in the perioperative period are important. Other comments on descending thoracic aortic surgery are noted in the next section.

G. Thoracic aneurysms

1. Thoracic aneurysms tend to develop in elderly patients with hypertension, chronic lung disease, and diffuse atherosclerosis, including cerebrovascular, coronary, and renovascular disease. Prevention or recognition of problems involving these organ systems is essential to achieve an uneventful recovery.

2. Repair of ascending aortic and arch aneurysms may involve use of deep hypothermic circulatory arrest, which is associated with a multitude of potential complications. Despite active rewarming to 37°C on bypass, significant temperature afterdrop is common and aggressive rewarming measures are necessary in the ICU. Coagulopathies are commonly present and require aggressive management to minimize mediastinal bleeding. Although antegrade or retrograde cerebral perfusion may extend the acceptable period of circulatory arrest, careful preoperative and postoperative neurologic evaluation is essential.[96,97]

3. Repair of descending thoracic and thoracoabdominal aneurysms involves a thoracotomy incision and often takedown of the diaphragm. The extensive incision can produce significant pain that can compromise a patient's ventilatory status and often requires high doses of analgesics. Furthermore, the patient's pulmonary function may be compromised by the use of massive transfusions of blood and blood components during surgery. These factors, superimposed on preexisting lung disease, may lead to a prolonged period of intubation. More than 10% of patients undergoing these repairs require tracheostomy for prolonged ventilatory support.[98]

4. A coagulopathy is frequently present after surgery and must be aggressively managed, including early surgical reexploration, if necessary.

5. Cross-clamping of the descending aorta can result in paraplegia or renal failure, even if distal perfusion is provided during the cross-clamp period. Cerebrospinal fluid (CSF) drainage is usually initiated in the operating room prior to surgery to improve spinal cord perfusion pressure and maintained for about 24 hours.[99–103] Particular attention to a pre- and postoperative neurologic evaluation for several days is important. Delayed onset of paraplegia occurring in the ICU may develop but, if recognized immediately, is usually reversible with elevation of the systemic blood pressure, high-dose steroids, and cerebrospinal fluid drainage.[104,105]

6. Cross-clamping may also produce renal failure, and measures should be taken during surgery to optimize renal perfusion. This may include use of mannitol, furosemide, or a fenoldopam infusion.[106] The incidence of renal failure after thoracoabdominal surgery is between 12% and 25% in major series.[98]

H. **Left ventricular aneurysms and ventricular arrhythmia surgery**

1. Patients undergoing resection of an LV aneurysm usually have markedly depressed LV function. Although ventricular size and geometry are better preserved using the endoaneurysmorrhaphy or endoventricular circular patch plasty techniques than with a linear closure, the stroke volume of the left ventricle after LV aneurysm repair is usually lower after surgery. Achieving adequate filling pressures (usually a PCWP around 20–25 mm Hg) is essential to optimize stroke volume. Filling pressures may rise precipitously with minimal volume infusion because of the small, noncompliant LV chamber. Many patients generate a satisfactory cardiac output by virtue of a faster heart rate that should not be reduced pharmacologically unless the stroke volume is satisfactory. Hemodynamic support and IABP insertion are frequently necessary to allow weaning from CPB.

2. Surgery for ventricular tachycardia usually involves a blind endocardial resection with cryoablation and is successful in about 80% of patients. To minimize the risk of postoperative ventricular arrhythmias, lidocaine can be used prophylactically for 24 hours. Most of these patients will be candidates for postoperative ICD placement with or without electrophysiologic testing.

3. ICDs are usually placed in the electrophysiology lab in patients with sustained ventricular tachycardia or other suspected life-threatening arrhythmias. If the patient has had heart surgery and had a preoperative indication for the device, the ICD is placed several days after surgery. Similarly, if the patient has poor ventricular function and develops nonsustained or sustained ventricular tachycardia after surgery, an ICD may be considered before hospital discharge. The device is tested and usually left in the active mode. There should be a card posted above the head of the patient's bed indicating the status of the ICD so that anyone who responds to an emergency knows whether the device is activated or not. If the patient required antiarrhythmic medication preoperatively and has not undergone an endocardial resection, the medication should be continued after ICD implantation. Generally, patients are maintained on either β-blockers or amiodarone if they have malignant ventricular arrhythmias.

References

1. Higgins TL, Yared JP, Ryan T. Immediate postoperative care of cardiac surgical patients. J Cardiothorac Vasc Anesth 1996;10:643–58.
2. Pande RU, Nader ND, Donias HW, D'Ancona G, Karamanoukian HL. Review: Fast-tracking cardiac surgery. Heart Surg Forum 2003;6244–8.
3. Nathan HJ. The potential benefits of perioperative hypothermia. Ann Thorac Surg 1999;68:1452–3.
4. Mora CT, Henson MB, Weintraub WS, et al. The effect of temperature management during cardiopulmonary bypass on neurologic and neuropsychologic outcomes in patients undergoing coronary revascularization. J Thorac Cardiovasc Surg 1996;112:514–22.
5. Jones T, Roy RC. Should patients be normothermic in the immediate postoperative period? Ann Thorac Surg 1999;68:1454–5.
6. Sessler DI. Perioperative heat balance. Anesthesiology 2000;92:578–96.
7. Grocott HP, Mathew JP, Carver EH, et al. A randomized controlled trial of the Arctic Sun Temperature Management System versus conventional methods for preventing hypothermia during off-pump cardiac surgery. Anesth Analg 2004;98:298–302.
8. Rajek A, Lenhardt R, Sessler DI, et al. Efficacy of two methods for reducing postbypass afterdrop. Anesthesiology 2000;92:447–56.
9. Tugrul M, Pembeci K, Camci E, Ozkan T, Telci L. Comparison of the effects of sodium nitroprusside and isoflurane during rewarming on cardiopulmonary bypass. J Cardiothorac Vasc Anesth 1997;11:712–7.
10. Rajek A, Lenhardt R, Sessler DI, et al. Tissue heat content and distribution during and after cardiopulmonary bypass at 31°C and 27°C. Anesthesiology 1998;88:1511–8.
11. Insler SR, O'Connor MS, Leventhal MJ, Nelson DR, Starr NJ. Association between postoperative hypothermia and adverse outcome after coronary artery bypass surgery. Ann Thorac Surg 2000; 70:175–81.
12. Sessler DI. Complications and treatment of mild hypothermia. Anesthesiology 2001;95:531–43.
13. De Witte J, Sessler DI. Perioperative shivering: physiology and pharmacology. Anesthesiology 2002;96:467–84.
14. Frank SM, Fleisher LA, Olson KF, et al. Multivariate determinants of early postoperative oxygen consumption in elderly patients. Anesthesiology 1995;83:241–9.
15. Valeri CR, Khabbaz K, Khuri SF, et al. Effect of skin temperature on platelet function in patients undergoing extracorporeal bypass. J Thorac Cardiovasc Surg 1992;104:108–16.
16. Brauer A, English MJ, Lorenz N, et al. Comparison of forced-air warming systems with lower body blankets using a copper manikin of the human body. Acta Anaesthesiol Scand 2003;47:58–64.
17. Cross MH, Davies JC, Shah MV. Post-operative warming in the cardiac patient: evaluation of the Bair Hugger convective warming system. J Cardiothorac Vasc Anesth 1994;8(suppl 3):80.
18. Pathi V, Berg GA, Morrison J, Cramp G, McLaren D, Faichney A. The benefits of active rewarming after cardiac operations: a randomized prospective trial. J Thorac Cardiovasc Surg 1996; 111:637–41.
19. Doufas AG, Lin CM, Suleman MI, et al. Dexmedetomidine and meperidine additively reduce shivering threshold in humans. Stroke 2003:34:1218–23.
20. Kranke P, Eberhart LH, Roewer N, Tramer MR. Pharmacological treatment of postoperative shivering: a quantitative systematic review of randomized controlled trials. Anesth Analg 2002;94:453–60.
21. Milne E, James KS, Nimmo S, Hickey S. Oxygen consumption after hypothermic cardiopulmonary bypass: the effect of continuing a propofol infusion postoperatively. J Cardiothorac Vasc Anesth 2002;16:32–6.
22. Kurz A, Go JC, Sessler DI, Kaer K, Larson MD, Bjorksten AR. Alfentanil slightly increases the sweating threshold and markedly reduces the vasoconstriction and shivering thresholds. Anesthesiology 1995;83:293–9.
23. Leslie K, Sessler DI, Bjorksten AR, et al. Propofol causes a dose-dependent decrease in the thermoregulatory threshold for vasoconstriction but has little effect on sweating. Anesthesiology 1994;81:353–60.

24. Despotis GJ, Hogue CW Jr. Pathophysiology, prevention, and treatment of bleeding after cardiac surgery: a primer for cardiologists and an update for the cardiothoracic team. Am J Cardiol 1999;83:15B–30.

25. Levi M, Cromheecke ME, de Jonge E, et al. Pharmacological strategies to decrease excessive blood loss in cardiac surgery: a meta-analysis of clinically relevant endpoints. Lancet 1999;354:1940–7.

26. Habbib R, Zacharias A, Engoren M. Determinants of prolonged mechanical ventilation after coronary artery bypass grafting. Ann Thorac Surg 1996;62:1164–71.

27. Gott JP, Cooper WA, Schmidt FE Jr, et al. Modifying risk for extracorporeal circulation: trial of four antiinflammatory strategies. Ann Thorac Surg 1998;66:747–54.

28. Meade MO, Guyatt G, Butler R, et al. Trials comparing early vs late extubation following cardiovascular surgery. Chest 2001;120(suppl 6):445S–53S.

29. Thomson IR, Harding G, Hudson RJ. A comparison of fentanyl and sufentanil in patients undergoing coronary artery bypass graft surgery. J Cardiothorac Vasc Anesth 2000;14:652–6.

30. Howie MB, Cheng D, Newman MF, et al. A randomized double-blinded multicenter comparison of remifentanil versus fentanyl when combined with isoflurane/propofol for early extubation in coronary artery bypass graft surgery. Anesth Analg 2001;92:1084–93.

31. Guarracino F, Penzo D, De Cosmo D, Vardanega A, De Stefani R. Pharmacokinetic-based total intravenous anaesthesia using remifentanil and propofol for surgical myocardial revascularization. Eur J Anaesthesiol 2003;20:385–90.

32. Alhan C, Toraman F, Karabulut EH, et al. Fast track recovery of high risk coronary bypass surgery patients. Eur J Cardiothorac Surg 2003;23:678–83.

33. Hall RI, Sandham D, Cardinal P, et al. Propofol vs midazolam for ICU sedation. A Canadian multicenter randomized trial. Chest 2001;119:1151–9.

34. Jacobi J, Fraser GL, Coursin DB, et al. Clinical practice guidelines for the sustained use of sedatives and analgesics in the critically ill adult. Crit Care Med 2002;30:119–41.

35. Ralley FE, Day FJ, Cheng DCH. Pro: Nonsteroidal anti-inflammatory drugs should be routinely administered for postoperative analgesia after cardiac surgery. J Cardiothorac Vasc Anesth 2000;14:731–4.

36. Hynninen MS, Cheng DC, Hossain I, et al. Non-steroidal anti-inflammatory drugs in treatment of postoperative pain after cardiac surgery. Can J Anaesth 2000;47:1182–7.

37. Herr DL, Sum-Ping ST, England M. ICU sedation after coronary artery bypass graft surgery: dexmedetomidine-based versus propofol-based sedation regimens. J Cardiothorac Vasc Anesth 2003;17:576–84.

38. Ready LB, Brown CR, Stahlgren LH, et al. Evaluation of intravenous ketorolac administered by bolus or infusion for treatment of postoperative pain. A double-blind, placebo-controlled, multicenter study. Anesthesiology 1994;80:1277–86.

39. Griffin MJ, Hines RL. Management of perioperative ventricular dysfunction. J Cardiothorac Vasc Anesth 2001;15:90–106.

40. Ley SJ, Miller K, Skov P, Preisig P. Crystalloid versus colloid fluid after cardiac surgery. Heart Lung 1990;19:31–40.

41. Gallagher JD, Moore RA, Kerns D, et al. Effects of colloid or crystalloid administration on pulmonary extravascular water in the postoperative period after coronary artery bypass grafting. Anesth Analg 1985;64:753–8.

42. Zerr KJ, Furnary AP, Grunkemeier GL, Bookin S, Kanhere V, Starr A. Glucose control lowers the risk of wound infection in diabetics after open heart operations. Ann Thorac Surg 1997;63:356–61.

43. Furnary AP, Gao G, Grunkemeier GL, et al. Continuous insulin infusion reduces mortality in patients with diabetes undergoing coronary artery bypass grafting. J Thorac Cardiovasc Surg 2003;125:1007–21.

44. Mekontso-Dessap A, Houel R, Soutstelle C, Kirsch M, Thebert D, Loisance DY. Risk factors for post-cardiopulmonary bypass vasoplegia in patients with preserved left ventricular function. Ann Thorac Surg 2001;71:1428–32.

45. Gomes WJ, Carvalho AC, Palma JH, et al. Vasoplegic syndrome after open heart surgery. J Cardiovasc Surg (Torino) 1998;39:619–23.

46. Gomes WJ, Erlichman MR, Batista-Filho ML, et al. Vasoplegic syndrome after off-pump coronary artery bypass surgery. Eur J Cardiothorac Surg 2003;23:165–9.

47. Aurigemma G, Battista S, Orsinelli D, Sweeney A, Pape L, Cuenoud H. Abnormal left ventricular intracavity flow acceleration in patients undergoing aortic valve replacement for aortic stenosis. A marker for high postoperative morbidity and mortality. Circulation 1992;86:926–36.

48. Bartunek J, Sys SU, Rodrigues AC, Scheurbeeck EV, Mortier L, de Bruyne B. Abnormal systolic intracavity flow velocities after valve replacement for aortic stenosis. Mechanisms, predictive factors, and prognostic significance. Circulation 1996;93:712–9.

49. Gordon G, Rastegar H, Khabbaz K, Schumann R, England M. Perioperative use of nesiritide in adult cardiac surgery. Anesth Analg 2004;98:SCA1–134.

50. Hill LL, De Wet C, Hogue CW Jr. Management of atrial fibrillation after cardiac surgery. Part II: Prevention and treatment. J Cardiothorac Vasc Anesth 2002;16:626–37.

51. Roffman JA, Fieldman A. Digoxin and propranolol in the prophylaxis of supraventricular tachydysrhythmias after coronary artery bypass surgery. Ann Thorac Surg 1981;31:496–501.

52. Speziale G, Ruvolo G, Fattouch K, et al. Arrhythmia prophylaxis after coronary artery bypass grafting: regimens of magnesium sulfate administration. Thorac Cardiovasc Surg 2000;48:22–6.

53. Bert AA, Reinert SE, Singh AK. A beta-blocker, not magnesium, is effective prophylaxis for atrial tachyarrhythmias after coronary artery bypass graft surgery. J Cardiothorac Vasc Anesth 2001;15:204–9.

54. Gavard JA, Chaitman BR, Sakai S, et al. Prognostic significance of elevated creatine kinase MB after coronary bypass surgery and after an acute coronary syndrome: results from the GUARDIAN trial. J Thorac Cardiovasc Surg 2003;126:807–13.

55. Alyanakian MA, Dehoux M, Chatel D, et al. Cardiac troponin I in diagnosis of perioperative myocardial infarction after cardiac surgery. J Cardiothorac Vasc Anesth 1998;12:288–94.

56. Stein PD, Schunemann HJ, Dalen JE, Gutterman D. Antithrombotic therapy in patients with saphenous vein and internal mammary artery grafts. The Seventh ACCP conference on antithrombotic and thrombolytic therapy. Chest 2004;126:600S–8S.

57. Ascione R, Caputo M, Angelini G. Off-pump coronary artery bypass grafting: not a flash in the pan. Ann Thorac Surg 2003;75:306–13.

58. Mack MJ. Pro: beating heart surgery for coronary revascularization: is it the most important development since the introduction of the heart-lung machine? Ann Thorac Surg 2000;70:1774–8.

59. Ngaage DL. Off-pump coronary artery bypass grafting: the myth, the logic and the science. Eur J Cardiothorac Surg 2003;24:557–70.

60. Puskas JD, Williams WH, Duke PG, et al. Off-pump coronary artery bypass grafting provides complete revascularization with reduced myocardial injury, transfusion requirements, and length of stay: a prospective randomized comparison of two hundred unselected patients undergoing off-pump versus conventional coronary artery bypass grafting. J Thorac Cardiovasc Surg 2003;125:797–808.

61. Nuttall GA, Erchul DT, Haight TJ, et al. A comparison of bleeding and transfusion in patients who undergo coronary artery bypass grafting via sternotomy with and without cardiopulmonary bypass. J Cardiothorac Vasc Anesth 2003;17:447–51.

62. Nader ND, Khadra WZ, Reich NT, Bacon DR, Salerno TA, Panos AL. Blood product use in cardiac revascularization: comparison of on-pump and off-pump techniques. Ann Thorac Surg 1999;68:1640–3.

63. Lee JD, Lee SJ, Tsushima WT, et al. Benefits of off-pump bypass on neurologic and clinical morbidity: a prospective randomized trial. Ann Thorac Surg 2003;76:18–26.

64. Athanasiou T, Al-Ruzzeh S, Kumar P, et al. Off-pump myocardial revascularization is associated with less incidence of stroke in elderly patients. Ann Thorac Surg 2004;77:745–53.

65. Taggart DP, Browne SM, Halligan PW, Wade DT. Is cardiopulmonary bypass still the cause of cognitive dysfunction after cardiac operations? J Thorac Cardiovasc Surg 1999;118:414–21.

66. Athanasiou T, Aziz O, Mangoush O, et al. Do off-pump techniques reduce the incidence of postoperative atrial fibrillation in elderly patients undergoing coronary artery bypass grafting? Ann Thorac Surg 2004;77:1567–74.

67. Salamon T, Michler RE, Knott KM, Brown DA. Off-pump coronary artery bypass grafting does not decrease the incidence of atrial fibrillation. Ann Thorac Surg 2003;75:505–7.

68. Michelsen LG, Horswell S. Anesthesia for off-pump coronary artery bypass grafting. Semin Thorac Cardiovasc Surg 2003;15:71–82.

69. Zimbler N, Ashley EM. Anaesthesia for coronary artery bypass: should it differ off-pump and on-pump? Hosp Med 2003;64:564.

70. Haaverstad R, Vitale N, Tjomsland O, Tromsdal A, Torp H, Samstad SO. Intraoperative color Doppler ultrasound assessment of LIMA-to-LAD anastomoses in off-pump coronary artery bypass grafting. Ann Thorac Surg 2002;74:S1390–4.

71. Suematsu Y, Ohtsuka T, Miyairi T, Motomura N, Takamoto S. Ultrasonic evaluation of graft anastomoses during coronary artery bypass grafting without cardiopulmonary bypass. Ann Thorac Surg 2002;74:273–5.

72. Cimen S, Ozkul V, Ketenci B, et al. Daily comparison of respiratory functions between on-pump and off-pump patients undergoing CABG. Eur J Cardiothorac Surg 2003;23:589–94.

73. Cumpeeravut P, Visudharom K, Jotisakulratana V, Pitigagool V, Banyatpiyaphod S, Pamornsing P. Off-pump coronary artery bypass surgery: evaluation of extubation time and predictors of failed early extubation. J Med Assoc Thai 2003;8(suppl I):S28–35.

74. Casati V, Valle PD, Benussi S et al. Effects of tranexamic acid on postoperative bleeding and related histochemical variables in coronary surgery: comparison between on-pump and off-pump techniques. J Thorac Cardiovasc Surg 2004;128:83–91.

75. Englberger L, Markart P, Eckstein FS, Immer FF, Berdat PA, Carrel TP. Aprotinin reduces blood loss in off-pump coronary artery (OPCAB) surgery. Eur J Cardiothorac Surg 2002;22:545–51.

76. Thomas JL, Dickstein RA, Parker FB, et al. Prognostic significance of the development of left bundle conduction defects following aortic valve replacement. J Thorac Cardiovasc Surg 1982;84:382–6.

77. Salem DN, Stein PD, Al-Ahmad A, et al. Antithrombotic therapy in valvular heart disease—native and prosthetic. The Seventh ACCP conference on antithrombotic and thrombolytic therapy. Chest 2004;126:457S–82S.

78. Mistiaen W, Van Cauwelaert Ph, Muylaert Ph, Sys SU, Harrisson F, Bortier H. Thromboembolic events after aortic valve replacement in elderly patients with a Carpentier-Edwards Perimount pericardial bioprosthesis. J Thorac Cardiovasc Surg 2004;127:1166–70.

79. Moinuddeen K, Quin J, Shaw R, et al. Anticoagulation is unnecessary after biological aortic valve replacement. Circulation 1998;98:II-95–9.

80. Orszulak TA, Schaff HV, Mullany CJ, et al. Risk of thromboembolism with the aortic Carpentier-Edwards bioprosthesis. Ann Thorac Surg 1995;59:462–8.

81. Bonow RO, Carabello B, de Leon Jr AC, et al. ACC/AHA guidelines for the management of patients with valvular heart disease. A report of the American College of Cardiology/American Heart Association task force on practice guidelines (Committee on management of patients with valvular heart disease). J Am Coll Cardiol 1998;32:1486–588.

82. Spinale FG, Smith AC, Carabello BA, Crawford FA. Right ventricular function computed by thermodilution and ventriculography. A comparison of methods. J Thorac Cardiovasc Surg 1990;99:141–52.

83. Camara ML, Aris A, Alvarez J, Padro JM, Caralps JM. Hemodynamic effects of prostaglandin E1 and isoproterenol early after cardiac operations for mitral stenosis. J Thorac Cardiovasc Surg 1992;103:1177–85.

84. Mahoney PD, Loh E, Blitz LR, Herrmann HC. Hemodynamic effects of inhaled nitric oxide in women with mitral stenosis and pulmonary hypertension. Am J Cardiol 2001;87:188–92.

85. De Wet CJ, Affleck DG, Jacobsohn E, et al. Inhaled prostacyclin is safe, effective, and affordable in patients with pulmonary hypertension, right heart dysfunction, and refractory hypoxemia after cardiothoracic surgery. J Thorac Cardiovasc Surg 2004;127:1058–67.

86. D'Ambra MN, LaRaia PJ, Philbin DM, Watkins WD, Hilgenberg AD, Buckley MJ. Prostaglandin E₁: a new therapy for refractory right heart failure and pulmonary hypertension after mitral valve replacement. J Thorac Cardiovasc Surg 1985;89:567–72.

87. Santini G, Gatti G, Borghetti V, Oppido G, Mazzucco A. Routine left atrial catheterization for the post-operative management of cardiac surgical patients: is the risk justified? Eur J Cardiothorac Surg 1999;16:218–21.

88. Garcia-Villarreal OA, Gonzalez-Oviedo R, Rodriguez-Gonzalez H, Martinez-Chapa HD. Superior septal approach for mitral valve surgery: a word of caution. Eur J Cardiothorac Surg 2003;24:862–7.

89. Tambuer L, Meyns B, Flameng W, Daenen W. Rhythm disturbances after mitral valve surgery: comparison between left atrial and extended transseptal approach. Cardiovasc Surg 1996;4:820–4.

90. Karlson KH, Ashraf MM, Berger RL. Rupture of the left ventricle following mitral valve replacement. Ann Thorac Surg 1988;46:590–7.

91. Passage J, Jalali H, Tam RKW, Harrocks S, O'Brien MF. BioGlue surgical adhesive: an appraisal of its indications in cardiac surgery. Ann Thorac Surg 2002;74:432–7.

92. de Figueiredo LFP, Coselli JS. Individual strategies of hemostasis for thoracic aortic surgery. J Cardiac Surg 1997;12(suppl):222–8.

93. Sundt TM III, Kouchoukos NT, Saffitz JE, Murphy SF, Wareing TH, Stahl DJ. Renal dysfunction and intravascular coagulation with aprotinin and hypothermic circulatory arrest. Ann Thorac Surg 1993;55:1418–24.

94. Smith CR, Spanier TB. Aprotinin in deep hypothermic circulatory arrest. Ann Thorac Surg 1999;68:278–86.

95. Royston D. Pro: aprotinin should be used in patients undergoing circulatory arrest. J Cardiothorac Vasc Anesth 2001;15:121–5.

96. Griepp RB. Cerebral protection during aortic arch surgery. J Thorac Cardiovasc Surg 2001;121:425–7.

97. Reich DL, Uysal S, Ergin MA, Griepp RB. Retrograde cerebral perfusion as a method of neuroprotection during thoracic aortic surgery. Ann Thorac Surg 2001;72:1774–82.

98. Cambria RP, Clouse WD, Davison JK, Dunn PF, Corey M, Dorer D. Thoracoabdominal aneurysm repair: results with 337 operations performed over a 15-year interval. Ann Surg 2002;236:471–9.

99. Estrera AL, Rubenstein FS, Miller CC III, Huynh TTT, Letsou GV, Safi HJ. Descending thoracic aortic aneurysm: surgical approach and treatment using the adjuncts cerebrospinal fluid drainage and distal aortic perfusion. Ann Thorac Surg 2001;72:481–6.

100. Estrera AL, Miller CC III, Huynh TTT, Porat E, Safi HJ. Neurologic outcome after thoracic and thoracoabdominal aortic aneurysm repair. Ann Thorac Surg 2001;72:1225–31.

101. LeMaire SA, Miller CC III, Conklin LD, Schmittling ZC, Coselli JC. Estimating group mortality and paraplegia rates after thoracoabdominal aortic aneurysm repair. Ann Thorac Surg 2003;75:508–13.

102. Plestis KA, Nair DG, Russo M, Gold JP. Left atrial femoral bypass and cerebrospinal fluid drainage decreases neurologic complications in repair of descending and thoracoabdominal aortic aneurysms. Ann Vasc Surg 2001;15:49–52.

103. Coselli JS, Lemaire SA, Koksoy C, Schmittling ZC, Curling PE. Cerebrospinal fluid drainage reduces paraplegia after thoracoabdominal aortic aneurysm repair: results of a randomized clinical trial. J Vasc Surg 2002;35:631–9.

104. Maniar HS, Sundt TM III, Prasad SM, et al. Delayed paraplegia after thoracic and thoracoabdominal aneurysm repair: a continuing risk. Ann Thorac Surg 2003;75:113–20.

105. Huynh TT, Miller CC, Safi HJ. Delayed onset of neurologic deficit: significance and management. Semin Vasc Surg 2000;13:340–4.

106. Sheinbaum R, Ignacio C, Safi HJ, Estrera A. Contemporary strategies to preserve renal function during cardiac and vascular surgery. Rev Cardiovasc Med 2003;4(suppl):S2–8.

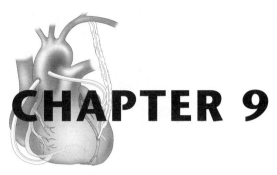

CHAPTER 9

Mediastinal Bleeding

Mediastinal Bleeding

I. Overview

A. The use of cardiopulmonary bypass (CPB) during cardiac surgical procedures causes a significant disruption of the coagulation system.[1,2] In addition to hemodilution from a crystalloid prime, contact of blood with the extracorporeal circuit activates platelets and several cascades that activate the extrinsic and intrinsic coagulation systems and trigger fibrinolysis.[3] In fact, systemic heparinization alone causes platelet dysfunction and induces fibrinolysis.[4] In addition, the use of cell-saving devices produces loss of platelets and coagulation factors. Thus, a myriad of factors can contribute to a coagulopathy that is present to varying degrees in all patients undergoing surgery on CPB.

B. Although off-pump coronary artery bypass (OPCAB) surgery avoids many of these problems and is associated with reduced usage of blood products,[5,6] the ability of the antifibrinolytic agents to reduce bleeding suggests that low-grade fibrinolysis, perhaps related to heparin, is still present.[7,8] Although a coagulopathy after OPCAB is very unusual, it may occur in patients who have sustained substantial blood loss with blood scavenged in and returned from the cell-saving device. This results in depletion of coagulation factors and platelets. The occurrence of substantial bleeding after an OPCAB procedure generally indicates a surgical source.

C. Postoperative bleeding gradually tapers over the course of several hours in the majority of patients, but about 1–3% of patients will require reexploration in the operating room for persistent mediastinal bleeding. Prompt and aggressive treatment upon arrival in the ICU may frequently arrest "medical bleeding," but evidence of persistent or increasing amounts of bleeding should prompt early exploration (see section VII).

D. Mediastinal bleeding can be a highly morbid and lethal problem. Although hypovolemia can be corrected by volume infusions, the bleeding patient tends to be hemodynamically unstable out of proportion to the degree of bleeding and fluid replacement. Bleeding invariably requires use of various blood products to maintain normovolemia, correct anemia, and correct a coagulopathy. Transfused blood is replete with vasoactive cytokines, provides hemoglobin that is less effective in transporting oxygen, and can potentially contribute to respiratory insufficiency, delayed extubation, right ventricular failure, transfusion reactions, and transmission of viral disease. Transfusions increase the risk of infection and renal dysfunction, and also increase operative and long-term mortality.[9–13] Most importantly, however, blood that accumulates around the heart can produce **cardiac tamponade** with severe hemodynamic compromise that can precipitously cause cardiac arrest. Vigilant attention to the degree of bleeding and to trends in hemodynamic parameters should allow steps to be taken to avert this problem.

E. All patients who have a median sternotomy incision for cardiac surgery have mediastinal drainage tubes placed at the conclusion of the operation. Pleural tubes are also placed if the pleural spaces have been entered. Although 32F or 34F chest tubes are commonly used, smaller Silastic (Blake) drains are also very effective in evacuating blood and are more comfortable for the patient.[14-16] Upon arrival in the surgical ICU, the chest tubes are connected to a thoracic drainage system and placed to 20 cm of H_2O suction. They are gently milked or stripped to maintain patency. Autotransfusion of shed blood can be considered to reduce the requirement for homologous transfusion, although it is not cost-effective when the amount of drainage is insignificant and, in fact, it may contribute to worsening of a coagulopathy.[17-19]

F. Some surgeons do not obligatorily place chest tubes into widely opened pleural spaces, especially after off-pump surgery. However, any bleeding that occurs in the pleural space will tend to accumulate and not be drained by the mediastinal tubes. This can produce a deceptive picture with insidious bleeding that can only be detected by chest x-ray.

G. A pleural tube is placed after a MIDCAB procedure performed through a left thoracotomy or after a mitral valve procedure performed through a right thoracotomy or parasternal incision. Mediastinal drains are placed after minimally invasive valve operations performed through either upper or transverse sternotomies or parasternal incisions.

II. Etiology of Mediastinal Bleeding (Box 9.1)

Mediastinal bleeding is somewhat arbitrarily categorized as surgical or medical in nature. Significant bleeding after uneventful surgery is usually surgical in nature, especially when initial coagulation studies are fairly normal. However, persistent bleeding depletes coagulation factors and platelets causing a coagulopathy that is self-perpetuating. In contrast, bleeding that is noted after complex operations with long durations of CPB is frequently associated with abnormal coagulation studies and is considered medical in nature. However, even after correction of coagulation abnormalities, discrete bleeding sites may be present that will not stop without reexploration. Thus, the initial approach to bleeding is to try to ascertain any contributing factors that can account for the degree of bleeding and then take the appropriate steps to correct them.[20,21]

A. Surgical bleeding is usually related to:

1. Anastomotic sites (suture lines)

2. Side branches of arterial or venous conduits

3. Substernal soft tissues, sternal suture sites, bone marrow, periosteum

4. Raw surfaces caused by previous surgery, pericarditis, or radiation therapy

---

Box 9.1 • Causes of Mediastinal Bleeding

1. Surgical bleeding sites
2. Heparin effect, residual or rebound
3. Platelet dysfunction
4. Thrombocytopenia
5. Clotting factor deficiency
6. Fibrinolysis

B. Anticoagulant effect related to heparin

1. Residual heparin effect may result from inadequate neutralization with protamine. Administering fully heparinized "pump" blood as the protamine infusion is being completed may reintroduce unneutralized heparin into the blood. Similarly, residual heparin in cell saver blood given after protamine administration may reintroduce unreversed heparin.

2. Heparin rebound may occur when heparin reappears from tissue stores after protamine administration. This is more common in patients receiving large amounts of heparin, especially obese patients.

C. Quantitative platelet defects

1. Preoperative thrombocytopenia may result from use of heparin, in which case testing for heparin antibodies is essential to rule out heparin-induced thrombocytopenia. Drug reactions (especially to antibiotics) and hypersplenism in patients with liver disease may be causative. Occasionally, mild thrombocytopenia is present for no identifiable reason.

2. Hemodilution on CPB and consumption in the extracorporeal circuit reduce the platelet count by about 30–50%; thrombocytopenia will be progressive as the duration of CPB lengthens.

3. Protamine administration transiently reduces the platelet count by about 30%.

D. Qualitative platelet defects are a major concern with the liberal use of antiplatelet agents in patients with acute coronary syndromes.

1. Preoperative platelet dysfunction may result from antiplatelet medications (aspirin, clopidogrel), glycoprotein IIb/IIIa inhibitors (abciximab, tirofiban, eptifibatide), herbal medications and vitamins (fish oils, ginkgo products, vitamin E), or uremia.

2. Exposure of platelets to the CPB circuit with α-granule release and alteration of platelet membrane receptors impairs platelet function. The degree of platelet dysfunction correlates with the duration of CPB and the degree of hypothermia after bypass.

E. Depletion of coagulation factors

1. Preoperative hepatic dysfunction, residual warfarin effect, vitamin K–dependent clotting factor deficiencies, von Willebrand's disease, and thrombolytic therapy reduce the level of clotting factors.

2. Hemodilution on CPB reduces most factors by 50% and factor V by 80%. This is most pronounced in patients with a small blood volume.

3. Loss of clotting factors results from use of intraoperative cell-saving devices.

F. Fibrinolysis causes clotting factor degradation and platelet dysfunction

1. Preoperative use of thrombolytic agents

2. Plasminogen activation during bypass

3. Heparinization itself induces a fibrinolytic state

III. Prevention of Perioperative Bleeding (Box 9.2)[22–24]

A. Preoperative assessment of the patient's coagulation system should entail measurement of a prothrombin time (PT), partial thromboplastin time (PTT), and platelet count. Any abnormality should be investigated and corrected, if possible, prior to surgery.

Box 9.2 • Methods of Minimizing Operative Blood Loss and Transfusion Requirements

1. Stop all anticoagulant and antiplatelet medications preoperatively.

2. Identify abnormal preoperative abnormalities (R/O HIT if thrombocytopenic) and transfuse patients requiring urgent surgery to a hematocrit > 30% preoperatively; place elective patients on iron and/or erythropoietin to optimize hematocrit.

3. Use antifibrinolytic therapy (aprotinin, ε-aminocaproic acid, or tranexamic acid).

4. Autologous blood withdrawal if satisfactory hematocrit.

5. Meticulous surgical technique with careful inspection of anastomotic sites and all artery and vein side branches before coming off bypass.

6. Consider off-pump coronary bypass grafting, if feasible.

7. Use a heparin-coated circuit, if available.

8. Consider retrograde autologous priming of the bypass circuit.

9. Avoid cardiotomy suction.

10. Complete neutralization of heparin with protamine to return ACT to baseline.

11. Salvage pump blood either via hemofiltration or cell saver and reverse any residual heparin with protamine.

12. Administer appropriate blood component therapy based on suspicion of the hemostatic defect (especially platelet dysfunction) or use point-of-care testing to direct blood component therapy.

13. Be patient.

B. **Heparin-induced thrombocytopenia (HIT)** may develop in patients receiving intravenous heparin for several days before surgery. Thus, it is very important to recheck the platelet count on a daily basis in these patients. If the patient develops thrombocytopenia and has confirmation of heparin antibodies by serologic testing or a serotonin release assay, an alternative means of anticoagulation will be necessary (see page 154).[25]

C. **Cessation of medications** with antiplatelet or anticoagulant effects is essential to allow their effects to dissipate in order to minimize blood loss. A more detailed discussion of these medications is presented in Chapter 4. Specific recommendations are as follows:

1. **Warfarin** should be stopped 4 days before surgery to allow for resynthesis of vitamin K–dependent clotting factors and normalization of the international normalized ratio (INR).[26] If interim anticoagulation is required, heparin is substituted. If the patient requires urgent surgery, vitamin K should be given (two doses of 5 mg IV should suffice) to normalize the INR. If emergency surgery is indicated, fresh frozen plasma (FFP) may be necessary.[27]

2. **Unfractionated heparin** is reversible with protamine and is commonly used for acute coronary syndromes. It can be continued up to the time of surgery without any increased morbidity during line placement.

3. **Low-molecular-weight heparin,** generally given in a dose of 1 mg/kg SC q12h for acute coronary syndromes, should be stopped at least 12 hours prior to surgery,

since it is only 80% reversible with protamine. Studies have shown increased bleeding when it is administered within 12 hours of surgery.[28]

4. **Aspirin** should be stopped at least 3 days prior to surgery to ensure adequate restoration of platelet function and reduce transfusion requirements.[29,30] Preoperative cessation of aspirin has become controversial because several studies have demonstrated reduced rates of infarction and mortality when aspirin is continued up to the time of surgery.[31,32] Aprotinin and tranexamic acid are useful in reducing bleeding associated with preoperative use of aspirin.[33,34]

5. **Clopidogrel** has antiplatelet effects that last for the life span of the platelet, and it should therefore be stopped 5–7 days prior to elective surgery.[35] However, it is commonly used in acute coronary syndromes and in anticipation of a stenting procedure. Although inhibition of platelet activity occurs about 2 hours after the drug is administered, achievement of a steady state with 50% inhibition of platelet aggregation occurs about 6 hours after a loading dose of 300 mg or after about 4–5 doses of 75 mg. If surgery is then required on an urgent basis, significant bleeding may be encountered. Aprotinin may be successful in reducing bleeding in patients receiving this medication (although this has not been studied), but platelets are often required. If the active metabolite of clopidogrel is still present in the bloodstream, exogenously administered platelets may be ineffective.

6. **Ticlopidine** has been replaced by clopidogrel in patients undergoing stenting, although some patients still receive it for the management of cerebrovascular disease. Since its activity also lasts the life span of the platelet, it should be stopped at least 7 days prior to surgery. If bleeding is encountered, platelets may be needed. An abnormal bleeding time caused by ticlopidine can be normalized within 2 hours by methylprednisolone 20 mg IV.[36]

7. **Tirofiban** (Aggrastat) and **eptifibatide** (Integrilin) are short-acting IIb/IIIa inhibitors that allow for recovery of 80% of platelet function within 4–6 hours of being discontinued.[37] They should be stopped about 4 hours prior to surgery. Some studies have shown that continuing these medications up to the time of surgery may preserve platelet function on pump, leading to increased platelet number and function after bypass with no adverse effects on bleeding.[38]

8. **Abciximab (Reopro)** is a long-acting IIb/IIIa inhibitor used for high-risk percutaneous coronary intervention that has a half-life of 12 hours. If surgery must be performed on an emergency basis, platelets are effective in producing hemostasis since there is very little circulating unbound drug. Ideally, surgery should be delayed for at least 12 hours and preferably for 24 hours since recovery of platelet function takes up to 48 hours. Although abnormal bleeding times and platelet aggregation tests are still abnormal in up to 25% of patients at this time, there is little hemostatic compromise at receptor blockade levels less than 50%.[39]

9. **Thrombolytic therapy** is an alternative to primary angioplasty in patients presenting with ST-segment elevation myocardial infarctions. Although currently used agents have short half-lives measured in minutes, the systemic hemostatic defects persist much longer. These effects include depletion of fibrinogen, reduction in factor II, V, and VIII levels, impairment of platelet aggregation, and the appearance of fibrin split products. If surgery is required for persistent ischemia after failed thrombolytic therapy, it should be delayed by at least 12–24 hours. If it is required emergently, plasma and cryoprecipitate will probably be necessary to correct the anticipated coagulopathy.

D. Antifibrinolytic therapy should be used to reduce intraoperative blood loss (see pages 149–152).[40,41]

1. **Aprotinin** is a serine protease inhibitor that is extremely effective in reducing blood loss and transfusion requirements. It preserves adhesive platelet receptors during the early period of CPB, exhibits antifibrinolytic properties by inhibiting plasmin, and also inhibits kallikrein, blocking the contact phase of coagulation and inhibiting the intrinsic coagulation cascade. Although it has been recommended for primary coronary bypass operations, it is very expensive and is usually reserved for complex operations and reoperations.[42–46] Doses and other concerns about use of aprotinin are discussed in Chapter 4.

2. **ε-aminocaproic acid** (Amicar) is an antifibrinolytic agent that may preserve platelet function by inhibiting the conversion of plasminogen to plasmin. It is effective in reducing blood loss and, because of its low cost, is usually the drug of choice for all first-time operations and anticipated uncomplicated reoperations. Most studies suggest it is not as effective as aprotinin.[44,47]

3. **Tranexamic acid** (Cyclokapron) has similar properties to ε-aminocaproic acid. It has also been shown to reduce perioperative blood loss. It is more expensive than ε-aminocaproic acid but much less expensive than aprotinin. Some studies have shown its efficacy to be equivalent to that of ε-aminocaproic acid; others have shown it to be as effective as aprotinin.[44–46]

E. Autologous blood withdrawal before instituting bypass protects platelets from the damaging effects of CPB. It has been demonstrated to preserve red cell mass and reduce transfusion requirements. However, its efficacy in reducing perioperative bleeding is controversial.[48–52] It can be considered when the calculated on-pump hematocrit after withdrawal remains satisfactory (greater than 20–22%). This can be calculated using the following equation: amount that can be withdrawn = EBV − [0.22 (EBV + PV + CV)]/HCT, where EBV is the estimated blood volume (70 × kg), PV is the priming volume, CV is the estimated cardioplegia volume, and HCT is the prewithdrawal hematocrit.

F. Platelet-rich plasmapheresis entails the withdrawal of platelet-rich plasma using a plasma separator at the beginning of the operation with its readministration after protamine infusion. This improves hemostasis and reduces blood loss. Although it might be beneficial in reoperations, it is expensive, time-consuming, and probably of little benefit when prophylactic antifibrinolytic medications are used.[53,54]

G. Meticulous surgical technique is the mainstay of hemostasis. Warming the patient to normothermia before terminating bypass improves the function of the coagulation system.

H. CPB considerations

1. The use of **heparin-coated circuits** during bypass allows for a reduction in heparin dosing and has been associated with reduced perioperative blood loss.[55]

2. **Retrograde autologous priming** of the extracorporeal circuit entails withdrawal of crystalloid prime to minimize hemodilution, thus maintaining a higher hematocrit and colloid oncotic pressure on pump. In some studies, this has been shown to reduce the rate of transfusion.[56]

3. **Avoidance of cardiotomy suction** may reduce perioperative bleeding. Blood aspirated from the pericardial space has been in contact with tissue factor and contains high levels of factor VIIa, procoagulant particles, and activated complement proteins, and exhibits fibrinolytic activity.[57–59]

IV. Assessment of Bleeding in the ICU

A. The appropriate assessment of bleeding in the ICU requires the following steps:

1. Frequent documentation of the amount of blood draining into the collection system and attention to tube patency

2. Determination of the color (arterial or venous) and pattern of drainage (sudden dump when turned or continuous drainage)

3. Monitoring of hemodynamic parameters with ongoing awareness of the possibility of cardiac tamponade

4. Identification of potential causative factors by review of coagulation studies

5. Suspicion of undrained blood in the mediastinum or pleural spaces by review of a chest x-ray, auscultating decreased breath sounds on examination, or noting elevation of peak inspiratory pressures on the ventilator

B. Quantitate the amount of chest tube drainage. Make sure that the chest tubes are patent because the extent of ongoing hemorrhage may be masked when the tubes have clotted or blood has drained into an open pleural space. **Note:** When patients are turned or moved, they occasionally drain a significant volume of blood that has been accumulating in the chest for several hours. This may suggest the acute onset of bleeding and the need for surgical exploration. The presence of dark blood and minimal additional drainage are clues that this does not represent active bleeding. Serial chest x-rays may be helpful in identifying residual blood.

C. Assess hemodynamics with the Swan-Ganz catheter. Maintenance of adequate filling pressures and cardiac output is essential and is generally accomplished using crystalloid or colloid solutions. However, in the bleeding patient, these will produce hemodilution and progressive anemia.

1. If filling pressures are decreasing and nonheme fluid is administered, one needs to anticipate a decrease in the hematocrit from hemodilution, but more so with ongoing bleeding. The administration of volume in the form of clotting factors and platelets to promote hemostasis must be accompanied by red cell transfusions to maintain a safe hematocrit. It should be reiterated that unstable hemodynamics are frequently seen in the bleeding patient even if filling pressures are maintained.

2. Evidence of rising filling pressures and decreasing cardiac outputs may suggest the development of cardiac tamponade. Equilibration of intracardiac pressures may be noted with postoperative tamponade, but, more commonly, accumulation of clot adjacent to the right or left atrium will produce variable elevation in intracardiac pressures that are also consistent with right or left ventricular failure, respectively.[60]

3. If hemodynamic measurements suggest borderline cardiac function and tamponade cannot be ruled out, **transesophageal echocardiography** (TEE) is invaluable in making the correct diagnosis. Tamponade should be suspected when hemodynamic compromise is associated with excessive bleeding, bleeding that has abruptly stopped, or even minimal chest tube drainage caused by clotted tubes or spillage into the pleural space. TEE is often more accurate than a transthoracic study in detecting clot around the heart because the latter may be compromised by inability to obtain acoustic windows necessary to adequately identify an effusion.

D. Obtain **coagulation studies** upon arrival in the ICU and **serial hematocrits** if the patient is bleeding. Coagulation studies need not be ordered if the patient has minimal mediastinal bleeding. However, if hemostasis was difficult to achieve in the operating room or hemorrhage persists (generally greater than 100 mL/h), lab tests may be helpful in assessing whether a coagulopathy is contributing to mediastinal bleeding. Tests for some of the more common nonsurgical causes of bleeding (residual heparin effect, thrombocytopenia, and clotting factor deficiency) are readily available, but documentation of platelet dysfunction requires additional technology.[61] Although no individual test correlates that well with the amount of bleeding, together they can usually direct interventions in a somewhat scientific manner.[62] No matter what the results of coagulation testing are, clinical judgment remains paramount in trying to ascertaining whether the bleeding is more likely to be of a surgical nature (which tends to persist) or due to a coagulopathy (which might improve).

1. **Prothrombin time** measured as the INR assesses the extrinsic coagulation cascade. The INR may be slightly prolonged after a standard pump run, but clotting factor levels exceeding 30% of normal should allow for satisfactory hemostasis. An abnormal INR can be corrected with FFP.

2. **Partial thromboplastin time** assesses the intrinsic coagulation cascade and can also detect residual or recurrent heparin effect ("heparin rebound"). As an isolated abnormality or with slight elevation of the INR, protamine is beneficial in correcting the PTT and controlling bleeding.

3. **Platelet count.** Although CPB reduces the platelet count by about 30–50% and also produces platelet dysfunction, platelet function is usually adequate to produce hemostasis. Platelet transfusions may be justified in the bleeding patient for thrombocytopenia (generally < 100,000/μL) or for suspicion of platelet dysfunction (usually for patients on aspirin or clopidogrel).

4. **Platelet function** can be assessed by a variety of available technologies, including those that measure platelet aggregometry and other sophisticated tests of clot formation and retraction.[61,63]

5. Additional tests may be considered for severe bleeding if a coagulopathy is suspected. However, if normal coagulation studies are present before or after the standard corrective measures are taken, surgical reexploration is generally indicated.

   a. Assessment for **fibrinolysis** entails measurement of D-dimer and fibrinogen levels. Fibrinolysis is associated with an elevation in the PT and PTT, and decreased levels of factor I (fibrinogen < 150 mg/dL) and factor VIII. However, an elevated D-dimer alone is not uncommon and may also be noted if shed blood is autotransfused.[64] Use of aprotinin may be considered if fibrinolysis is confirmed, even if one of the other antifibrinolytic medications had been used during surgery, although it may contribute to a prothrombotic state.

   b. **Thromboelastography** (Figure 9.1) gives a qualitative measurement of clot strength. It is used to evaluate the interaction of platelets with the coagulation cascade from the onset of clot formation through clot lysis. The thromboelastogram shows a distinct contour in patients with fibrinolysis.[65]

   c. **Sonoclot analysis** (Figure 9.2) is another viscoelastic method for evaluating clot formation and retraction that allows for assessment of coagulation factors, fibrinogen, and platelet activity. The device measures the changing impedance to movement imposed by the developing clot on a small probe that vibrates at an ultrasonic frequency within a blood sample. Studies have suggested that both a thromboelastogram and a Sonoclot are more predictive of bleeding than routine coagulation studies. This modality has seen limited use but can direct appropriate therapy in patients with persistent bleeding.[66]

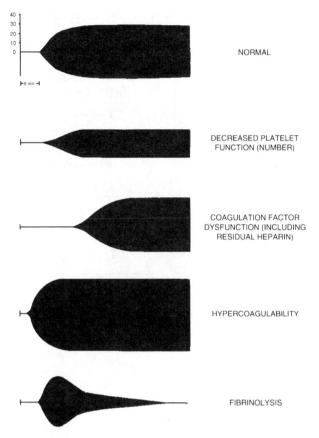

Figure 9.1 • Representative thromboelastographic tracings. *(Reproduced with permission from Tuman KJ, McCarthy RJ, Ivankovich AD. The thromboelastograph: is it the solution to coagulation problems? Cardiothorac Vasc Anesth update 1991;2; chapter 8:1–13.)*

E. **Repeat a chest x-ray**

1. Note the overall width of the mediastinum. A widened mediastinum may suggest undrained clotted blood accumulating within the pericardial cavity that could cause cardiac tamponade. Comparison with preoperative films can be misleading because of differences in technique, but any difference noted between the immediate postoperative supine film and a repeat film should be noted.

2. Note the distance between the edge of the Swan-Ganz catheter in the right atrium or the location of the right atrial pacing wires (if placed on the right atrial free wall) and the edge of the mediastinal silhouette. If this distance widens, suspect clot accumulation adjacent to the right atrium.

3. Note any accumulation of blood within the pleural spaces that has not drained through the pleural chest tubes. This can be difficult to assess since fluid will layer out on a supine film, so a discrepancy in the haziness of the two pleural spaces should be sought.

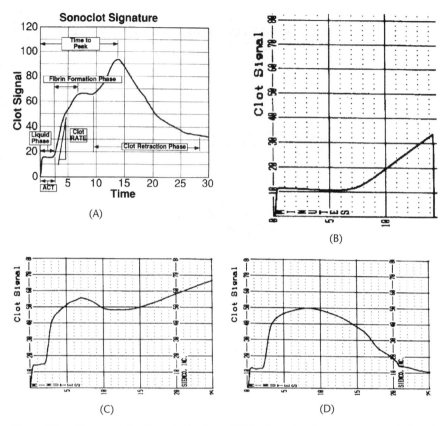

Figure 9.2 • Representative Sonoclot tracings. (A) The Sonoclot signature assesses the liquid phase of initial clot formation, the rate of fibrin and clot formation, further fibrinogenesis and platelet-fibrin interaction, a peak impedance after completion of fibrin formation, and a downward slope as platelets induce contraction of the completed clot. (B) Heparinization. (C) Poor platelet function (slow clot retraction). (D) Hyperfibrinolysis (no tightening associated with clot retraction). *(Images courtesy of Sienco, Inc.)*

V. Management of Mediastinal Bleeding (Box 9.3)

Although there is no role for prophylactic blood product transfusions in the prevention of bleeding following open-heart surgery, persistent bleeding must be treated immediately and aggressively based on the suspected cause of hemorrhage. It is a truism that the longer a patient bleeds, the worse the coagulopathy becomes. In general, the most benign and least invasive treatments should be considered first. If a patient was "dry" at the time of closure and suddenly starts to bleed, the source is usually surgical in nature and requires reexploration. In contrast, the patient with persistent bleeding may have a surgical or medical cause for the bleeding.[24,67]

    A. Ensure chest tube patency. Ongoing bleeding without drainage leads to tamponade. Gently milk the tubes to remove clot. Aggressive stripping is not necessary. There is no particular advantage to any of the common practices (milking, stripping, fan folding, or tapping) in maintaining chest tube patency.[68]

Box 9.3 • Management of Postoperative Mediastinal Bleeding

1. Explore early for significant ongoing bleeding or tamponade
2. Ensure that chest tubes are patent
3. Warm patient to normothermia
4. Control hypertension and shivering
5. Check results of coagulation studies (PT, PTT, platelet count)
6. Protamine 25 mg IV for two doses
7. Consider use of 10 cm PEEP with caution
8. Packed cells if hematocrit <26%
9. Platelets, one unit/10 kg
10. Fresh frozen plasma, 2–4 units
11. Aprotinin 2 million KIU IV over 20 minutes
12. Cryoprecipitate, one unit/10 kg
13. Desmopressin (DDAVP) 0.3 µg/kg IV over 20 minutes (if suspect platelet dysfunction from uremia or aspirin)
14. **Transesophageal echocardiography** if concerned about tamponade

---

B. Warm the patient to 37°C. Hypothermia produces a generalized suppression of the coagulation mechanism and also impairs platelet function.[69] The use of a heated humidifier in the ventilator circuit, a warming blanket, or a radiant heat shield is beneficial and will reduce the tendency to shiver. All blood products should be delivered through blood-warming devices.

C. Control hypertension with vasodilators (nitroprusside) or β-blockers (esmolol for the hyperdynamic heart) (see Chapter 11).

D. Control agitation if the patient is awake with short-acting sedatives.
   1. Propofol 25–50 µg/kg/min
   2. Midazolam 2.5–5.0 mg IV q1–2h
   3. Morphine sulfate 2.5–5 mg IV q1–2h

E. Control shivering with:
   1. Meperidine 25–50 mg IV
   2. Pancuronium 0.1 mg/kg IV over 5–10 minutes, then 0.01 mg/kg q1h or a continuous infusion of 2–4 mg/h (always with sedation)

F. Use of increasing level of positive end-expiratory pressure (PEEP) to augment mediastinal pressure has been shown to reduce bleeding.[70] However, prophylactic PEEP at levels of either 5 or 10 cm H_2O has not been found effective in reducing bleeding or transfusion requirements.[71] If it is elected to increase PEEP to control bleeding, careful attention to its effects on hemodynamics is essential.

G. Use of blood components to manage early significant bleeding should be based on suspicion of the hemostatic defect. This is often necessary before the results of coagulation studies are available. For example, the patient who has received aspirin, clopidogrel, or IIb/IIIa inhibitors or is uremic is likely to have platelet dysfunction and will benefit primarily from platelet transfusions, even if the platelet count is normal. In contrast, the patient who has recently been on warfarin or has hepatic dysfunction is more likely to have clotting factor deficiencies and may benefit more from an initial transfusion of FFP. Both platelets and FFP may be necessary in patients who have had a long duration of CPB (> 3 hours) or who have received multiple blood products during surgery. Aggressive treatment with blood components should be provided as soon as possible for significant hemorrhage because persistent bleeding causes progressive depletion of clotting factors and platelets ("coagulopathy begets coagulopathy").

H. Once the results of coagulation studies become available, there is more objective information on which to base therapy. If coagulation studies were obtained while in the operating room, these results may be available even before the patient's arrival in the ICU and appropriate therapy can be initiated in the operating room. If bleeding persists despite corrective measures, clotting studies can be repeated to reassess the status of the coagulation system.

1. An elevated PT implies the need for clotting factors provided by FFP and/or cryoprecipitate.

2. An elevated PTT suggests a problem with the intrinsic coagulation cascade or persistent heparin effect. Additional protamine should be given first; FFP and/or cryoprecipitate may also be indicated.

3. A platelet count below 100,000/µL suggests the need for platelet transfusions. Because CPB induces platelet dysfunction, suspicion of a qualitative defect in the actively bleeding patient should be treated with platelets even if the platelet count is adequate.

4. Note: Abnormal results need not be treated if the patient has minimal bleeding. Blood samples are frequently drawn from heparinized lines, so they should be repeated if results are markedly abnormal or inconsistent with the amount of bleeding. Platelet transfusions are not indicated in the nonbleeding patient until the count approaches 30,000, although most patients in the immediate postoperative period tend to bleed at platelet counts less than about 60,000.

5. Note: Blood transfusions are often neglected in the bleeding patient when anemia may be progressive and exacerbated by hemodilution from the administration of FFP and platelet transfusions. A borderline hematocrit in the bleeding patient necessitates concomitant blood transfusion to maintain a hematocrit at a reasonable level (> 26–28%) to maintain satisfactory tissue oxygenation. Notably, platelet function is impaired in the profoundly anemic patient.[72] Red cells increase platelet-to-platelet interaction and facilitate the interaction of platelets with the subendothelium to improve hemostasis.

I. Protamine should be given in a dose of 25–50 mg if the PTT is elevated. Although the activated clotting time generally returns to baseline after protamine administration in the operating room, reinfusion of cell saver blood or release of heparin from tissue stores can leave residual unneutralized heparin that contributes to bleeding. This may occur because the half-life of protamine is only about 5 minutes.[73] If the PTT remains elevated after additional protamine, unneutralized heparin is usually not the problem, and excessive use of protamine should be avoided because protamine itself can cause anticoagulation.[74] Protamine is given slowly (5 mg/min) in the ICU. Adverse reactions are very rare if protamine was well tolerated in the operating room (see pages 161–162 for a discussion of protamine reactions).

J. Aprotinin given in a dose of 2 million units over 20 minutes may be effective in reducing bleeding due to its antifibrinolytic activity and other ill-defined hemostatic effects. Several studies have demonstrated its efficacy in reducing postoperative blood loss and blood product usage when given only postoperatively, both in patients taking and not taking preoperative aspirin, independent of the degree of bleeding at the time of administration.[75–78] Other studies have demonstrated benefits of postoperative aprotinin in bleeding patients,[78,79] but not when doses lower than 2 million units are used.[80,81] One of these studies showed no reduction in D-dimer levels, suggesting that fibrinolysis was not inhibited.[81] Most studies, however, have shown a potential benefit to using postoperative aprotinin with few adverse effects aside from transient reversible renal dysfunction. Thus, since ongoing fibrinolysis in the pericardial cavity may contribute to postoperative bleeding, use of aprotinin should be considered in the patient with persistent bleeding that may be nonsurgical in origin.[67]

K. Desmopressin (DDAVP) can be given at a dosage of 0.3–0.4 μg/kg IV over 20 minutes. A slow infusion may attenuate the peripheral vasodilatation and hypotension that often follows DDAVP infusion.[82] Peak effects are seen in 30–60 minutes.

1. Bleeding following cardiac surgery is often secondary to an acquired defect in the formation of the platelet plug caused by a deficiency in von Willebrand's factor. DDAVP increases the level of procoagulant activity (VIII:c) and raises the level of von Willebrand's factor (VIII:vWF) by approximately 50% by releasing it from tissue stores. These factors are responsible for promoting platelet adhesion to the subendothelium.

2. Desmopressin has not been found to have much benefit in reducing bleeding in routine cardiac surgical procedures.[83] However, it may be beneficial in patients with von Willebrand's disease and other disorders affecting platelet function, including uremia and use of antiplatelet medications.[84] It has been shown to improve hemostasis in patients with significant intraoperative bleeding, especially if there is evidence of severe platelet dysfunction.[85,86] Thus it can be recommended as an adjunct to blood component therapy in this situation, although it is difficult to prove whether it is of much benefit.

L. Calcium chloride 1 g IV (10 mL of 10% solution) over 15 minutes may be administered if the patient has received multiple transfusions of citrate-phosphate-dextrose (CPD) preserved blood during a short period of time (e.g., more than 10 units within 1–2 hours). The citrate used as a preservative in CPD blood binds calcium, but hypocalcemia is unusual because of the rapid metabolism of citrate by the liver. However, calcium administration is not necessary when adenine-saline (AS-1) is used as the preservative. If hypocalcemia is present, as it often is following CPB, calcium chloride is preferable to calcium gluconate because it provides three times more ionized calcium.

VI. Blood Components, Colloids, and Blood Substitutes

A. Red cell transfusions are indicated in the severely anemic patient, especially when there is persistent hemorrhage. Tissue oxygen delivery depends on the cardiac output and the hemoglobin level and is commonly reduced by at least 25% postoperatively. The safe lower limit for the hematocrit in the stable postoperative patient following open-heart surgery is probably around 22–24%.[87–89] In fact, one study showed that such a low hematocrit was associated with a lower incidence of Q-wave infarctions and mortality.[90] Nonetheless, extra vigilance is essential in the bleeding patient to maintain a satisfactory hematocrit to ensure adequate tissue oxygenation, minimize myocardial ischemia, and prevent hemodynamic compromise. It is therefore safest in the bleeding patient to administer blood when the hematocrit is less than 26%. This can maintain a margin of safety, especially when there is ongoing blood loss and hemodilution from the administration of blood components that provide platelets and clotting factors.

1. Blood transfusions are not benign. They contain proinflammatory mediators and cytokines, are immunosuppressive, and are associated with an increased risk of wound infection, sepsis, respiratory insufficiency, and renal dysfunction.[10–13] Use of blood transfusions increases operative mortality and lowers long-term survival.[9] Transfusions carry the risk of viral transmission.[91,92] Although the risks of hepatitis C and human immunodeficiency virus (HIV) are extremely low (about 1/100,00 and 1/200,000–1/2,000,000 units, respectively), the risk of cytomegalovirus is high (50% of units). Leukocyte depletion by the blood bank can reduce the risk of cytomegalovirus and may reduce the overall incidence of infection.[93]

2. Use of blood filters is beneficial in removing microaggregates of blood. Blood filters of at least 170 μm pore size must be used for all blood transfusions. Filters of 20–40 μm pore size are more effective in removing microaggregates of fibrin, platelet debris, and leukocytes that accumulate in stored blood. These filters have been shown to decrease the incidence of nonhemolytic febrile transfusion reactions and may reduce the adverse effects of multiple transfusions on pulmonary function. Micropore filters must always be used with autotransfused blood. One of the drawbacks, however, is that blood usually cannot be transfused rapidly through these filters. Blood lines should be primed with isotonic solutions (preferably normal saline). Ringer's lactate should not be used because it contains calcium and can theoretically precipitate clotting in intravenous tubing. D5W is hypotonic and will produce significant red cell hemolysis.

3. **Note:** Care should be taken to avoid transfusing cold blood products. Blood warmers should generally be used if the patient receives rapid transfusions. If one unit is to be transfused, it should be allowed to sit at ambient room temperature or under a heating hood for several minutes to warm.

4. **Packed red blood cells** have an average hematocrit of 70%, and 1 unit will raise the hematocrit of a 70 kg man by 3%. At least 70% of transfused cells survive 24 hours, and these cells have a normal life span. Since packed cells contain no clotting factors, administration of FFP should be considered to replace clotting factors if a large number of units (generally more than 5) is given over a short period of time.

5. **Fresh whole blood** (less than 6 hours old) has a hematocrit of about 35% and contains clotting factors and platelets. One unit has been shown to provide equivalent, if not superior, hemostasis to that of 10 units of platelets.[94] It is probably the best replacement product, but most blood banks fractionate blood into components, and fresh whole blood is usually not available for use.

6. **Cell saver blood** (shed and washed in the operating room) is rinsed with heparinized saline and is devoid of clotting factors and platelets. Up to 12% of the heparin may be retained after centrifugation. If returned to the patient in large quantities, administration of additional protamine may be necessary. The survival, function, and hemolysis of washed red blood cells is equivalent to that of nonprocessed blood.[95,96] Leukocyte filtration of centrifuged cell saver blood

removes activated leukocytes, reducing the inflammatory response and improving lung function after surgery.[97]

7. **Hemofiltration blood** is obtained by placing a hemofilter in the extracorporeal circuit. This provides concentrated red cells and also preserves platelets and clotting factors. Studies have shown superior blood salvage and hemostasis with use of a hemofilter than with cell-saving devices.[98]

8. **Autotransfusion** of shed mediastinal blood can be used as a means of volume resuscitation and, to a lesser degree, as a means of blood salvage. It has been shown to reduce the use of red cell transfusions in some, but not all, studies.[17–19] Infusion of this blood can produce a coagulopathy because it has low levels of factor I and VIII, a low level of platelets that are dysfunctional, and elevated levels of fibrin split products and D-dimers.[64,99] Although one study showed that minimal bacterial contamination occurs in blood collected in standard drainage systems for up to 18 hours,[100] others have noted an increased risk of wound infection with autotransfusion, especially if given after 6 hours.[101,102] Generally, autotransfusion should be limited to the first 6–8 hours to minimize the risk of infection.

   a. Blood may be reinfused from soft plastic collection bags or directly from the plastic shell via a pump and a 20–40 μm filter. The blood is returned to the patient filtered but unwashed. Washing can eliminate the high-titers of fibrin split products in the blood.[103]

   b. Autotransfusion is not cost-effective if small amounts of blood are returned to the patient. Given in large amounts, it may be deleterious because it produces a coagulopathy that is associated with an elevation in PT, PTT, and D-dimers and a reduction in fibrinogen.[103] However, when moderate amounts are retransfused (about 500–1000 mL), it appears to be cost-effective in reducing transfusion requirements and does not produce significant abnormalities in coagulation parameters.[17]

B. **Platelets** should be given to the bleeding patient if the platelet count is less than 100,000/μL. Furthermore, since platelets are dysfunctional in patients receiving antiplatelet medications and IIb/IIIa inhibitors, and following a long duration of CPB, one should not hesitate to administer platelets for ongoing bleeding even if the platelet count exceeds 100,000/μL. Platelets are not indicated if the patient is not bleeding unless the count is perilously low (<20,000–30,000/μL).

1. Platelets are provided as a pooled preparation from one or several donors, usually as a 6 unit bag. Generally, this is the amount that is initially provided to the average-size adult patient (ideally 1 unit/10 kg). Each unit transfused should increase the platelet count by 7–10,000/μL. One unit of platelets contains 70% of the platelets in a unit of fresh blood, although platelets lose some of their functional capacity during storage. Platelets stored at room temperature can be used for up to 5 days and have a life span of 8 days. Those stored at 4°C are useful for only 24 hours (only 50–70% of total platelet activity is present at 6 hours) and have a life span of only 2–3 days.

2. **Note:** Platelet function is also impaired when the hematocrit is less than 30%. Thus, raising the hematocrit toward 30% should be considered to improve platelet function.[22,72]

3. Patients receiving clopidogrel may be less responsive to platelet transfusions if there is any remaining active metabolite in the bloodstream. In patients who

have received abciximab within 12 hours of surgery, exogenous platelets should be effective since virtually all of the abciximab should be bound to platelets, leaving little unbound drug in the bloodstream.

4. ABO compatibility should be observed for platelets but is not essential. For each donor used there is a similar risk of transmitting hepatitis and HIV as one unit of blood.

5. Platelets should be administered through a 170 μm filter. Several filters are available (such as the Pall LRF 10 filter) that can be used to remove leukocytes from platelet transfusions. Use of these filters may be beneficial in reducing the risk of allergic reactions caused by red and white cells present in platelet packs. Pretreatment with diphenhydramine (50 mg IV), cimetidine (300 mg IV) (H_1 and H_2 blockers) and steroids (hydrocortisone 100 mg IV) might also attenuate these reactions but is usually not necessary.

C. **Fresh frozen plasma** (FFP) contains all clotting factors except platelets and should be considered the colloid of choice when significant mediastinal bleeding is present. Only 30% of the normal level of most clotting factors is essential to provide hemostasis, but due to the hemodilutional effects of CPB and the progressive loss of clotting factors during ongoing bleeding, one should not hesitate to administer FFP to improve hemostasis, even if the INR is normal.

1. One unit of FFP contains about 250 mL of volume. The amount given is usually 2–4 units for the average adult.

2. FFP should be ABO compatible, transfused within 2 hours of thawing, and given through a 170 μm filter. Since each unit is derived from one donor, FFP has a similar risk of transmitting hepatitis or HIV as one unit of blood.

3. FFP may be given to patients with antithrombin III (AT III) deficiency, which may only be recognized when significant heparin resistance is noted in the operating room.[104] To minimize the amount of volume infused, a concentrated source of AT III is commercially available (Thrombate III).[105]

4. **Note:** The administration of plasma and platelets not only provides clotting factors but also raises filling pressures. These blood products will therefore lower the hematocrit and can precipitate fluid overload. If the hematocrit is less than 26% or not yet available and the patient is bleeding, anticipate the need for blood if other volume is being administered. Remember that the hematocrit does not change with acute blood loss until replacement fluids are administered.

D. **Cryoprecipitate**

1. One bag of cryoprecipitate contains about 20–25 mL and is derived from one donor. It provides approximately 40–50% of the original plasma content of factor VIII and von Willebrand's factor and is also a source of factors I (fibrinogen) and XIII. It is usually pooled from several donors into a larger bag of 10 units (200–250 mL). The amount given is usually 0.1 unit/kg (e.g., 7 units to a 70 kg patient).

2. Cryoprecipitate is especially beneficial for patients with von Willebrand's disease or documented hypofibrinogenemia. It may also benefit patients requiring surgery soon after thrombolytic therapy, which significantly reduces fibrinogen levels.

3. Cryoprecipitate should be given through a 170 μm filter within 6 hours of thawing. ABO compatibility should be observed but is not essential.

E. **Recombinant factor VIIa (rFVIIa)** is a drug approved for use in hemophiliacs that has been used successfully in arresting bleeding in patients with severe uncontrollable coagulopathies after various of open-heart surgery. It combines with tissue factor and activates the extrinsic coagulation system via factor X. This results in thrombin generation and prompt correction of the prothrombin time. rFVIIa is able to promote localized hemostasis at the site of tissue injury, and although tissue factor and activated platelets are present systemically after CPB, systemic thrombosis has not been noted to occur. It has been given in a dose of 20 to 90 µg/kg in several case reports and a second dose may be given after 2 hours, if necessary (half-life is 2.9 hours).[106-110]

F. **Hetastarch** 6% in saline (Hespan), hetastarch in balanced electrolyte solution (Hextend), and 5% **albumin** are colloid solutions that are used as volume expanders. They should generally be avoided in the bleeding patient unless the patient is hypovolemic and blood components are not available. Their dilutional effect on clotting factors can be minimized by limiting infusion volume to 1500 mL/day (about 20–25 mL/kg). Hydroxyethyl starch in saline (not in balanced electrolyte solution), in particular, can produce a coagulopathy by reducing levels of factor VIII, von Willebrand's factor, and fibrinogen, impairing fibrinogen polymerization and clot strength. These factors, as well as reduced availability of the platelet IIb/IIIa receptor, contribute to the antiplatelet effects of this solution.[111-115]

G. **Blood substitutes.** Extensive research has been carried out into the development of red blood cell substitutes that consist of hemoglobin-based oxygen carriers (HBOCs). A study of one such compound, HBOC-201, a polymerized bovine hemoglobin solution (Hemopure, Biopure Corporation, Cambridge, MA), found that it preserved oxygen transport and eliminated the need for transfusions in 34% of patients after cardiac surgery, although substantial doses of this short-acting product were required.[116]

VII. Guidelines for Mediastinal Reexploration

A. The presence of untapering mediastinal bleeding or suspected cardiac tamponade is an indication for urgent mediastinal reexploration. Emergency reexploration in the ICU is indicated for exsanguinating hemorrhage or tamponade with incipient cardiac arrest. Surgical exploration should be considered when there is acute onset of rapid bleeding (> 300 mL/h) after minimal blood loss, or persistent bleeding above arbitrary threshold levels at various times after surgery. General guidelines for reexploration include hourly bleeding rates of approximately:[117]

   1. More than 400 mL/h for 1 hour (> 200 mL/m^2)
   2. More than 300 mL/h for 2–3 hours (> 150 mL/m^2/h × 2–3 hours)
   3. More than 200 mL/h for 4 hours (> 100 mL/m^2/h × 4 hours)

B. Reexploration for bleeding is associated with increased operative mortality and morbidity, often because of a delay in returning the patient to the operating room and the necessity for open-chest resuscitation in the ICU.[118,119] Early reexploration for persistent hemorrhage may reduce the requirement for homologous transfusions, reduce the risk of respiratory insufficiency, and may also lower the wound infection rate associated with an undrained mediastinal hematoma.[120-122] Emergency exploration in the ICU for tamponade or bleeding is associated with a high survival rate, in contrast to emergency thoracotomy for malignant arrhythmias or a myocardial infarction.[123]

C. The diagnosis of cardiac tamponade is suggested by hemodynamic compromise with elevated filling pressures, usually in a patient with significant mediastinal bleeding or significant bleeding that has stopped. The following findings should heighten the suspicion of cardiac tamponade:

1. Sudden cessation of significant mediastinal bleeding.

2. Low cardiac output and hypotension with respiratory variation and narrowing of the pulse pressure. Note that positive-pressure ventilation reverses and accentuates the blood pressure response to respiration. During early inspiration, compression of pulmonary capacitance vessels augments left heart filling and blood pressure; however, in late inspiration, decreased left heart filling and blood pressure occur. This is in contradistinction to the fall in blood pressure noted with spontaneous inspiration. Thus classic pulsus paradoxus is not an applicable sign of tamponade in the ventilated patient.

3. Equilibration of intracardiac pressures with right atrial = PCW = left atrial pressure resulting from increased intrapericardial pressure. **Note:** It is not unusual for clot to accumulate next to the right or left atrium and cause unequal elevations of right atrial and left atrial pressures.[124,125]

4. Radiographic findings of a widened mediastinum or displacement of the right heart border from the cardiac silhouette (suggesting clot adjacent to the right atrium).

5. Compensatory tachycardia

6. Dysrhythmias

7. Decreased electrocardiographic voltage

8. Electromechanical dissociation

D. The diagnosis of tamponade can occasionally be very difficult to make. The scenario of hypotension, tachycardia, and elevated filling pressures with moderate mediastinal bleeding is not an uncommon scenario in a patient with marginal myocardial function. If hemodynamics do not improve after volume infusion and inotropic support, tamponade may be present. If time allows, **echocardiography** should be performed to differentiate ventricular failure from tamponade. Transthoracic echocardiography can usually detect blood compressing the atria and ventricles, but occasionally is unable to do so when satisfactory acoustical windows cannot be obtained. Thus, in equivocal situations, a transesophageal study should be performed to make the diagnosis. The presence of left or right ventricular diastolic collapse is a reliable sign of tamponade.[126] When echocardiography is not available or the patient has very tenuous hemodynamics, emergency mediastinal exploration may be necessary to make the appropriate diagnosis. Computed tomography is very sensitive in the detection of hemopericardium but cannot provide an assessment of tamponade physiology; furthermore, it requires moving an unstable patient out of the monitoring environment of the ICU.

VIII. Technique of Emergency Resternotomy

A. Emergency reexploration is indicated for exsanguinating hemorrhage or tamponade with incipient cardiac arrest. Every member of the house staff must be thoroughly familiar with the location and use of emergency thoracotomy equipment as he or she may be the only individual available to perform an emergency sternotomy and save a patient's life. A small subxiphoid incision may initially relieve some of the pressure around the heart, but in dire circumstances it is easier and more expeditious to open the entire sternotomy wound.

B. An emergency resternotomy pack must be available and readily accessible in all cardiac surgical ICUs. This must include all the essential equipment to perform the procedure, including gowns, gloves, and masks, antiseptic solutions and drapes to prep and drape the patient expeditiously, and a preselected assortment of essential instruments. Having a separate small kit with instruments essential to open the chest (knife, heavy needle holder and wire cutter, sponges) is helpful while the larger pack of instruments is being opened.

C. Technique of emergency resternotomy

1. Remove the dressing.

2. Pour antiseptic on skin.

3. Place four towels around the sternotomy incision.

4. Open the wound down to the sternum with a knife. If skin staples are present, make the incision adjacent to the staples.

5. If sternal wires were used, cut with a wire cutter; if a wire cutter is not available, untwist the wires with a heavy needle holder until they fatigue and break. If the sternum was not closed with wire, simply cut the sutures with the knife.

6. Place the sternal retractor to expose the heart (a one-piece retractor is essential).

7. Place a finger over the bleeding site if it can be identified and suction the remainder of the chest to improve exposure.

8. Resuscitate with volume through central or peripheral lines.

9. Initiate internal massage if the chest is opened for cardiac arrest or marginal blood pressure. Commonly, improvement in cardiac activity and blood pressure will be noted upon relief of tamponade (and often from the bolus of epinephrine given as the patient is deteriorating). An experienced individual can achieve satisfactory compression using one-hand massage (usually the left hand), placing the fingers behind the heart and compressing against the thenar eminence. Use of the right hand may result in perforation of the right ventricular outflow tract and is more difficult to perform. Therefore, it is generally recommended that two hands be used, compressing the heart between the left hand, placed behind and around the left ventricular apex, and the palm and flattened fingers of the right hand anteriorly. Attention to the location of all bypass grafts is critical, especially the left internal thoracic artery graft.

10. Control major and then minor bleeding sites. Manual control of a bleeding site should be obtained while the chest is suctioned and the patient receives volume resuscitation. Only then should specific attention be given to placing sutures or ties to control bleeding. Manual control can usually minimize bleeding and "buys time" until a more experienced person arrives or the operating room can be made available. **Note:** If the patient remains hemodynamically unstable, it is preferable to resuscitate him or her in the ICU rather than rush to the operating room. Invariably the bleeding site can be controlled and the patient stabilized.

11. If the patient has arrested, but tamponade is not present, an intraaortic balloon usually should be placed and the patient brought back to the operating room as soon as possible.

12. Irrigate the mediastinum extensively with warm saline or antibiotic solution and consider leaving drainage catheters for postoperative antibiotic irrigation.

References

1. Czer LSC. Mediastinal bleeding after cardiac surgery: etiologies, diagnostic considerations, and blood conservation methods. J Cardiothorac Anesth 1989;3:760–75.

2. Woodman RC, Harker LA. Bleeding complications associated with cardiopulmonary bypass. Blood 1990;76:1680–97.

3. Paramo JA, Rifon J, Llorens R, Casares J, Paloma MJ, Rocha E. Intra- and postoperative fibrinolysis in patients undergoing cardiopulmonary bypass surgery. Haemostasis 1991;21:58–64.

4. Khuri SF, Valeri CR, Loscalzo J, et al. Heparin causes platelet dysfunction and induces fibrinolysis before cardiopulmonary bypass. Ann Thorac Surg 1995;60:1008–14.

5. Nuttall GA, Erchul DT, Haight TJ, et al. A comparison of bleeding and transfusion in patients who undergo coronary artery bypass grafting via sternotomy with and without cardiopulmonary bypass. J Cardiothorac Vasc Anesth 2003;17:447–51.

6. Nader ND, Khadra WZ, Reich NT, Bacon DR, Salerno TA, Panos AL. Blood product use in cardiac revascularization: comparison of on-pump and off-pump techniques. Ann Thorac Surg 1999;68:1640–3.

7. Casati V, Valle PD, Benussi S, et al. Effects of tranexamic acid on postoperative bleeding and related histochemical variables in coronary surgery: comparison between on-pump and off-pump techniques. J Thorac Cardiovasc Surg 2004;128:83–91.

8. Englberger L, Markart P, Eckstein FS, Immer FF, Berdat PA, Carrel TP. Aprotinin reduces blood loss in off-pump coronary artery (OPCAB) surgery. Eur J Cardiothorac Surg 2002;22:545–51.

9. Engoren MC, Habib RH, Zacharias A, Schwann TA, Riordan CJ, Durham SJ. Effect of blood transfusion on long-term survival after cardiac operation. Ann Thorac Surg 2002;74:1180–6.

10. Chelemer SB, Prato BS, Cox PM Jr, O'Connor GT, Morton JR. Association of bacterial infection and red blood cell transfusion after coronary artery bypass surgery. Ann Thorac Surg 2002;73:138–42.

11. Leal-Noval S, Rincon-Ferrari MD, Garcia-Curiel A, et al. Transfusion of blood components and postoperative infection in patients undergoing cardiac surgery. Chest 2001;119:1461–8.

12. Habib RH, Zacharias A, Engoren M. Determinants of prolonged mechanical ventilation after coronary artery bypass grafting. Ann Thorac Surg 1996;62:1164–71.

13. Fransen E, Maessen J, Dentener M, Senden N, Buurman W. Impact of blood transfusions on inflammatory mediator release in patients undergoing cardiac surgery. Chest 1999;116:1233–9.

14. Obney JA, Barnes MJ, Lisagor PG, Cohen DJ. A method for mediastinal drainage after cardiac procedures using small silastic drains. Ann Thorac Surg 2000;70:1109–10.

15. Frankel TL, Hill PC, Stamou SC, et al. Silastic drains vs conventional chest tubes after coronary artery bypass. Chest 2003;124:108–13.

16. Lancey RA, Gaca C, Vander Salm TJ. The use of smaller, more flexible chest drains following open-heart surgery: an initial evaluation. Chest 2001;119:19–24.

17. Murphy GJ, Allen SM, Unsworth-White J, Lewis CT, Dalrymple-Hay MJ. Safety and efficacy of perioperative cell salvage after coronary artery bypass grafting: a randomized trial. Ann Thorac Surg 2004;77:1553–9.

18. Axford TC, Dearani JA, Ragno G, et al. Safety and therapeutic effectiveness of reinfused shed blood after open heart surgery. Ann Thorac Surg 1994;57:615–22.

19. Martin J, Robitaille D, Perault LP, et al. Reinfusion of mediastinal blood after heart surgery. J Thorac Cardiovasc Surg 2000;120:499–504.

20. Mammen EF, Koets MH, Washington BC, et al. Hemostasis changes during cardiopulmonary bypass surgery. Semin Thromb Hemost 1985;11:281–92.

21. Kalter RD, Saul CM, Wetstein L, Soriano C, Reiss RF. Cardiopulmonary bypass. Associated hemostatic abnormalities. J Thorac Cardiovasc Surg 1979;77:427–35.

22. Hardy JF, Bélisle S, Janvier G, Samama M. Reduction in requirements for allogeneic blood products: nonpharmacologic means. Ann Thorac Surg 1996;62:1935–43.

23. Levy JH. Pharmacologic preservation of the hemostatic system during cardiac surgery. Ann Thorac Surg 2001;72:S1814–20.

24. Despotis GJ, Hogue CW Jr. Pathophysiology, prevention, and treatment of bleeding after cardiac surgery: a primer for cardiologists and an update for the cardiothoracic team. Am J Cardiol 1999;83:15B–30B.

25. Warkentin TE, Greinacher A. Heparin-induced thrombocytopenia and cardiac surgery. Ann Thorac Surg 2003;76:2121–31.

26. White RH, McKittrick T, Hutchinson R, Twitchell J. Temporary discontinuation of warfarin therapy: changes in the international normalized ratio. Ann Intern Med 1995;122:40–2.

27. Hirsh J, Fuster V, Ansell J, Halperin JL. American Heart Association/American College of Cardiology Foundation guide to warfarin therapy. Circulation 2003;41:1633–52.

28. Jones HU, Muhlestein JB, Jones KW, et al. Preoperative use of enoxaparin compared with unfractionated heparin increases the incidence of re-exploration for postoperative bleeding after open-heart surgery in patients who present with an acute coronary syndrome. Clinical investigation and reports. Circulation 2002;106(suppl I):I-19–22.

29. Gibbs NM, Weightman WM, Thackray NM, Michalopoulos N, Weidmann C. The effects of recent aspirin ingestion on platelet function in cardiac surgical patients. J Cardiothorac Vasc Anesth 2001;15:55–9.

30. Weightman WM, Gibbs NM, Weidmann CR, et al. The effect of preoperative aspirin-free interval on red blood cell transfusion requirements in cardiac surgical patients. J Cardiothorac Vasc Anesth 2002;16:54–8.

31. Dacey LJ, Munoz JJ, Johnson ER, et al. Effects of preoperative aspirin use on mortality in coronary artery bypass grafting patients. Ann Thorac Surg 2000;70:1986–90.

32. Mangano DT for the multicenter study of perioperative ischemia research group. Aspirin and mortality from coronary bypass surgery. N Engl J Med 2002;347:1309–17.

33. Bidstrup BP, Hunt BJ, Sheikh S, Parratt RN, Bidstrup JM, Sapsford RN. Amelioration of the bleeding tendency of preoperative aspirin after bypass grafting. Ann Thorac Surg 2000;69:541–7.

34. Pleym H, Stenseth R, Wahba A, Bjella L, Karevold A, Dale A. Single-dose tranexamic acid reduces postoperative bleeding after coronary surgery in patients treated with aspirin until surgery. Anesth Analg 2003;96:923–8.

35. Kam PCA, Nethery CM. The thienopyridine derivatives (platelet adenosine diphosphate receptor antagonists), pharmacology, and clinical developments. Anaesthesia 2003;58:28–35.

36. Thomson Physician's Desk Reference, 2004, 58th edition: page 2964.

37. Chun R, Orser BA, Madan M. Platelet glycoprotein IIb/IIIa inhibitors: overview and implications for the anesthesiologist. Anesth Analg 2002;95:879–88.

38. Bizzari F, Scolletta S, Tucci E, et al. Perioperative use of tirofiban hydrochloride (Aggrastat) does not increase surgical bleeding after emergency or urgent coronary artery bypass grafting. J Thorac Cardiovasc Surg 2001;122:1181–5.

39. Silvestry SC, Smith PK. Current status of cardiac surgery in the Abciximab-treated patient. Ann Thorac Surg 2000;70:S12–9.

40. Levi M, Cromheecke ME, de Jonge E, et al. Pharmacological strategies to decrease excessive blood loss in cardiac surgery: a meta-analysis of clinically relevant endpoints. Lancet 1999;354:1940–7.

41. Laupacis A, Fergusson D. Drugs to minimize perioperative blood loss in cardiac surgery: meta-analyses using perioperative blood transfusions as the outcome. The International Study of Perioperative Transfusions (ISPOT) Investigators. Anesth Analg 1997;85:258–67.

42. Rich JB. The efficacy and safety of aprotinin use in cardiac surgery. Ann Thorac Surg 1998;66:S6–11.

43. Lemmer JH Jr, Dilling EW, Morton JR, et al. Aprotinin for primary coronary artery bypass grafting: a multicenter trial of three dose regimens. Ann Thorac Surg 1996;62:1659–68.

44. Casati V, Guzzon D, Oppizzi M, et al. Hemostatic effects of aprotinin, tranexamic acid and epsilon-aminocaproic acid in primary cardiac surgery. Ann Thorac Surg 1999;68:2252–7.

45. Casati V, Guzzon D, Oppizzi M, et al. Tranexamic acid compared with high-dose aprotinin in primary elective heart operations: effects on perioperative bleeding and allogeneic transfusions. J Thorac Cardiovasc Surg 2000;120:520–7.

46. Wong BI, McLean RF, Fremes SE, et al. Aprotinin and tranexamic acid for high transfusion risk cardiac surgery. Ann Thorac Surg 2000;69:808–16.

47. Daily PO, Lamphere JA, Dembitsky WP, Adamson RM, Dans NF. Effect of prophylactic epsilon-aminocaproic acid on blood loss and transfusion requirements in patients undergoing first-time coronary artery bypass grafting. A randomized, prospective, double-blind study. J Thorac Cardiovasc Surg 1994;108:99–108.

48. Schonberger JP, Bredee JJ, Tjian D, Everts PA, Wildervuur CR. Intraoperative predonation contributes to blood saving. Ann Thorac Surg 1993;56:893–8.

49. Petry AF, Jost J, Sievers H. Reduction of homologous blood requirements by blood-pooling at the onset of cardiopulmonary bypass. J Thorac Cardiovasc Surg 1994;107:1210–4.

50. Helm RE, Klemperer JD, Rosengart TK, et al. Intraoperative autologous blood donation preserves red cell mass but does not decrease postoperative bleeding. Ann Thorac Surg 1996;62:1431–41.

51. Flom-Halvorsen HI, Ovrum E, Oystese R, Brosstad F. Quality of intraoperative autologous blood withdrawal for retransfusion after cardiopulmonary bypass. Ann Thorac Surg 2003;76:744–8.

52. Ramnath AN, Naber HR, de Boer A, Leusink JA. No benefit of intraoperative whole blood sequestration and autotransfusion during coronary artery bypass grafting: results of a randomized clinical trial. J Thorac Cardiovasc Surg 2003;125:1432–7.

53. Shore-Lesserson L, Reich DL, DePerio M, Silvay G. Autologous platelet-rich plasmapheresis: risk versus benefit in repeat cardiac operations. Anesth Analg 1995;81:229–35.

54. Christenson JT, Reuse J, Badel P, Simonet F, Schmuziger M. Plateletpheresis before redo CABG diminishes excessive blood transfusion. Ann Thorac Surg 1996;62:1373–9.

55. McCarthy PM, Yared JPP, Foster RC, Ogella DA, Borsh JA, Cosgrove DM III. A prospective randomized trial of Duraflo II heparin-coated circuits in cardiac reoperations. Ann Thorac Surg 1999;67:1268–73.

56. Balachandran S, Cross MH, Karthikeyan S, Mulpur A, Hansbro SD, Hobson P. Retrograde autologous priming of the cardiopulmonary bypass circuit reduces blood transfusion after coronary artery surgery. Ann Thorac Surg 2002;73:1912–8.

57. Johnell M, Elgue G, Larsson R, Larsson A, Thelin S, Siegbahn A. Coagulation, fibrinolysis, and cell activation in patients and shed mediastinal blood during coronary artery bypass grafting with a new heparin-coated surface. J Thorac Cardiovasc Surg 2002;124:321–32.

58. Chung JH, Gikakis N, Rao AK, Drake TA, Colman RW, Edmunds LH Jr. Pericardial blood activates the extrinsic coagulation pathway during clinical cardiopulmonary bypass. Circulation 1996;93:2014–8.

59. Tabuchi N, De Hann J, Gallendat HRCG, Boonstra PAW, van Oeveren W. Activation of fibrinolysis in the pericardial cavity during cardiopulmonary bypass surgery. J Thorac Cardiovasc Surg 1993;106:828–33.

60. Russo AM, O'Connor WH, Waxman HL. Atypical presentations and echocardiographic findings in patients with cardiac tamponade occurring early and late after cardiac surgery. Chest 1993;104:71–8.

61. Shore-Lesserson L. Point-of-care coagulation monitoring for cardiovascular patients: past and present. J Cardiothorac Vasc Anesth 2002;16:99–106.

62. Gelb AB, Roth RI, Levin J, et al. Changes in blood coagulation during and following cardiopulmonary bypass. Lack of correlation with clinical bleeding. Am J Clin Pathol 1996;106:87–99.

63. Raman S, Silverman NA. Clinical utility of the platelet function analyzer (PFA-100) in cardiothoracic procedures involving extracorporeal circulation. J Thorac Cardiovasc Surg 2001;122:190–1.

64. Vertrees RA, Conti VR, Lick SD, Zwischenberger JB, McDaniel LB, Schulman G. Adverse effects of postoperative infusion of shed mediastinal blood. Ann Thorac Surg 1996;62:717–23.

65. Tuman KJ, Spiess BD, McCarthy RJ, Ivankovich AD. Comparison of viscoelastic measures of coagulation after cardiopulmonary bypass. Anesth Analg 1989;69:69–75.

66. Hett DA, Walker D, Pilkington SN, Smith DC. Sonoclot analysis. Brit J Anaesth 1995;75:771–6.

67. Hartstein G, Janssens M. Treatment of excessive mediastinal bleeding after cardiopulmonary bypass. Ann Thorac Surg 1996;62:1951–4.

68. Wallen M, Morrison A, Gillies D, O'Riordan R, Bridge C, Stoddard F. Mediastinal chest drain clearance for cardiac surgery. Cochrane Database Syst Rev 2002;2:CD003042.

69. Valeri CR, Khabbaz K, Khuri SF, et al. Effect of skin temperature on platelet function in patients undergoing extracorporeal bypass. J Thorac Cardiovasc Surg 1992;104:108–16.

70. Ilabaca PA, Oschner JL, Mills NL. Positive end-expiratory pressure in the management of the patient with a postoperative bleeding heart. Ann Thorac Surg 1980;30:281–4.

71. Collier B, Kolff J, Devineni R, Gonzalez LS III. Prophylactic positive end-expiratory pressure and reduction of postoperative blood loss in open-heart surgery. Ann Thorac Surg 2002;74:1191–4.

72. Fernandez F, Goudable C, Sie P, et al. Low haematocrit and prolonged bleeding time in uremic patients: effect of red cell transfusions. Br J Haematol 1985;59:139–48.

73. Butterworth J, Lin YA, Prielipp RC, Bennett J, Hammon JW, James RL. Rapid disappearance of protamine in adults undergoing cardiac operation with cardiopulmonary bypass. Ann Thorac Surg 2002;74:1589–95.

74. Nuttall GA, Oliver WC, Ereth MH, et al. Protamine-induced anticoagulation following coronary bypass. Proc Am Acad Cardiovasc Perfusion 1986;7:94–7.

75. Alvarez JM, Jackson LR, Chatwin C, Smolich JJ. Low-dose postoperative aprotinin reduces mediastinal drainage and blood product use in patients undergoing primary coronary artery bypass grafting who are taking aspirin: a prospective, randomized, double-blind, placebo-controlled trial. J Thorac Cardiovasc Surg 2001;122:457–63.

76. Cicek S, Demirkilic U, Kuralay E, Ozal E, Tatar H. Postoperative aprotinin: effect on blood loss and transfusion requirements in cardiac operations. Ann Thorac Surg 1996;61:1372–6.

77. Cicek S, Demirkilic U, Ozal E, et al. Postoperative use of aprotinin in cardiac operations: an alternative to its prophylactic use. J Thorac Cardiovasc Surg 1996;112:1462–7.

78. Kallis P, Tooze JA, Talbot S, Cowans D, Bevan DH, Treasure T. Aprotinin inhibits fibrinolysis, improves platelet adhesion and reduces blood loss: results of a double-blind randomized clinical trial. Eur J Cardiothorac Surg 1994;8:315–23.

79. Angelini GD, Cooper GJ, Lamarra M, Bryan AJ. Unorthodox use of aprotinin to control life-threatening bleeding after cardiopulmonary bypass. Lancet 1990;335:799–800.

80. Ray MJ, Hales MM, Brown L, O'Brien MF, Stafford EG. Postoperatively administered aprotinin or epsilon aminocaproic acid after cardiopulmonary bypass has limited benefit. Ann Thorac Surg 2001;72:521–6.

81. Forestier F, Belisle S, Robitaille D, Martineau R, Perrault LP, Hardy JF. Low-dose aprotinin is ineffective to treat excessive bleeding after cardiopulmonary bypass. Ann Thorac Surg 2000;69:452–6.

82. Frankville DD, Harper GB, Lake CL, Johns RA. Hemodynamic consequences of desmopressin administration after cardiopulmonary bypass. Anesthesiology 1991;74:988–96.

83. Ozkisacik E, Islamoglu F, Posacioglu H, et al. Desmopressin usage in elective cardiac surgery. J Cardiovasc Surg (Torino) 2001;42:741–7.

84. Gratz I, Koehler J, Olsen D, et al. The effect of desmopressin acetate on postoperative hemorrhage in patients receiving aspirin therapy before coronary artery bypass operations. J Thorac Cardiovasc Surg 1992;104:1417–22.

85. Cattaneo M, Harris AS, Stromberg U, Mannucci PM. The effect of desmopressin on reducing blood loss in cardiac surgery: a meta-analysis of double-blind, placebo-controlled trials. Thromb Haemost 1995;74:1064–70.

86. Czer LSC, Bateman TM, Gray RJ, et al. Treatment of severe platelet dysfunction and hemorrhage after cardiopulmonary bypass: reduction in blood product usage with desmopressin. J Am Coll Cardiol 1987;9:1139–47.

87. Johnson RG, Thurer RL, Kruskal MS, et al. Comparison of two transfusion strategies after elective operations for myocardial revascularization. J Thorac Cardiovasc Surg 1992;104:307–14.

88. Doak GJ, Hall RI. Does hemoglobin concentration affect perioperative myocardial lactate flux in patients undergoing coronary artery bypass surgery? Anesth Analg 1995;80:910–6.

89. Baron JG. Which lower value of haematocrit or haemoglobin concentration should guide the transfusion of red blood cell concentrates during and after extracorporeal circulation? Ann Fr Anesth Réanim 1995;14(suppl):21–7.

90. Spiess BD, Ley C, Body SC, et al. Hematocrit value on intensive care unit entry influences the frequency of Q-wave myocardial infarction after coronary artery bypass grafting. J Thorac Cardiovasc Surg 1998;116:460–7.

91. Goodnough LT, Brecher ME, Kanter MH, AuBuchon JP. Transfusion medicine. First of two parts. Blood transfusion. N Engl J Med 1999;340:438–47.

92. Chamberland ME. Emerging infectious agents: do they pose a risk to the safety of transfused blood and blood products? Clin Infect Dis 2002;34:797–805.

93. van de Watering LMG, Hermans J, Houbiers JGA, et al. Beneficial effects of leukocyte depletion of transfused blood on postoperative complications in patients undergoing heart surgery: a randomized clinical trial. Circulation 1998;97:562–8.

94. Mohr R, Martinowitz U, Lavee J, Amroch D, Ramot B, Goor DA. The hemostatic effects of transfusing fresh whole blood versus platelet concentrates after cardiac operations. J Thorac Cardiovasc Surg 1988;96:530–4.

95. Ansell J, Parilla N, King M, et al. Survival of autotransfused red blood cells recovered from the surgical field during cardiovascular operations. J Thorac Cardiovasc Surg 1982;84:387–91.

96. Valeri CR, Dennis RC, Ragno G, Pivacek LE, Hechtman HB, Khuri SF. Survival, function, and hemolysis of shed red blood cells processed or nonwashed and washed red blood cells. Ann Thorac Surg 2001;72:1598–602.

97. Gu YJ, deVries AJ, Boonstra PW, van Oeveren W. Leukocyte depletion results in improved lung function and reduced inflammatory response after cardiac surgery. J Thorac Cardiovasc Surg 1996;112:494–500.

98. Boldt J, Zickmann B, Fedderson B, Herold C, Dapper F, Hempelmann G. Six different hemofiltration devices for blood conservation in cardiac surgery. Ann Thorac Surg 1991;51:747–53.

99. Hartz R, Smith JA, Green D. Autotransfusion after cardiac operation. Assessment of hemostatic factors. J Thorac Cardiovasc Surg 1988;96:178–82.

100. Andreasen AS, Schmidt H, Jarlov JO, Skov R. Autologous transfusion of shed mediastinal blood after coronary artery bypass grafting and bacterial contamination. Ann Thorac Surg 2001;72:1327–30.

101. Body SC, Birmingham J, Parks R, et al. Safety and efficacy of shed mediastinal blood transfusion after cardiac surgery: a multicenter observational study. Multicenter Study of Perioperative Ischemia Research Group. J Cardiothorac Vasc Anesth 1999;13:410–6.

102. Dial S, Nguyen D, Menzies D. Autotransfusion of shed mediastinal blood. A risk factor for mediastinitis after cardiac surgery? Results of a cluster investigation. Chest 2003;124:1847–51.

103. Griffith LD, Billman GF, Daily PO, Lane TA. Apparent coagulopathy caused by infusion of shed mediastinal blood and its prevention by washing of the infusate. Ann Thorac Surg 1989;47:400–6.

104. Sabbagh AH, Chung GK, Shuttleworth P, Applegate BJ, Gabrhel W. Fresh frozen plasma: a solution to heparin resistance during cardiopulmonary bypass. Ann Thorac Surg 1984;37:466–8.

105. Lemmer JH Jr, Despotis GJ. Antithrombin III concentrate to treat heparin resistance in patients undergoing cardiac surgery. J Thorac Cardiovasc Surg 2002;123:213–7.

106. Al Douri M, Shafi T, Al Khudairi D, et al. Effect of the administration of recombinant activated factor VII (rFVIIa; Novoseven) in the management of severe uncontrolled bleeding in patients undergoing heart valve replacement surgery. Blood Coagul Fibrinolysis 2000;11(suppl1):S121–7.

107. Hendriks HG, van der Maaten JM, de Wolf J, et al. An effective treatment of severe intractable bleeding after valve repair by one single dose of activated recombinant factor VII. Anesth Analg 2001;93:287–9.

108. Von Heymann C, Hotz H, Konertz W, et al. Successful treatment of refractory bleeding with recombinant factor VIIa after redo coronary artery bypass graft surgery. J Cardiothorac Vasc Anesth 2002;16:615–6.

109. Stratman G, Russell IA, Merrick SH. Use of recombinant factor VIIa as a rescue treatment for intractable bleeding following repeat aortic arch repair. Ann Thorac Surg 2003;76:2094–7.

110. Murkin JM. A novel hemostatic agent: the potential role of recombinant activated factor VII (rFVIIa) in anesthetic practice. Can J Anaesth 2002;49:S21–6.

111. Kirklin JK, Lell WA, Kouchoukos NT. Hydroxyethylstarch versus albumin for colloid infusion following cardiopulmonary bypass in patients undergoing myocardial revascularization. Ann Thorac Surg 1984;37:40–6.

112. Wilkes NJ, Woolf RL, Powanda MC, et al. Hydroxyethyl starch in balanced electrolyte solution (Hextend™)—pharmacokinetic and pharmacodynamic profiles in healthy volunteers. Anesth Analg 2002;94:538–44.

113. Franz A, Braunlich P, Gamsjager T, Felfernig M, Gustorff B, Kozek-Langernecker SA. The effects of hydroxyethyl starches of varying molecular weights on platelet function. Anesth Analg 2001;92:1402–7.

114. Jamnicki M, Bombeli T, Seifert B, et al. Low- and medium-molecular weight hydroxyethyl starches. Comparison of their effect on blood coagulation. Anesthesiology 2000;93:1231–7.

115. Innerhofer P, Fries D, Margreiter J, et al. The effects of perioperative administered colloids and crystalloids on primary platelet-mediated hemostasis and clot formation. Anesth Analg 2002;95:858–65.

116. Levy JH, Goodnough LT, Greilich PE, et al. Polymerized bovine hemoglobin solution as a replacement for allogeneic red blood cell transfusion after cardiac surgery: results of a randomized, double-blind trial. J Thorac Cardiovasc Surg 2002;124:35–42.

117. Parolari A, Antona C, Gerometta P, et al. The effect of "high dose" aprotinin and other factors on bleeding and revisions for bleeding in adult coronary and valve operations: an analysis of 2190 patients during a five-year period (1987–1991). Eur J Cardiothorac Surg 1995;9:77–82.

118. Unsworth-White MJ, Herriot A, Valencia O, et al. Resternotomy for bleeding after cardiac operation: a marker for increased morbidity and mortality. Ann Thorac Surg 1995;59:664–7.

119. Moulton MJ, Creswell LL, Mackey ME, Cox JL, Rosenbloom M. Reexploration for bleeding is a risk factor for adverse outcomes after cardiac operations. J Thorac Cardiovasc Surg 1996;111:1037–46.

120. Karthik S, Grayson AD, McCarron EE, Pullan, DM, Desmond MJ. Reexploration for bleeding after coronary artery bypass surgery: risk factors, outcomes, and the effect of time delay. Ann Thorac Surg 2004;78:527–34.

121. Fiser SM, Tribble CG, Kern JA, Long SM, Kaza AK, Kron IL. Cardiac reoperation in the intensive care unit. Ann Thorac Surg 2001;71:1888–93.

122. McKowen RL, Magovern GJ, Liebler GA, Park SB, Burkholder JA, Maher TD. Infectious complications and cost-effectiveness of open resuscitation in the surgical intensive care unit after cardiac surgery. Ann Thorac Surg 1985;40:388–92.

123. Anthi A, Tzelepis GE, Alivizatos P, Michalis A, Palatianos GM, Geroulanos S. Unexpected cardiac arrest after cardiac surgery. Incidence, predisposing causes, and outcome of open chest cardiopulmonary resuscitation. Chest 1998;113:15–9.

124. Bateman T, Gray R, Chaux A, et al. Right atrial tamponade complicating cardiac operation. Clinical, hemodynamic, and scintigraphic correlates. J Thorac Cardiovasc Surg 1982;84:413–9.

125. Torelli J, Marwick TH, Salcedo EE. Left atrial tamponade: diagnosis by transesophageal echocardiography. J Am Soc Echocardiogr 1991;4:413–4.

126. Schwartz SL, Pandian NG, Cao QL, Hsu TL, Aronovitz M, Diehl JT. Left ventricular diastolic collapse in regional left heart tamponade. An experimental echocardiographic and hemodynamic study. J Am Coll Cardiol 1993;22:907–13.

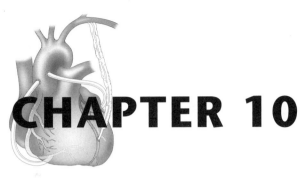

CHAPTER 10

Respiratory Management

10 Respiratory Management

I. General Comments

A. Virtually all patients undergoing open-heart surgery have some element of postoperative pulmonary dysfunction. However, in the vast majority of patients, it is well tolerated with minimal impairment in oxygenation and ventilation. Thus, it is possible and desirable in most patients to achieve early endotracheal extubation within the first 12 hours after surgery. This has been shown in multiple studies to reduce pulmonary complications, encourage earlier mobilization, and shorten the hospital stay.[1-9]

B. General anesthesia and a median sternotomy incision are used for the vast majority of patients undergoing open-heart surgery, and the internal thoracic artery (ITA) is used in virtually all coronary bypass operations. These factors have significant adverse effects on pulmonary function and chest wall mechanics.[10-12] Although the use of cardiopulmonary bypass (CPB) is associated with a systemic inflammatory response that has been incriminated as the major cause of postoperative pulmonary dysfunction, studies comparing postoperative pulmonary function in patients undergoing on- and off-pump surgery have not demonstrated a significant difference, except perhaps in patients with advanced pulmonary disease.[13-16] Thus, anesthetic management and ICU protocols to achieve early extubation should be the goal after both types of operations.

C. Despite the myriad of potential adverse effects of open-heart surgery on pulmonary function delineated in the next section, most patients have adequate pulmonary reserve to tolerate these insults quite well. Postoperative respiratory impairment and the likelihood of "delayed extubation" can be predicted fairly reliably based on clinical variables.[17-31] These should be analyzed for each patient to see if there are any modifiable factors that can be addressed to reduce these risks. Nonetheless, standard protocols for ventilatory management and early extubation can be applied to all but the very highest risk patients with excellent results. In approximately 5% of patients, mechanical ventilatory support beyond 48 hours is necessary because of marked hemodynamic compromise, poor oxygenation, or inadequate ventilation.

D. An understanding of the postoperative changes in pulmonary function, basic concepts in oxygenation and ventilation, routine pulmonary management, and contributing factors to respiratory dysfunction allows for the early identification and management of problems that can optimize the recovery of pulmonary function.

II. Postoperative Changes in Pulmonary Function

A. During the early postoperative period, the principal mechanisms underlying poor gas exchange with borderline oxygenation are ventilation/perfusion (V/Q) mismatch and intrapulmonary shunting.[11,32] Contributing factors include the following:

    1. General anesthetics, neuromuscular relaxants, and narcotics decrease the central respiratory drive and contribute to decreased respiratory muscle function.

2. The median sternotomy incision produces chest wall splinting and reduces most pulmonary function testing variables; the presence of chest tubes for mediastinal or pleural drainage also impairs respiratory function.[33]

3. Harvesting of the ITA with pleural entry is associated with a decrease in chest wall compliance and deterioration of pulmonary function tests to a greater degree than when no ITA is harvested.

   a. Significant reductions in peak expiratory flow rates (forced expiratory volume in 1 second [FEV_1], forced vital capacity [FVC]), functional residual capacity (FRC), and expiratory reserve volume have been documented and may be exacerbated by the presence of pleural chest tubes.[33–39]

   b. ITA harvesting is associated with a higher incidence of pleural effusions and perhaps atelectasis.[36–38]

   c. There is the potential for phrenic nerve injury and devascularization during ITA harvesting, the latter being more common in diabetic patients.[40–42]

   d. Interestingly, one study showed that the incidence of respiratory complications and the degree of respiratory impairment are no greater if bilateral, rather than just unilateral, ITA harvesting is performed.[37]

4. Effects of cardiopulmonary bypass[10,43]

   a. Cardiogenic pulmonary edema from hemodilution, fluid overload, and reduction in oncotic pressure.

   b. Noncardiogenic interstitial pulmonary edema from the "systemic inflammatory response" that produces an increase in endothelial permeability and accumulation of extravascular lung water; this also decreases lung surfactant contributing to atelectasis. Contributory factors to this syndrome include:

      i. Complement activation

      ii. Release of cytokines and other inflammatory mediators

      iii. Pulmonary sequestration of neutrophils activated by blood contact with the extracorporeal circuit; this results in release of proteolytic enzymes, such as neutrophil elastase, that may damage tissue and increase alveolar-endothelial permeability.

   c. Hyperoxia may increase oxygen free-radical damage

   d. Imbalance of arachidonic acid metabolites

   e. Hypothermia, cardiopulmonary ischemia, or failure to ventilate the lungs may impair pulmonary function.[44]

5. Compromised hemodynamic status: impairment in left ventricular (LV) function with elevation in pulmonary artery (PA) pressures may contribute to pulmonary edema; this may lead to impairment of right ventricular (RV) function by increasing pulmonary vascular resistance (PVR).

6. Blood transfusions may cause microembolization, and transfusion of proinflammatory mediators that may elevate the PVR and PA pressures, increase inspiratory pressures, impair oxygenation, and reduce RV function. Transfusions also increase the risk of wound infection and pneumonia.

7. Preexisting comorbidities may impair postoperative pulmonary function, such as preexisting lung disease (especially chronic obstructive pulmonary disease [COPD] with any active bronchitic component) and obesity, which produces V/Q imbalance and impairs oxygenation.[22]

8. Diaphragmatic dysfunction from phrenic nerve injury may result from the use of iced saline slush in the pericardial well or from direct injury or devascularization from harvesting of the ITA.[40,41]

9. Studies have shown that impairment of pulmonary function persists for several months after surgery. One study showed that the values for FEV_1, forced expiratory flow at 50% of FVC (FEF_{50}), and maximal voluntary ventilation remained more than 25% less than preoperative values at 3.5 months after surgery.[44]

III. Routine Ventilator, Sedation, and Analgesia Management (Box 10.1)

A. For open-heart surgery, patients generally receive a balanced anesthetic regimen consisting of a narcotic (fentanyl, sufentanil, or remifentanil), an inhalational anesthetic, a neuromuscular blocker, and a sedative, such as midazolam or propofol.[45,46] In addition to their selection based on the patient's underlying cardiac disease, the use and dosing of these medications should be modified based on the plans for postoperative extubation.

B. Upon arrival in the ICU, patients are placed on a volume-cycled respirator for full ventilator support either in the synchronized intermittent mandatory ventilation (SIMV) or assist/control (A/C) modes. They remain anesthetized from the residual effects of narcotics, anxiolytic medications, and muscle relaxants given during surgery.

1. Before the patient can initiate and achieve adequate spontaneous ventilation, controlled ventilation will provide efficient gas exchange and decrease oxygen consumption by reducing the work of breathing. This may be very important during the first few postoperative hours when hypothermia, acid-base and electrolyte disturbances, and hemodynamic instability are most pronounced.

Box 10.1 • Initial Respiratory Orders

1. Initial ventilator settings:
   a. Tidal volume: 8–10 mL/kg
   b. Respiratory rate: 8–10/min
   c. FIO_2: 1.0
   d. PEEP: 5 cm H_2O
   e. Pressure support: 5–8 cm H_2O
2. Display pulse oximetry on bedside monitor
3. Chest x-ray after arrival in ICU (or in OR)
4. Check ABGs 15–30 minutes after arrival
5. Reduce FIO_2 to 0.4 as long as $PaO_2 > 100$ torr or O_2 saturation $> 95\%$
6. Adjust ventilator settings to maintain $PaCO_2 > 30$ torr with pH 7.30–7.50
7. Propofol 25–50 µg/kg/min; gradually decrease dose once standard weaning criteria are present and then initiate weaning when patient is mentally alert with reversal of neuromuscular blockade.

2. Several studies have evaluated the effects of A/C ventilation, SIMV, and biphasic intermittent positive airway pressure (BiPAP) in the early postoperative period. All three modes of ventilation were found to have comparable effects on hemodynamics and gas exchange, but BiPAP reduced the use of analgesics and sedatives and the duration of ventilation. BiPAP allows for unrestricted spontaneous breathing during all phases of respiration and may be more comfortable for the patient during the early return of spontaneous ventilation.[47,48]

C. Initial ventilator settings are as follows:

Tidal volume: 8–10 mL/kg

IMV rate: 8–10 breaths/min

Fraction of inspired oxygen (FIO_2): 1.0

Positive end-expiratory pressure (PEEP): 5 cm H_2O

Pressure support of 5–8 cm H_2O

D. The tidal volume and respiratory rate are selected to achieve a minute ventilation of approximately 100 mL/kg/min. Patients with COPD often benefit from lower respiratory rates and higher tidal volumes with increased inspiratory flow rates. The latter allows more time for the expiratory phase and can reduce the potential for the development of high levels of "auto-PEEP" and air trapping that may adversely affect hemodynamics.[49] Lower tidal volumes with higher respiratory rates are often beneficial for patients with restrictive lung disease.

E. A low level (5 cm H_2O) of PEEP is routinely added to the respiratory circuit to prevent atelectasis. Despite this common practice, studies suggest that this level of PEEP does not reopen atelectatic lung and produces no significant improvement in oxygenation over zero PEEP.[50] A PEEP level of 10 cm H_2O or higher is usually necessary to improve lung recruitment, but it must be used judiciously because it may reduce venous return and impair right and left ventricular function.[51–53] Caution is required especially when the patient is hypovolemic from peripheral vasodilatation or when impaired RV function is already present.

F. Continuous pulse oximetry is used during mechanical ventilation with display of the arterial oxygen saturation (SaO_2) on the bedside monitor. This can bring attention to abrupt changes in oxygenation and should obviate the need to obtain arterial blood gases (ABGs) on a frequent basis in the stable patient. Concern should be raised when the SaO_2 is < 95%.

G. Although not commonly used in the ICU, capnography (end-tidal CO_2) can be used to provide a relative assessment of the level of $PaCO_2$, although it is inaccurate when V/Q mismatch is present. For example, the end-tidal CO_2 will be much lower than the $PaCO_2$ when there is an increase in physiologic dead space (increased V/Q). It is also affected by the degree of CO_2 production, the minute ventilation, and the cardiac output. Nonetheless, an abrupt change in the contour of the capnogram signifies an acute problem with the patient's ventilatory status, hemodynamics, or metabolic state.

H. A chest x-ray should be checked after the patient's arrival in the ICU. The position of the endotracheal tube, Swan-Ganz catheter or any central line, and intraaortic balloon pump (IABP) should be identified. The lung fields should be evaluated for lung expansion/atelectasis, pneumothorax, undrained pleural effusion, pulmonary edema, or infiltrates. Attention should be paid to the width of the mediastinum, primarily for later comparison in the event of postoperative hemorrhage.

I. An initial ABG should be checked about 15–20 minutes after the patient's arrival in the ICU. The F_{IO_2} is gradually reduced to 0.40 and the tidal volume and respiratory rate are adjusted to maintain the ABGs within a normal range. The extent of hypothermia should be taken into consideration when making these adjustments, anticipating that the P_{CO_2} will rise as the patient warms. The metabolic demand and CO_2 production are decreased 10% for every degree less than 37°C. Acceptable ABGs include:

P_{aO_2} > 80 torr (S_{aO_2} > 95%)

P_{aCO_2} 32–48 torr

pH 7.32–7.48

J. Adequate sedation and analgesia must be provided in the early postoperative period to minimize anxiety, pain, and hemodynamic stress that may contribute to myocardial ischemia and hypertension.[54] This often seems difficult when the goal is to have an awake patient with an indwelling endotracheal tube who is comfortable, yet does not have hypertension or tachycardia.

1. Upon arrival in the ICU, most patients will remain sedated from narcotics and propofol (usually at a dose of 25 µg/kg/min) used at the conclusion of surgery. Dexmedetomidine is a very useful medication that provides analgesic and anxiolytic properties without sedation, allows for use of lower doses of other medications, and can be continued after extubation. This α_2-adrenergic agonist may be started in the operating room or later with a loading dose of 1 µg/kg over 10 minutes followed by a continuous infusion of 0.2–0.7 mg/kg/h.[55] If early extubation is contemplated, midazolam is best avoided after CPB is terminated because it has a half-life of more than 10 hours after surgery.[56]

2. Suctioning should be performed only as needed because it can produce endobronchial trauma and a transient bronchoconstrictor response.[57]

3. Once standard criteria for weaning are met, the patient is weaned from propofol over a short period of time. Most patients awaken within 20 minutes of termination of a propofol infusion, although it may take several more hours before they can be extubated.

4. Optimal pain management consists of a continuous infusion of a low-dose narcotic, such as morphine sulfate (0.01–0.02 mg/kg/h), to blunt the sympathetic response and alleviate pain. Such a protocol avoids the respiratory depression and pain associated with the peaks and valleys of bolus doses of medication. It may also be given safely after the patient is extubated. Ketorolac (Toradol) 30 mg IV can be used for breakthrough pain during the IV morphine infusion or later to decrease oral narcotic requirements.[58] Its use should be limited to 72 hours, and it should be avoided in patients with renal dysfunction. Other nonsteroidal antiinflammatory medications may be administered safely without concerns about renal dysfunction.[59] Some groups administer indomethacin 50 mg PR just before stopping the propofol infusion and find that few patients require additional narcotics.[60]

K. ABGs should be checked if there is a significant change in the patient's clinical picture or if noninvasive monitoring (pulse oximetry or end-tidal CO_2) suggests a problem.

A cautious approach is to check the ABGs after 4–6 hours, before initiating weaning, and just before extubation. Once criteria for weaning have been met, the IMV rate is gradually decreased, and if satisfactory mechanics and ABGs are present, the patient is extubated (Boxes 10.2 to 10.4).

IV. Basic Concepts of Oxygenation

A. The first of the two primary goals of mechanical ventilation is the achievement of satisfactory arterial oxygenation. Although this is usually assessed by the arterial Pao_2, it should be remembered that the Pao_2 is a measurement of the partial pressure of oxygen dissolved in the bloodstream; it indirectly reflects oxygen saturation of hemoglobin (Hb) in the blood and does not measure the oxygen content of the blood.

B. Blood oxygen content is determined primarily by the amount of oxygen bound to Hb (the arterial oxygen saturation or Sao_2) and to a minimal extent by that dissolved in solution (the Pao_2). Each gram of Hb can transport 1.39 mL of oxygen per 100 mL of blood (vol%), whereas each 100 torr of Pao_2 transports 0.031 vol%. Thus, correction of anemia does significantly more to improve blood oxygen content than does raising the level of dissolved oxygen (Pao_2) by increasing the Fio_2.

   1. The oxygen-Hb dissociation curve demonstrates the relationship between Pao_2 and O_2 saturation (Figure 10.1). The amount of oxygen delivered to tissues depends on a number of factors that can affect this relationship. A shift to the left, as noted with hypothermia and alkalosis, indicates more avid binding of oxygen and less release to the tissues, whereas a shift to the right, noted with acidosis, improves tissue oxygen delivery.

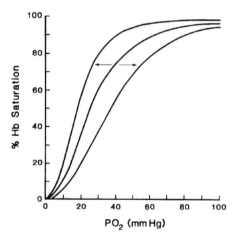

Figure 10.1 • Oxygen-hemoglobin dissociation curve. The sigmoid curve delineates the saturation of hemoglobin at increasing levels of PO_2. Note that a PO_2 of 65 torr corresponds to a saturation of 90%. Higher levels of O_2 produce only small increments in blood oxygen content, but a PO_2 below this level results in a precipitous fall in O_2 saturation. A shift of the curve to the left, as is noted with alkalosis and hypothermia, increases the affinity of hemoglobin for oxygen and decreases tissue oxygen delivery. A shift to the right occurs with acidosis and improves tissue oxygen delivery.

2. Note that a Pao_2 of 65 torr corresponds to an O_2 saturation of 90%, but this lies at the shoulder of the sigmoid curve. Below this level, a small decrease in Pao_2 causes a precipitous fall in O_2 saturation. Therefore, although a Pao_2 of 60–70 torr is certainly acceptable, there is little margin of safety in the event of a sudden change in hematocrit, cardiac output, or ventilator function.

3. The relationship between Pao_2 and oxygen saturation also dissociates when methemoglobinemia is present. This occurs when more than 1% of available Hb is in an oxidized form and unable to bind oxygen. It has been noted in patients receiving high-dose IV nitroglycerin (over 10 μg/kg/min for several days), especially when hepatic or renal dysfunction is present. [61] When methemoglobinemia is present, the Pao_2 may be high but the true O_2 saturation measured directly by oximetry is very low. Thus, ischemia may be exacerbated by undetected hypoxemia. It should be remembered that the O_2 saturation reported back from the blood gas laboratory is usually calculated from a nomogram based on the Pao_2, pH, and temperature; it is not measured directly.

4. Pulse oximetry is beneficial in measuring O_2 saturations continuously when the PO_2 is low, but because it measures several forms of hemoglobin, it will overestimate the oxyhemoglobin content when methemoglobinemia is present.

5. The amount of oxygen available to tissues depends not only on the Sao_2, pH, and the blood Hb content but also on the cardiac output. An attempt to improve oxygen saturation at the expense of a decrease in cardiac output is counterproductive. This may be noted when increasing levels of PEEP are applied in the hypovolemic patient.

C. The Pao_2 is generally used to assess the adequacy of oxygenation, but its relationship to the Fio_2 should be examined. The Pao_2/Fio_2 ratio is a reliable predictor of pulmonary dysfunction and can also be used to assess whether weaning is feasible. [62] The calculation of the alveolar-arterial oxygen difference $[D(A - a)O_2]$ also takes the Fio_2 into consideration and is a very sensitive index of the efficiency of gas exchange. This is calculated according to the following equation:

$$D(A - a)O_2 = (Fio_2)(713) - Pao_2 - Paco_2 / 0.8$$

D. In patients with normal pulmonary function, the Pao_2 may be well over 500 torr on 100% oxygen immediately after surgery. The Fio_2 should be gradually decreased to 0.40 as tolerated to prevent adsorption atelectasis and oxygen toxicity. However, it should not be lowered any further even if the Pao_2 seems high in order to maintain a safety margin for oxygenation in the event that hypotension, dysrhythmias, bleeding, or a pneumothorax should suddenly develop.

E. Suboptimal oxygenation is considered to be present when the Pao_2 is less than 350 torr or the $D(A - a)O_2$ is greater than 350 on 100% oxygen. A postoperative Pao_2/Fio_2 ratio of less than 350 is more likely to be noted in patients with low preoperative PO_2, hypertension, and a history of smoking. [62] However, Pao_2 values such as these are not uncommon after open-heart surgery and should not cause much alarm. However, concern should be raised when the PO_2 remains less than 80 torr with an Fio_2 greater than 50%.

F. Some patients with chronic pulmonary disease have a relatively "fixed shunt" with a Pao_2 of 60–70 torr despite a high Fio_2 and moderate levels of PEEP. It is best to avoid an Fio_2 greater than 0.5 for more than a few days, if possible, to avoid complications associated with oxygen toxicity. Keep in mind that a Pao_2 of 65 torr corresponds to an O_2 saturation of 90% and is acceptable in these patients.

V. Basic Concepts of Alveolar Ventilation

A. The second goal of mechanical ventilation is that of alveolar ventilation, which regulates the level of Pco_2. This is controlled by setting the tidal volume and the respiratory rate on the ventilator and should provide a minute ventilation of approximately 8–10 L/min. The level of Pco_2 is determined most reliably by the ABGs. Noninvasive monitoring with end-tidal CO_2 gives a reasonably accurate assessment of $Paco_2$, although the correlation depends on the amount of physiologic dead space.

B. Hypocarbia

1. Mild hypocarbia (Pco_2 of 30–35 torr) is quite acceptable in the immediate postoperative period, especially when the patient is hypothermic. It produces a mild respiratory alkalosis that:

   a. Decreases the patient's respiratory drive.

   b. Allows for increased CO_2 production to occur from the increased metabolic rate associated with warming and shivering without producing respiratory acidosis. Remember that the metabolic rate is decreased 10% for every degree below 37°C and most patients return to the ICU from the operating room with a core temperature around 35–36°C.

   c. Compensates for the mild metabolic acidosis that frequently develops from hypoperfusion and peripheral vasoconstriction when the patient is still hypothermic.

2. A more profound respiratory alkalosis has potential detrimental effects and must be avoided.

   a. It leads to hypokalemia and may predispose to ventricular arrhythmias.

   b. It shifts the oxygen-hemoglobin dissociation curve to the left, decreasing oxygen release to the tissues.

   c. Note: Hypocarbia with a normal pH is masking a metabolic acidosis that may need to be evaluated and addressed.

3. **Management** of hypocarbia is best accomplished by lowering the IMV rate. The amount of dead space in the tubing can also be increased. Adding 10% of the tidal volume in mL/kg to the tubing will raise the Pco_2 approximately 5 torr.

   a. Although the addition of PEEP to the ventilator circuit usually prevents alveolar collapse by maintaining volume in the lungs above the critical closing volume, alveolar hypoventilation and atelectasis are best prevented by maintaining an adequate tidal volume of 8–10 mL/kg. The tidal volume can be lowered but usually should be decreased only if peak inspiratory pressures are excessively high (over 35–40 cm H_2O).

   b. Occasionally, hypocarbia may develop in a patient who is "fighting the ventilator" with repeated triggering. These patients seem unable to breathe in synchrony with delivered breaths. This may be noted in patients with hypoxia, mental confusion or delirium, anxiety, or inadequate sedation. Some patients become very agitated when spontaneous breaths are initiated against high levels of PEEP.

      i. It is important to assess the adequacy of ventilation and oxygenation first.

      ii. If these are satisfactory, additional sedation and/or paralysis should be used to minimize the patient's respiratory drive. Full ventilation is then resumed in the controlled mandatory ventilation (CMV) mode. PEEP levels should be decreased to 5 cm H_2O or less if Pao_2 permits.

   iii. Pressure support ventilation (PSV) (see page 326) increases the comfort of the spontaneously breathing patient and may reduce the work of breathing.

C. Hypercarbia

  1. Hypercarbia indicates that the minute ventilation provided by the ventilator is inadequate to meet ventilatory demands. Adjustment of ventilator settings must accommodate the progressive increase in Pco_2 that occurs during the early postoperative period as the metabolic rate increases from warming and postanesthetic shivering. During the weaning process, a slightly elevated Pco_2 in the range of 48–50 torr is usually acceptable, since the patient is still somewhat sedated. Higher levels of Pco_2 usually mean that the patient is not awake enough to maintain adequate ventilation.

  2. A lower tidal volume may be requested by the surgeon to minimize tension on a short ITA pedicle. In these patients, it is preferable to increase the IMV rate rather than the tidal volume to compensate for an elevated Pco_2.

  3. During weaning from mechanical ventilation, hypercarbia may represent compensatory hypoventilation in response to a metabolic alkalosis. This frequently results from aggressive diuresis in the early postoperative period. Use of acetazolamide (Diamox) 250–500 mg IV q8–12h in conjunction with other diuretics is beneficial in correcting a primary metabolic alkalosis. However, the metabolic component should only be partially corrected in patients with chronic CO_2 retention.

  4. Manifestations of significant hypercarbia and respiratory acidosis include:

    a. Tachycardia

    b. Hypertension

    c. Arrhythmias

    d. Increasing PA pressures

  5. Treatment

    a. Moderate hypercarbia in the fully ventilated patient is corrected by increasing either the respiratory rate or tidal volume, as long as the peak inspiratory pressure is less than 40 cm H_2O.

    b. Significant hypercarbia usually indicates a mechanical problem such as ventilator malfunction, endotracheal tube malposition, or a pneumothorax. The latter may still be present even when bilateral breath sounds seem to be heard above all the other extraneous noises of the ICU setting. Temporary handbag ventilation, adjustment of ventilator settings, repositioning of the endotracheal tube, or insertion of a chest tube will usually resolve the problem.

    c. Sedation can be obtained with short-acting narcotics or other sedatives. These include:

      i. Propofol 25–75 µg/kg/min

      ii. Morphine sulfate 2.5–5 mg IV q1–2h

      iii. Midazolam 2.5–5.0 mg IV q1h or 2 mg/h as a continuous infusion. This can reduce the total narcotic requirement but will delay extubation.

      iv. Fentanyl drip can be used when a more prolonged period of sedation is indicated. The usual dosage is a 50–100 µg IV bolus over 5 minutes followed by a drip of 50–200 µg/h of a 2.5 mg/250 mL mix.

d. Shivering is best controlled using meperidine 25–50 mg IV.[63] More persistent and refractory shivering that is deleterious to hemodynamics may need to be controlled with pharmacologic paralysis. **It is important never to paralyze an awake patient without also administering sedation.** Paralytic agents, including pancuronium, vecuronium, or atracurium, can be used if meperidine fails to control the shivering (see Appendix 7 for dosages).

6. If the patient becomes hypercarbic because of "fighting the ventilator" and is receiving inadequate tidal volumes, the steps noted above (sedation and conversion to PSV) will allow for improved ventilation.

7. The persistence of hypercarbia despite standard therapeutic measures usually indicates significant ventilatory failure. This will be discussed later in this chapter.

VI. Considerations to Achieve Early Extubation

A. Although an initial period of sedation is usually beneficial to allow for evaluation of bleeding, the achievement of hemodynamic stability, and warming to normothermia, early extubation soon thereafter is preferable for most patients. This improves hemodynamic performance, decreases pulmonary complications, requires less medication, and allows for more rapid mobilization and a faster recovery.[64] Virtually all studies have demonstrated the safety and efficacy of early extubation, with documentation of decreased length of stay and hospital costs.[1–9] The important concept is that this should represent "early" extubation once certain criteria are met; it should never represent "premature" extubation, when discontinuation of mechanical ventilation may prove deleterious to the patient's recovery. The advantages of extubation in the operating room or within the first few hours have not been defined, but in high likelihood they do not reduce the length of stay in the ICU or the overall hospital stay.[65–67]

B. The potential disadvantages of early extubation must always be taken into consideration. These include:

1. Increased sympathetic tone causing tachycardia and hypertension that can adversely affect myocardial recovery and can contribute to myocardial ischemia during the first 4–6 hours in the ICU.[68]

2. Increased risk of bleeding if hypertension develops.

3. More chest pain and splinting if less analgesia is given; this may cause hypoventilation and atelectasis, potentially contributing to oxygen desaturation and the necessity for reintubation.

4. Compromise of ventilatory status if there is significant fluid overload.

C. The selection of patients for early extubation should not be overly restrictive, but it does depend on an understanding of potential risk factors for pulmonary dysfunction and delayed extubation. Some of these factors can be modified or influenced by therapeutic measures, whereas others cannot. The Society of Thoracic Surgeons has developed a risk model for predicting prolonged ventilation beyond 48 hours.[17] In addition, numerous publications have identified risk factors that increase respiratory morbidity and increase the duration of ventilation.[18–31] All of these factors must be taken into consideration when deciding whether early extubation is feasible or whether more prolonged support will be in the patient's best interest.

Table 10.1 • Exclusionary Criteria for Early Extubation

Preoperative Criteria	Intraoperative Criteria	Postoperative Criteria
Pulmonary edema	Deep hypothermic circulatory arrest	Mediastinal bleeding
Intubated	Coagulopathy	Hemodynamic instability/need for an IABP
Cardiogenic shock	Severe myocardial dysfunction	Respiratory failure/hypoxia
Sepsis	Long pump run > 4–6 h	Stroke

1. **Preoperative factors:** older patient age, females, lower body surface area, preexisting impairment of cardiac (New York Heart Association [NYHA] class IV/ congestive heart failure [CHF], poor LV function, shock), respiratory (smoking, COPD) and renal subsystems (elevated creatinine), obesity, urgent or emergent surgery with hemodynamic instability.

2. **Intraoperative factors:** reoperations, long durations of CPB, requirement for multiple blood products, significant fluid administration, elevated blood glucose on CPB, poor hemodynamic performance requiring inotropes or IABP support, perioperative myocardial infarction.

3. **Postoperative factors:** excessive mediastinal bleeding, use of multiple blood products, reexploration for bleeding, sepsis, pneumonia, renal dysfunction, stroke or depressed level of consciousness, gastrointestinal bleeding.

D. In general, the pharmacologic protocol for postoperative sedation should be similar for most patients, although more liberal use of longer-acting medications (such as morphine, fentanyl, or midazolam) can be considered in patients at very high risk for requiring prolonged ventilation (Table 10.1). Use of standard protocols and criteria for weaning should allow for extubation when clinically indicated, even if it takes a little longer than desired. The duration of intubation should not be based on risk factors alone or dictated by a rigid time schedule. Of interest, since smoking is a significant risk factor for postoperative morbidity, one study showed that it is advantageous to extubate smokers earlier rather than later to reduce the risk of respiratory morbidity.[69]

VII. Therapeutic Interventions to Optimize Postoperative Respiratory Performance

A. Recognition of risk factors for pulmonary dysfunction can direct attention to potential therapeutic steps to optimize postoperative performance. The management of modifiable factors, performance of a proficient operation, and aggressive postoperative management of all subsystems are essential to achieve early extubation and minimize the risk of postoperative respiratory failure.

B. Preoperative considerations

1. Attempt to convince the patient to stop cigarette smoking at least one month prior to surgery.

2. Treat all active cardiopulmonary disease processes, such as pneumonia, bronchospasm, and CHF, to optimize oxygenation and ventilatory status.

3. Transfuse patients to a hematocrit greater than 30% prior to surgery to minimize the degree of hemodilution during surgery and the requirement for blood and blood components.

4. Optimize hemodynamic performance and renal function as well as possible prior to surgery.

C. Intraoperative considerations

1. Modify the CPB circuit to minimize the inflammatory response, hemodilution, and bleeding: use membrane oxygenators, centrifugal pumps, and heparin-coated circuits; consider retrograde autologous priming and use of leukocyte-depleting filters.[70,71]

2. Minimize fluid administration during CPB or off-pump surgery.

3. Use aprotinin selectively to decrease the inflammatory response and minimize perioperative bleeding.[72]

4. Perform an expeditious, technically proficient operation with excellent myocardial protection to achieve complete revascularization or satisfactory valve function with fastidious attention to hemostasis.

5. Use inotropic support or an IABP as necessary to achieve satisfactory hemodynamic performance (cardiac index > 2 L/min/m^2) and avoid excessively high filling pressures.

6. Consider use of steroids (methylprednisolone or dexamethasone) to decrease the inflammatory response.[73–75]

7. Control blood glucose on CPB with intravenous insulin (keep blood sugar < 180 mg/dL).

8. Consider ventilating the lungs during bypass (shown to improve postpump oxygenation).[76,77]

9. Use fenoldopam for patients with renal dysfunction (creatinine > 1.5 mg/dL) to optimize renal function during CPB.[78,79]

10. Consider hemofiltration to remove fluid in patients with preoperative CHF or with renal dysfunction and to remove inflammatory mediators.[80]

11. Use short-acting narcotics and propofol for sedation to allow for early extubation.

D. Postoperative considerations

1. Initiate aggressive management of postoperative bleeding with low threshold for reexploration to minimize use of blood products.

2. Administer volume judiciously to optimize hemodynamics; then use aggressive diuresis once hemodynamics have stabilized to eliminate extravascular lung water.

3. Initiate hyperglycemia protocol to reduce risk of sternal wound infection[81] (see Appendix 6).

4. Select medications to provide short-acting anxiolysis and sedation (propofol) that allow the patient to awaken within hours of its discontinuation.

5. Provide adequate analgesia without producing respiratory depression (continuous IV morphine, nonsteroidal antiinflammatory drugs).

6. Use antihypertensive medications, rather than sedatives, to control hypertension.

7. Have a higher threshold for blood transfusions (hematocrit in the low 20s), except in elderly patients or those with hypotension, tachycardia, or oxygenation issues in whom a higher hematocrit may be beneficial.

VIII. Ventilatory Weaning and Extubation in the Immediate Postoperative Period

A. **Criteria for weaning** (see Box 10.2). Weaning a patient from the ventilator depends on the ability and desire of the nursing and medical staffs to identify when the patient is ready to be weaned and their willingness to initiate weaning

---

Box 10.2 • Criteria for Weaning from Mechanical Ventilation

I. Initial Postoperative Period

1. Awake with stimulation

2. Adequate reversal of neuromuscular blockade

3. Chest tube drainage < 50 mL/h

4. Core temperature > 35.5°C

5. Hemodynamic stability

   a. Cardiac index > 2.2 L/min/m²
   b. Blood pressure stable at 100–120 systolic on/off medications
   c. Heart rate < 120/min
   d. No arrhythmias

6. Satisfactory ABGs on full ventilation

   a. $Pao_2/Fio_2 > 150$ ($PO_2 > 75$ torr on Fio_2 of 0.5)
   b. $Paco_2 < 50$ torr
   c. pH 7.30–7.50

II. Prolonged Ventilation

1. Underlying disease process has resolved

2. Awake, oriented with adequate mental alertness to initiate an inspiratory effort

3. Hemodynamic stability on no vasoactive drugs

4. Hemoglobin and metabolic status are optimized

5. Satisfactory ABGs as above (many studies recommend $Pao_2/Fio_2 > 200$) with respiratory rate < 35/min

6. Rapid shallow breathing index < 100

when indicated, no matter what time of the day or night, not when it is convenient to do so. The criteria include:

1. Patient awake with stimulation
2. Chest tube drainage < 50 mL/h
3. Hemodynamic stability
   a. Cardiac index > 2.2 L/min/m^2 on minimal inotropic support
   b. Blood pressure stable at 100–140 mm Hg systolic on/off medications
   c. No arrhythmias
4. Core temperature > 35.5°C
5. Evidence of reversal of neuromuscular blockade
6. Satisfactory oxygenation (Pao_2 > 75 torr with an Fio_2 ≤ 0.5 and 5 cm of PEEP) and ventilation (Pco_2 < 50 torr)

B. **Method of weaning after short-term ventilation**
   1. Minimize sedation.
   2. Maintain the Fio_2 at 0.5 or below with a PEEP of no more than 5–7.5 cm H_2O. If the patient still requires a higher level of PEEP, weaning is usually not indicated. If oxygenation is satisfactory, lower the PEEP in 2.5–5 cm H_2O intervals to 5 cm H_2O and initiate weaning.
   3. Weaning is usually accomplished in the SIMV mode. The IMV rate is reduced by two breaths every 30 minutes with observation of the Sao_2. If the ABGs and respiratory mechanics are acceptable after a 30–60 minute spontaneous breathing trial (SBT) on either T-piece or continuous positive airway pressure (CPAP) of 5 cm H_2O (see extubation criteria below), the endotracheal tube is removed.[82]
   4. Weaning should be stopped and ventilation resumed at a higher rate when there are clinical signs that it is not being tolerated. These signs are noted in Box 10.3.
   5. **Note:** A rise in PA pressures is often the first hemodynamic abnormality noted in the patient who is not tolerating weaning very well. Tachypnea is the first clinical sign of ineffective weaning.

Box 10.3 • Failure Criteria During Weaning from the Ventilator

1. Somnolence, agitation, or diaphoresis
2. Systolic blood pressure increases by more than 20/min or to over 160/min
3. Heart rate changes by more than 20% in either direction or to over 140
4. Acute need for vasoactive medications
5. Arrhythmias develop or become more frequent
6. Respiratory rate increases more than 10 breaths/min or to over 35/min for 5 minutes
7. Pao_2 falls to less than 60 torr on Fio_2 of 0.5 or Sao_2 falls to less than 90%
8. Pco_2 rises above 50 torr with respiratory acidosis (pH < 7.30)

Box 10.4 • Extubation Criteria

I. Initial Postoperative Period
1. Awake without stimulation
2. Acceptable respiratory mechanics
   a. Negative inspiratory force > 25 cm H_2O
   b. Tidal volume > 5 mL/kg
   c. Vital capacity > 10–15 mL/kg
   d. Spontaneous respiratory rate < 24/min
3. Acceptable arterial blood gases on 5 cm or less of CPAP or PSV
   a. Pao_2 > 70 torr on Fio_2 of 0.5 or less
   b. $Paco_2$ < 48 torr
   c. pH 7.32–7.45

II. Prolonged Ventilation
1. Comfortable breathing pattern without diaphoresis, agitation or anxiety; respiratory rate < 35/min
2. Adequate mental status to protect the airway, initiate a cough, and raise secretions
3. Hemodynamic tolerance of the weaning process as delineated in Box 10.3
4. Respiratory mechanics and ABGs as above
5. A cuff leak > 110 mL with the cuff deflated

C. Extubation criteria (see Box 10.4) include the weaning criteria listed above, as well as:

1. Patient awake without stimulation
2. Acceptable respiratory mechanics
   a. Vital capacity > 10–15 mL/kg
   b. Negative inspiratory force > 25 cm H_2O
   c. Spontaneous respiratory rate < 24/min
   d. Rapid shallow breathing index (respiratory rate/tidal volume in liters) < 100
3. Acceptable ABGs on 5 cm or less of CPAP
   a. Pao_2 > 70 torr on an FIO_2 less than 0.5
   b. Pco_2 < 48 torr
   c. pH 7.32–7.45

D. Extubation may be accomplished from CPAP or T-piece. Although oxygenation may be slightly better during a CPAP than a T-piece trial, postextubation oxygenation is frequently better in patients weaned with T-piece because the Pao_2 declines less than in patients who were extubated from CPAP.[83,84]

E. Additional considerations
1. Some patients get very agitated when sedatives are weaned. Even though adequate ABGs may be maintained, agitated patients are frequently given more sedation throughout the night with another attempt at weaning in the

morning. Gradual weaning from sedation, communication from the nurses, and then a very rapid wean to CPAP and extubation is often the best course for these patients.

2. If the patient was very difficult to intubate in the operating room, it is essential to ensure that the ABGs and respiratory mechanics are satisfactory before extubation. Early extubation in the middle of the night should be performed cautiously in these patients. An individual experienced in difficult intubations should be present. A flexible laryngoscope or bronchoscope should also be available.

3. Elderly patients and those with more advanced cardiac disease or hepatic dysfunction often take longer to awaken from anesthesia even if sedatives are not administered. This may reflect slow metabolism of medications administered intraoperatively or may occasionally represent transient obtundation from borderline cerebral hypoperfusion during surgery or other causes. It is important to resist the temptation to reverse narcotic effect with naloxone. This medication can precipitate severe pain, anxiety, hypertension, dysrhythmias, and bleeding, and may result in recurrent respiratory depression when its effects have worn off. Similarly, flumazenil to reverse benzodiazepines should be avoided early in the postoperative period.

4. However, if a patient fails to awaken after 24–36 hours and the question arises as to whether this represents a stroke, encephalopathy, or simply residual sedation, one might consider the cautious use of a reversal agent to sort out the nature of the problem. Naloxone (Narcan) may be given in 0.1–0.2 mg IV increments every 3 minutes. Flumazenil is given in a dose of 0.2 mg IV over 30 seconds, followed by doses of 0.3 mg, then 0.5 mg every 30 seconds, if necessary, to a maximum of 3 mg in one hour.

5. Many patients, especially those who have received supplemental narcotics, demonstrate excellent respiratory mechanics when stimulated, but then drift off to sleep and become apneic. Constricted pupils may be noted in patients with persistent narcotic effect. These patients are not yet ready for weaning and extubation. Do not confuse comfortable breathing with persistent narcotic or sedative effect.

IX. Postextubation Respiratory Care (Box 10.5)

A. After extubation, the patient's breathing pattern, Sao_2, and hemodynamics must be observed carefully. Occasionally, especially in patients who were difficult to intubate, laryngeal stridor may be prominent and may require use of racemic epinephrine, steroids (dexamethasone 4 mg IV), or even reintubation. Failure to demonstrate a "cuff leak" during positive-pressure ventilation when the cuff is deflated usually indicates laryngotracheal edema, which may cause upper airway obstruction after extubation. This phenomenon is uncommon after short-term intubation but may be noted after several days of mechanical ventilation.

B. Because the median sternotomy incision is associated with moderate discomfort and decreased chest wall compliance, patients tend to splint, take shallow breaths, and cough poorly. Oxygenation may be compromised by fluid overload and atelectasis from poor inspiratory effort. It is advisable to supply 40–70% humidified oxygen by face mask for a few days. If the patient has borderline oxygenation, use of a BiPAP mask often proves beneficial in improving oxygenation and avoiding reintubation.[85]

Box 10.5 • Postextubation Respiratory Care

1. Pulse oximetry
2. Face mask, nasal cannula, or BiPAP mask to achieve $Sao_2 > 90\%$
3. Adequate analgesia (morphine, ketorolac)
4. Chest x-ray after pleural tubes are removed
5. Incentive spirometer/deep breaths q1–2h; use cough pillow
6. Mobilization as soon as possible; frequent repositioning in bed
7. Antiembolism stockings for DVT prophylaxis; consider Venodyne boots or SC heparin if high-risk
8. Aggressive diuresis once hemodynamically stable
9. Bronchodilators for bronchospasm (consider steroids if severe COPD)
10. Antibiotics for a positive sputum culture

BiPAP noninvasive ventilation has been demonstrated to be superior to incentive spirometry in improving oxygenation in the first few postoperative days.[86] It has also been shown to prevent the increase in extravascular lung water associated with the weaning process that is noted in patients placed on nasal cannula after extubation.[87] Mask CPAP may be sufficient if pulmonary edema is the primary cause of respiratory distress.[85]

C. Upon transfer to the floor, most patients benefit from the use of supplemental oxygen with nasal cannula for a few days. Monitoring of Sao_2 by pulse oximetry is helpful in patients with borderline oxygenation, especially during ambulation.

D. Although swallowing difficulties are uncommon in patients who are intubated for less than 48 hours, such problems are not uncommon with longer durations of intubation. Careful attention must be paid to the patient's initial oral intake to observe for potential aspiration. Patients who require longer periods of intubation frequently require a full swallowing evaluation before initiating oral intake.[88,89]

E. Once the patient is hemodynamically stable and no longer needs volume administration to maintain intravascular volume, aggressive diuresis with intravenous furosemide, either as intermittent bolus doses or a continuous infusion, should be initiated to eliminate excess extravascular lung water. Diuretics are continued until the patient has reached his or her preoperative weight and can be weaned from nasal cannula with an acceptable Sao_2 (> 90% on room air).

F. The patient should be mobilized and encouraged to cough and take deep breaths.[90] An incentive spirometer is very beneficial in maintaining the FRC and preventing atelectasis, although objective evidence of its efficacy in preventing postoperative pulmonary complications is fairly weak.[91] In fact, one study showed that the same benefit could be derived from taking 30 deep breaths without mechanical assistance as from use of a blow bottle device or inspiratory resistance positive expiratory pressure mask.[92] A "cough pillow" should be used to brace the chest during deep breathing and coughing to minimize discomfort and splinting. Chest physical therapy usually is not indicated but may be helpful in patients with significant underlying lung disease, borderline pulmonary function, or copious secretions. Albuterol administered via nebulizer is frequently beneficial.

G. Satisfactory narcotic analgesia is very helpful in improving the patient's respiratory effort. Initially, continuous or intermittent intravenous morphine infusions may be used with conversion to patient-controlled analgesia pumps for 1–2 days for patients having significant pain. Use of ketorolac after extubation is very effective in reducing or eliminating the narcotic requirement in patients with moderate to severe pain for the first few days.

H. Antiembolism stockings should be used routinely for patients after surgery to reduce the risk of deep venous thrombosis and pulmonary embolism. Mobilization is probably more important in reducing this risk. If the patient remains in the ICU and is sedated or poorly mobilized, graded compression devices, such as the Venodyne system, should be used. Subcutaneous heparin 5000 units SC bid may prove of benefit in patients considered at high risk for deep venous thrombosis, but must be used cautiously to minimize the risk of delayed tamponade.[93,94]

X. Acute Respiratory Insufficiency/Short-Term Ventilatory Support

A. Prolonged mechanical ventilation beyond 48 hours is necessary in about 5% of patients undergoing open-heart surgery. It may be provided while hemodynamic issues or transient pleuropulmonary insults, such as pulmonary edema, are being treated.[95] It may also be indicated for patients without intrinsic pulmonary problems who are sedated, obtunded, or have sustained neurologic insults. These patients may have adequate gas exchange but need an endotracheal tube for airway protection.

B. Acute respiratory insufficiency characterized by inadequate oxygenation ($PO_2 < 60$ torr on 0.5 FIO_2) or ventilation ($Pco_2 > 50$ torr) during mechanical ventilatory support occurs in about 1% of patients undergoing surgery on CPB. This usually results from a severe perioperative cardiopulmonary insult (usually hypotension, shock, or sepsis) that is often superimposed on preexisting lung disease. Predisposing factors to this problem include advanced age, significant COPD, active smoking history, depressed LV function and clinical CHF, obesity, and diabetes.[96,97] Overly vigorous fluid administration, both intraoperatively and postoperatively in hemodynamically unstable patients, is a common cause of poor oxygenation.

C. "Acute lung injury" with poor oxygenation has been defined as a Pao_2/FIO_2 ratio < 300, the extreme of which is the acute respiratory distress syndrome (ARDS), defined as a Pao_2/FIO_2 ratio < 200.[43,98] This is a very serious problem that may lead to multisystem organ failure and carries a mortality rate exceeding 50%. This should be differentiated from the transient poor oxygenation related to lung edema (often with ratios < 200) that can be readily managed with diuretics and not associated with a high mortality rate. Acute lung injury may progress to a more chronic phase of ventilator dependence and will be discussed in the next section on chronic respiratory insufficiency/ventilator dependence.

D. **Etiology.** During the first 48 hours, oxygenation problems predominate and can produce tissue hypoxia. Inadequate ventilation (hypercapnia) at this time is usually the result of a mechanical problem.

1. Inadequate O_2 delivery and ventilation (mechanical problems)
    a. Ventilator malfunction
    b. Improper ventilator settings: low FIO_2, tidal volume, or respiratory rate
    c. Endotracheal tube problems: cuff leak, incorrect endotracheal tube placement (larynx, mainstem bronchus, esophagus), kinking or occlusion of the tube
2. Low cardiac output states leading to mixed venous desaturation, venous admixture, and hypoxemia
3. Pulmonary problems
    a. Atelectasis or lobar collapse
    b. Pulmonary edema
        i. Cardiogenic from fluid overload and/or LV dysfunction, hemodilution on pump with reduced colloid oncotic pressure.[99]
        ii. Noncardiogenic from pulmonary endothelial injury with increased microvascular permeability. This may be related to activation of complement, neutrophils, or release of other inflammatory mediators associated with extracorporeal circulation. This problem is more prominent as the duration of bypass lengthens and is more common in patients receiving multiple blood transfusions.[100]
    c. Pneumonia
    d. Intrinsic pulmonary disease (COPD), bronchospasm, or air trapping
    e. Blood transfusions: microembolization, transfusion of proinflammatory mediators
4. Intrapleural problems
    a. Pneumothorax
    b. Hemothorax or pleural effusion
5. Metabolic problems: shivering leading to increased peripheral oxygen extraction
6. Pharmacologic causes: drugs that inhibit hypoxic pulmonary vasoconstriction (nitroglycerin, nitroprusside, calcium channel blockers, ACE inhibitors)[101]
E. The acute development of shortness of breath or an abrupt change in ABGs after an uneventful early postoperative course should raise suspicion of the following problems:
    1. Pneumothorax, possibly tension
    2. Atelectasis or lobar collapse from poor inspiratory effort or mucous plugging
    3. Aspiration pneumonia
    4. Cardiac tamponade
    5. Acute pulmonary edema (from ischemia, LV dysfunction, or undetected renal insufficiency)
    6. Pulmonary embolism
F. **Manifestations**
    1. Tachypnea (rate > 30 breaths/min) with shallow breaths
    2. Paradoxical inward movement of the abdomen during inspiration ("abdominal paradox")
    3. Agitation, diaphoresis, obtundation, or mental status changes
    4. Tachycardia or bradycardia
    5. Arrhythmias
    6. Hypertension or hypotension

Box 10.6 • Management of Acute Ventilatory Insufficiency

1. Examine patient, ventilator settings and function, ABGs, and chest x-ray
2. Hand ventilate with 100% oxygen; increase F_{IO_2} on ventilator until problem is sorted out
3. Ensure alveolar ventilation by correcting mechanical problems (adjust ventilator, reposition endotracheal tube, insert chest tube)
4. Assess and optimize hemodynamics
5. Add PEEP in 2.5- to 5-cm H_2O increments while decreasing F_{IO_2} to 0.5 or less; serially evaluate cardiac output at higher levels of PEEP to ensure optimal systemic oxygen delivery
6. Consider sedation or paralysis if patient–ventilator dyssynchrony
7. Treat identifiable pr1oblems:
   a. Diuretics for pulmonary edema
   b. Antibiotics for pneumonia
   c. Bronchodilators for bronchospasm
   d. Transfusion for low hematocrit (< 26%)
8. Institute chest physiotherapy
9. Begin nutritional supplementation

G. **Assessment and management** of acute respiratory insufficiency during mechanical ventilation (Box 10.6)

1. **Examine the patient:** auscultate for bilateral breath sounds and listen over the stomach to make sure the tube has not slipped into the larynx or been placed in the esophagus.

2. **Increase the F_{IO_2} to 1.0** until the causative factors have been identified. **Manually ventilate** with a resuscitation bag (Ambu®) if ventilator malfunction is suspected. This not only provides ventilation but also permits an assessment of pulmonary compliance. **Note:** Make sure the gas line on the bag is attached to the oxygen (green) and not the room air (yellow) connector and that the gas has been turned on.

3. **Ensure adequate alveolar ventilation**
   a. **Check ventilator function** and settings. Optimize the following:
      i. Tidal volume
      ii. Ventilator trigger sensitivity
      iii. Inspiratory flow rate; patients with COPD may have significant air trapping that produces an autoPEEP effect; increasing the inspiratory flow rate decreases the inspiration/expiration ratio, allowing more time to exhale the delivered breath; this can also be accomplished by decreasing the respiratory rate.
   b. **Obtain a chest x-ray** looking for any of the potential etiologic factors listed above; specifically note any mechanical problems that can be corrected by simple repositioning of the endotracheal tube or chest tube insertion.

  c. Repeat the ABGs.

  d. Note: An acute increase in peak inspiratory pressure may signify the development of a pneumothorax, although it can also result from severe bronchospasm, flash pulmonary edema, mainstem intubation, or an obstructed airway (copious secretions, the patient biting the endotracheal tube).

4. Assess and optimize hemodynamic status. A Swan-Ganz pulmonary artery catheter should be inserted to assess the patient's fluid status and cardiac output. A low cardiac output reduces oxygen delivery, lowers the mixed venous oxygen saturation, and increases venous admixture, further decreasing the Pao_2. Inotropic support or diuresis may be indicated. An echocardiogram may be helpful in identifying a contributory problem, such as significant LV or RV dysfunction, cardiac tamponade, mitral regurgitation, or a recurrent ventricular septal defect.

5. Add **PEEP** to the respiratory circuit to improve oxygenation and to allow weaning of the Fio_2 to less than 0.5. An Fio_2 of greater than 0.5 improves Pao_2 to a very minimal extent if the intrapulmonary shunt exceeds 20%. This is true because it is not possible to oxygenate perfused but nonventilated alveoli to eliminate venous admixture. Furthermore, maintenance of an Fio_2 exceeding 0.5 for several days can produce alveolar-capillary damage, alveolar collapse, and stiff, noncompliant lungs (so-called "oxygen toxicity").

  a. PEEP recruits previously closed alveoli to increase the surface area for oxygen exchange, thus increasing the FRC and preventing early airway closure. PEEP decreases intrapulmonary shunting by causing a redistribution of lung water from the alveoli to the perivascular interstitial space, although it does not decrease extravascular lung water content.

  b. A baseline level of 5 cm H_2O of PEEP is usually added to the circuit for all patients admitted to the ICU. This substitutes for the loss of the "physiologic PEEP" of normal breathing caused by the endotracheal tube. This level of PEEP is well tolerated by the heart but probably does little to improve oxygenation.[50] Thus, PEEP should be added in increments of 2.5–5 cm H_2O to a level of 10 cm H_2O or greater to improve oxygenation.

  c. Caution must be exercised when using high levels of PEEP because it creates high positive airway and intrathoracic pressures. This may compromise hemodynamic performance, thus impairing oxygen transport and tissue oxygenation. The optimal level of PEEP can be determined by observation of the arterial waveform and serial assessments of cardiac function. Improving oxygenation with PEEP while depressing the cardiac output is counterproductive because a low cardiac output not only reduces oxygen delivery but also lowers the mixed venous oxygen saturation, increasing venous admixture and further decreasing the Pao_2.

   i. PEEP decreases venous return and increases pulmonary vascular resistance (PVR) and RV afterload, resulting in depressed RV output in the presence of hypovolemia. The decrease in right-sided filling reduces LV end-diastolic volume and cardiac output. Volume infusion is necessary to counteract this effect before increasing the level of PEEP.

   ii. In patients with intrinsic pulmonary disease and especially ARDS, the PVR may be elevated. Increasing levels of PEEP may produce RV failure and dilatation, shifting the interventricular septum and compromising filling and compliance of the left ventricle. In these patients, volume infusion must be given cautiously.

iii. Adding high levels of PEEP to patients with severe COPD may cause overdistention of alveoli that are highly compliant and poorly perfused, resulting in increased V/Q shunting and producing endothelial damage and progressive hypoxia.

d. High levels of PEEP can result in "barotrauma" (pneumothorax, pneumomediastinum), which can compromise ventilation and produce acute hemodynamic embarrassment. Barotrauma is caused by alveolar overdistention and is attributable more directly to the severity of the underlying lung disease than to the peak airway pressure.[102] Nonetheless, modes of ventilation that provide lower tidal volumes have been used in patients with ARDS to improve oxygenation.[103]

e. **Note:** Care must be exercised when suctioning a patient on high levels of PEEP. Oxygenation can become very marginal when PEEP has been temporarily discontinued. A PEEP valve should be used during manual ventilation if the patient's oxygenation is dependent on PEEP.

f. The interpretation of pressure tracings from a pulmonary artery catheter is influenced by PEEP. The measured CVP, PA, and left atrial pressures are elevated, but transmural filling pressures, which determine the gradient for venous return, are decreased because pressure is transmitted through the lungs to the pleural space. A general rule is that the true pulmonary capillary wedge pressure (PCWP) is equal to the measured pressure minus half of the PEEP level at end-expiration. In situations in which the alveolar pressure exceeds that in the pulmonary vessels (e.g., during hypovolemia), the PCWP will reflect the intraalveolar pressure and not the left atrial pressure. If ventilation is discontinued to obtain PA pressure measurements in the hypovolemic patient, hypoxemia may develop and persist for up to one hour.[104]

6. **Sedation** with/without paralysis often improves gas exchange by improving the efficiency of ventilation. It can relax the diaphragm and chest wall and reduce the energy expenditure or "oxygen cost" of breathing.

7. Additional supportive measures

a. **Diuresis** (usually with IV furosemide) usually improves oxygenation in the early postoperative period when pulmonary interstitial edema may impair gas exchange. Depending on the patient's hemodynamic stability and renal function, a continuous infusion of IV furosemide (10–20 mg/h) can be used to promote a steady diuresis.

b. The patient's chest x-ray should be reviewed and cultures obtained of pulmonary secretions. Indiscriminate use of antibiotics should be discouraged, but broad-spectrum antibiotics can be initiated if there is suspicion of an infectious component to the patient's borderline pulmonary function. The antibiotics should then be modified depending on culture sensitivities.

c. **Bronchodilators**, such as albuterol, are useful for patients with increased airway resistance that may be compromising their ventilatory or hemodynamic status. Steroids may be useful for patients with severe COPD (see page 330).

d. Patients with intrinsic lung disease or postoperative respiratory failure are more predisposed to the development of atrial and ventricular arrhythmias, which can compromise hemodynamic performance. Although amiodarone has seen increasing acceptance as a first-line drug for a variety of arrhythmias, it has been reported to cause severe oxygenation problems even when used on a short-term basis.[105,106] An alternative medication might be considered in patients with significant respiratory issues.

e. **Blood transfusions** can be given to treat anemia if the hematocrit is less than 26–28% and may improve tissue oxygenation. Despite the intuitive logic that blood transfusions should improve blood oxygen content, improve tissue oxygen delivery, and potentially reduce the duration of mechanical ventilation, numerous studies have demonstrated little benefit, and even a detriment, to a liberal transfusion policy.[107,108] Transfused red cells do not have good oxygen-carrying capacity, they transmit proinflammatory mediators that can worsen pulmonary function, and they are immunosuppressive, increasing the risk of nosocomial infection.

f. **Bronchoscopy** may be beneficial when postural drainage and suctioning fail to resolve atelectasis because of the presence of tenacious secretions.

8. Methods of mechanical ventilation for patients requiring prolonged ventilatory support are discussed in section XII.

XI. Chronic Respiratory Failure/Ventilator Dependence

A. **Etiology.** The inability to wean the patient from the ventilator within a few days after surgery may be caused by problems that impair oxygenation ("hypoxemic respiratory failure)" and/or produce primary ventilatory insufficiency ("hypercapneic respiratory failure"). Although many patients can be weaned after a few days of additional ventilatory support once contributing factors have been addressed, a few will progress to a phase of ventilator dependence.[17,109] The mortality rate associated with the need for prolonged ventilation over 5 days is approximately 25% and commonly results from multiorgan system failure.[110]

1. **Hypoxia.** The persistence of oxygenation problems beyond 48 hours usually indicates severe hemodynamic compromise or an acute parenchymal lung problem. These are frequently superimposed on preexisting problems, such as preoperative acute pulmonary edema, pulmonary hypertension, or COPD. The primary causes of hypoxemia are:

a. Hemodynamic instability, especially a low cardiac output state that requires multiple pressors. This increases the oxygen cost of breathing and can produce both hypoxemia and hypercarbia.

b. Parenchymal problems

   i. Interstitial pulmonary edema, either noncardiogenic (capillary leak or sepsis) or cardiogenic (CHF)

   ii. Pneumonia

   iii. Lower airway obstruction (bronchitis, secretions, bronchospasm) often associated with COPD

2. **ARDS** represents a nonspecific diffuse acute lung injury with inflammation of the lung parenchyma. It is associated with noncardiogenic pulmonary edema from increased microvascular permeability. The lungs become stiff and noncompliant with severe impairment to gas exchange from alveolar-capillary damage, interstitial edema, and atelectasis. ARDS can produce both oxygenation and ventilatory failure.[111–113]

a. CPB has been implicated as a causative factor of ARDS because it produces a systemic inflammatory response. Neutrophil-initiated pulmonary dysfunction with oxygen free-radical generation is suspected to be the mechanism of this injury. However, since ARDS develops in fewer than 1% of patients undergoing open-heart surgery, other important contributory factors must be present. Factors such as older age, smoking, and hypertension have been associated with the development of ARDS, but they are very common comorbidities in surgical patients.[111]

b. Although the pathophysiologic process causing ARDS appears to be noncardiogenic in nature, most patients developing the syndrome have preexisting compromise of cardiac function. The major predictors of ARDS include reoperations, perioperative shock, increasing number of blood transfusions, emergency surgery, poor LV function, and advanced NYHA class. It might be inferred that the capillary leak associated with CPB may be worse in patients in poor clinical condition, especially if there is perioperative hemodynamic compromise, and these patients are more prone to develop this highly lethal syndrome. Subsequently, any additional insult, such as pneumonia, sepsis, cardiogenic pulmonary edema from LV dysfunction or renal failure, or multiple transfusions, will lead to progressive respiratory deterioration, multisystem organ failure, and death.

3. **Hypercarbia.** Primary ventilatory failure is caused by an imbalance between ventilatory capacity and demand and is the most common reason for failure to wean from the ventilator.[114] The patient is incapable of generating the respiratory effort necessary to sustain the "work of breathing," a term that refers to the work necessary to overcome the impedance to ventilation produced by the disease process and the resistance of the ventilator circuitry. Contributory factors include:

a. Increased ventilatory demand with increased CO_2 production and O_2 demand
    i. Sepsis (which also impairs oxygen uptake), fever, chills
    ii. Pain, anxiety
    iii. Catabolic states
    iv. Carbohydrate overfeeding
    v. Increased dead space (COPD)
    vi. Reduced lung compliance: pneumonia, pulmonary edema
    vii. Increased resistance: bronchospasm, airway inflammation

b. Decreased respiratory drive
    i. Altered mental status from medications, stroke, or encephalopathy
    ii. Sleep deprivation

c. Decreased respiratory muscle function
    i. Significant obesity
    ii. Ventilatory muscle weakness from protein malnutrition, medications (neuromuscular blockers, aminoglycosides, steroids), dynamic hyperinflation, or critical illness polyneuropathy (see page 547)[115,116]
    iii. Metabolic abnormalities (hypophosphatemia, hyper- or hypomagnesemia, hypokalemia, hypocalcemia, hypothyroidism)[117]
    iv. Diaphragmatic paralysis from phrenic nerve injury. This may be caused by the use of iced slush within the pericardial well during cardioplegic arrest. Unilateral paralysis usually does not cause ventilatory insufficiency unless there is severe underlying lung disease. Bilateral paralysis may

---

Box 10.7 • Supportive Measures in Patients with Chronic Ventilatory Failure

1. Select appropriate mode of ventilatory support
2. Suction PRN and prevent aspiration
3. Optimize hemodynamic status
4. Provide adequate analgesia but avoid oversedation and neuromuscular blockers
5. Provide adequate nutrition, preferably with low-carbohydrate enteral feedings
6. Optimize metabolic and electrolyte status (thyroid, hematocrit, sugar, magnesium, phosphate)
7. Specific considerations:
   a. Give bronchodilators/steroids for bronchospasm
   b. Give antibiotics for infections/antipyretics for fever
   c. Institute diuresis if fluid overload
   d. Drain any pleural effusions
8. Institute physical therapy and reposition to prevent decubitus ulcers
9. Stress ulcer prophylaxis with sucralfate or a proton pump inhibitor
10. Consider tracheostomy if prolonged ventilatory support (longer than 2 weeks) is anticipated

---

require prolonged ventilatory support, although recovery can usually be anticipated within a year.[118,119]

  d. The transition from mechanical to spontaneous ventilation with conversion from positive to negative intrapleural pressure increases LV afterload. This increases metabolic and cardiac demands and may not be tolerated by patients with limited cardiac reserve.

B. Clinical manifestations of ventilator dependence that often indicate inability to wean include:

  1. Tachypnea (rate > 30 breaths/min) with shallow breaths
  2. Paradoxical inward movement of the abdomen during inspiration ("abdominal paradox")

C. Management involves selecting an appropriate means of ventilation (see next section) while identifying the factors that may be contributing to ventilator dependence. Measures should be taken to optimize cardiac performance, improve the respiratory drive and neuromuscular competence, and reduce the respiratory load by improving intrinsic pulmonary function and reducing the minute ventilation requirement.[114,120,121] As these issues are being addressed, it is important to identify when a patient is ready for weaning or discontinuation of ventilatory support (Box 10.7).

  1. Improve hemodynamic status with inotropic support. Pulmonary vasodilators, such as nitroprusside and nitroglycerin, should generally be avoided because they can increase intrapulmonary shunting by preventing hypoxic vasoconstriction.

The phosphodiesterase inhibitors, including inamrinone and milrinone, are beneficial in providing inotropic, lusitropic (relaxant), and vasodilator effects. In patients with severe ventricular dysfunction and elevated PA pressures, nesiritide may be of benefit (see Chapter 11).

2. **Improve respiratory drive and neuromuscular competence.**

a. Avoid oversedation and neuromuscular blockers.

b. Provide adequate nutrition to achieve positive nitrogen balance and improve respiratory muscle strength and immune competence. Overfeeding with carbohydrates or fats can increase CO_2 production and the respiratory quotient (RQ). The RQ represents the CO_2 output/O_2 uptake and is normally 0.8. Excessive carbohydrate may raise the RQ to 1.0 and adds to the ventilatory burden. A tube feeding such as Pulmocare should be considered.

c. Select the appropriate mode of ventilatory support to reduce the work of breathing and train the respiratory muscles to support spontaneous ventilation (see next section). Avoid prolonged periods of spontaneous ventilation until the patient appears ready for a weaning trial. In patients with severe oxygen desaturation, use of the prone position may improve oxygenation and allow for earlier weaning.[122]

d. Optimize acid-base, electrolyte, and endocrine (thyroid) status. Metabolic alkalosis and hypothyroidism inhibit the central respiratory drive. Correct potassium, magnesium, and phosphate levels. Correct profound anemia.

e. Initiate physical therapy.

f. Evaluate diaphragmatic motion during fluoroscopy ("sniff test"). Diaphragmatic plication may improve respiratory function in patients with ventilator dependence caused by unilateral diaphragmatic dysfunction.[123]

3. **Reduce the respiratory load.**

a. Reduce impedance to ventilation.

   i. Give bronchodilators or steroids for bronchospasm (see last section of this chapter).

   ii. Employ chest physical therapy, frequent repositioning, and suctioning to mobilize and aspirate secretions and prevent atelectasis.

   iii. Consider tracheostomy (see section C.4 below).

b. Improve lung compliance.

   i. Give antibiotics for pneumonia.

   ii. Give diuretics for fluid overload and pulmonary edema.

   iii. Use thoracentesis or tube thoracostomy for pleural effusions.

   iv. Prevent abdominal distention with nasogastric suction or metoclopramide.

c. Reduce the minute ventilation requirement.

   i. Provide adequate analgesia for pain and sedatives for anxiety. Excessive sedation must be avoided because it inhibits the central respiratory drive.

   ii. Administer antipyretics for fever to reduce metabolic demand.

   iii. Treat infections (sepsis, pneumonia) with appropriate antibiotics to minimize antibiotic resistance.

   iv. Avoid overfeeding to lower CO_2 production.

   v. Prevent ventilator-associated pneumonia (VAP). This problem is multifactorial and a number of preventive strategies should be employed. Basic strategies involve using oral intubation and attempting extubation as soon as feasible, ensuring adequate hand washing by the health care team, keeping the patient semirecumbent, avoiding gastric overdistention, draining condensates from the ventilator circuit, maintaining adequate cuff pressure to prevent aspiration, providing adequate nutritional support, and using continuous subglottic suctioning.[124,125]

vi. Stress ulcer prophylaxis should be achieved using sucralfate rather than antacids or H_2 antagonists that raise gastric pH. Proton pump inhibitors have been found to be very effective in reducing the risk of stress-related bleeding with no documentation of any increase in the risk of VAP.[126–128]

vii. The use of selective digestive decontamination to reduce the incidence of lower respiratory tract infection is controversial. There is evidence that the combination of topical oropharyngeal agents, drugs given down the nasogastric tube (tobramycin, polymyxin, and amphotericin), and intravenous antibiotics (broad-spectrum cephalosporins) can reduce the incidence of VAP in surgical patients, but this strategy may lead to the emergence of antibiotic-resistant strains.[129]

4. **Tracheostomy** should be performed if it is anticipated that the patient may require mechanical ventilatory support for more than 2 weeks.[114] Persistent laryngotracheal intubation leads to laryngeal damage and swallowing dysfunction.[130] Tracheostomy reduces airway resistance and glottic trauma, improves the ability to suction the lower airways, lowers the risk of sinusitis (although probably does not reduce the risk of VAP), improves patient comfort and mobility, often allows the patient to eat, and generally makes the patient look and feel better. It commonly leads to earlier decannulation than standard endotracheal intubation.

a. The traditional concept had been that tracheostomy should be delayed for at least 2–3 weeks after a median sternotomy incision to decrease the risk of mediastinitis. This remains controversial, with some studies confirming and others refuting any relationship between early surgical tracheostomy and mediastinitis.[131,132]

b. The most common and preferred method of tracheostomy in recent years has been the Ciaglia "percutaneous dilatational tracheostomy" (see Appendix 13).[133–136] This can be performed safely at the bedside and, with bronchoscopic guidance, has a complication rate of less than 10%. Complications include bleeding, posterior tracheal laceration, tube obstruction from hematoma or edema of the posterior tracheal wall, and stomal infection.[136,137] The risk of cross-contamination of a median sternotomy wound is low, even if performed within a few days of surgery.[133,134] The incidence of late tracheal stenosis is lower than that of a surgical tracheostomy.[137]

c. An alternative approach is the Fanconi translaryngeal tracheostomy, which gives comparable results with perhaps fewer complications.[138]

XII. Methods of Ventilatory Support[114,120,139]

A. Full ventilatory support is required when the patient remains anesthetized and sedated after surgery. It is also required for the patient with acute or chronic respiratory failure while underlying disease processes are managed and nutrition is optimized.

Ventilatory support is provided using volume-preset modes or pressure-controlled ventilation (PCV). Full support can reduce the work of breathing and improve the efficiency of gas exchange in the patient who is sedated and/or paralyzed. Subsequently, partial ventilatory support should be initiated to wean the patient from the ventilator.

B. **Volume-preset modes.** Most patients are placed on "volume ventilators" that deliver a preset tidal volume. A limit is set on the peak pressure to avoid barotrauma. Patients with noncompliant, stiff lungs or bronchospastic airways can be difficult to ventilate in this mode because some of the preset tidal volume may not be delivered once the peak pressure limit is reached. This system is best for patients with normal or increased compliance (emphysema).

1. **Assist-control (A/C) ventilation** delivers a preset tidal volume when triggered by the patient's inspiratory effort or at preset intervals if no breath is taken. If the patient is out of synchrony with the ventilator or hyperventilates, a significant respiratory alkalosis or acidosis may occur. This mode of ventilation is best used only when the patient requires full ventilation and should not be used for weaning. In fact, the patient's efforts may persist despite the machine's superimposed breath, leading to increased respiratory muscle fatigue.

2. **Controlled mandatory ventilation (CMV)** will provide a positive-pressure breath to the patient at a preset volume and rate. This should be used only during the temporary period of full ventilator support because it will lead to respiratory muscle deconditioning.

   a. **Intermittent mandatory ventilation (IMV).** In the IMV mode, the patient's spontaneous inspiration will generate a tidal volume consistent with his or her effort and the machine will deliver a full tidal volume at a designated rate. Spontaneous breaths require opening of a demand valve that can increase the work of breathing, a problem that can be overcome by the use of a continuous-flow or flow-by system.

   b. **Synchronized intermittent mandatory ventilation (SIMV).** In the SIMV mode, the patient breathes spontaneously and, at preset intervals, the next spontaneous breath is augmented by a full tidal volume from the ventilator. Since the ventilator's breath is synchronized to the patient's efforts, high peak pressures are avoided and breathing is more comfortable. Because many of the patient's efforts are not augmented, initial use of this system is not recommended during the early phase of ventilatory support because it increases the work of breathing more than A/C ventilation. A low level of pressure support can be added to decrease the work of spontaneous breathing.

C. **Pressure-preset or volume-variable modes.** Pressure ventilators deliver gas flow up to a set pressure limit. The amount of gas flow delivered (the tidal volume) depends on the compliance of the lungs and airway resistance. This system ensures delivery of a more consistent tidal volume to patients with increased airway resistance (bronchospasm, restrictive lung disease). It is best avoided in patients with emphysema, in whom overinflation of the lungs can occur at low pressures.

1. **Pressure-controlled ventilation** is a time-cycled mode of ventilation that allows the clinician to preset the peak airway pressure and the inspiratory time. A breath is then delivered at predetermined intervals. PCV at a level of

20 cm H_2O provides full ventilatory support with a tidal volume of about 8–10 mL/kg.

2. **Pressure support ventilation** differs from other ventilator modes in that the patient's inspiratory effort is augmented by a selected level of inspiratory pressure rather than volume. The patient's efforts determine the respiratory rate, flow rate, and inspiratory time. The tidal volume is determined by the level of pressure support, the patient's inspiratory effort, lung compliance, and the resistance of the circuitry and the patient's airway. This mode is flow-cycled, not time-cycled. It is used to provide partial support as the patient is weaned from the ventilator (see below).

D. No matter which mode of ventilation is selected, attention must be paid to avoiding high peak inspiratory pressures. This can produce barotrauma as well as hemodynamic compromise by impeding venous return and impairing ventricular function. The inspiratory plateau pressure (IPP) is the peak pressure at the end of inspiration and should be maintained at less than 35 cm H_2O. Means of lowering the IPP include lowering of the level of PEEP, lowering the tidal volume, or decreasing the inspiratory flow rate to increase the I/E ratio.

1. The concept of low tidal volume ventilation has been studied in patients with ARDS. It is believed that alveolar overdistention can produce changes in endothelial cell permeability and produce barotrauma and noncardiogenic pulmonary edema. Use of low tidal volume ventilation (5–6 mL/kg) may improve oxygenation with permissive hypercapnia and has been associated with reduced mortality in patients with ARDS.[103,140]

2. Decreasing the inspiratory flow rate increases the inspiratory flow time and may decrease peak pressures. However, if the expiratory time is too short to allow for full exhalation, as may occur in patients with bronchospastic airways, the next breath may be "stacked" on top of the previous one, producing lung hyperinflation and the autoPEEP effect. This can have harmful hemodynamic effects and can produce barotrauma. Thus, increasing the inspiratory flow rate or reducing the respiratory rate may be necessary to avoid this effect.

E. **Noninvasive positive-pressure ventilation** can be used as a means of avoiding intubation in patients with acute respiratory decompensation.[85,141–145] It can also facilitate earlier extubation in patients in whom standard criteria are not quite met. The primary advantage is the avoidance of the risks of intubation, including laryngotracheal trauma, sinusitis, and respiratory tract infections.

1. Generally, an oronasal mask with a soft silicone seal is used to improve patient comfort, although it can make the patient feel claustrophobic. A bilevel device (BiPAP) is commonly used because it is leak tolerant, allows for rebreathing, and is more effective in lowering the Pco_2.

2. The oxygen flow rate is adjusted to achieve an $Sao_2 > 90\%$. Generally, it is not possible to exceed an Fio_2 of 0.5, so if the patient is severely hypoxic, intubation will usually be necessary.

3. The ventilator is set in a pressure-limited mode with an initial pressure of 8–10 cm H_2O and gradually increased to a maximum of 20 cm H_2O. This limits the maximal inspiratory time and improves patient-ventilator synchrony. The expiratory pressure is set at 5 cm H_2O.

XIII. Weaning from the Ventilator[146-152]

A. Once it is decided that a patient no longer requires full ventilatory support, a means of weaning the patient from the ventilator should be selected. Intuitively, the gradual reduction of ventilatory support should allow for strengthening of the respiratory muscles and a successful wean. However, studies of weaning modalities have shown that this strategy does not expedite the weaning process and in fact may delay it.[114,120]

B. The most effective means of assessing the potential for successful extubation is to attempt either one daily 30-minute or 2-hour T-piece trial, both of which have equal efficacy to multiple short-piece trials.[147-149] Extubation outcome is comparable using spontaneous breathing trials (SBT) with either T-piece or PSV up to 7 cm H_2O.[150] If the patient does not satisfy extubation criteria after this trial, 24 hours of full ventilation is recommended before another attempt at weaning. If the next attempt is unsuccessful, PSV weaning should be used. PSV weaning is equal or superior to T-piece weaning, which, in turn, is better than SIMV weaning.[151,152] It is estimated that about 10% of patients will still require reintubation even if they meet extubation criteria.

C. The most sensitive predictor of a successful ventilatory wean is a rapid shallow breathing index (RSBI) of less than 100 breaths/min. The RSBI is the ratio of the respiratory rate/tidal volume in liters during spontaneous ventilation for one minute. If the RSBI is less than 100, a weaning trial should be attempted because the estimated rate of successful weaning is greater than 80%. An RSBI that exceeds 100 does not preclude weaning, since about 50% of such patients can be weaned and extubated. Generally, however, if the RSBI exceeds 100 and the patient's respiratory rate is greater than 38 during a brief SBT, the likelihood of a successful wean is quite low.[114,120,153-155]

D. Practical aspects of weaning and extubation

   1. It is essential to address and manage all the potentially correctable causes of respiratory failure. Once this has been accomplished, weaning can be initiated if the criteria noted in Box 10.2 are met.

   2. The use of sedatives during mechanical ventilation is often essential to reduce the patient's anxiety and minute ventilation requirements. However, the use of continuous IV sedation depresses the patient's sensorium and respiratory drive and can delay the weaning process.[156] Stopping the sedatives and reinitiating them only if necessary should expedite the weaning process.[157]

   3. No matter which technique is used for weaning (T-piece, SIMV, or PSV), an SBT is performed using a T-piece or a low level of CPAP or PSV for up to 2 hours. Although there may be a theoretical advantage to each of these techniques (increased FRC with CPAP or less resistance to breathing with PSV), studies have suggested that all have similar outcomes.[114,146,150]

   4. Several factors must be evaluated in assessing a patient's tolerance of an SBT prior to considering extubation. If the failure criteria noted in Box 10.3 are noted, the SBT should not be continued for more than 2 hours. PSV should be titrated to achieve a respiratory rate <25/min and an additional period of support should be provided before another attempt at weaning. However, if the patient appears to be weaning satisfactorily and satisfies the extubation criteria listed in Box 10.4, extubation can usually be accomplished. Specific concerns are the following:

a. The patient should be able to breathe comfortably with a stable respiratory rate and have no diaphoresis, agitation, or anxiety during the weaning process.

b. The patient must have an adequate mental status to protect the airway, initiate a cough, and raise secretions. The necessity to suction more than every 2 hours for excessive secretions may preclude extubation. Notably, approximately 30% of patients with ventilator dependence have difficulty swallowing and will be prone to aspiration.[89]

c. There must be hemodynamic tolerance of the weaning technique and adequate ABGs, as noted in Boxes 10.3 and 10.4.

d. A cuff leak >110 mL with the cuff deflated should be documented to ensure adequate airway diameter. If this cannot be demonstrated, there may be significant tracheobronchial edema (or perhaps just encrusted secretions) that must be managed prior to attempting extubation. Use of steroids, such as dexamethasone, may be beneficial.[158]

5. Noninvasive positive-pressure ventilation using BiBAP can improve oxygenation in many patients after extubation. It may be used to provide ventilatory support if extubation has been performed even though standard criteria have not been met.[141–144] If the patient has evidence of pulmonary edema, mask CPAP usually suffices.[85]

E. T-piece weaning

1. T-piece weaning involves alternating periods of full support (rest) with increasing periods of independent spontaneous ventilation (stress). A gradual increase in the duration of independent breathing can increase the strength and endurance of the respiratory muscles. This technique is generally not recommended except for a brief SBT. The sudden transition to a complete workload is usually not well tolerated in the early phase of recovery from severe ventilatory failure and may result in profound respiratory muscle fatigue.

2. Generally, once the contributing factors to a patient's ventilatory dependence are addressed and the RSBI is less than 125, an SBT of 30 minutes to 2 hours can be used to see if the patient satisfies the criteria for extubation.[147] T-piece weaning in this fashion appears to be the most rapid method of achieving extubation.[148]

F. SIMV weaning

1. With SIMV, the mandatory breaths are patient-triggered, thus avoiding overinflation and improving the patient's comfort. The work of breathing with an IMV system (as well as with CPAP) is reduced using a continuous-flow or flow-by system.[159] During the weaning process, the IMV rate is gradually decreased and the patient assumes a greater proportion of the minute ventilation. Since the energy expenditure of the respiratory muscles increases as the IMV rate is lowered, lowering of the IMV rate during the day can be coupled with complete rest at night to avoid muscle fatigue. Of concern is that respiratory muscle rest does not occur during the mandatory breath and this may induce respiratory muscle fatigue. When the patient can maintain

spontaneous ventilation for a prolonged period and satisfies standard criteria, extubation can be accomplished.

2. The use of pressure support concomitantly with IMV can also reduce the work of breathing during the patient's spontaneous respirations. Weaning can be accomplished by initially reducing the IMV rate and subsequently reducing the level of pressure support. The duration of spontaneous ventilation on progressively lower levels of pressure support or CPAP is then extended and the patient is extubated.

3. Rapid SIMV weaning is usually used immediately after surgery to achieve early extubation. However, most studies have shown that SIMV weaning is the least effective means of weaning a chronically ventilated patient.[114,120,149–151]

G. Pressure support ventilation[160,161]

1. With PSV, the patient's spontaneous inspiration triggers the ventilator to deliver gas flow to the circuit until a selected amount of inspiratory pressure is achieved ("patient-triggered" and "pressure-limited"). Airway pressure remains constant by automatic adjustment of the flow rate as long as the patient maintains an inspiratory effort. Gas flow stops when the flow rate demand decreases below 25% of the initial peak inspiratory flow rate, and exhalation is then allowed to occur passively. Modifications of this system include "volume support," with which the PSV level is automatically adjusted to provide a preset tidal volume, and "volume-assured pressure support," with which additional volume is provided to provide a preset tidal volume, even if the pressure rises.

2. The patient's own effort determines the respiratory rate, the inspiratory time and flow rate (tidal volume/inspiratory time), and the expiratory time. The eventual inspired tidal volume depends on the level of PSV, the patient's respiratory effort, and the resistance of the airway, which may be elevated if a small endotracheal tube is being used or if secretions, bronchospasm, and decreased lung compliance are present. Because the patient controls most of the parameters during the respiratory cycle, PSV results in more comfortable breathing for the patient.

3. The advantage of PSV is that it reduces the work of breathing by overcoming the impedance of the ventilatory circuitry and supplying some of the pressure work required to initiate ventilation. PSV reconditions the respiratory muscles to assume more spontaneous ventilation without producing excessive energy expenditure. It thus may expedite the weaning process.

4. PSV results in lower peak airway pressures, lower respiratory rates, and higher tidal volumes than other modes of ventilation. Thus, it is beneficial for the patient who is out of synchrony with the ventilator ("fighting the ventilator"). However, if the patient has COPD with increased airway resistance and increased compliance, the inspiratory phase may be prolonged but will terminate when the patient attempts to exhale. This may induce patient discomfort. Such discomfort can be counteracted by reducing the level of pressure support or converting to pressure control to provide a shorter inspiratory phase.

5. Weaning is accomplished by progressively lowering the levels of PSV and observing the patient for fatigue and other parameters indicative of intolerance of the weaning process (see Box 10.3). Weaning options include:

    a. Increasing the duration of spontaneous ventilation with lower levels of PSV during the daytime ("sprinting") with full support of higher levels of PSV at night. If the patient tolerates PSV for 12 hours, the level of PSV is gradually reduced by 2 cm H_2O intervals daily or every other day, and the tidal volume and respiratory rate are assessed. Extubation is accomplished when the patient is able to breathe comfortably for 2 hours at low levels of PSV (around 6–8 cm H_2O support).

    b. PSV with IMV. A level of partial PSV support is selected and the IMV rate is gradually decreased. When the IMV rate has been reduced to less than 4 breaths/min, the PSV level is then decreased as discussed above.

    6. Potential disadvantages of PSV

a. PSV requires an intact respiratory drive to trigger the ventilator. Inadequate ventilation will result if the patient is apneic or has an unstable neurologic status, respiratory drive, or mechanics.

b. Cardiac output may be compromised because airway pressure is always positive. With IMV weaning, there is a phase of negative intrathoracic pressure that can augment venous return.

c. Shallow tidal volumes from poor inspiratory effort may lead to atelectasis.

d. A gas leak in the system may prevent PSV from being terminated, producing persistently high airway pressures and hemodynamic compromise.

e. In-line nebulizers (for bronchodilators) are in the inspiratory limb and may make it difficult for the patient to initiate a breath to trigger PSV.

XIV. Other Respiratory Complications

    A. Respiratory complications can occur during the period of mechanical ventilation, soon after extubation, or later during convalescence on the postoperative floor. The management of these complications must be individualized, taking the patient's overall medical condition, the extent and nature of the surgical procedure, the precipitating factors, and the phase of recovery into consideration. The management of pneumothorax, pleural effusions, and bronchospasm are discussed here. Pulmonary embolism, diaphragmatic dysfunction, and pneumonia are discussed in Chapter 13.

    B. Pneumothorax. If the pleural space is entered at the time of surgery, there is generally free communication with the pericardial space. Although some surgeons may only place mediastinal tubes in this situation (through which air should exit), most will place mediastinal and pleural tubes. Occasionally, a small opening into the pleural space may not be detected intraoperatively, usually caused by the passage of a sternal wire through the pleura. An immediate postoperative chest x-ray usually demonstrates a pneumothorax, and a chest tube should be placed at this time, regardless of the size of the pneumothorax, if the patient is to remain on positive-pressure ventilation. Less commonly, a pneumothorax is absent on the initial x-ray but evident on subsequent films. Small pneumothoraces noted after extubation can generally be observed and monitored by serial x-rays if the patient is asymptomatic.

    1. Always consider the possibility of a pneumothorax (possibly tension) when ABGs deteriorate or hemodynamic instability develops for no obvious reason after several hours of stability. Often the first sign is a sudden increase in the peak inspiratory pressure, indicated by repeated alarming of the ventilator.

2. Evidence of an air leak in the chest drainage system may indicate loose connections, rather than a leak from the lung. However, chest tubes should never be removed until it is confirmed that an air leak is not the result of an intrapleural or parenchymal problem. Air leaks gradually resolve within a few days in the vast majority of patients. If not, placement of a new pleural tube through the lateral chest wall and use of a Heimlich valve may allow the patient to be discharged with an active air leak.

3. Progressive subcutaneous emphysema may develop if air exits under positive pressure where the pleura has been violated. In patients with severe emphysema or bronchospastic airways, it may result from alveolar rupture. However, it may result from visceral pleural injury at the time of surgery, no matter how small. Subcutaneous emphysema may occur when the chest tubes are still in place, but it more commonly occurs after they have been removed. A pneumothorax may or may not be present. Management usually requires placement of unilateral or bilateral chest tubes (or unkinking of indwelling tubes that might have caused the problem) and, if the emphysema is severe, decompressing skin incisions in the upper chest or neck.

4. A chest x-ray should always be obtained after the removal of pleural chest tubes. A small pneumothorax (< 20%) can be observed with serial films. However, aspiration of the pleural space or placement of a new chest tube is indicated if the pneumothorax exceeds 20% or the patient is symptomatic.

C. **Pleural effusions** are noted postoperatively in approximately 60% of patients undergoing cardiac surgery and are more common when the pleural cavity has been entered for ITA takedown.[162] This usually results from oozing of blood and serous fluid from the chest wall. However, a hemothorax may develop if blood spills over from the pericardial space. An effusion developing on the right side is more commonly serous in nature from fluid overload.

1. **Prevention.** Leaving a Silastic (Blake) drain in the pleural cavity for several days after surgery has been shown to lower the incidence of late pleural effusions.[163] Adequate drainage of opened pleural cavities at the time of surgery should reduce the incidence of bloody effusions but cannot always be accomplished when minimally invasive incisions are made.[164]

2. **Presentations and treatment**

   a. A hemothorax may develop if a patient with significant mediastinal bleeding drains blood into an opened pleural cavity. This may prove beneficial in avoiding cardiac tamponade,[165] but should be suspected in the patient with hemodynamic instability, a falling hematocrit, filling pressures that fail to rise with volume (although they may rise if tamponade is also developing), and increasing peak inspiratory pressures on the ventilator. A supine chest x-ray may demonstrate more opacification on one side than the other, but the degree of hemothorax may be difficult to determine. Computed tomography is helpful in assessing the size of an effusion. Echocardiography can also identify a large effusion.

   b. A large pleural effusion can produce atrial or ventricular diastolic collapse and cardiac tamponade even in the absence of a pericardial effusion.[166-169] These findings can be confirmed by echocardiography.

   c. Most patients with pleural effusions are asymptomatic, and in the vast majority of cases small effusions resolve within a few months either with use of diuretics (especially right-sided effusions) or spontaneously. However, patients with underlying lung disease or moderate effusions may develop dyspnea. In these situations, a thoracentesis is indicated either in the hospital or during a follow-up visit. Chest tube placement may be considered for large effusions in the early postoperative period, when blood is more likely to have accumulated.

    d. Postpericardiotomy syndrome may contribute to the development of recurrent serous or serosanguineous effusions. This should be managed initially by use of nonsteroidal antiinflammatory drugs or steroids, but may require thoracentesis for symptom relief.

D. Bronchospasm can occur at the termination of surgery and can produce difficulty with sternal closure. Severe bronchospasm and air trapping developing in the ICU can produce difficulties with mechanical ventilation as well as hemodynamic problems that can mimic cardiac tamponade. Modification of the ventilator circuit to increase the inspiratory flow rate will decrease the inspiration/expiration ratio, allowing more time for exhalation, and should decrease the autoPEEP effect. Bronchospasm can be precipitated by fluid overload, drug reactions, blood product transfusions, or the use of β-blockers, and it can occur in patients with or without known COPD or bronchospastic airways. Treatment involves the following:

1. Inhalational bronchodilators delivered by nebulizer or metered dose inhaler are helpful during mechanical ventilation as well as after extubation.

    a. The combination of albuterol and ipratropium (Combivent, DuoNeb) provides the best bronchodilation.[170] This is available as an inhalation aerosol. One actuation provides around 20 μg of ipratropium and 100 μg of albuterol.

    b. Albuterol (Ventolin, Proventil) 0.5 mL of 0.5% solution (2.5 mg) in 2.5 mL normal saline q6h or 2 puffs q6h

    c. Ipratropium (Atrovent) 2.5 mL of 0.02% solution in 2.5 mL normal saline q6–8h or 2 puffs q4–6h

    d. Metaproterenol (Alupent, Metaprel) 0.2–0.3 mL of 5% solution in 2.5 mL normal saline q4–6h

    e. Racemic epinephrine 0.5 mL of 0.25% solution in 3.5 mL normal saline q4h

2. Intravenous aminophylline has several beneficial effects. It is a bronchodilator and a mild diuretic, increases the respiratory drive, improves respiratory muscle function, and may decrease the PA pressures and improve RV function. However, it is arrhythmogenic and chronotropic and must be used cautiously in patients with tenuous hemodynamics. Nonetheless, the tachycardia that may be present frequently improves when bronchospasm resolves.

    a. IV aminophylline is given as a 5–8 mg/kg load over 30 minutes followed by a continuous infusion. The maintenance dosage in mg/kg ideal body weight per hour should be 0.6 for nonsmokers, 0.9 for smokers, and 0.3 for patients with cardiac decompensation or liver disease.

    b. When PO theophylline is substituted for IV aminophylline, the appropriate dose can be calculated from either of the following formulas:

Total daily dose = (mg/h IV aminophylline)(24 h)(0.8)

or

10 × (mg/h IV aminophylline) = dose of theophylline bid

The IV infusion is stopped immediately after the first oral dose.

    c. The dosage of sustained-release theophylline is 200–300 mg q8–12h.

    d. Therapeutic levels are 10–20 μg/mL.

3. Epinephrine can be selected as an inotrope if cardiac output is marginal because it is an excellent bronchodilator. Since it is also a strong positive chronotrope, it must be used cautiously when sinus tachycardia is present.

4. Corticosteroids are frequently beneficial when bronchospasm is refractory to the above measures. They may increase airway responsiveness to other β-agonists. Dosing regimens can be extrapolated from those used for patients with acute exacerbations of COPD.[171–174] Two of these protocols are the following:

    a. Methylprednisolone (Solu-Medrol) 0.5 mg/kg IV q6h × 3 days, then prednisone 0.5 mg/kg q12h × 3 days, then 0.5 mg/kg qd × 4 days (10 day total course)[172]

    b. Methylprednisolone 125 mg IV q6h × 4 days, then prednisone 60 mg qd × 4 days, then 40 mg qd × 4 days, then 20 mg qd × 4 days (15 day total course)[173]

5. Note: β-blockers are generally contraindicated during episodes of bronchospasm. However, patients with a history of bronchospastic airways can frequently tolerate the selective β-blockers, such as esmolol, metoprolol, and atenolol.[175]

References

1. Meade MO, Guyatt G, Butler R, et al. Trials comparing early vs late extubation following cardiovascular surgery. Chest 2001;120:445S–53.
2. Cheng DCH, Karski J, Peniston C, et al. Early tracheal extubation after coronary artery bypass graft surgery reduces costs and improves resource use. A prospective, randomized, controlled trial. Anesthesiology 1996;85:1300–10.
3. Lee TWR, Jacobsohn E. Pro: tracheal extubation should occur routinely in the operating room after cardiac surgery. J Cardiothorac Vasc Anesth 2000;14:603–10.
4. Peragallo RA, Cheng DCH. Con: tracheal extubation should not occur routinely in the operating room after cardiac surgery. J Cardiothorac Vasc Anesth 2000;14:611–3.
5. Cheng DCH, Karski J, Peniston C, et al. Morbidity outcome in early versus conventional tracheal extubation after coronary artery bypass grafting: a prospective randomized controlled trial. J Thorac Cardiovasc Surg 1996;112:755–64.
6. Konstantakos AK, Lee JH. Optimizing timing of early extubation in coronary artery bypass surgery patients. Ann Thorac Surg 2000;69:1842–5.
7. Reis J, Mota JC, Ponce P, Costa-Pereira A, Guerreiro M. Early extubation does not increase complication rates after coronary artery bypass graft surgery with cardiopulmonary bypass. Eur J Cardiothorac Surg 2002;21:1026–30.
8. Guller U, Anstrom KJ, Holman WL, Allman RM, Sansom M, Peterson ED. Outcomes of early extubation after bypass surgery in the elderly. Ann Thorac Surg 2004;77:781–8.
9. Higgins TL. Safety issues regarding early extubation after coronary artery bypass surgery. J Cardiothorac Vasc Anesth 1995;9(suppl):24–9.
10. Ng CSH, Wan S, Yim APC, Arifi AA. Pulmonary dysfunction after cardiac surgery. Chest 2002;121:1269–77.
11. Matthay MA, Wiener-Kronish JP. Respiratory management after cardiac surgery. Chest 1989;95:424–34.
12. Shapira N, Zabatino SM, Ahmed S, Murphy DMF, Sullivan D, Lemole GM. Determinants of pulmonary function in patients undergoing coronary bypass operations. Ann Thorac Surg 1990;50:268–73.
13. Roosens C, Heerman J, De Somer F, et al. Effects of off-pump coronary surgery on the mechanics of the respiratory system, lung, and chest wall: comparison with extracorporeal circulation. Crit Care Med 2002;30:2430–7.
14. Cox CM, Ascione R, Cohen AM, Davies IM, Ryder IG, Angelini GD. Effect of cardiopulmonary bypass on pulmonary gas exchange: prospective randomized study. Ann Thorac Surg 2000;69:140–5.
15. Taggart DP. Respiratory dysfunction after cardiac surgery: effects of avoiding cardiopulmonary bypass and the use of bilateral internal mammary arteries. Eur J Cardiothorac Surg 2000;18:31–7.
16. Covino E, Santise G, Di Lello F, et al. Surgical myocardial revascularization (CABG) in patients with pulmonary disease: beating heart versus cardiopulmonary bypass. J Cardiovasc Surg (Torino) 2001;42:23–6.
17. Shroyer ALW, Coombs LP, Peterson ED, et al. The Society of Thoracic Surgeons: 30-day mortality and morbidity risk models. Ann Thorac Surg 2003;75:1856–64.
18. Canver CC, Chanda J. Intraoperative and postoperative risk factors for respiratory failure after coronary bypass. Ann Thorac Surg 2003;75:853–8.
19. Legare JF, Hirsch GM, Buth KJ, MacDougall C, Sullivan JA. Preoperative prediction of prolonged mechanical ventilation following coronary artery bypass grafting. Eur J Cardiothorac Surg 2001;20:930–6.
20. Suematsu Y, Sato H, Ohtsuka T, Kotsuka Y, Araki S, Takamoto S. Predictive risk factors for delayed extubation in patients undergoing coronary artery bypass grafting. Heart Vessels 2000;15:214–20.
21. Branca P, McGaw P, Light R. Factors associated with prolonged mechanical ventilation following coronary artery bypass surgery. Chest 2001;119:537–46.
22. Yamagishi T, Ishikawa S, Ohtaki A, Takahashi T, Ohki S, Morishita Y. Obesity and postoperative oxygenation after coronary artery bypass grafting. Jpn J Thorac Cardiovasc Surg 2000;48:632–6.

23. Bezanson JL, Deaton C, Craver J, Jones E, Guyton RA, Weintraub WS. Predictors and outcomes associated with early extubation in older adults undergoing coronary artery bypass surgery. Am J Crit Care 2001;10:383–90.

24. Yende S, Wunderink R. Causes of prolonged mechanical ventilation after coronary artery bypass surgery. Chest 2002;122:245–52.

25. Hawkes CA, Dhileepan S, Foxcroft D. Early extubation for adult cardiac surgical patients. Cochrane Database Syst Rev 2003;4:CD003587.

26. Naughton C, Reilly N, Powroznyk A, et al. Factors determining the duration of tracheal intubation in cardiac surgery: a single-centre sequential patient audit. Eur J Anaesthesiol 2003;20:225–33.

27. Alhan C, Toraman F, Karabulut EH, et al. Fast track recovery of high risk coronary bypass surgery patients. Eur J Cardiothorac Surg 2003;23:678–83.

28. Habib RH, Zacharias A, Engoren M. Determinants of prolonged mechanical ventilation after coronary artery bypass grafting. Ann Thorac Surg 1996;62:1164–71.

29. Bando K, Sun K, Binford RS, Sharp TG. Determinants of longer duration of endotracheal intubation after adult cardiac operations. Ann Thorac Surg 1997;63:1026–33.

30. Cohen AJ, Katz MG, Frenkel G, Medalion B, Geva D, Schachner A. Morbid results of prolonged intubation after coronary artery bypass surgery. Chest 2000;118:1724–31.

31. Arom KV, Emery RW, Petersen RJ, Schwartz M. Cost-effectiveness and predictors of early extubation. Ann Thorac Surg 1995;60:127–32.

32. Hachenberg T, Tenling A, Nystrom SO, Tyden H, Hedenstierna G. Ventilation-perfusion inequality in patients undergoing cardiac surgery. Anesthesiology 1994;80:509–19.

33. Hagl C, Harringer W, Gohrbandt B, Haverich A. Site of pleural drain insertion and early postoperative pulmonary function following coronary artery bypass grafting with internal mammary artery. Chest 1999;115:757–61.

34. Berrizbeitia LD, Tessler S, Jacobowitz IJ, Kaplan P, Budzilowicz L, Cunningham JN. Effect of sternotomy and coronary bypass surgery on postoperative mechanics. Comparison of internal mammary and saphenous vein bypass grafts. Chest 1989;96:873–6.

35. Vargas FS, Terra-Filho M, Hueb W, Teizeira LR, Cukier A, Light RW. Pulmonary function after coronary bypass surgery. Respir Med 1997;91:629–33.

36. Hurlbut D, Myers ML, Lefcoe M, Goldbach M. Pleuropulmonary morbidity: internal thoracic artery versus saphenous vein graft. Ann Thorac Surg 1990;50:959–64.

37. Daganou M, Dimopoulou I, Michalopoulos N, et al. Respiratory complications after coronary artery bypass surgery with unilateral or bilateral internal mammary artery grafting. Chest 1998;113:1285–9.

38. Gilbert TB, Barnas GM, Sequeira AJ. Impact of pleurotomy, continuous positive airway pressure, and fluid balance during cardiopulmonary bypass on lung mechanics and oxygenation. J Cardiothorac Vasc Anesth 1996;10:844–9.

39. Shenkman Z, Shir Y, Weiss YG, Bleiberg B, Gross D. The effects of cardiac surgery on early and late pulmonary functions. Acta Anaesthesiol Scand 1997;41:1193–9.

40. Tripp HF, Bolton JW. Phrenic nerve injury following cardiac surgery: a review. J Card Surg 1998;13:218–23.

41. O'Brien JW, Johnson SH, VanSteyn SJ, et al. Effects of internal mammary artery dissection on phrenic nerve perfusion and function. Ann Thorac Surg 1991;52:182–8.

42. Yamazaki K, Kato H, Tsujimoto S, Kitamura R. Diabetes mellitus, internal thoracic artery grafting, and the risk of an elevated hemidiaphragm after coronary artery bypass surgery. J Cardiothorac Vasc Anesth 1994;8:437–40.

43. Asimakopoulos G, Smith PLC, Ratnatunga CP, Taylor KM. Lung injury and acute respiratory distress syndrome after cardiopulmonary bypass. Ann Thorac Surg 1999;68:1107–15.

44. Insler SR, O'Connor MS, Leventhal MJ, Nelson DR, Starr NJ. Association between postoperative hypothermia and adverse outcome after coronary artery bypass surgery. Ann Thorac Surg 2000;70:175–81.

45. Olivier P, Sirieix D, Dassier P, D'Attellis N, Baron JF. Continuous infusion of remifentanil and target-controlled infusion of propofol for patients undergoing cardiac surgery: a new approach for scheduled early extubation. J Cardiothorac Vasc Anesth 2000;14:29–35.

46. Walder B, Borgeat A, Suter PM, Romand JA. Propofol and midazolam versus propofol alone for sedation following coronary artery bypass grafting: a randomized, placebo-controlled trial. Anaesth Intensive Care 2002;30:171–8.

47. Rathgeber J, Schorn B, Falk V, Kazmaier S, Speigel T, Burchardi H. The influence of controlled mandatory ventilation (CMV), intermittent mandatory ventilation (IMV) and biphasic intermittent positive airway pressure (BIPAP) on the duration of intubation and consumption of analgesics and sedatives. A prospective analysis of 596 patients following adult cardiac surgery. Eur J Anaesthesiol 1997;14:576–82.

48. Kazmaier S, Rathgeber J, Buhre W, et al. Comparison of ventilatory and haemodynamic effects of BIPAP and S-IMV/PSV for postoperative short-term ventilation in patients after coronary artery bypass grafting. Eur J Anaesthesiol 2000;17:601–10.

49. Pepe PE, Marini JJ. Occult positive end-expiratory pressure in mechanically ventilated patients with airflow obstruction. The Auto-PEEP effect. Am Rev Respir Dis 1982;126:166–70.

50. Michalopoulos A, Anthi A, Rellos K, Geroulanos S. Effects of positive end-expiratory pressure (PEEP) in cardiac surgery patients. Respir Med 1998;92:858–62.

51. Valta P, Takala J, Elissa NT, Milic-Emili J. Effects of PEEP on respiratory mechanics after open heart surgery. Chest 1992;102:227–33.

52. Van Trigt P, Spray TL, Pasque MK, et al. The effect of PEEP on left ventricular diastolic dimensions and systolic performance following myocardial revascularization. Ann Thorac Surg 1982;33:585–92.

53. Boldt J, King D, von Bormann B, Scheld H, Hempelmann G. Influence of PEEP ventilation immediately after cardiopulmonary bypass on RV function. Chest 1988;94:566–71.

54. Mangano DT, Siciliano D, Hollenberg M, et al. Postoperative myocardial ischemia. Therapeutic trials using intensive analgesia following surgery. Anesthesiology 1992;76:342–53.

55. Herr DL, Sum-Ping ST, England M. ICU sedation after coronary artery bypass graft surgery: dexmedetomidine-based versus propofol-based sedation regimens. J Cardiothorac Vasc Anesth 2003;17:576–84.

56. Maitre PO, Funk B, Crevoisier C, Ha HR. Pharmacokinetics of midazolam in patients recovering from cardiac surgery. Eur J Clin Pharmacol 1989;37:161–6.

57. Guglielminotti J, Desmonts JM, Dureuil B. Effects of tracheal suctioning on respiratory resistances in mechanically ventilated patients. Chest 1998;113:1335–8.

58. Ready LB, Brown CR, Stahlgren LH, et al. Evaluation of intravenous ketorolac administered by bolus or infusion for treatment of postoperative pain. A double-blind, placebo-controlled, multicenter study. Anesthesiology 1994;80:1277–86.

59. Lee A, Cooper MG, Craig JC, Knight JF, Keneally JP. Effects of nonsteroidal anti-inflammatory drugs on post-operative renal function in adults. Cochran Database Syst Rev 2000;4:CD002765.

60. Karski JM. Practical aspects of early extubation in cardiac surgery. J Cardiothorac Vasc Anesth 1995;9(Suppl 1):30–3.

61. Bojar RM, Rastegar H, Payne DD, et al. Methemoglobinemia from intravenous nitroglycerin: a word of caution. Ann Thorac Surg 1987;43:332–4.

62. Suematsu Y, Sato H, Ohtsuka T, Kotsuka Y, Araki S, Takamoto S. Predictive risk factors for pulmonary oxygen transfer in patients undergoing coronary artery bypass grafting. Jpn Heart J 2001;42:143–53.

63. De Witte J, Sessler DI. Perioperative shivering. Anesthesiology 2002;96:467–84.

64. Gall SA Jr, Olsen CO, Reves JG, et al. Beneficial effects of endotracheal extubation on ventricular performance. Implications for early extubation after cardiac operations. J Thorac Cardiovasc Surg 1988;95:819–27.

65. Reis J, Mota JC, Ponce P, Costa-Pereira A, Guerreiro M. Early extubation does not increase complication rates after coronary artery bypass graft surgery with cardiopulmonary bypass. Eur J Cardiothorac Surg 2002;21:1026–30.

66. Montes FR, Sanchez SI, Giraldo JC, et al. The lack of benefit of tracheal extubation in the operating room after coronary artery bypass surgery. Anesth Analg 2000;91:776–80.

67. Nicholson DJ, Kowalski SE, Hamilton GA, Meyers MP, Serrette C, Duke PC. Postoperative pulmonary function in coronary artery bypass graft surgery patients undergoing early tracheal

extubation: a comparison between short-term mechanical ventilation and early extubation. J Cardiothorac Vasc Anesth 2002;16:27–31.

68. Waltall H, Ray S, Robson D. Does extubation result in haemodynamic instability in patients following coronary artery bypass grafts? Intensive Crit Care Nurs 2001;17:286–93.

69. Ngaage DL, Martins E, Orkell E, et al. The impact of the duration of mechanical ventilation on the respiratory outcome in smokers undergoing cardiac surgery. Cardiovasc Surg 2002;10:345–50.

70. Redmond JM, Gillinov AM, Stuart RS, et al. Heparin-coated bypass circuits reduce pulmonary injury. Ann Thorac Surg 1993;56:474–8.

71. Karaiskos TE, Palatianos GM, Triantafillou CD, et al. Clinical effectiveness of leukocyte filtration during cardiopulmonary bypass in patients with chronic obstructive pulmonary disease. Ann Thorac Surg 2004;78:1339–44.

72. Landis RC, Asimakopoulos G, Poullis M, Haskard DO, Taylor KM. The antithrombotic and anti-inflammatory mechanisms of action of aprotinin. Ann Thorac Surg 2001;72:2169–75.

73. Schurr UP, Zund G, Hoerstrup SP, et al. Preoperative administration of steroids: influence on adhesion molecules and cytokines after cardiopulmonary bypass. Ann Thorac Surg 2001;72:1316–20.

74. Chaney MA, Durazo-Arvizu RA, Nikolov MP, Blakeman BP, Bakhos M. Methylprednisolone does not benefit patients undergoing coronary artery bypass grafting and early tracheal extubation. Thorac Cardiovasc Surg 2001;121:561–9.

75. Tassani P, Richter JA, Barankay A, et al. Does high-dose methylprednisolone in aprotinin-treated patients attenuate the systemic inflammatory response during coronary artery bypass grafting procedures? J Cardiothorac Vasc Anesth 1999;13:165–72.

76. Loekinger A, Kleinsasser A, Lindner KH, Margreiter J, Keller C, Hoerman C. Continuous positive airway pressure at 10 cm H_2O during cardiopulmonary bypass improves postoperative gas exchange. Anesth Analg 2000;91:522–7.

77. Chaney MA, Kikolov MP, Blakeman BP, Bakhos M. Protective ventilation attenuates postoperative pulmonary dysfunction in patients undergoing cardiopulmonary bypass. J Cardiothorac Vasc Anesth 2000;14:514–8.

78. Garwood S, Swamidoss CP, Davis EA, Samson L, Hines RL. A case series of low-dose fenoldopam in seventy cardiac surgical patients at increased risk of renal dysfunction. J Cardiothorac Vasc Anesth 2003;17:17–21.

79. Caimmi PP, Pagani L, Micalizzi E, et al. Fenoldopam for renal protection in patients undergoing cardiopulmonary bypass. J Cardiothorac Vasc Anesth 2003;17:491–4.

80. Huang H, Yao T, Wang W, et al. Continuous ultrafiltration attenuates the pulmonary injury that follows open heart surgery with cardiopulmonary bypass. Ann Thorac Surg 2003;76:136–40.

81. Furnary AP, Zerr KJ, Grunkemeier GL, Starr A. Continuous intravenous insulin infusion reduces the incidence of deep sternal wound infection in diabetic patients after cardiac surgical procedures. Ann Thorac Surg 1999;67:352–60.

82. Tomlinson JR, Miller KS, Lorch DG, Smith L, Reines HD, Sahn SA. A prospective comparison of IMV and T-piece weaning from mechanical ventilation. Chest 1989;96:348–52.

83. Jones DP, Byrne P, Morgan C, Fraser I, Hyland R. Positive end-expiratory pressure vs T-piece. Extubation after mechanical ventilation. Chest 1991;100:1655–9.

84. Annest SJ, Gottlieb M, Paloski WH, et al. Detrimental effects of removing end-expiratory pressure prior to endotracheal extubation. Ann Surg 1980;191:539–45.

85. Liesching T, Kwok H, Hill NS. Acute applications of noninvasive positive pressure ventilation. Chest 2003;124:699–713.

86. Matte P, Jacquet L, Van Dyck M, Goenen M. Effects of conventional physiotherapy, continuous positive airway pressure and non-invasive ventilatory support with bilevel positive airway pressure after coronary artery bypass grafting. Acta Anaesthesiol Scand 2000;44:75–81.

87. Gust R, Gottschalk A, Schmidt H, Bottiger BW, Bohrer H, Martin E. Effects of continuous (CPAP) and bi-level positive airway pressure (BiPAP) on extravascular lung water after extubation of the trachea in patients following coronary artery bypass grafting. Intensive Care Med 1996;22:1345–50.

88. Barquist E, Brown M, Cohn S, Lundy D, Jackowski J. Postextubation fiberoptic endoscopic evaluation of swallowing after prolonged endotracheal intubation: a randomized, prospective trial. Crit Care Med 2001;29:1710–13.

89. Tolep K, Getch CL, Criner GJ. Swallowing dysfunction in patients receiving prolonged mechanical ventilation. Chest 1996;109:167–72.

90. Stiller K, Montarello J, Wallace M, et al. Efficacy of breathing and coughing exercises in the prevention of pulmonary complications after coronary artery surgery. Chest 1994;105:741–7.

91. Overend TJ, Anderson CM, Lucy SD, Bhatia C, Jonsson BI, Timmermanns C. The effect of incentive spirometry on postoperative pulmonary complications. A systematic review. Chest 2001;120:971–8.

92. Westerdahl E, Lindmark B, Eriksson T, Hedenstierna G, Tenling A. The immediate effects of deep breathing exercises on atelectasis and oxygenation after cardiac surgery. Scand Cardiovasc J 2003;37:336–7.

93. Shammas NW. Pulmonary embolus after coronary artery surgery: a review of the literature. Clin Cardiol 2000;23:639–44.

94. Ramos R, Salem BI, Pawlikowski MP, Coordes C, Eisenberg S, Leindenfrost R. The efficacy of pneumatic compression stockings in the prevention of pulmonary embolism after cardiac surgery. Chest 1996;109:82–5.

95. Louagie Y, Gonzalez E, Jamart J, Bulliard G, Schoevaerdts JC. Postcardiopulmonary bypass lung edema. A preventable complication? Chest 1993;103:86–95.

96. Cohen A, Katz M, Katz R, Hauptman E, Schachner A. Chronic obstructive pulmonary disease in patients undergoing coronary artery bypass grafting. J Thorac Cardiovasc Surg 1995;109:574–81.

97. Bevelaqua F, Garritan S, Haas F, Salazar-Schicchi J, Axen K, Reggiani JL. Complications after cardiac operations in patients with severe pulmonary impairment. Ann Thorac Surg 1990;50:602–6.

98. Bernard GR, Artigas A, Brigham KL, et al. The American-European Consensus Conference on ARDS: definitions, mechanisms, relevant outcomes, and clinical trial coordination. Am J Respir Crit Care Med 1994;149:818–24.

99. Klancke KA, Assey ME, Kratz JM, Crawford FA. Postoperative pulmonary edema in postcoronary artery bypass graft patients. Relationship of total serum protein and colloid oncotic pressures. Chest 1983;84:529–34.

100. Maggart M, Stewart S. The mechanisms and management of noncardiogenic pulmonary edema following cardiopulmonary bypass. Ann Thorac Surg 1987;43:231–6.

101. Tsai BM, Wang M, Turrentine MW, Mahomed Y, Brown JW, Meldrum DR. Hypoxic pulmonary vasoconstriction in cardiothoracic surgery: basic mechanisms to potential therapies. Ann Thorac Surg 2004;78:360–8.

102. Marcy TW. Barotrauma: detection, recognition and management. Chest 1993;104:578–84.

103. The ARDS Network. Ventilation with lower tidal volumes as compared with traditional tidal volumes for acute lung injury and ARDS. N Engl J Med 2000;342:1301–8.

104. Schwartz SZ, Shoemaker WC, Nolan-Avila LS. Effects of blood volume and discontinuance of ventilation on pulmonary vascular pressures and blood gases in patients with low levels of positive end-expiratory pressure. Crit Care Med 1987;15:671–5.

105. Kaushik S, Hussein A, Clarke P, Lazar HL. Acute pulmonary toxicity after low-dose amiodarone therapy. Ann Thorac Surg 2001;72:1760–1.

106. Ashrafian H, Davey P. Is amiodarone an underrecognized cause of acute respiratory failure in the ICU? Chest 2001;120:275–82.

107. Hebert PC, Blajchman MA, Cook DJ, et al. Do blood transfusions improve outcomes related to mechanical ventilation? Chest 2001;119:1850–7.

108. Spiess BD. Blood transfusions: the silent epidemic. Ann Thorac Surg 2001;72:S1832–7.

109. Marini JJ. The physiologic determinants of ventilator dependence. Respir Care 1986;31:271–82.

110. Kollef MH, Wragge T, Pasque C. Determinants of mortality and multiorgan dysfunction in cardiac surgery patients requiring prolonged mechanical ventilation. Chest 1995;107:1395–1401.

111. Milot J, Perron J, Lacasse Y, Letourneau L, Cartier PC, Maltais F. Incidence and predictors of ARDS after cardiac surgery. Chest 2001;19:884–8.

112. Asimakopoulos G, Taylor KM, Smith PL, Ratnatunga CP. Prevalence of acute respiratory distress syndrome after cardiac surgery. J Thorac Cardiovasc Surg 1999;117:620–1.

113. Ware LB, Matthay MA. The acute respiratory distress syndrome. N Engl J Med 2000;342:1334–49.

114. MacIntyre NR, Cook DJ, Ely EW Jr, et al. Evidence-based guidelines for weaning and discontinuing ventilatory support. A collective task force facilitated by the American College of Chest Physicians. The American Association for Respiratory Care; and the American College of Critical Care Medicine. Chest 2001;120:375S–95S.

115. Hund E. Critical illness polyneuropathy. Curr Opin Neurol 2001;14:649–53.

116. Piper SN, Koetter KP, Triem JG, et al. Critical illness polyneuropathy following cardiac surgery. Scand Cardiovasc J 1998;32:309–12.

117. Otero M, Santomauro EA, Alexander JC et al. Hypophosphatemia associated weaning failure in open heart patients. Chest 1999;11:385S–6.

118. Chandler KW, Rozas CJ, Kory RC, Goldman AL. Bilateral diaphragmatic paralysis complicates local cardiac hypothermia during open heart operation. Am J Med 1984;77:243–9.

119. Wilcox PG, Pare PD, Pardy RL. Recovery after unilateral phrenic injury associated with coronary artery revascularization. Chest 1990;98:661–6.

120. Manthous CA, Schmidt GA, Hall JB. Liberation from mechanical ventilation. A decade of progress. Chest 1998;114:886–901.

121. Brower RG, Ware LB, Berthiaume Y, Matthay MA. Treatment of ARDS. Chest 2001;120:1347–67.

122. Firodiya M, Mehta Y, Juneja R, Trehan N. Mechanical ventilation in the prone position: a strategy for acute respiratory failure after cardiac surgery. Indian Heart J 2001;53:83–6.

123. Graham DR, Kaplan D, Evans CC, Hind CRK, Donnelly RJ. Diaphragmatic plication for unilateral diaphragmatic paralysis: a 10-year experience. Ann Thorac Surg 1990;49:248–52.

124. Kollef MH. The prevention of ventilator-associated pneumonia. N Engl J Med 1999;340:627–34.

125. Kollef MH, Skubas NJ, Sundt TM. A randomized clinical trial of continuous aspiration of subglottic secretions in cardiac surgery patients. Chest 1999;116:1339–46.

126. Steinberg KP. Stress-related mucosal disease in the critically ill patient: risk factors and strategies to prevent stress-related bleeding in the intensive care unit. Crit Care Med 2002;30(6 Suppl):S362–4.

127. Yang YX, Lewis JD. Prevention and treatment of stress ulcers in critically ill patients. Semin Gastrointest Dis 2003;14:11–9.

128. Jung R, MacLaren R. Proton-pump inhibitors for stress ulcer prophylaxis in critically ill patients. Ann Pharmacother 2002;36:1929–37.

129. Kollef MH. Selective digestive decontamination should not be routinely employed. Chest 2003;123:464S–8.

130. Stone DJ, Bogdonoff DL. Airway considerations in the management of patients requiring long-term endotracheal intubation. Anesth Analg 1992;74:276–87.

131. Stamenkovic SA, Morgan IS, Pontefract DR, Campanella C. Is early tracheostomy safe in cardiac patients with median sternotomy incisions? Ann Thorac Surg 2000;69:1152–4.

132. Curtis J, Clark NC, McKenney CA, et al. Tracheostomy: risk factor for mediastinitis after cardiac operations. Ann Thorac Surg 2001;72:731–4.

133. Byhahn C, Rinne T, Halbig S, et al. Early percutaneous tracheostomy after median sternotomy. J Thorac Cardiovasc Surg 2000;120:329–34.

134. Hubner N, Rees W, Seufert K, Bockelmann M, Christmann U, Warner X. Percutaneous dilatational tracheostomy done early after cardiac surgery – outcome and incidence of mediastinitis. Thorac Cardiovasc Surg 1998;46:89–92.

135. Freeman BD, Isabella K, Lin N, Buchman TG. A meta-analysis of prospective trials comparing percutaneous and surgical tracheostomy in critically ill patients. Chest 2000;118:1412–8.

136. Polderman KH, Spijkstra JJ, de Bree R, et al. Percutaneous dilatational tracheostomy in the ICU. Optimal organization, low complication rates, and description of a new complication. Chest 2003;123:1595–1602.

137. van Heurn LWE, Goei R, de Pleog I, Ramsey G, Brink PRG. Late complications of percutaneous dilatational tracheotomy. Chest 1996;110:1572–6.

138. Westphal K, Byhahn C, Rinne T, Wilke HJ, Wimmer-Greinecker G, Lischke V. Tracheostomy in cardiosurgical patients: surgical tracheostomy versus Ciaglia and Fantoni methods. Ann Thorac Surg 1999;68:486–92.

139. Tobin MJ. Advances in mechanical ventilation. N Engl J Med 2001;344:1986–96.

140. Brower RG, Rubenfeld GD. Lung-protective ventilation strategies in acute lung injury. Crit Care Med 2003;31(Suppl):S312–6.

141. Rabatin JT, Gay PC. Noninvasive ventilation. Mayo Clin Proc 1999;74:817–20.

142. Antonelli M, Conti G, Rocco M, et al. A comparison of noninvasive positive-pressure ventilation and conventional mechanical ventilation in patients with acute respiratory failure. N Engl J Med 1998;339:429–35.

143. Girault C, Daudenthum I, Chevron V, Tamion F, Leroy J, Bonmarchand G. Noninvasive ventilation as a systematic extubation and weaning technique in acute on chronic respiratory failure: a prospective, randomized controlled study. Am J Crit Care Med 1999;160:86–92.

144. Nava S, Ambrosino N, Clini E, et al. Noninvasive mechanical ventilation in the weaning of patients with respiratory failure due to chronic obstructive pulmonary disease: a randomized controlled trial. Ann Intern Med 1998;128:721–8.

145. Antonelli M, Conti G, Moro ML, et al. Predictors of failure of noninvasive positive pressure ventilation in patients with acute hypoxemic respiratory failure: a multicenter study. Intensive Care Med 2001;27:1718–28.

146. Hess D. Ventilator modes used in weaning. Chest 2001;120:474S–76.

147. Esteban E, Alia I, Tobin MJ, et al. Effect of spontaneous breathing trial duration on outcome of attempts to discontinue mechanical ventilation. Am J Respir Crit Care Med 1999;159:512–8.

148. Esteban A, Frutos F, Tobin MJ, et al. A comparison of four methods of weaning patients from mechanical ventilation. N Engl J Med 1995;332:345–50.

149. Meade M, Guyatt G, Sinuff T, et al. Trials comparing alternative weaning modes and discontinuation assessments. Chest 2001:120:425S–37.

150. Esteban A, Alia I, Gordo F, et al. Extubation outcome after spontaneous breathing trials with T-tube or pressure support ventilation. Am J Respir Crit Care Med 1997;156:459–65.

151. Brochard L, Rauss A, Benito S, et al. Comparison of three methods of gradual withdrawal from ventilatory support during weaning from mechanical ventilation. Am J Respir Crit Care Med 1994;150:896–903.

152. Marelich GP, Murin S, Battistella F, Inciardi J, Vierra T, Roby M. Protocol weaning of mechanical ventilation in medical and surgical patients by respiratory care practitioners and nurses. Effect on weaning time and incidence of ventilation-associated pneumonia. Chest 2000;118:459–67.

153. Meade M, Guyatt G, Cook D, et al. Predicting success in weaning from mechanical ventilation. Chest 2001;120:400S–24.

154. Yang KL, Tobin MJ. A prospective study of indexes predicting the outcome of trials of weaning from mechanical ventilation. N Engl J Med 1991;324:1445–50.

155. Lee KH, Hui KP, Chan TB, Tan WC, Lim TK. Rapid shallow breathing (frequency-tidal volume ratio) did not predict extubation outcome. Chest 1994;105:540–3.

156. Kollef MH, Levy NT, Ahrens TS, Schaiff R, Prentice D, Sherman G. The use of continuous IV sedation is associated with prolongation of mechanical ventilation. Chest 1998;114:541–8.

157. Schweickert WD, Gehlbach BK, Pohlman AS, Hall JB, Kress JP. Daily interruption of sedative medications and complications of critical illness in mechanically ventilated patients. Crit Care Med 2004;32:1272–6.

158. Meade MO, Guyatt G, Cook DJ, Sinuff T, Butler R. Trials of corticosteroids to prevent postextubation airway complications. Chest 2001;120:464S–8.

159. Sassoon CSH, Giron AE, Ely EA, Light RW. Inspiratory work of breathing in flow-by and demand-flow continuous positive airway pressure. Crit Care Med 1989;17:1108–14.

160. Banner MJ, Kirby RR, MacIntyre NR. Patient and ventilator work of breathing and ventilatory muscle loads at different levels of pressure support ventilation. Chest 1991;100:531–3.

161. Brochard L, Harf A, Lorino H, Lemaire F. Inspiratory pressure support prevents diaphragmatic fatigue during weaning from mechanical ventilation. Am Rev Respir Dis 1989;139:513–21.

162. Light RW, Rogers JT, Moyers JP, et al. Prevalence and clinical course of pleural effusions at 30 days after coronary artery and cardiac surgery. Am J Respir Crit Care Med 2002;166:1567–71.

163. Payne M, Magovern GJ Jr, Benckart DH, et al. Left pleural effusion after coronary artery bypass decreases with a supplemental pleural drain. Ann Thorac Surg 2002;73;149–52.

164. Ricci M, Salerno TA, D'Ancona G, Bergsland J, Karamanoukian HL. A peril of minimally invasive surgery. J Card Surg 1999;14:482–3.

165. Ali IM, Lau P, Kinley CE, Sanalla A. Opening the pleura during internal mammary artery harvesting: advantages and disadvantages. Can J Surg 1996;39:42–5.

166. Sadaniantz A, Anastacio R, Verma V, Aprahamian N. The incidence of diastolic right atrial collapse in patients with pleural effusion in the absence of pericardial effusion. Echocardiography 2003;20:211–5.

167. Traylor JJ, Chan K, Wong I, Roxas JN, Chandraratna PA. Large pleural effusions producing signs of cardiac tamponade resolved by thoracentesis. Am J Cardiol 2002;89:106–8.

168. Alam HB, Levitt A, Molyneaux R, Davidson P, Sample GA. Can pleural effusions cause cardiac tamponade? Chest 1999;116:1820–2.

169. Kaplan LM, Epstein SK, Schwartz SL, Cao QL, Pandian NG. Clinical, echocardiographic, and hemodynamic evidence of cardiac tamponade caused by large pleural effusions. Am J Respir Crit Care Med 1995;151:904–8.

170. The COMBIVENT Inhalation Solution Study Group. Routine nebulized ipratropium and albuterol together are better than either alone in COPD. Chest 1997;112:1514–21.

171. Stoller JK. Acute exacerbations of chronic obstructive pulmonary disease. N Engl J Med 2002;346:988–94.

172. Saymer A, Aytemur ZA, Cirit M, Unsal I. Systemic glucocorticoids in severe exacerbations of COPD. Chest 2001;119:726–30.

173. Niewoehner DE, Erbland ML, Deupree RH, et al. Effect of systemic glucocorticoids on exacerbations of chronic obstructive pulmonary disease. N Engl J Med 1999;340:1941–7.

174. McCrory DC, Brown C, Gelfand SE, Bach PB. Management of acute exacerbations of COPD. A summary and appraisal of published evidence. Chest 2001;119:1190–1209.

175. Gold MR, Dec GW, Cocca-Spofford D, Thompson BT. Esmolol and ventilatory function in cardiac patients with COPD. Chest 1991;100:1215–8.

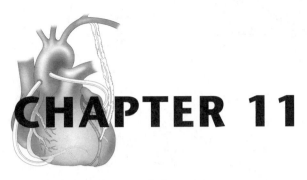

Cardiovascular Management

Cardiovascular Management

The achievement of satisfactory hemodynamic performance is the primary objective of postoperative cardiac surgical management. Optimal cardiac function ensures adequate perfusion and oxygenation of other organ systems and improves the chances for an uneventful recovery from surgery. Even brief periods of cardiac dysfunction can result in impairment of organ system function, leading to potentially life-threatening complications. This chapter presents the basic concepts in cardiovascular management and then reviews the evaluation and management of the low cardiac output syndrome, hypertension, and rhythm disturbances that can contribute to compromised cardiovascular function.

I. Basic Principles

The important concepts of postoperative cardiac care are those of cardiac output, tissue oxygenation, and the ratio of myocardial oxygen supply and demand. Ideally, one should strive to obtain a cardiac index greater than 2.2 L/min/m² with a normal mixed venous oxygen saturation while optimizing the oxygen supply/demand ratio.

A. **Cardiac output** is determined by the stroke volume and heart rate ($CO = SV \times HR$). The stroke volume is equal to the left ventricular end-diastolic volume (LVEDV) minus the left ventricular end-systolic volume (LVESV) and is calculated by dividing the cardiac output by the heart rate. The three major determinants of stroke volume are preload, afterload, and contractility.

1. **Preload** refers to the LV end-diastolic fiber length or end-diastolic volume. This can be estimated most precisely by two-dimensional echocardiography, which provides real-time imaging of ventricular dimensions and function during the cardiac cycle. However, the status of LV volume is more commonly assessed by a measurement of left-sided filling pressures. These include the pulmonary artery diastolic (PAD) pressure and pulmonary capillary wedge pressure (PCWP), which can be measured with a Swan-Ganz or pulmonary artery (PA) catheter, and the left atrial pressure (LAP), which is measured from a line placed directly into the left atrium. The relationship between filling pressures and volumes is determined by ventricular compliance.

a. Generally, the closer the site of assessment to the left ventricle, the closer the correlation to the LVEDP. Thus, the correlation is best for LAP > PCWP > PAD pressure. The PAD pressure generally correlates with the PCWP, but is frequently higher in patients with preexisting pulmonary hypertension or intrinsic pulmonary disease. In these patients, there is an increased transpulmonary gradient (equal to the PA mean pressure minus the PCWP). Thus, in these situations, the PAD may significantly overestimate the true LV volume.

b. Filling pressures must be interpreted cautiously in the early postoperative period.[1,2] The PAD and PCW pressures often correlate poorly with the LVEDV early after surgery because of altered ventricular compliance from myocardial edema resulting from cardiopulmonary bypass (CPB) and the use of cardioplegia solutions. Furthermore, the release of various inflammatory substances during bypass and the administration of blood products may increase the pulmonary vascular resistance (PVR).

   c. The patient with a stiff, hypertrophied left ventricle from hypertension or aortic stenosis may require high filling pressures to achieve adequate ventricular filling. In contrast, the dilated, volume-overloaded heart may be highly compliant, with an elevated LVEDV at lower pressures.

   d. For patients with relatively normal ventricular function, many centers do not use Swan-Ganz catheters and rely on central venous pressure (CVP) measurements to assess preload. Although this is an inaccurate means of assessing preload in the diseased heart, it gives a fairly good approximation of left heart filling in the normal heart.[3,4] Generally, if the CVP exceeds 15–18 mm Hg, inotropic support is indicated. If the patient has other signs of low cardiac output (poor oxygenation, tapering urine output, acidosis), insertion of a Swan-Ganz catheter will allow for a more objective evaluation of the problem.

2. **Afterload** refers to the LV wall tension during systole. It is determined by both the preload (Laplace's law relating radius to wall tension) and the systemic vascular resistance (SVR) against which the heart must eject after the period of isovolumic contraction. The SVR can be calculated from measurements obtained from the Swan-Ganz catheter (Table 11.1). It should be kept in mind that the equation to calculate SVR is based on the cardiac output, not the cardiac index. Thus, it will be higher in the smaller patient at a comparable cardiac index. The use of vasodilators to lower the SVR may improve the stroke volume, often in combination with volume infusions and inotropic agents.

3. **Contractility** is the intrinsic strength of myocardial contraction at constant preload and afterload. However, it can be improved by increasing the preload or heart rate, decreasing the afterload, or using inotropic medications.[5] Contractility is generally assessed by the ejection fraction and is best determined by echocardiography. However, the heart's inotropic state is usually inferred from an analysis of the cardiac output and filling pressures.

   a. In cardiac surgery patients, the cardiac output is usually obtained by thermodilution technology using a Swan-Ganz catheter and bedside computer. A measured aliquot of volume is infused into the CVP port of the catheter, and the thermistor near the tip measures the pattern of temperature change from which the computer calculates the cardiac output. A continuous cardiac output catheter is frequently used during off-pump surgery and can provide frequent on-line assessments of the cardiac output.[6]

   b. Alternative means of measuring cardiac output are the esophageal Doppler, thoracic bioimpedance, and pulse contour analysis.[7-13] The esophageal Doppler provides Doppler flow velocity waveforms that include flow time and peak velocity. These allow for assessment of left ventricular contractility, filling, and systemic vascular resistance (Figure 7.2). Bioimpedance measures the resistivity of the body to an electrical current. Since this current is distributed primarily in the blood and extracellular fluid, the change in body resistivity over time is related to the dynamic changes of the blood which correlates with the stroke volume.[11] The pulseCO device is a system that calculates the cardiac output from the energy of the arterial pressure waveform.[12,13] The arterial blood passes through a lithium sensor and an algorithm calculates the stroke volume and

Table 11.1 • Hemodynamic Formulas

Formula	Normal Values
Cardiac output (CO) and index (CI)	
CO = SV × HR	4–8 L/min
CI = CO/BSA	2.2–4.0 L/min/m^2
Stroke volume (SV)	
$SV = \dfrac{CO\ (L/min) \times 1000\ (mL/L)}{HR}$	60–100 mL/beat (1 mL/kg/beat)
Stroke volume index (SVI)	
SVI = SV/BSA	33–47 mL/beat/m^2
Mean arterial pressure (MAP)	
$MAP = DP + \dfrac{(SP - DP)}{3}$	70–100 mm Hg
Systemic vascular resistance (SVR)	
$SVR = \dfrac{MAP - CVP}{CO} \times 80$	800–1200 dynes-s/cm^5
Pulmonary vascular resistance (PVR)	
$PVR = \dfrac{PAP - PCWP}{CO} \times 80$	50–250 dynes-sec/cm^5
Left ventricular stroke work index (LVSWI)	
LVSWI = SVI × (MAP − PCWP) × 0.0136	45–75 mg-M/beat/m^2

BSA = body surface area; HR = heart rate; DP = diastolic pressure; SP = systolic pressure; CVP = central venous pressure; PAP = mean pulmonary arterial pressure; PCWP = pulmonary capillary wedge pressure.

cardiac output. All of these technologies provide comparable cardiac output measurements to those obtained by thermodilution with the Swan-Ganz catheter.

4. The presence of a low cardiac output does not necessarily imply that ventricular function is impaired. It may be noted with slow heart rates, hypovolemia, and with a small, stiff ventricular chamber. In contrast, a satisfactory cardiac output may accompany significant ventricular dysfunction when the left ventricle is dilated, especially if a significant tachycardia is present. Thus, management of a low cardiac output state must take into account all of the factors mentioned above to determine the appropriate treatment.

B. Tissue oxygenation

1. Oxygen transport to tissues is the basic principle on which hemodynamic support should be based. It is determined by the cardiac output, the hemoglobin (Hb) level, and the arterial oxygen saturation (SaO_2). This is represented by the equation:

$$O_2 \text{ delivery} = CO \text{ (Hb} \times \% \text{ sat)}(1.39) + (PaO_2)(0.0031)$$

where 1.39 is milliliters of oxygen transported per gram of Hb and 0.0031 is the solubility coefficient of oxygen dissolved in solution (mL/torr of PaO_2).

2. It should be noted in this equation that the majority of oxygen transported to the tissues is in the form of oxygen bound to Hb, not that dissolved in solution. Thus, one of the major factors lowering O_2 delivery in the postoperative period is a low hematocrit. Increasing the Hb level by 1 g/dL can increase blood oxygen content by 1.39 vol%, whereas an increase in PaO_2 of 100 torr will only transport an additional 0.3 vol% of oxygen.

3. Studies have suggested that the safe lower limit for hematocrit in the early postoperative period to maintain adequate tissue oxygenation in the stable, elective patient is probably around 22–24%.[14-16] Since this may reduce tissue oxygen delivery to less than 60% of normal, it is imperative that arterial oxygen saturation be close to 100% and cardiac output be optimized to achieve adequate O_2 delivery. Once an arterial saturation of 95–100% has been achieved, there is little additional benefit of maintaining a high FiO_2 and PaO_2.

4. The threshold for administering blood transfusions has increased with the understanding that patients may fare better postoperatively with hematocrits under 30%.[17] Furthermore, the morbidity associated with blood transfusions has also become more apparent. Transfusions contain proinflammatory cytokines, low levels of 2,3-diphosphoglycerate (2,3-DPG) with increased Hb affinity for oxygen, and are associated with an increased risk of respiratory complications, wound infections, and mortality.[18-20] Despite these issues as well as the lingering concern about the transmission of HIV and hepatitis viruses, it is fairly universal practice to transfuse patients to a hematocrit over 25% when they are elderly, frail, have poor ventricular function, borderline respiratory function, hypotension, tachycardia, or ischemic ECG changes.

5. **Mixed venous oxygen saturation** (SvO_2) can be used to assess the adequacy of tissue perfusion and oxygenation. PA catheters using reflective fiberoptic oximetry are available to monitor the SvO_2 in the PA on a continuous basis and are commonly used during off-pump surgery to provide early signs of hemodynamic deterioration. Intermittent SvO_2 measurements can be measured from blood samples obtained from the distal PA port of the Swan-Ganz catheter. A change of 10% in the SvO_2 can occur before any change is noted in hemodynamic parameters. Despite its theoretical benefit, several studies have suggested that SvO_2 is an unreliable and insensitive predictor of the cardiac output. However, when analyzed in conjunction with other hemodynamic parameters, following trends in the SvO_2 does offer insight into cardiac performance and tissue oxygen delivery.[21,22]

   a. In the postoperative cardiac surgical patient, a fall in SvO_2 generally reflects decreased oxygen delivery or increased oxygen extraction by tissues and is suggestive of a reduction in cardiac output. However, other constantly changing factors that affect oxygen supply and demand may also influence SvO_2 and must be taken into consideration. These include shivering, temperature, anemia, alteration in F_{IO_2}, and the efficiency of alveolar gas exchange. The Fick equation, which uses the arteriovenous oxygen content difference to determine cardiac output, can be rearranged as follows:

$$Svo_2 = Sao_2 - \frac{\dot{V}O_2}{Hb \times 1.39 \times CO} \times 10$$

where:

Svo_2 = mixed venous oxygen saturation

Sao_2 = arterial oxygen saturation

$\dot{V}O_2$ = oxygen consumption

normal Pvo_2 = 40 torr and Svo_2 = 75%

normal Pao_2 = 100 torr and Sao_2 = 99%

   b. This equation indicates that a decrease in Svo_2 may result from a decrease in Sao_2, cardiac output, or Hb level, or an increase in oxygen consumption.

   c. When the arterial O_2 saturation is normal ($Sao_2 > 95\%$), a $Pvo_2 < 30$ torr or an $Svo_2 < 60$–65% suggests the presence of a decreased cardiac output and the need for further assessment and therapeutic intervention. Conversely, a rise in Svo_2 reflects less oxygen extraction as seen during hypothermia, sepsis, or intracardiac or significant peripheral arteriovenous shunting. When an elevated Svo_2 is noted, oxygen delivery or utilization may be impaired and an otherwise "normal" cardiac output may be insufficient to provide adequate tissue oxygenation.

   6. When the cardiac index exceeds 2.2 L/min/m² and the arterial oxygen saturation is adequate ($> 95\%$), it may be inferred that oxygen delivery to the tissues is satisfactory. Thus, Svo_2 measurements to assess oxygen delivery are not necessary. However, there are a few situations when calculation of tissue oxygenation may be valuable in assessing cardiac function.

   a. The thermodilution cardiac output is unreliable (tricuspid regurgitation, improperly positioned Swan-Ganz catheter) or not available (Swan-Ganz catheter has not been placed or cannot be placed, such as in the patient with a mechanical tricuspid valve or central venous thrombosis).[23]

   b. The thermodilution cardiac output may seem spuriously low and inconsistent with the clinical scenario (malfunctioning Swan-Ganz catheter or incorrect calibration of computer). A normal Svo_2 indicates that the cardiac output is sufficient to meet tissue metabolic demands.

   c. The patient has a marginal cardiac output and online assessment of trends in the mixed venous oxygen saturation can provide up-to-date information on the relative status of cardiac function.

C. Myocardial oxygen supply and demand

   1. Myocardial O_2 demand (mvO_2) is influenced by factors similar to those that determine the cardiac output (afterload, preload, heart rate, and contractility). Reducing afterload will generally improve cardiac output with a decrease in mvO_2, whereas an increase in any of the other three factors will improve cardiac output at the expense of an increase in mvO_2. *Preoperative* management of the patient with ischemic heart disease is primarily directed towards minimizing O_2 demand.[24]

2. **Myocardial O_2 supply** is determined by coronary blood flow (which may be influenced by stenosis, thrombus, or spasm in a native vessel or bypass graft), the duration of diastole, the coronary perfusion pressure, the Hb level, and the arterial oxygen saturation. When complete revascularization has been achieved, *postoperative* management is directed towards optimizing factors that improve O_2 supply and, to a lesser degree, minimize any increase in O_2 demand.

   a. A heart rate of 80–90/min should be achieved, and excessive tachycardia and arrhythmias must be avoided.

   b. An adequate perfusion pressure (mean pressure 80–90 mm Hg) should be maintained, taking care to avoid both hypotension and hypertension.

   c. Ventricular distention and wall stress (afterload) should be minimized by avoiding excessive preload, reducing the SVR, and using inotropic medications to improve contractility.

   d. The hematocrit should be maintained at a safe level. Although an increased level of Hb always improves oxygen delivery, transfusions carry inherent risks and their risks and benefits must be weighed. In general, myocardial ischemia should not occur in the well-protected, revascularized heart unless the hematocrit drops to the low 20s.[14–16]

II. Low Cardiac Output Syndrome

A. General comments

1. The achievement of a satisfactory cardiac output is the primary objective of postoperative cardiovascular management. Hemodynamic norms for the patient recovering uneventfully from cardiac surgery are a cardiac index greater than 2.2 L/min/m², a PCWP or PAD pressure below 20 mm Hg, and a heart rate below 100/min. The patient should have warm, well-perfused extremities with an excellent urine output.[25]

2. Low cardiac output states are more common in patients with compromised LV systolic or diastolic function (low ejection fraction, cardiomegaly, elevated LVEDP), longer durations of cardiopulmonary bypass, and in women.[26,27] Increased lactate release after 5 minutes of reperfusion is more common in these patients and is an independent predictor of a low cardiac output. It suggests that there is delayed recovery of aerobic metabolism, perhaps as a result of inadequate myocardial protection.[28]

3. Myocardial function generally declines for about 6–8 hours following surgery, presumably from ischemic/reperfusion injury with use of cardioplegic arrest, before returning to baseline within 24 hours.[29] Temporary inotropic support is often required during this period to optimize hemodynamic performance. Drugs used to provide support at the conclusion of CPB should generally be continued for this brief period of time and can be weaned once the cardiac output is satisfactory.

4. When marginal ventricular function is present, compensatory mechanisms include sympathetic autonomic stimulation and endogenous catecholamine production. These increase heart rate, contractility, and arterial and venous tone, elevating both preload and afterload. All of these factors may improve cardiac output or systemic blood pressure, but they may also increase myocardial oxygen demand at a time when asymptomatic ischemia is commonly present.[30]

5. When compensatory mechanisms are exhausted, the advanced clinical manifestations of the low cardiac output syndrome will be noted. These include:

   a. Poor peripheral perfusion with pale, cool extremities and diaphoresis
   b. Pulmonary congestion and poor oxygenation
   c. Impaired renal perfusion and oliguria
   d. Metabolic acidosis

6. The use of invasive monitoring to continuously evaluate a patient's hemodynamic status allows for appropriate therapeutic interventions to be undertaken before these advanced clinical signs become apparent. Nonetheless, subtle findings, such as a progressive tachycardia or cool extremities, should alert the astute clinician to the fact that the patient needs more intensive management. Intervention is indicated for a low cardiac output state, defined as a cardiac index below 2.0 L/min/m², usually associated with left-sided filling pressures exceeding 20 mm Hg and an SVR exceeding 1500 dyne-s/cm⁵. It cannot be overemphasized that observing trends in hemodynamic parameters, rather than absolute numbers, is important when evaluating a patient's progress or deterioration.

7. A general scheme for the management of postoperative hemodynamic problems is presented in Table 11.2.

B. **Etiology.** A low cardiac output state may result from abnormal preload, contractility, heart rate, or afterload. It may also be noted in patients with satisfactory systolic function but marked left ventricular hypertrophy (LVH) and diastolic dysfunction.[31]

   1. Decreased LV preload

      a. Hypovolemia (bleeding, vasodilatation from warming, vasodilators, narcotics, or sedatives)
      b. Cardiac tamponade

Table 11.2 • Management of Hemodynamic Problems

BP	PCW	CO	SVR	Plan
↓	↓	↓	↓	Volume
N	↑	N	↑	Venodilator or diuretic
↓	↑	↓	↑	Inotrope
↑	↑	↓	↑	Vasodilator
↑↓	↑	↓	↑	Inotrope/vasodilator/IABP
↓	N	N↑	↓	α-agent

↑ = increased; ↓ = decreased; N = normal; ↑↓ = variable.

    c. Positive-pressure ventilation and PEEP

    d. Right ventricular (RV) dysfunction (RV infarction, pulmonary hypertension)

    e. Tension pneumothorax

  2. Decreased contractility

    a. Low ejection fraction

    b. Myocardial "stunning" from transient ischemic/reperfusion injury, myocardial ischemia or infarction

        i. Poor intraoperative myocardial protection

        ii. Incomplete myocardial revascularization

        iii. Evolving infarction at time of surgery

        iv. Native coronary artery or graft spasm

    c. Hypoxia, hypercarbia, acidosis

  3. Tachy- and bradyarrhythmias

    a. Tachycardia with reduced cardiac filling time

    b. Bradycardia

    c. Atrial arrhythmias with loss of atrial contraction

    d. Ventricular arrhythmias

  4. Increased afterload

    a. Vasoconstriction

    b. Fluid overload and ventricular distention

    c. LV outflow tract obstruction following mitral valve repair or replacement (from struts or retained leaflet tissue)

  5. Diastolic dysfunction with impaired relaxation and high filling pressures

  6. Syndromes associated with cardiovascular instability and hypotension

    a. Sepsis (hypotension from a reduction in SVR; hyperdynamic with a high cardiac output early and myocardial depression at a later stage)

    b. Anaphylactic reactions (blood products, drugs)

    c. Adrenal insufficiency (primary or in the patient on preoperative steroids)

    d. Protamine reactions

C. Assessment (concerns noted in parentheses)

  1. Bedside physical examination (breath sounds, murmurs, warmth of extremities, peripheral pulses)

  2. Hemodynamic measurements: assess filling pressures and determine cardiac output with a Swan-Ganz PA catheter; calculate SVR; measure Svo_2 (low cardiac output, high filling pressures, high SVR, low Svo_2)

  3. Arterial blood gases (hypoxia, hypercarbia, acidosis/alkalosis), hematocrit (anemia), and serum potassium (hypo- or hyperkalemia)

  4. Electrocardiogram (ischemia, arrhythmias, conduction abnormalities)

  5. Chest x-ray (pneumothorax, hemothorax, position of endotracheal tube or intraaortic balloon)

  6. Urinary output (oliguria)

  7. Chest tube drainage (mediastinal bleeding)

  8. Two-dimensional echocardiography is very helpful when the cause of a low cardiac output syndrome is difficult to determine. Along with hemodynamic measurements, it can help identify whether it is related to LV systolic or diastolic

---

Box 11.1 • Management of Low Cardiac Output Syndrome

1. Look for noncardiac correctable causes (respiratory, acid-base, electrolyte)
2. Treat ischemia or coronary spasm
3. Optimize preload (PCWP or LA pressure of 18–20 mm Hg)
4. Optimize heart rate at 90–100/min with pacing
5. Control arrhythmias
6. Assess cardiac output and start inotrope if cardiac index is less than 2.0 L/min/m²
   * Epinephrine unless arrhythmias or tachycardia
   * Dopamine (if low SVR) or dobutamine (if high SVR)
   * Inamrinone/milrinone
   * Insert IABP
   * Nesiritide if low cardiac index and high filling pressures
7. Calculate SVR and start vasodilator if SVR over 1500
   * Nitroprusside if high filling pressures, SVR, and blood pressure
   * Nitroglycerin if high filling pressures or evidence of coronary ischemia or spasm
8. If blood pressure is low with a low SVR:
   * Norepinephrine if marginal cardiac output
   * Phenylephrine if satisfactory cardiac output
   * Vasopressin if refractory to the above
9. Give blood transfusion if hematocrit is less than 26%

---

dysfunction, RV systolic dysfunction, or cardiac tamponade. **Transesophageal echocardiography (TEE)** provides better and more complete information than a transthoracic study and can be readily performed in the intubated patient. It should always be considered when the clinical picture is consistent with tamponade but a transthoracic study is inconclusive.[32]

D. **Treatment** (Box 11.1)[25]

1. Ensure satisfactory **oxygenation** and **ventilation** (see Chapter 10).

2. Treat **ischemia** or **coronary spasm** if suspected. Myocardial ischemia often responds to intravenous nitroglycerin (IV NTG) but may require further investigation if it persists. Coronary spasm (see page 407) can be difficult to diagnose but usually responds to IV NTG and/or a calcium channel blocker, such as sublingual nifedipine or IV diltiazem.

3. Optimize **preload** by raising filling pressures with volume infusion to a PCWP or PAD pressure of about 18–20 mm Hg. This may be all that is necessary to achieve a satisfactory cardiac output. Volume infusion is preferable to atrial pacing for improving cardiac output because it places less metabolic demand on the recovering myocardium.[33]

   a. The ideal left-sided filling pressures can be determined from a review of pre- and intraoperative hemodynamic data and an understanding of the patient's cardiac pathophysiology. Data obtained before the induction of anesthesia tend to be misleading (all values tend to be elevated), as can data after the patient is anesthetized due to alterations in loading conditions and autonomic tone. Direct visual inspection of the heart, TEE, and measurement of cardiac outputs at the termination of CPB will usually indicate the appropriate filling pressures for optimal ventricular filling and cardiac performance.

b. For example, a PCWP around 15–18 mm Hg is usually best for patients with preserved LV function. In contrast, a PCWP in the low 20s may be necessary to achieve adequate preload in patients with poor LV function, a stiff hypertrophied ventricle with diastolic dysfunction, a small LV chamber (mitral stenosis or after resection of an LV aneurysm), or preexisting pulmonary hypertension from mitral valve disease. Ventricular size and compliance should be kept in mind when deciding whether additional volume is the next appropriate step in the patient with marginal cardiac function.

c. The response to volume infusion may be variable. Failure of filling pressures to rise with volume may result from the capillary leak that is present during the early postoperative period. It may also result from vasodilatation associated with rewarming or the use of medications with vasodilator properties, such as propofol or narcotics. However, it may also reflect the beneficial attenuation of peripheral vasoconstriction that is attributable to an improvement in cardiac output caused by the volume infusion. As the SVR and afterload gradually decrease, the cardiac output may improve further without an increase in preload.

d. A rise in filling pressures without improvement in cardiac output may adversely affect myocardial performance as well as the function of other organ systems. At this point, inotropic support is usually necessary. Thus, careful observation of the response to volume infusion is imperative.

    i. Excessive preload increases LV wall tension and may exacerbate ischemia by increasing myocardial oxygen demand and decreasing the transmyocardial gradient (aortic diastolic pressure minus LV diastolic pressure) for coronary blood flow. It may also impair myocardial contractility.

    ii. Excessive preload may lead to interstitial edema of the lungs, resulting in increased extravascular lung water, ventilation/perfusion abnormalities, and hypoxemia.

    iii. Excessive preload in the patient with RV dysfunction may impair myocardial blood flow to the right ventricle resulting in progressive ischemia. A distended right ventricle may contribute to LV dysfunction because of overdistention and septal shift that impairs LV distensibility and filling.

    iv. The presence of RV or biventricular dysfunction may also cause systemic venous hypertension, which may reduce perfusion pressure to other organ systems. This may affect the kidneys (causing oliguria), the gastrointestinal (GI) tract (splanchnic congestion, jaundice, ileus), or the brain (contributing to altered mental status).

    v. Thus, the temptation must be resisted to administer additional volume to the failing heart with high filling pressures. **Excessive preload *must* be avoided because it may lead to deterioration, rather than improvement, in ventricular function.**

4. Stabilize the **heart rate and rhythm.** All attempts should be made to achieve atrioventricular (AV) synchrony with a heart rate of 90–100/min. This may require atrial (AOO or AAI) or AV (DDD or DVI) pacing. These modalities take advantage of the 20–30% improvement in cardiac output provided by atrial contraction that will not be achieved with ventricular pacing alone. This is especially important in the hypertrophied ventricle. Antiarrhythmic drugs should be used as necessary to control ventricular ectopy or slow the response to atrial fibrillation (AF).

5. **Improve contractility** with inotropic agents. This should be based on an understanding of the α, β, or nonadrenergic hemodynamic effects of vasoactive medications and their anticipated influence on preload, afterload, heart rate, and contractility. These medications and a strategy for their selection are noted on pages 358–371.

    a. The use of inotropic agents in the early postoperative period may seem paradoxical in that augmented cardiac output is being achieved at the expense of an increase in oxygen demand (e.g., increased heart rate and contractility). However, the *major* determinant of oxygen demand is the pressure work that the left ventricle must perform. This is reflected by the afterload, which is determined by preload and SVR. Inotropic drugs that are used to increase contractility do not necessarily increase oxygen demand in the failing heart because they reduce preload, afterload, and frequently the heart rate as a result of improved cardiac function.

    b. If the cardiac output remains low, physiologic support with an **intraaortic balloon pump (IABP)** should be strongly considered. If the patient cannot be weaned from bypass or has hemodynamic evidence of severe ventricular dysfunction despite maximal medical therapy and the IABP, use of **a circulatory assist device** should be considered. This is discussed on pages 377–389.

6. **Reduce afterload** with vasodilators if the cardiac output is marginal while carefully monitoring systemic blood pressure to avoid hypotension (see page 389). Vasodilators must be used cautiously when the cardiac index is very poor because an elevated SVR from intense vasoconstriction is often a compensatory mechanism in low cardiac output states to maintain central perfusion. If the calculated SVR exceeds 1500, vasodilators may be indicated either alone or in combination with inotropic medications.

7. It is essential to integrate all hemodynamic parameters when concluding that a patient is or is not doing well. For example, the blood pressure may be high when the heart is not performing well, the cardiac output may be acceptable when the heart is struggling, and the cardiac output can be low even when ventricular function is normal.

    a. The presence of a satisfactory or elevated blood pressure is not necessarily a sign of good cardiac performance. Blood pressure (BP) is related directly to the cardiac output and the SVR (BP = CO × SVR). In the early postoperative period, myocardial function may be marginal despite normal or elevated blood pressure because of an elevated SVR resulting from augmented sympathetic tone and peripheral vasoconstriction. Vasodilators can be used to reduce afterload in the presence of elevated filling pressures, thus reducing myocardial ischemia and improving myocardial function. However, **withdrawal of inotropic support in the hypertensive patient should be considered**

only after a satisfactory cardiac output has been documented. Otherwise, acute deterioration may ensue.

b. One should not be deceived into concluding that myocardial function is satisfactory when the cardiac output is "adequate" but is being maintained by fast heart rates at low stroke volumes.

   i. Tachycardia is often an ominous sign of acute myocardial ischemia or infarction, and it may render the borderline heart ischemic. The stroke volume index (SVI) is an excellent method of assessing myocardial function because it assesses how much blood the heart is pumping each beat. Unless the patient is hypovolemic, a low SVI (less than 30 mL/beat/m²) indicates poor myocardial function for which inotropic support is usually indicated. Although β-blockers would theoretically be beneficial to control tachycardia in the injured or ischemic heart, they are poorly tolerated in the presence of LV dysfunction and must be avoided.

   ii. Sinus tachycardia may represent a beneficial compensatory mechanism for a small stroke volume in patients with a small LV chamber (following LV aneurysm resection or mitral valve replacement for mitral stenosis). In these situations, an attempt to slow the heart rate pharmacologically may compromise the cardiac output significantly. Not infrequently, sinus tachycardia is a means of compensating for hypovolemia and quickly resolves after fluid administration.

   iii. Tachycardia may also be present in patients with marked LVH and diastolic dysfunction, especially after aortic valve replacement for aortic stenosis. In these situations, the cardiac output may be low despite preserved ventricular function because of a small noncompliant LV chamber. β-blockers or calcium channel blockers can be used to slow the heart rate after adequate volume replacement has been achieved, but they must be used with extreme caution. Use of a medication with lusitropic (relaxant) properties, such as inamrinone/milrinone or nesiritide, may be helpful.

   iv. Tachycardia accompanying a large stroke volume is often seen in young patients with preserved ventricular function. It can be managed safely with a β-blocker, such as esmolol.

c. The cardiac output may be marginal when the patient is hypovolemic (even if LV function is normal) and does not develop a compensatory tachycardia. This is noted in patients who were well β-blocked prior to surgery and in those who require pacing at the conclusion of the operation. Pacing up to a rate of 90/min and a moderate volume infusion are invariably successful in improving the cardiac output in this situation. If the cardiac output is not acceptable once the filling pressures are satisfactory, an inotrope should be added. The common temptation to continue to administer fluid once the filling pressures are elevated may be more harmful than helpful to the struggling heart.

8. **Maintain blood pressure**

a. If the patient has **a satisfactory cardiac output but a low systemic resistance and low blood pressure**, the filling pressures are often low and a moderate volume infusion may improve the blood pressure. This scenario is common in sedated patients receiving medications that have potent vasodilator properties. It is also common in patients who had been taking certain medications preoperatively, such as the angiotensin-converting enzyme (ACE) inhibitors (which block the renin-angiotensin system), calcium channel blockers, angiotensin receptor blockers, and amiodarone (which blocks sympathetic stimulation by α and β blockade).

   i. If hypotension persists, an α-agent should be used to increase the SVR. Norepinephrine is the preferred drug when the cardiac output is marginal because it has β-agonist properties, whereas phenylephrine is a pure α-agonist and is best used if the cardiac output is satisfactory. Although one study showed that norepinephrine had little adverse effect on renal function, most studies suggest that it produces some degree of renal vasoconstriction.[34,35] Some patients respond better to norepinephrine than phenylephrine, and others just the reverse.

   ii. When refractory hypotension persists despite a satisfactory cardiac output and use of phenylephrine or norepinephrine, it may represent a condition of autonomic failure termed "vasoplegia." This may be a consequence of the systemic inflammatory response and may be related to nitric oxide (NO)–induced vasodilatation. It has been shown that levels of vasopressin are low in most normotensive patients after bypass but are inappropriately low in patients with vasodilatory "shock." **Arginine vasopressin** acts on vasomotor V1 and renal V2 receptors and, given in a dosage of 0.1–0.4 U/min, can restore blood pressure in these patients. Such low dosages may suffice because patients with vasodilatory shock tend to be hypersensitive to its effects. It also improves renal perfusion in that it constricts the efferent rather than the afferent arterioles, in contradistinction to the effects of α-agents on renal perfusion.[36–39]

   iii. An alternative to the use of vasopressin is **methylene blue** 1.5 mg/kg, which inhibits guanylate cyclase elicited by nitric oxide. It has been reported to be beneficial in reducing morbidity and mortality in patients with postbypass vasoplegia.[40,41]

   b. **If the blood pressure and the cardiac output remain low** after adequate filling pressures are restored, inotropic support should be initiated, anticipating a rise in systemic blood pressure. If this does not occur, an IABP may be required to improve the cardiac output. Frequently, an α-agent must also be added, and norepinephrine is preferable because it provides some β effects. Sometimes, use of an α-agent to improve coronary perfusion pressure leads to an improvement in cardiac output. Vasopressin is best avoided when the cardiac output is marginal because it may compromise splanchnic blood flow more than norepinephrine due to the fact that it is a pure vasoconstrictor with no inotropic properties.[42]

9. Correct **anemia** with blood transfusions. The hematocrit is usually maintained above 24% in the postoperative period, but transfusions should be considered for hemodynamic instability or evidence of myocardial ischemia.

E. **Right ventricular failure and pulmonary hypertension**

   1. A low cardiac output state may be the result of RV failure, producing inadequate filling of the left heart. Patients may be predisposed to RV dysfunction because of preexisting conditions, such as:

      a. Right coronary artery (RCA) disease or severe coronary disease in a left-dominant circulation.

    b. RV infarction secondary to a proximal RCA occlusion.

    c. Pulmonary hypertension associated with mitral/aortic disease or severe LV dysfunction in patients undergoing heart transplantation. In the latter patients, the donor heart may not be able to acutely adapt to long-standing pulmonary hypertension, especially if undersized with a prolonged ischemic time, and RV failure will ensue.

2. However, RV systolic dysfunction may also occur in patients with no known preexisting RV problems. It may be attributable to:

    a. Poor myocardial protection, usually due to poor collateral circulation with an occluded RCA or due to exclusive use of retrograde cardioplegia

    b. Prolonged ischemic times/myocardial stunning

    c. Inadvertent RCA distribution ischemia (kinking of the RCA in aortic root replacements)

    d. Coronary embolism of air (usually in valve operations), thrombi, or particulate matter (in reoperative coronary artery bypass grafting [CABG] or valve operations)

    e. Systemic hypotension and RV hypoperfusion

    f. Acute pulmonary hypertension (increased PVR and RV afterload) from:
- Vasoactive substances associated with blood product transfusions and CPB
- Severe LV dysfunction
- Protamine reaction ("catastrophic pulmonary vasoconstriction")
- Hypoxemia and acidosis
- Tension pneumothorax

    g. RV pressure overload: intrinsic pulmonary disease, acute respiratory distress syndrome, pulmonary embolism

3. Isolated RV dysfunction is characterized by a high RA/PCW pressure ratio, although this is usually unreliable when LV dysfunction is also present. RV ejection fraction thermodilution catheters and echocardiography are very helpful in assessing the status of RV function.[43,44] However, the presence of significant tricuspid regurgitation in these patients may render thermodilution cardiac outputs unreliable. Thus, alternative means of assessing cardiac output, such as a mixed venous oxygen saturation, rapid response RV catheter, or noninvasive test (pulse contour analysis, bioimpedance, or esophageal Doppler) may be necessary.

4. RV dysfunction may contribute to progressive LV dysfunction due to ventricular independence. When the RV dilates, it shifts the interventricular septum leftward, impairing LV distensibility. Progressive LV dysfunction may then reduce systemic perfusion pressure, causing RV ischemia, and may elevate PA pressures and RV afterload.

5. The goals of treatment are to optimize RV preload, ensure AV conduction, maintain systemic perfusion pressure, improve RV contractility, reduce RV afterload by reducing PVR, and optimize LV function (Box 11.2).

    a. RV preload must be raised cautiously to avoid the adverse effects of RV dilatation on RV myocardial blood flow and LV function. It is generally taught that cardiac output can be improved by volume infusions in patients sustaining RV infarctions with compromised RV function. However, the RA pressure should not be increased to more than 20 mm Hg. If no improvement in cardiac output ensues when volume is given to reach this pressure,

---

Box 11.2 • Treatment of Right Ventricular Failure

1. Optimize preload with CVP of 18–20 mm Hg
2. Ensure AV conduction
3. Maintain adequate systemic perfusion pressure with vasoactive mediations or an IABP
4. Lower RV afterload (PVR) and improve RV contractility
   a. Correct hypothermia, hypoxemia, hypercarbia, acidosis
   b. Select inotropes with vasodilator properties (inamrinone, milrinone, low-dose epinephrine, dobutamine)
   c. Use a pulmonary vasodilator
      i. Nesiritide
      ii. Inhaled nitric oxide
      iii. Inhaled prostacyclin
      iv. IV prostaglandin E_1
      v. Adenosine
      vi. Endothelin antagonists? (bosentan PO, tezosentan IV)
5. Optimize left ventricular function
6. Mechanical circulatory assist (RVAD) if no response to the above

---

additional volume infusions should be avoided. Volume overload of the right ventricle contributes to progressive deterioration of RV function, impairment of LV filling, and systemic venous hypertension.

b. AV conduction is essential.

c. Systemic perfusion pressure must be maintained while trying to avoid medications that can also increase PVR. Maintaining adequate perfusion of the RV may require intraaortic balloon pump support.

d. Correction of hypothermia, hypoxemia, hypercarbia, and respiratory acidosis by hyperventilation will decrease PVR (acidosis rather than hypercarbia is most deleterious).

e. Inotropic medications that can support RV and LV function and also reduce the PA pressure should be selected.

    i. The phosphodiesterase (PDE) inhibitors **inamrinone and milrinone** are very beneficial in improving RV contractility and reducing PA pressures, although they are usually associated with systemic hypotension that may require α-agents to support the SVR. Unfortunately, the use of α-agents may also increase the PVR. Dobutamine may produce effects similar to those of the PDE inhibitors.

    ii. Isoproterenol, while effective in improving RV contractility, is usually accompanied by a significant tachycardia and is rarely used today, except in patients undergoing cardiac transplantation.

f. Pulmonary vasodilators should also be considered.

    i. Nesiritide is a synthetic β-type natriuretic peptide that has no direct inotropic effect, but is a powerful balanced vasodilator that lowers preload and afterload. This reduces PA and systemic pressures and indirectly improves the cardiac output. It also improves renal perfusion and provides a powerful diuretic effect that is synergistic when given with a loop diuretic.[45,46] It is given as a 2 μg/kg IV bolus over one minute followed by an infusion of 0.01–0.03 μg/kg/min.

    ii. Inhaled nitric oxide (iNO) is a selective pulmonary vasodilator with minimal effect on SVR.[47–49] It can decrease RV afterload and augment RV performance while maintaining systemic perfusion pressure. The usual dose is 10–40 ppm administered via the ventilatory circuit. The circuit must be designed to optimally mix O_2 and NO to generate a low level of NO_2, which is toxic to lung tissue. Measurements of the concentration of NO in the inhaled limb and NO_2 in the exhalation limb of the ventilatory circuit by chemiluminescence are essential during delivery. Ideally, a scavenger system should be attached to the exhaust port of the ventilator. Although iNO is quite effective, it is very expensive, somewhat cumbersome to use, and potentially toxic if not appropriately monitored.

- NO does not increase intrapulmonary shunting. It may reverse the hypoxic vasoconstriction that is frequently noted with other pulmonary vasodilators (such as nitroprusside) and may improve the Pao_2/Fio_2 ratio.[49,50]
- The greater the degree of pulmonary hypertension, the greater the percentage reduction in PVR.[51]
- When pulmonary hypertension is refractory to NO, as may be noted in valve patients, the addition of dipyridamole 0.2 mg/kg IV may reduce RV afterload.[52–54] Dipyridamole blocks the hydrolysis of cyclic guanosine monophosphate in vascular smooth muscle and may also attenuate rebound pulmonary hypertension noted after NO withdrawal. This phenomenon may be the result of elevated endothelin-1 levels induced by NO administration.[55]
- NO in the bloodstream is rapidly metabolized to methemoglobin (metHb) and levels should be monitored. Methemoglobinemia is rarely noted in adults but can be a significant problem in young children.
- NO should be weaned slowly to prevent a rebound increase in PVR. A general guideline is to decrease the dose by no more than 20% every 30 minutes. Inhalation can be stopped once 6 ppm is reached.
- A comparative study of iNO and milrinone used for patients with pulmonary hypertension upon separation from bypass showed that iNO was associated with lower heart rates, better RV ejection fraction, and less requirement for phenylephrine to support systemic resistance.[56]

    iii. Prostaglandin E$_1$ (PGE$_1$) and its analogs **(epoprostenol [prostacyclin] and iloprost)** are potent pulmonary vasodilators that have been used primarily to assess vascular reactivity in patients awaiting heart transplantation. However, they are also beneficial in reducing PA pressure and improving RV function in patients with severe pulmonary hypertension during and after various types of cardiac surgery (usually mitral valve surgery and cardiac transplantation).

- **PGE$_1$** is given at a dosage of 0.03–0.2 µg/kg/min to achieve pulmonary vasodilation, but generally must be given at a dosage of less than 0.1 µg/kg/min to avoid systemic hypotension.[57] Higher dosages may necessitate an infusion of norepinephrine to counteract the decrease in SVR. To minimize adverse effects on the pulmonary vasculature, norepinephrine should be given directly into a left atrial line.[58]

- **Epoprostenol** (prostacyclin, PGI$_2$) administered intravenously is not inactivated by the lungs and is 10 times more potent a systemic vasodilator than PGE$_1$. However, inhaled PGI$_2$ is a very effective short-acting selective pulmonary vasodilator that can improve RV performance without affecting SVR.[59-61] It may also improve oxygenation by decreasing ventilation/perfusion mismatch. Studies have reported use of a single 60 µg inhalation in the operating room or a continuous inhalation using either a weight-based protocol (up to 50 ng/kg/min at which dose some systemic vasodilatation may occur) or a concentration-based protocol, giving 8 mL/h of a 20 µg/mL solution. There is complete reversal of effect about 25 minutes after inhaled PGI$_2$ is stopped. The advantages of this medication over iNO are that it is significantly less expensive, has no toxic metabolites, and is easy to administer and monitor.

- **Iloprost** is a prostacyclin analog that also reduces PVR and increases cardiac output with little effect on blood pressure or SVR. It can be given in an aerosolized dose of 12.5–50 µg during and after surgery.[62,63] Its hemodynamic effect lasts 1–2 hours after a single administration.

iv. A comparative study of iNO (40 ppm), PGE$_1$ (0.1 µg/kg/min), and NTG (3–5 µg/kg/min) in patients with pulmonary hypertension after cardiac surgery showed that all three medications were capable of reducing PVR. However, iNO increased cardiac output without systemic vasodilatation, PGE$_1$ increased cardiac output and improved RV performance with systemic vasodilatation, and NTG reduced SVR without any hemodynamic improvement.[64,65] This study demonstrated the advantages of the inhaled pulmonary vasodilators over several systemically administered medications.

v. **Adenosine** administered at a rate of 500 µg/kg/min produces significant selective pulmonary vasodilatation with subsequent increase in cardiac output.[66]

vi. **Endothelin-receptor antagonists** have been used in patients with primary pulmonary hypertension and may also prove beneficial in postoperative patients with elevated PA pressures and RV dysfunction. The utility and role of these medications have yet to be delineated. Available medications include bosentan, which can be taken orally, and tezosentan, which was available intravenously in Europe in mid-2004.

g. If RV dysfunction persists despite use of inotropic support, pulmonary vasodilators, and an intraaortic balloon pump, implementation of mechanical assistance, such as a right ventricular assist device, may be necessary.

F. Diastolic dysfunction is a common cause of congestive heart failure (CHF) in hypertensive patients. It can pose hemodynamic problems after surgery due to the additional impact of CPB and cardioplegia on myocardial edema and compliance. It is most prominent after a prolonged period of cardioplegic arrest, especially in the small hypertrophied heart.

1. Diastolic dysfunction may be caused by impaired systolic relaxation or decreased diastolic compliance, often with an inappropriate tachycardia.[67] The end result is a low cardiac output syndrome with a small LV chamber at end-diastole yet high left-sided filling pressures (see page 247). The stiffness of the heart is usually evident on the echocardiogram, which will often confirm normal systolic function even though the patient is in a low output state.

2. This problem can be difficult to manage and often results in end-organ dysfunction, such as renal failure, that progresses until the diastolic dysfunction improves. Although inotropic drugs are frequently given, they are of little benefit. In contrast, ACE inhibitors may improve diastolic compliance; lusitropic drugs, such as the calcium channel blockers, nesiritide, and inamrinone/milrinone, may improve relaxation; and bradycardic drugs, such as β-blockers or calcium channel blockers, can be used for an inappropriate tachycardia. Aggressive diuresis may also be beneficial in reducing myocardial edema that might contribute to reduced compliance.

III. Inotropic and Vasoactive Drugs

A. General comments

1. A variety of vasoactive medications are available to provide hemodynamic support for the patient with marginal myocardial function. They should be chosen carefully to achieve a satisfactory cardiac index (> 2.2 L/min/m²) and blood pressure once adequate filling pressures have been achieved. The selection of a particular drug depends on an understanding of its mechanism of action and limitations to its use. The catecholamines exert their effects on α- and β-adrenergic receptors. They elevate levels of intracellular cyclic AMP (cAMP) by β-adrenergic stimulation of adenylate cyclase. In contrast, the PDE inhibitors (inamrinone, milrinone) elevate cAMP levels by inhibiting cAMP degradation. Elevation of cAMP augments calcium influx into myocardial cells and increases contractility.[25]

   - α_1 and α_2 stimulation results in increased SVR and PVR. Cardiac α_1 receptors increase contractility and decrease the heart rate.
   - β_1 stimulation results in increased contractility (inotropy), heart rate (chronotropy), and conduction (dromotropy).
   - β_2 stimulation results in peripheral vasodilatation and bronchodilatation.

2. The net effects of medications that share α and β properties usually depend on the dosage level and are summarized in Table 11.3.

3. Concomitant use of several medications with selective effects may minimize the side effects of higher doses of individual medications. For example:

Table 11.3 • Hemodynamic Effects of Vasoactive Medications

Medication	SVR	HR	PCW	CI	MAP	MVO$_2$
Dopamine	↓↑	↑↑↑	↓↑	↑	↓↑	↑
Dobutamine	↓	↑↑↑	↓	↑	↓↔↑	↑↔
Epinephrine	↓↑	↑↑	↓↑	↑	↑	↑
Inamrinone/milrinone	↓↓	↑	↓	↑	↓	↑↓
Isoproterenol	↓↓	↑↑↑↑	↓	↑	↓↑	↑↑
Calcium chloride	↑	↔	↑	↑	↑↑	↑
Norepinephrine	↑↑	↑↑	↑↑	↑	↑↑↑	↑
Phenylephrine	↑↑	↔	↑	↔	↑↑	↔↑
Nesiritide	↓↓	↔	↓↓	↑*	↓↓	↓↓

↑ = increased; ↓ = decreased; ↔ = no change; ↓↑ = variable effect; * = indirect effect.

Note:
1. The effect may vary with dosage level (particularly dopamine and epinephrine, in which case the effect seen at low dosage is indicated by the first arrow).
2. The relative effect is indicated by the number of arrows.
3. For some medications, an improvement in MAP may occur from the positive inotropic effect despite a reduction in SVR.
4. The effects of inamrinone, milrinone, and calcium are not mediated by α- and β-receptors.

- Inotropes with vasoconstrictive (α) properties can be combined with vasodilators to improve contractility while avoiding an increase in SVR.
- Inotropes with vasodilator properties can be combined with α-agonists to maintain SVR.
- Catecholamines can be combined with the PDE inhibitors to provide synergistic inotropic effects while achieving pulmonary and systemic vasodilatation.
- α-agents can be infused directly into the left atrium to maintain SVR while a pulmonary vasodilator is infused into the right heart.

4. The benefits of most vasoactive medications are noted when adequate blood levels are achieved in the systemic circulation. Thus, these medications should be given into the central circulation via controlled infusion pumps rather than peripherally. Nonetheless, higher levels can be reached by drug infusion into the

Table 11.4 • Mixes and Dosage Ranges for Vasoactive Medications

Medication	Mix	Dosage Range
Dopamine	400 mg/250 mL	2–20 µg/kg/min
Dobutamine	500 mg/250 mL	5–20 µg/kg/min
Epinephrine	1 mg/250 mL	1–4 µg/min (0.01– 0.05 µg/kg/min)
Inamrinone	200 mg/200 mL	0.75 mg/kg bolus, then 10–15 µg/kg/min
Milrinone	20 mg/200 mL	50 µg/kg bolus, then 0.375–0.75 µg/kg/min
Isoproterenol	1 mg/250 mL	0.5–10 µg/min (0.01–0.1 µg/kg/min)
Norepinephrine	4 mg/250 mL	1–50 µg/min (0.015–0.5 µg/kg/min)
Phenylephrine	40 mg/250 mL	5–150 µg/min (0.05–1.5 µg/kg/min)

Note: X mg placed in 250 mL gives an infusion rate of X µg (milligrams divided by 100) in 15 drops of solution. For example, a 200-mg/250-mL mix gives a drip of 200 µg in 15 drops. 60 microdrops = 1 mL; 15 drops/min = 15 mL/h.

Note: the final volume of the mix reflects the total volume; thus, for amrinone, 50 mL of amrinone is added to 150 mL to achieve a total volume of 200 mL. For all of the other medications, the drug volume is very small.

left atrium rather than the central venous circulation, which results in partial removal or inactivation of these drugs by the lungs. Furthermore, infusion of medications, such as norepinephrine or epinephrine, through a left atrial line minimizes elevation of the PVR, which may contribute to RV dysfunction.[68]

5. The standard mixes and dosage ranges are listed in Table 11.4.

B. Epinephrine

1. **Hemodynamic effects**

a. Epinephrine is a potent β_1 inotropic agent that increases cardiac output by an increase in heart rate and contractility. At doses less than 2 µg/min (<0.03 µg/kg/min), it has a β_2 effect that produces mild peripheral vasodilatation, but the blood pressure is usually maintained or elevated by the increase in cardiac output. At doses greater than 2 µg/min (>0.03 µg/kg/min), α effects will increase the SVR and raise the blood pressure. Metabolic acidosis may also be noted at low doses of epinephrine when α effects are not evident.

b. Epinephrine has strong β_2 properties that produce bronchodilatation.

    c. Although epinephrine may contribute to arrhythmias or tachycardia, studies have shown that epinephrine given at a dosage of 2 μg/min causes less tachycardia than dobutamine given at a dosage of 5 μg/kg/min.[69]

    d. Epinephrine delivered through a left atrial line produces a higher cardiac index with lower pulmonary pressures and PVR than when delivered through a central venous line. This may be beneficial in the patient with RV dysfunction in whom an increase in RV afterload would not be well tolerated.[68] In this situation, however, the PDE inhibitors are preferable.

2. Indications

    a. Epinephrine is usually the first-line drug for a **borderline cardiac output** in the absence of tachycardia or ventricular ectopy. It is very helpful in the hypertrophied heart that often takes several minutes to recover adequate systolic function after cardioplegic arrest. Epinephrine is extremely effective and has very low cost.

    b. It is especially helpful in **stimulating the sinus node** mechanism when the intrinsic heart rate is slow. It is frequently beneficial in improving the atrium's responsiveness to pacing at the conclusion of bypass.

    c. **Bronchospasm** may respond well to epinephrine, especially when an inotrope is also required.

    d. **Anaphylaxis** (protamine reaction).

    e. Resuscitation from cardiac arrest.

3. Dosage: starting dose is 1 μg/min (about 0.01 μg/kg/min) with a mix of 1 mg/250 mL. Dosage can be increased to 4 μg/min (about 0.05 μg/kg/min). Higher doses are rarely indicated in patients following cardiac surgery.

C. Dopamine

1. Hemodynamic effects depend on the dosage, although plasma levels and effects may not correlate with the infused dose.[70]

    a. At doses of 2–3 μg/kg/min, dopamine has a selective "dopaminergic" effect that reduces afferent arteriolar tone in the kidney, with an indirect vasoconstrictive effect on efferent arterioles. The net effect is an increase in renal blood flow, glomerular filtration rate, and urine output. A mild β_2 effect decreases peripheral resistance and may reduce blood pressure. Even at this low dosage level, there is activation of α_1 and β_1 receptors. The latter may produce a profound tachycardia. **Note:** Dopamine's diuretic effect may also be attributable to its effects on renal tubular function as well as some inotropic effect at this level. It has not been shown to prevent or alter the natural history of acute tubular necrosis once it develops.[71]

    b. At doses of 3–8 μg/kg/min, dopamine exhibits a β_1 inotropic effect that improves contractility and, to a variable degree, a chronotropic effect that increases heart rate and the potential for arrhythmogenesis. It also has a dromotropic effect that increases AV conduction during AF/atrial flutter.[72]

    c. At doses greater than 8 μg/kg/min, there are increasing inotropic effects, but also a predominant α effect that occurs directly and by endogenous release of norepinephrine. This raises the SVR, systemic blood pressure, and filling pressures, and may adversely affect myocardial oxygen consumption and ventricular function. Concomitant use of a vasodilator, such as nitroprusside, to counteract these α effects allows for the best augmentation of cardiac output. The dopaminergic effect may still be present despite the vasoconstrictive effects.[25]

2. **Indications**

  a. Dopamine may be considered a first-line drug for a **low cardiac output state**, especially when the SVR is low and the blood pressure is marginal. Its use may be limited by the development of a profound tachycardia, even at very low dosages, and occasionally by excessive urine output. In these situations, another inotrope should be selected.

  b. It is beneficial in **improving urine output** in patients with or without preexisting renal dysfunction. Nonetheless, the "renoprotective" effect of dopamine during open-heart surgery and in the early postoperative course is controversial, with most studies suggesting it has no demonstrable benefit in preserving renal function.[73,74]

3. **Starting dose** is 2 μg/kg/min with a mix of 400 mg/250 mL. Dosage can be increased to 20 μg/kg/min.

D. **Dobutamine**

1. **Hemodynamic effects**

  a. Dobutamine is a positive inotropic agent with a strong β_1 effect that increases heart rate in a dose-dependent manner and also increases contractility. It also exhibits mild vasoconstrictive α_1 and mild vasodilatory β_2 effects that may influence SVR. In one study, the α_1 effect predominated over the β_2 effect causing an increase in SVR at the termination of CPB.[75] Diastolic filling pressures are usually reduced. Blood pressure is generally maintained by improved cardiac performance.

  b. Dobutamine has been compared with other inotropic agents in several studies.

    i. Dobutamine and dopamine increase myocardial oxygen demand to a comparable degree, but only dobutamine can match this increase with augmented myocardial blood flow.[76] This favorable effect on the myocardial supply-to-demand ratio is offset to some degree, however, by the development of tachycardia. Other studies have shown that, in contrast to dopamine, dobutamine reduces LV wall stress and oxygen demand by lowering preload and afterload.[77] This is particularly evident in volume-overloaded hearts (valve replacement for mitral or aortic regurgitation).[78]

    ii. Dobutamine causes more tachycardia than epinephrine.[69]

    iii. Dobutamine and the PDE inhibitors provide comparable hemodynamic support, although dobutamine is associated with more hypertension, tachycardia, and a greater chance of triggering AF.[79,80]

2. **Indications**

  a. Dobutamine is most useful when **the cardiac output is marginal and there is a mild elevation in SVR.** Its use is usually restricted by development of a tachycardia.

  b. It has a moderate **pulmonary vasodilator** effect and may be helpful in improving RV function and lowering RV afterload.

  c. It has a synergistic effect in improving cardiac output when used with a PDE inhibitor (inamrinone/milrinone). This combination is commonly used in patients awaiting cardiac transplantation.

3. **Starting dose** is 5 µg/kg/min using a mix of 500 mg/250 mL. Dosage can be increased to 20 µg/kg/min.

E. **Inamrinone (Inocor) and Milrinone (Primacor)**

1. **Hemodynamic effects**

a. These are phosphodiesterase (PDE) III inhibitors that can best be described as "inodilators."[81] They improve cardiac output by reducing systemic and pulmonary vascular resistance and by exerting a moderate positive inotropic effect. There is usually a modest increase in heart rate, a lowering of filling pressures, and a moderate reduction in systemic blood pressure. Thus, they generally are associated with a reduction in myocardial oxygen demand. Although the unloading effect produced by the decrease in SVR may contribute a great deal to their efficacy, an α-agent (phenylephrine or norepinephrine) is frequently required to maintain systemic blood pressure. They also have lusitropic (relaxant) properties.

b. Additive effects on ventricular performance are noted when used with one of the catecholamines, such as dobutamine, dopamine, or epinephrine, due to differing sites of action.[82–84]

c. Inamrinone and milrinone provide comparable hemodynamic effects[85] and have been compared with dobutamine in several studies. The increase in cardiac output is similar to that achieved with dobutamine, but dobutamine is associated with a greater increase in heart rate and a higher incidence of atrial and ventricular arrhythmias.[79,80] Consequently, dobutamine may increase myocardial oxygen demand and the risk of perioperative infarction. In addition, the PDE inhibitors, but not dobutamine, lower coronary vascular resistance.[86]

d. The tachycardia produced by the PDE inhibitors may be offset by the use of β-blockers without compromising the beneficial inotropic effects.[87]

2. **Indications**

a. These medications are generally second-line medications that should be used for a **persistent low cardiac output state** despite use of one of the catecholamines or when their use is limited by tachycardia. However, one study did show that a preemptive bolus of milrinone on pump significantly reduced the need for any catecholamine in the immediate perioperative period.[88]

b. They are particularly valuable in patients with **RV dysfunction** associated with an elevation in PVR, such as patients with pulmonary hypertension from mitral valve disease or those awaiting and following cardiac transplantation.

c. Their lusitropic (relaxant) properties may be of value in patients with significant **diastolic dysfunction** that may contribute to a low-output state, even with preserved systolic function.

3. **Advantages and disadvantages**

a. PDE inhibitors have long elimination half-lives (3.6 hours for inamrinone and 2.3 hours for milrinone), which are even longer in patients in low cardiac output states. Thus, an intraoperative bolus can be used to terminate bypass and provide a few hours of additional inotropic support without the need for continuous infusion. This should be considered due to the expense of these medications.

   b. Because the hemodynamic effects persist for several hours after the drug infusion is discontinued (in contrast to the short duration of action of the catecholamines), the patient must be observed carefully for deteriorating myocardial function for several hours as the drug effects wear off.
   c. Inamrinone has been associated with the development of thrombocytopenia. Therefore, platelet counts must be monitored on a daily basis. In contrast, thrombocytopenia is very rare with milrinone, which is often used for weeks at a time in patients awaiting transplantation.[89]
   d. PDE inhibitors vasodilate arterial conduits. Thus, they may prove beneficial in a patient with suspected coronary spasm who requires inotropic support.[90,91]

4. Starting dosages

   a. Inamrinone: 0.75 mg/kg bolus over 10 minutes followed by a continuous infusion of 10–15 μg/kg/min with a mix of 200 mg/200 mL of normal saline. When given during surgery, a 1.5 mg/kg bolus is usually required to achieve a satisfactory plasma concentration.[92]
   b. Milrinone: 50 μg/kg IV bolus over 10 minutes, followed by a continuous infusion of 0.375–0.75 μg/kg/min of a 20 mg/200 mL solution.

F. Isoproterenol

1. Hemodynamic effects

   a. Isoproterenol has a strong β_1 effect that increases cardiac output by a moderate increase in contractility and a marked increase in heart rate. Although it also has a β_2 effect that lowers SVR to a slight degree, the increased myocardial O_2 demand caused by the tachycardia limits its usefulness in coronary bypass patients. Isoproterenol may produce ischemia out of proportion to its chronotropic effects, and it also predisposes to ventricular arrhythmias.
   b. Isoproterenol's β_2 effect lowers PVR and reduces right heart afterload.
   c. There is a strong β_2 bronchodilator effect.

2. Indications

   a. **RV dysfunction** associated with an elevation in PVR. Isoproterenol is both an inotrope and a pulmonary vasodilator and thus is helpful in supporting RV function following mitral valve surgery in patients with preexisting pulmonary hypertension. Because it causes such a profound tachycardia, it has generally been replaced by the PDE inhibitors.[57] However, it is still commonly used following heart transplantation to reduce PVR, improve RV function, and produce ventricular relaxation.
   b. **Bronchospasm** when an inotrope is required.
   c. **Bradycardia** in the absence of functioning pacemaker wires. It is commonly used after heart transplantation to maintain a heart rate of 100–110/min.

3. Starting dose is 0.5 μg/min with a mix of 1 mg/250 mL. It can be increased to about 10 μg/min (usual dosage range is 0.01–0.1 μg/kg/min).

G. Norepinephrine (Levophed)

1. Hemodynamic effects

   a. Norepinephrine is a powerful catecholamine with both α- and β-adrenergic properties. Its predominant α effect raises SVR and blood pressure, while the β_1 effect increases both contractility and heart rate.
   b. By increasing afterload and contractility, norepinephrine increases myocardial oxygen demand and may prove detrimental to the ischemic or marginal

myocardium. It may also cause regional redistribution of blood flow away from the splanchnic circulation, reducing organ system perfusion and increasing the risk of visceral ischemia. One study showed that it may induce renal vasoconstriction, but another suggested that it did not impair renal function.[34,35]

   c. Note: There is a tendency to think that norepinephrine is providing only an α effect, but it does have strong β properties. Thus, it should be anticipated that both the cardiac output and heart rate will fall when the drug is weaned.

2. Indications

   a. Norepinephrine is primarily indicated when the patient has a marginally **low cardiac output with a low blood pressure caused by a low SVR.** This is often noted when the patient warms and vasodilates. Use of a pure α-agent is feasible if the cardiac index exceeds 2.5 L/min/m², but norepinephrine can provide some inotropic support if the cardiac index is borderline. If the cardiac index is below 2.0 L/min/m², another inotrope should probably be used in addition to or in place of norepinephrine.

   b. Norepinephrine is frequently effective in raising the blood pressure when little effect has been obtained from phenylephrine (and vice versa).

   c. It has been used as an inotrope to improve cardiac output in conjunction with a vasodilator, such as phentolamine or sodium nitroprusside (SNP), to counteract its α effects, but this combination is used infrequently.[93]

3. Starting dose is 1 µg/min (about 0.015 µg/kg/min) with a mix of 4 mg/250 mL. The dosage may be increased as necessary to achieve a satisfactory blood pressure. Higher dosages (probably > 20 µg/min or > 0.2 µg/kg/min) reduce visceral and peripheral blood flow, frequently producing a metabolic acidosis.

H. Phenylephrine (Neo-Synephrine)

1. Hemodynamic effects

   a. Phenylephrine is a pure α-agent that increases SVR and may cause a reflex decrease in heart rate. Myocardial function may be compromised if an excessive increase in afterload is produced by phenylephrine; however, it is frequently improved by an elevation in coronary perfusion pressure that resolves myocardial ischemia.

   b. Phenylephrine has no direct cardiac effects.

2. Indications

   a. Phenylephrine is indicated only to **increase the SVR when hypotension coexists with a satisfactory cardiac output.** This is commonly noted at the termination of bypass or in the ICU when the patient warms and vasodilates. If the blood pressure remains low after volume infusions, yet the cardiac output is satisfactory, phenylephrine can be used to maintain a systemic blood pressure around 100–110 mm Hg. Significantly higher pressures should be avoided to minimize the adverse effects of an elevated SVR on myocardial function.

   b. Phenylephrine can be used **preoperatively to manage ischemia** by maintaining perfusion pressure while NTG is used to reduce preload.

3. Advantages and disadvantages

   a. Patients often become refractory to the effects of phenylephrine after several hours of use, necessitating a change to norepinephrine. Conversely, some patients respond very poorly to norepinephrine and have an immediate blood pressure response to low-dose phenylephrine.

b. By providing no cardiac support other than an increase in central perfusion pressures, phenylephrine has limited indications.

c. **Note:** Be very careful when administering α-agents to patients whose entire revascularization procedure is based on arterial grafts.

4. **Starting dose** is 5 μg/min with a mix of 40 mg/250 mL. The dosage can be increased as necessary to maintain a satisfactory blood pressure. The usual dosage range is 0.05–1.5 μg/kg/min.

I. Calcium chloride

1. **Hemodynamic effects.** Calcium chloride's primary effect is to increase the SVR and the mean arterial pressure. It has little effect on the heart rate. It produces a transient improvement in systolic function at the termination of CPB, although it may increase ventricular stiffness, suggesting that it produces transient diastolic dysfunction.[94]

   a. One study showed that $CaCl_2$ produces a transient inotropic effect if hypocalcemia is present and a more sustained increase in SVR, independent of the calcium level.[95]

   b. A study that compared epinephrine and calcium chloride upon emergence from CPB showed that both increased the mean arterial pressure, but only epinephrine increased the cardiac output, suggesting that calcium did not provide any inotropic support.[96] Although this study did not find any beneficial or negative effect of combining these two medications, another one suggested that the calcium salts may attenuate the cardiotonic effects of catecholamines, such as dobutamine or epinephrine, but have little effect on the efficacy of inamrinone.[97]

2. **Indications**

   a. Frequently used **at the termination of CPB to augment systemic blood pressure** by either its positive inotropic or vasoconstrictive effect.

   b. **To support myocardial function or blood pressure on an emergency basis** until further assessment and intervention can be undertaken. **Note:** Calcium is not recommended for routine use during a cardiac arrest.

   c. **Hyperkalemia** ($K^+ > 6.0$ mEq/L)

3. **Usual dosage** is 0.5–1 g slow IV bolus.

J. Triiodothyronine

1. **Hemodynamic effects**

   a. Most patients have been found to have reduced levels of free triiodothyronine (T_3) and thyroxine at the conclusion of CPB, but a relationship to impaired myocardial performance is not clear.[98,99] Administration of T_3 has been shown to increase cardiac output and lower SVR in patients with depressed ventricular function. Its positive inotropic effect results from increased aerobic metabolism and synthesis of high-energy phosphates. It causes a dose-dependent increase in myocyte contractile performance that is independent of and additive to β-adrenergic stimulation.

   b. Randomized studies have produced conflicting results on whether the intraoperative administration of T_3 improves ventricular function, decreases inotropic requirements, and improves overall outcome. However, significant improvement in hemodynamics has been demonstrated in patients with impaired ventricular function, many of whom could not be weaned from bypass on multiple inotropes until T_3 was administered.[100-104]

   c. Note: Calcium channel blockers have been shown to interfere with the action of T_3.[104]

   d. There is some evidence that T_3 may reduce the incidence of postoperative AF through an unknown mechanism.[105]

2. Indications

   a. T_3 may be indicated to provide inotropic support as a salvage step when bypass cannot be terminated with maximal inotropic support and the IABP.

   b. T_3 is helpful in improving donor heart function in brain-dead patients when ventricular function is depressed.

3. Usual dosage is 0.2–0.8 µg/kg IV, which may be followed by an infusion of 0.12 µg/kg/h for 6 hours.

K. Other modalities to manage low cardiac output

   1. Nesiritide is a recombinant B-type natriuretic peptide that has been used primarily in patients with decompensated heart failure. It decreases sympathetic stimulation and inhibits the neurohormonal response (i.e., activation of the renin-angiotensin-aldosterone system and endothelin) noted in patients with heart failure. By inference, these same changes may be seen in patients with postcardiotomy ventricular dysfunction and elevated PA pressures.[45,46,106]

   a. Nesiritide produces balanced vasodilatation resulting in a decrease in preload (PA pressure) and afterload (SVR). It indirectly increases cardiac output and does so with no increase in heart rate or myocardial oxygen demand. It exhibits lusitropic (relaxant) properties, dilates native coronary arteries and arterial conduits, and has no proarrhythmic effects.

   b. Nesiritide dilates the renal afferent and efferent arterioles, producing an increase in glomerular filtration. It thus has a strong diuretic and natriuretic effect that is synergistic with that of the loop diuretics.

   c. Indications: In the cardiac surgical patient, nesiritide is useful in conditions of diastolic dysfunction, and when postcardiotomy systolic dysfunction is accompanied by elevated PA pressures. Such conditions are noted in patients with cardiogenic shock preoperatively or severe ventricular dysfunction upon weaning from bypass or in patients with pulmonary hypertension associated with mitral valve disease, before and after cardiac transplantation, with use of assist devices, or with fluid overload secondary to postoperative renal failure.

   d. Dosage: Nesiritide is given in a dose of 2 µg/kg over one minute followed by an infusion of 0.01–0.03 µg/kg/min. It has a rapid onset of action with most of its hemodynamic effects noted within the first 30 minutes. Although its half-life is only 18 minutes, hypotension may persist for hours after the infusion is discontinued. It may be given through a peripheral IV and does not require intensive monitoring.

   2. Glucose-insulin-potassium (GIK). GIK has been demonstrated to have an inotropic effect on the failing myocardium after cardioplegic arrest. It provides metabolic support to the myocardium by increasing anaerobic glycolysis, lowering free fatty acid levels, preserving intracellular glycogen stores, and stabilizing membrane function. The mixture contains 50% glucose, 80 units/L of regular insulin, and 100 mEq/L of potassium infused at a rate of 1 mL/kg/h.[107]

3. **Dopexamine** is a synthetic catecholamine that stimulates dopaminergic receptors as well as β_2, and to a lesser extent, β_1-adrenergic receptors. It provides an inotropic effect by inhibiting neuronal uptake of catecholamines, and it also increases heart rate in a dose-related manner. It decreases SVR and improves renal and splanchnic perfusion. It also decreases PVR and can improve RV function. Its effects are fairly equivalent to those of dobutamine, although it may cause more tachycardia. It is given as an infusion of 1–4 µg/kg/min.[108]

4. **Enoximone** is a PDE inhibitor with hemodynamic effects similar to those of inamrinone. It decreases systemic, pulmonary, and coronary resistance and has a positive inotropic effect with minimal alteration in heart rate. Its vasodilating properties may be less than those of inamrinone, but it still usually requires a vasoconstrictor to offset the vasodilatory effects of the bolus injection. It also has an additive effect when given with a catecholamine. It is not associated with the development of thrombocytopenia. It is given as a 0.5–1.0 mg/kg bolus at the termination of bypass.[109]

5. **Levosimendan** is a new calcium-sensitizing "inodilator." It provides a positive inotropic effect by sensitizing myofilaments to calcium without increasing intracellular calcium levels. It also has vasodilator effects by opening ATP-dependent potassium channels in vascular smooth muscle. It improves cardiac output by increasing both stroke volume and heart rate and reduces preload and afterload by its vasodilating effects. It has been used for patients with acute exacerbations of heart failure in Europe and is being investigated for use in low cardiac output syndromes after cardiac surgery.[110] Postoperatively, it has been given as a 12 µg/kg loading dose over 10 minutes, followed by a continuous infusion of 0.1 µg/kg/min. The active metabolite has a very long half-life (80 hours), so a 24-hour infusion may provide benefits for up to a week. Thus, its role in the short-term management of postcardiotomy dysfunction has yet to be defined.

L. Recommended strategy for selection of vasoactive medications

1. The selection of a vasoactive medication should be based on several factors:

   a. An adequate understanding of the underlying cardiac pathophysiology derived from hemodynamic measurements and often echocardiography.

   b. Knowledge of the α, β, or nonadrenergic hemodynamic effects of the medications and their anticipated influence on preload, afterload, heart rate, and contractility.

2. Vasoactive medications are usually started in the operating room and maintained for about 6–12 hours while the heart recovers from the period of ischemia/reperfusion. The dosages are adjusted as the patient's hemodynamic parameters improve. Occasionally, when the heart demonstrates persistent "stunning" or has sustained a perioperative infarction, pharmacologic support and/or an IABP may be necessary for several days.

3. When the cardiac index is satisfactory (> 2.2 L/min/m²) but the blood pressure is low, an α-agent should be selected. Phenylephrine is commonly used in the operating room, but norepinephrine is probably a better drug to use in that it provides some β effects that are beneficial during the early phase of myocardial recovery. Systolic blood pressure need only be maintained around 100 mm Hg (mean pressure > 80 mm Hg) to minimize the increase in afterload. If neither of these medications suffices, vasopressin should be utilized.[36-39]

4. When the cardiac index remains marginal (< 2.0 L/min/m²) after optimizing volume status, heart rate, and rhythm, an inotropic agent should be selected. The first-line drugs are usually epinephrine, dobutamine, or dopamine. The major limitation to their use is the development of tachycardia, which tends to be less prominent with low-dose epinephrine. At inotropic levels, dopamine and epinephrine tend to raise SVR, whereas dobutamine's effect on SVR is variable but usually not significant. If a satisfactory cardiac output has been achieved and the blood pressure is elevated, addition of a vasodilator is beneficial. If the blood pressure is low, an α-agent can be added.

5. If the cardiac output still remains suboptimal despite moderate doses of drugs (epinephrine 2–3 μg/min [0.03–0.05 μg/kg/min], dobutamine 10 μg/kg/min, or dopamine 10 μg/kg/min), a second drug should be selected. The PDE inhibitors exhibit additive effects to those of the catecholamines and should be selected. These medications lower the SVR and may cause a modest tachycardia. They commonly require the use of norepinephrine to maintain SVR, although blood pressure may be maintained by the improvement in cardiac function. If norepinephrine is used, its β effect may further improve contractility, but it can also increase the heart rate. Its α effect may reduce organ system perfusion and may compromise flow in arterial conduits (such as the internal thoracic artery [ITA] or radial artery).[111] If the cardiac index remains marginal despite the use of two medications, an IABP should be inserted.

6. If the patient cannot be weaned from bypass and has hemodynamic evidence of persistent cardiogenic shock (PCWP >20 mm Hg, cardiac index <1.8 L/min/m²) despite medications and the IABP, a circulatory assist device should be considered.

7. Note: It is not uncommon for the cardiac output to fall to below 1.8 L/min/m² during the first 4–6 hours after surgery, which represents the time of maximal myocardial depression. The dose of an inotrope may have to be increased transiently or, less frequently, another one added. However, it is the **persistence of a low output state** beyond this time that raises concern, especially if there is any evidence of ischemia, continually rising filling pressures, oliguria, or a progressive metabolic acidosis. An IABP may need to be inserted in the ICU if these problems are present. However, in the absence of any specific identifiable problem, most patients gradually improve, and one should not be overly alarmed by or be excessively aggressive in response to transient drops in cardiac output. Echocardiography is helpful in assessing whether ventricular dysfunction or cardiac tamponade is causing the low output state and may often direct management appropriately.

8. Note: Use of α-agents can be dangerous in patients receiving radial artery grafts or in whom multiple grafts are based on ITA inflow. It is preferable to reduce the dose of the vasodilating drug (diltiazem or NTG used to prevent spasm) rather than increase the dose of a vasoconstricting medication.

M. Vasoactive medications provide specific hemodynamic benefits, but their use may be limited by the development of adverse effects. Nearly all of the catecholamines increase myocardial oxygen demand by increasing heart rate and contractility. Other side effects that may necessitate changing to or addition of another medication include:

1. Arrhythmogenesis and tachycardia (epinephrine, isoproterenol, dobutamine, dopamine)
2. Vasoconstriction and poor renal, splanchnic, and peripheral perfusion (norepinephrine, phenylephrine)
3. Vasodilatation that requires α agents to support systemic blood pressure with potential adverse effects on renal perfusion (inamrinone/milrinone)
4. Excessive urine output (dopamine)
5. Thrombocytopenia (inamrinone)
6. Cyanide and thiocyanate toxicity (nitroprusside)
7. Methemoglobinemia (nitroglycerin)

N. **Weaning from vasoactive medications**

1. Once the cardiac output and blood pressure have stabilized for a few hours, vasoactive medications should be weaned. α-agents should generally be weaned first. Their use should ideally be restricted to increasing the SVR to support blood pressure when the cardiac output is satisfactory. However, there are circumstances when α-agents are required to maintain cerebral and coronary perfusion in the face of a poor cardiac output. In these desperate life-saving situations, the resultant intense peripheral vasoconstriction can compromise organ system and peripheral perfusion, causing renal, mesenteric, and peripheral ischemia, acidosis, and frequently death.

   a. In the routine patient, SVR and blood pressure increase when myocardial function improves, narcotic effects abate, and sedatives, such as propofol, are discontinued. As the patient awakens and develops increased intrinsic sympathetic tone, α-agents can be stopped.

   b. When inamrinone/milrinone or the IABP is used to support myocardial function, an α-agent is frequently required to counteract the excellent unloading and decrease in SVR that is achieved. It may not be possible to wean the α-agent before the patient has been weaned from the medication or IABP because he or she may become hypotensive despite an excellent cardiac output. It is usually necessary to wean the α-agent in conjunction with weaning of the other modalities.

   c. Occasionally, a patient who has sustained a small perioperative infarction will have an excellent cardiac output but a low SVR. This requires temporary α support until the blood pressure improves spontaneously. Such support may be required for several days.

2. The stronger positive inotropes with the most potential detrimental effects on myocardial metabolism should be weaned next. Those that possess α properties should be decreased to doses at which these effects do not occur. If an IABP is present, it should not be removed until the patient is on a low dose of only one inotrope, unless complications of the IABP develop. Otherwise, weaning of the IABP should usually be deferred.

   a. The catecholamines should be weaned first to low doses. If the patient is on multiple drugs, epinephrine should be weaned to a low dose (2 μg/min or less) to avoid any α effects. Then dobutamine (which lacks significant α effects) and dopamine should be weaned to doses less than 10 μg/kg/min. At this dosage, the α effects of dopamine should dissipate but the β effects will be maintained.

b. Inamrinone/milrinone are second-line drugs and are usually weaned off with the patient still supported by low doses of catecholamines. These medications have few deleterious effects on myocardial function but often require the use of α-agents, which may have adverse effects on organ system perfusion. Thus, concomitant weaning of these medications is generally recommended before terminating the infusion of a catecholamine.

  i. Because of their long half-lives, the PDE inhibitors should be stopped several hours before the withdrawal of other major support modalities (IABP). The dosage is halved and then discontinued a few hours later if hemodynamics remains stable. The cardiac output must be monitored to observe for potential deterioration in myocardial function that may occur several hours after the infusion has been stopped. Not infrequently, the patient may require the reinstitution of inotropic support at that point.

  ii. Early discontinuation of inamrinone (or conversion to milrinone) should also be considered if the patient develops progressive thrombocytopenia. It is not always clear whether this is caused by this medication or other coexisting problems, such as heparin-induced thrombocytopenia or IABP-induced platelet destruction.

  iii. If the patient has a significant tachycardia from a catecholamine, the PDE inhibitor may be used exclusively (although often with an α-agent), and thus would be the last medication discontinued.

c. IABP removal may be performed once the patient is on low doses of inotropic support, such as epinephrine at 1 μg/min or dobutamine or dopamine at 5 μg/kg/min.

d. The use of vasoactive medications in patients on circulatory assist devices depends on the extent of support provided and the function of the unsupported ventricle. In patients receiving univentricular support, inotropic medications may be necessary to improve the function of the unassisted ventricle. Patients with biventricular support are usually given only α-agents to support systemic resistance. If the device is being used for temporary support rather than as a bridge to transplantation, inotropes may be given to assess ventricular function and reserve when flows are transiently reduced. If ventricular function is recovering, an inotrope, such as milrinone, may be given to provide support after removal of the device.

3. Vasodilators are commonly used during the early phase of postoperative recovery to reduce blood pressure when the patient is hypothermic, vasoconstricted, and hypertensive. They are weaned off as the patient vasodilates to maintain a systolic blood pressure of 100–120 mm Hg. Vasodilators may also be used alone or in conjunction with inotropic medications to improve myocardial function by lowering the SVR. In this situation, they are weaned concomitantly with the inotropes, depending on the cardiac output and the blood pressure. Continued use of antihypertensive medications is usually required in patients with a history of hypertension or those who have undergone aortic valve replacement for aortic stenosis. The most commonly used medication is sodium nitroprusside, which is then converted to oral medications (see section VII).

IV. Intraaortic Balloon Counterpulsation

Intraaortic balloon counterpulsation provides hemodynamic support and/or control of ischemia both before and after surgery.[112,113] In contrast to most inotropic agents, the IABP provides physiologic assistance to the failing heart by decreasing myocardial oxygen demand and improving coronary perfusion. Although it is an invasive device with several potential complications, it has proven invaluable in improving the results of surgery in high-risk patients and allowing for the survival of many patients with postcardiotomy ventricular dysfunction. The survival rate of patients requiring intraoperative IABP support approximates 60–70%.

A. **Indications**

1. Ongoing ischemia refractory to medical therapy or hemodynamic compromise prior to urgent surgery.

2. Prophylactic placement for high-risk patients with critical coronary disease (usually left main disease) or severe LV dysfunction—usually preoperatively, but occasionally at the beginning of an operation.[114]

3. High-risk patients undergoing off-pump surgery to maintain hemodynamic stability during lateral wall or posterior wall grafting.[115,116]

4. Unloading for cardiogenic shock or mechanical complications of myocardial infarction (MI), such as acute mitral regurgitation and ventricular septal rupture.

5. Postoperative low cardiac output syndrome unresponsive to moderate doses of inotropic agents.

6. Postoperative myocardial ischemia.

7. Acute deterioration of myocardial function to provide temporary support or a bridge to transplantation.

B. **Contraindications**

1. Aortic insufficiency

2. Aortic dissection

3. Severe aortic and peripheral vascular atherosclerosis (balloon can be inserted via the ascending aorta during surgery)

C. **Principles**

1. It reduces the impedance to LV ejection ("unloads the heart") by rapid deflation just before ventricular systole.

2. It increases diastolic coronary perfusion pressure by rapid inflation just after aortic valve closure.

3. This sequence reduces the time-tension index (systolic wall tension) and increases the diastolic pressure–time index, favorably altering the myocardial oxygen supply-demand ratio.

4. The IABP may also improve LV diastolic function after surgery.[117]

D. **Insertion techniques**

1. The IABP is placed through the femoral artery with the balloon situated just distal to the left subclavian artery so as not to impair flow to the left ITA (Figure 11.1). Generally, a 40 cc balloon is selected for most patients, using the 30 cc balloon in smaller patients, usually women. The ACS Supracor IABP (Abiomed, Danvers, MA) has been developed for positioning in the ascending aorta. In an animal model it was found to improve myocardial blood flow more

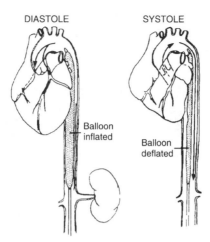

Figure 11.1 • The intraaortic balloon is positioned just distal to the left subclavian artery. Balloon inflation occurs in early diastole and improves coronary perfusion pressure. Deflation occurs just before systole to reduce the impedance to left ventricular ejection. *(Reproduced with permission from Maccioli GA, Lucas WJ, Norfleet EA. The intra-aortic balloon pump: a review. J Cardiothorac Anesth 1988;2:365–73.)*

than the standard descending aortic balloon without any impairment in cerebral blood flow.[118]

2. Percutaneous insertion is performed by the Seldinger technique, placing the balloon through a sheath and over a guidewire. The sheath can be left in place or removed from the artery (especially if the femoral artery is small). Some systems are sheathless to minimize occlusion of the femoral vessels, but these can cause shearing of the balloon in patients with significant aortoiliac atherosclerosis. Percutaneous insertion is associated with a significant risk of limb ischemia in patients with known peripheral vascular disease. Although insertion of the IABP can be performed blindly in the operating room or at the bedside, preoperative placement is usually performed in the cardiac cath lab using fluoroscopy to visualize the wire and the eventual location of the balloon. This may allow for placement through a tortuous iliofemoral system that otherwise might be fraught with danger.

3. Surgical insertion can be accomplished by exposing the femoral artery and placing the balloon through a sidearm graft or directly into the vessel through an arteriotomy or a percutaneous sheath. Transthoracic balloon placement via the ascending aorta may be necessary if severe aortoiliac disease is present.

E. **IABP timing** is performed from the ECG or the arterial waveform.

1. ECG: input to the balloon console is provided from skin leads or the bedside monitor. Inflation is set for the peak of the T wave at the end of systole with deflation set just before or on the R wave. The use of bipolar pacing eliminates the interpretation of pacing spikes as QRS complexes by the console.

2. Arterial waveform: inflation should occur at the dicrotic notch with deflation just before the onset of the aortic upstroke. This method is especially useful in the operating room where electrocautery may interfere with the ECG signal.

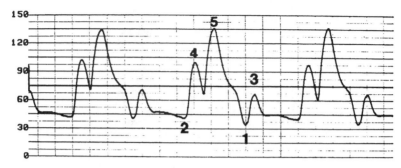

Figure 11.2 • Intraaortic balloon tracing at 1:2 inflation ratio. Note that the balloon aortic end-diastolic pressure (1) is lower than the patient's aortic end-diastolic pressure (2) and that the balloon-assisted peak systolic pressure (3) is lower than the systolic pressure that is generated without a preceding assisted beat (4). These changes reflect decreased impedance to ejection during systole. Coronary perfusion pressure is increased by diastolic augmentation achieved by balloon inflation (5).

3. A typical arterial waveform during a 1:2 ratio of IABP inflation is demonstrated in Figure 11.2. This shows the systolic unloading (decrease in the balloon-assisted systolic and diastolic pressures) and the diastolic augmentation that are achieved with the IABP.

F. **IABP problems and complications**

1. **Inability to balloon.** Once the balloon is situated properly and has unwrapped, satisfactory ballooning should be achieved by proper timing of inflation and deflation. However, unsatisfactory ballooning can occur in the following situations.

a. Unipolar atrial pacing. This produces a large atrial pacing spike that can be interpreted by the console as a QRS complex leading to inappropriate inflation. Use of bipolar pacing eliminates this problem. Most monitoring equipment suppresses pacing signals.

b. Rapid rates. Some balloon consoles are incapable of inflating and deflating fast enough to accommodate heart rates over 150 (usually when there is a rapid ventricular response to AF). Augmentation can be performed with a 1:2 ratio.

c. Arrhythmias. Atrial and ventricular ectopy can disrupt normal inflation and deflation patterns and must be managed.

d. Volume loss from the balloon detected by the console monitor alarms. This indicates a leak in the system, either at the connectors or from the balloon itself. Volume loss may also indicate that the balloon has not unwrapped properly, preventing proper inflation.

e. Balloon rupture. When blood appears in the balloon tubing, the balloon has perforated. Escape of gas (usually helium) from the balloon into the bloodstream can occur. **The balloon must be removed immediately.** Difficulty with removal (balloon entrapment) may be encountered if thrombus has formed within the balloon. Most consoles have alarms that will call attention to this problem and will prevent the device from inflating.

2. **Vascular complications**

   a. Catastrophic complications, such as aortic dissection or rupture of the iliac artery or aorta, are very uncommon. Paraplegia can result from development of a periadventitial aortic hematoma or embolization of atherosclerotic debris.[119]

   b. Embolization to visceral vessels, especially the mesenteric and renal arteries, can occur in the presence of significant aortic atherosclerosis.[120,121] In fact, cerebral embolization can occur if there are mobile atheroma in the proximal descending thoracic aorta.[122] Renal ischemia may occur if the balloon is situated too low and inflates below the level of the diaphragm.[123] This apparently does not affect mesenteric flow.[124]

   c. Distal ischemia is the most common complication of indwelling balloons, occurring in about 5–10% of patients. It is more common with percutaneous placement, although it has become less common with improvements in balloon technology that have reduced the diameter of most balloon cables to 7.5–8F. Nonetheless, ischemia is more likely to occur in the patient with a small body surface area and small femoral vessels or severe iliofemoral occlusive disease. Thrombosis near the insertion site or distal thromboembolism can also occur. Use of intravenous heparin (maintaining a partial thromboplastin time of 1.5–2 times control) is advisable to minimize ischemic and thromboembolic problems if the balloon remains in place for more than a few days after surgery. Generally, patients have a low-grade coagulopathy immediately after surgery and anticoagulation is not necessary for the first few days.

   d. The presence of distal pulses or Doppler signals must be assessed in all patients with an IABP. This should be compared with the peripheral pulse examination that should have been documented prior to surgery. Not infrequently, cool extremities with weak signals are noted in the early postoperative period from peripheral vasoconstriction that may be associated with a low cardiac output state, hypothermia, or use of vasopressors. This should resolve when the patient warms and myocardial function improves. However, persistent ischemia jeopardizes the viability of the distal leg. Options at this time include:

      i. Removing the sheath from the femoral artery if the balloon has been placed percutaneously.

      ii. Removing the balloon if the patient appears to be hemodynamically stable. If adequate distal perfusion cannot be obtained, femoral exploration is indicated.

      iii. Removing the balloon and placing it in the contralateral femoral artery (if that leg has adequate perfusion) if the patient is IABP-dependent. Using as small a caliber balloon as possible with sheath removal is essential.

      iv. Considering placement of a transthoracic balloon.

3. **Thrombocytopenia.** The mechanical action of persistent inflation and deflation destroys circulating platelets. It is not always clear whether progressive thrombocytopenia is caused by the IABP or medications that the patient may be receiving, such as heparin or inamrinone. Platelet counts must be checked at least on a daily basis.

G. Weaning of the IABP

1. IABP support can be withdrawn when the cardiac output is satisfactory on minimal inotropic support (usually less than 5 μg/kg/min of either dopamine or dobutamine or 1 μg/min of epinephrine). However, earlier removal may be indicated if complications develop, such as leg ischemia, balloon malfunction, thrombocytopenia, or infection.

2. Weaning is initiated by decreasing the inflation ratio from 1:1 to 1:2 for about 2–4 hours, and then to 1:3 or 1:4 (depending on which console device is used) for 1–2 more hours. Once it is determined that the patient can tolerate a low inflation ratio, the IABP should be removed. If there is an anticipated delay in removal of more than a few hours for manpower reasons or need to correct a coagulopathy, the ratio should be increased to at least 1:2 to prevent thrombus formation.

3. Removal can be achieved if hemodynamics remain stable when the inflation ratio is reduced. Serial measurements of filling pressures and cardiac outputs should be evaluated. Remember that the IABP produces efficient unloading, and the blood pressure noted on the monitor is lower during balloon assistance than with an unassisted beat (actually the diastolic pressure is higher, but the true systolic pressure is lower). Thus, visual improvement in blood pressure with weaning of the IABP is not by itself a sensitive measure of the patient's progress.

4. The operative mortality for patients receiving a prophylactic IABP is less than 5% but rises to about 30–40% for patients requiring an IABP for postcardiotomy support.[113,125] One study showed that the most significant correlate of operative mortality was a serum lactate level more than 10 mmol/L during the first 8 hours of support (100% mortality). Additional poor prognostic signs were a metabolic acidosis (base deficit > 10 mmol/L), mean arterial pressure < 60 mm Hg, urine output less than 30 mL/h for 2 hours, and the requirement for high dosages of epinephrine or norepinephrine (> 10 μg/min) during the early postoperative period.[126]

H. IABP removal techniques

1. Balloons inserted by the percutaneous technique can usually be removed percutaneously. This is performed by compressing the groin distal to the insertion site as the balloon is removed, allowing blood to flush out the skin wound for several heartbeats, and then compressing just proximal to the skin hole where the arterial puncture site is located (Figure 11.3). Pressure must be maintained for at least 45 minutes to ensure satisfactory thrombus formation at the puncture site. **Note:** It is important to resist the temptation to remove manual pressure and peek to see if hemostasis is achieved. This can be counterproductive and flush away immature clot that is sealing the vessel.

2. **Note:** Coagulation parameters must be checked and corrected before percutaneous removal or the patient may require groin exploration for persistent hemorrhage or a false aneurysm.

3. Surgical removal should be considered in patients with small or diseased vessels and in those with very weak pulses or Doppler signals with the balloon in place. The need for a thrombectomy and embolectomy may be anticipated in these patients. If the IABP has been in place for more than 5 days, percutaneous removal can be performed, but there is a greater chance that surgical repair of the femoral artery may be required.

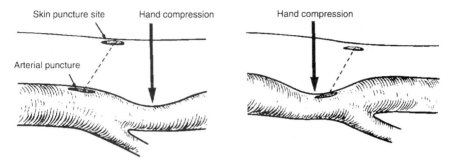

Skin puncture site   Hand compression   Hand compression

Arterial puncture

Figure 11.3 • Technique of percutaneous balloon removal. Initial compression is held below the level of the arterial puncture site to allow for flushing of blood. However, subsequent pressure should be maintained over the arterial puncture site to prevent bleeding. Note that the hole in the artery lies more cephalad than the hole in the skin.

V. Circulatory Assist Devices

A. If a patient cannot be weaned from CPB despite maximal pharmacologic support and use of the IABP, consideration should be given to placement of a circulatory assist device.[127,128] These devices provide flow to support the systemic or pulmonary circulation while resting the heart, allowing it to undergo metabolic and functional recovery.

1. Some devices are used for short-term support, anticipating recovery of ventricular function. These include the centrifugal pumps, the Abiomed BVS® 5000, and extracorporeal membrane oxygenation (ECMO). If recovery does not occur, these devices should be changed to those capable of providing long-term support (Thoratec pneumatic LVAD, Thoratec HeartMate, Abiomed AB5000™ ventricles, or Novacor LVAS) if cardiac transplantation is an option.

2. When chances for recovery are remote, often due to extensive perioperative infarction or biventricular failure, one of the Thoratec devices should be considered from the outset. However, use of these devices is generally restricted to suitable candidates for cardiac transplantation, although destination therapy has now become an option in patients who are not candidates for transplantation.[129] Use of pulsatile pumps can usually improve multiorgan system function and improve the clinical status of potential transplant recipients. Newer nonpulsatile pumps (DeBakey Micromed and the Jarvik 2000) can also be used for bridging and potentially for destination therapy. As of late 2004, there were more than 30 pumps in various stages of development to provide ventricular assist.

B. **Left ventricular assist devices (LVADs)**

1. LVADs provide systemic perfusion while decompressing the left ventricle. LV wall stress is reduced by about 80% with a 40% decrease in myocardial oxygen demand. LVAD flow is dependent on adequate intravascular volume and RV function. Although volume unloading is superior with pulsatile pumps, LV pressure unloading is comparable with pulsatile and nonpulsatile (centrifugal or axial flow) pumps.[130]

2. **Indications** (Box 11.3). The general indications for LVAD insertion are the presence of a cardiac index < 1.8 L/min/m^2 with a systolic BP < 80 mm Hg and

---

Box 11.3 • Indications for Circulatory Assist Devices

1. Complete and adequate cardiac surgical procedure
2. Correction of all metabolic problems (ABGs, acid-base, electrolytes)
3. Inability to wean from bypass despite maximal pharmacologic therapy and use of the IABP
4. Cardiac index < 1.8–2 L/min/m²

LVAD	RVAD	BiVAD
Systolic BP < 80 mm Hg	Mean RAP > 20 mm Hg	LAP > 20 mm Hg
LAP > 20 mm Hg	LAP < 15 mm Hg	RAP > 20–25 mm Hg
SVR > 2100 dynes-s/cm⁵	No TR	No TR
Urine output < 20 mL/h		Inability to maintain LVAD flow > 2.0 L/min/m² with RAP > 20 mm Hg

---

a PCWP or LAP > 20 mm Hg on maximal medical support.[131] This may be noted in the immediate postcardiotomy period or following an MI or other acute or chronic cardiac condition producing a severe cardiomyopathy. Malignant ventricular arrhythmias can also be managed by VAD insertion.

3. **Contraindications.** When the indications for LVAD placement are present, a critical element of decision-making is whether the patient is a candidate for transplantation and whether the patient's cardiac and noncardiac comorbidities contraindicate the placement of a VAD. A risk factor model predictive of poor survival after LVAD insertion has been devised by the Columbia-Presbyterian group. This includes, in decreasing order of significance, oliguria, CVP > 20 cm H_2O, mechanical ventilation, an elevated international normalized ratio (INR), reoperative status, WBC > 15,000, and a fever > 101.5°C. Generally, one must consider RV function, other cardiac disease (valve or coronary disease), noncardiac organ system function (neurologic, pulmonary, renal, hepatic), and other medical issues (infectious, vascular disease, diabetes) when making this critical decision.[132,133]

4. **Technique.** Drainage is provided from the left atrium or LV apex with return of blood to the aorta (Figure 11.4). A left atrial catheter may be inserted for accurate monitoring of left-sided filling pressures.

5. **Management** during LVAD support

   a. LVAD flow is initiated to achieve a systemic flow of 2.2 L/min/m² with an LA pressure of 10–15 mm Hg. All approved devices have an automatic mode that ejects a full stroke volume once the reservoir or bladder is full, although other triggering modes are available. Inability to achieve satisfactory flow

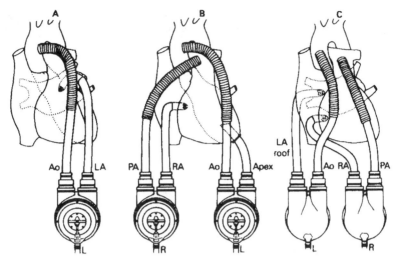

Figure 11.4 • Cannulation techniques for ventricular assist devices. (A) LVAD with left atrial and aortic cannulation. (B) BiVAD setup. The RVAD consists of right atrial and pulmonary artery cannulation. The LVAD cannulation sites are the left ventricular apex (the most common site) and the aorta. (C) BiVAD setup with LVAD drainage from the roof of the left atrium. The Thoratec device is demonstrated in this diagram, but the cannulation sites are similar for nearly all assist devices. *(Reprinted from Farrar DJ, Hill JD, Gray LA Jr, et al. Heterotopic prosthetic ventricles as a bridge to cardiac transplantation. A multicenter study in 29 patients. N Engl J Med 1988;318:333–40. Copyright © 1988 Massachusetts Medical Society. All rights reserved.)*

indicates either hypovolemia, improper position of the drainage catheter, or RV failure. Adequacy of tissue perfusion can be assessed by mixed venous oxygen saturations.

  b. Inotropic support should be stopped to decrease myocardial oxygen demand, but it may be required to support RV dysfunction. Use of α-agents may be necessary to support systemic resistance, aiming to maintain a mean arterial pressure > 75 mm Hg. Patients receiving LVADs commonly manifest "vasodilatory shock" and require use of vasopressin to maintain systemic pressure.[134]

  c. Heparinization to achieve an activated clotting time (ACT) of 175–200 seconds is recommended for most assist devices (Abiomed BVS® 5000 and the Thoratec pneumatic VAD system) once perioperative bleeding has ceased. An infusion of 500 U/h of heparin usually suffices, although most patients become heparin resistant. If pump flow is transiently decreased to less than 1.5 L/min, additional heparinization is recommended to achieve an ACT of 200–250 seconds. The Thoratec HeartMate VE LVAD does not require anticoagulation other than aspirin. Anticoagulation is mandatory, however, for any patient with a mechanical prosthetic valve and for those with biologic mitral or tricuspid valves to avoid thromboembolism, occlusion of the inflow conduit, or valvular incompetence.[135]

  d. For patients in whom temporary support is anticipated, LV function is assessed by TEE during partial support after at least 48 hours of support. If there is recovery of function, flow may be reduced to a minimal flow rate of 2 L/min (to minimize the risk of thromboembolism) with careful observation of hemodynamic parameters (cardiac output, filling pressures, and systemic pressure). Low-dose inotropic support can be initiated during the weaning process. Soon thereafter, the patient can be brought to the operating room and the heart observed for a short period of time at low flow. If the heart can sustain adequate hemodynamics and appears by TEE to have recovered adequate function, the device is removed. If an IABP was used (in patients with nonpulsatile devices), it can generally be removed the day following LVAD removal.

6. **Overall results.** Weaning has been accomplished in about 50% of patients receiving LVADs for postcardiotomy support with 25–30% of patients surviving to be discharged from the hospital. Improved survival is noted in patients with preserved RV function, no evidence of a perioperative MI, and recovery of LV function within 48–72 hours. If ventricular function does not recover after a week of support with a short-term device, a longer-term device should be placed as a bridge to transplantation. In patients receiving the HeartMate device, more commonly for clinical deterioration while awaiting a heart transplant, 65–75% of patients survive to be successfully transplanted, with a transplant survival greater than 60% at 5 years. This is similar to that noted in patients not requiring mechanical assist.[136]

C. **Right ventricular assist devices (RVADs)**

1. RVADs provide pulmonary blood flow while decompressing the right ventricle. RV failure may result from RV infarction, worsening of preexisting RV dysfunction caused by pulmonary hypertension, or poor intraoperative protection. One of the main contributing factors to RV dysfunction is an elevation in PVR, which can often be attributed to the proinflammatory cytokines and microembolization from multiple blood product transfusions. Achieving satisfactory systemic flow depends on adequate volume status and LV function. Although isolated RV failure may occur, it more commonly is associated with LV failure in the postcardiotomy period and may be evident after an LVAD has been implanted.[137]

2. **Indications.** See Box 11.3.

3. **Technique.** Drainage is provided from the right atrium with return of desaturated blood to the pulmonary artery (see Figure 11.4). The Abiomed BVS® 5000 and Thoratec pneumatic VAD are the only two devices approved to provide temporary RV support, although the Jarvik 2000 may be adaptable to provide biventricular support.[138]

4. **Management** during RVAD support

   a. RVAD flow is initiated to achieve a flow rate of 2.2 L/min/m², increasing the LA pressure to 15 mm Hg while maintaining a right atrial pressure of 5–10 mm Hg. Comparable to LVAD support, most devices function automatically, ejecting the full stroke volume once the device reservoir is full. Inability to achieve satisfactory flow rates may indicate hypovolemia, improper position of the drainage catheter, or cardiac tamponade that compresses the right atrium. If intravascular volume is adequate and tamponade is not present, systemic hypotension may be the result of impaired LV function that may require inotropic, IABP, or LVAD support. It may also result from systemic vasodilatation that requires use of an α-agent or vasopressin. TEE is helpful in evaluating the status of LV function in patients on RVAD support.

   b. Inhaled nitric oxide or prostacyclin is beneficial in reducing PA pressures and RV afterload.[47,61,139] They may allow for improved flow rates on the device and for better RV function upon weaning of the device.

   c. The requirement for heparinization is similar to that for LVADs.

   d. Assessment of myocardial recovery by TEE and weaning from the device are similar to LVADs. Thermodilution cardiac outputs can be used to determine RV recovery when the flow rate is transiently reduced to low levels of support.

  5. Overall results. Patients receiving RVADs for postcardiotomy support have a poor prognosis. Weaning has been accomplished in about 35% of patients, with 25% of patients surviving to be discharged from the hospital.[140]

D. Biventricular assist devices (BiVADs)

  1. Biventricular failure is noted in about 10% of patients who require assist devices for postcardiotomy dysfunction. BiVADs provide support of both the pulmonary and systemic circulations and can function during periods of ventricular fibrillation (VF). Although the need for biventricular assistance may not be evident from the outset, LV decompression often unmasks RV dysfunction by increasing septal shift and RV stroke work. Other factors that contribute to RV dysfunction include an increase in PVR from blood transfusions or acid-base abnormalities, LV dysfunction, vasopressors, and RV ischemia from systemic hypotension.

   a. Several studies have examined predictors of RV dysfunction after LVAD implantation. Reports from the Cleveland Clinic have shown that RVAD use was more likely to be necessary in small women with nonischemic etiologies and patients who required preoperative mechanical ventilation and circulatory support before LVAD insertion.[141,142] Although an initial study suggested that a dilated RV with increased RV preload and afterload predisposed to RV dysfunction after LVAD,[143] subsequent studies showed that elevated PA pressures and PVR were not risk factors; rather a low PA pressure and low RV stroke work index, reflecting impaired RV contractility, were significant risk factors for RVAD use after LVAD implantation.[141,142]

   b. The Columbia-Presbyterian group also found that patients requiring an RVAD had lower RV stroke work indices. In addition, they had worse hepatic (increased bilirubin) and renal function (often requiring dialysis), and had received more red cell and platelet transfusions.[144]

   c. iNO is very beneficial in reducing RV afterload after LVAD implantation and may obviate the need to place an RVAD.[139]

  2. Indications. See Box 11.3.

  3. Technique. BiVAD support incorporates the techniques noted above for LVAD and RVAD connections (see Figure 11.4). Usually BiVAD support is provided using either the Abiomed BVS® 5000 system, the Abiomed AB5000™ ventricles, or the Thoratec VAD system. Occasionally, the HeartMate device is placed anticipating the need for only LV assist, only to find that another device may be needed subsequently for RV failure or intractable arrhythmias. A hybrid system works well, although anticoagulation with heparin may prevent some of the endothelialization considered essential in the HeartMate to minimize thromboembolism.

4. **Management** during BiVAD support
   a. Sequential manipulations of RVAD and LVAD flow are used to achieve a systemic flow rate of 2.2 L/min/m². The RVAD flow is increased to raise the LA pressure to 15–20 mm Hg, and then the LVAD flow is increased to reduce the LA pressure to 5–10 mm Hg. Once filling of the devices is accomplished, the devices function on a fill-to-empty mode. Inability to achieve satisfactory flow rates usually indicates hypovolemia, tamponade, or catheter malposition on either side. Left- and right-sided flow rates may differ because of varying contributions of the native ventricles to pulmonary or systemic flow.
   b. Heparin requirements are similar to those noted above.
   c. Assessment of recovery and weaning is similar to the methods described for RVAD and LVAD devices.

5. **Overall results.** Weaning has been accomplished in about 35% of patients, with only 20% of patients surviving to be discharged from the hospital. These poor results reflect the adverse impact of biventricular failure on survival. In a report from Cedars-Sinai Medical Center of 19 patients receiving Thoratec BiVADs for cardiogenic shock, nearly 60% were successfully bridged to transplantation with a 90% posttransplantation survival.[145]

E. **Extracorporeal membrane oxygenation**

1. ECMO is a form of extracorporeal life support (ECLS) that serves as an alternative to ventricular assist devices. The system employs a membrane oxygenator, centrifugal pump, heat exchanger, oxygen blender, and a heparin-coated circuit. The latter provides a more biocompatible surface that minimizes platelet activation and the systemic inflammatory response, and reduces or eliminates the heparin requirement. This allows the ECMO circuit to be used for several days.[146]

2. **Indications.** ECMO is indicated for the short-term management of severe postcardiotomy ventricular dysfunction with or without hypoxemia. Criteria for use are similar to those of LVADs or biventricular assist. In many patients requiring VAD support, the duration of CPB is quite long due to the delay in deciding to proceed with VAD support, often resulting in both cardiogenic and noncardiogenic pulmonary edema that impairs oxygenation. If the heart does not recover after several days of ECMO support but the patient is otherwise considered a candidate for transplantation, it can be used as a bridge to a longer-term support device in anticipation of transplantation.[147–150] It can also be used emergently in patients sustaining cardiac arrest and in patients with severe hypoxemic acute respiratory distress syndrome, while the lung recovers from the inciting pathologic insult.[151,152]

3. **Technique.** At the conclusion of surgery, the same cannulation setup used for CPB is maintained (right atrium, aorta). If ECMO is considered subsequently, it may be established with venous drainage from the internal jugular vein or femoral vein with return of blood to the femoral artery through a side graft to allow for distal perfusion or to the carotid artery. An IABP is frequently inserted as well to improve coronary perfusion since the ECMO circuit is providing nonpulsatile flow.[153] Percutaneous femorofemoral bypass may be used to resuscitate a patient from cardiac arrest.

4. **Management.** Maximal medical support is essential to optimize the results of ECMO. Some of the essential elements are:[154]

   a. Optimizing preload to provide pulmonary perfusion and supporting SVR with α-agents or vasopressin

   b. Aggressive use of iNO for pulmonary hypertension

   c. Early and aggressive use of continuous venovenous hemofiltration (CVVH) for renal dysfunction

   d. Avoidance of anticoagulation

   e. Use of low tidal volume ventilation

   If the patient has suffered a severe neurologic insult or is not considered a candidate for transplantation, ECMO is usually terminated after 48 hours.[155] Otherwise, if there is recovery of organ system function within 5 days of implantation, discontinuation of ECMO or conversion to a longer-term LVAD system should be considered. Careful assessment of neurologic, pulmonary, hepatic, and renal status is essential. It is sometimes difficult to ascertain whether the patient has survivable or nonsurvivable organ system dysfunction that might contraindicate LVAD implantation.

5. **Results.** The results of ECMO depend on the indication for its use and the degree of organ system failure at the time it is initiated. Patients in whom it is implanted for a cardiac arrest fare poorly, although one report found a 31% survival in patients undergoing emergent ECMO for prolonged cardiac arrest.[151] Patients who develop multiorgan system failure before ECMO is initiated or who develop acute renal failure requiring dialysis have a very high mortality rate.[156,157] Of patients receiving ECMO for postcardiotomy cardiogenic shock, approximately 40–50% will die on ECMO support. Although the rest may be weanable from the device, only about half of these will survive the hospital stay. If a strategy of using ECMO as a bridge to longer-term assist devices and transplantation is employed, 30% of patients may survive to transplantation with favorable results.[147–150,157,158]

F. **Devices available to provide ventricular assist**

1. **Nonpulsatile pumps**

   a. Nonpulsatile centrifugal pumps (BioMedicus, Sarns) are the most readily available and easy-to-use systems for uni- or biventricular support. They are labor intensive in that they require fairly constant attention to flow rates. They are usually used for short-term support (about 7–10 days) because of concerns that hemolysis and end-organ damage may develop with longer term use. However, further research into nonpulsatile pumps has shown that end-organ changes do not necessarily occur with longer use of such pumps, which has led to the development of several permanently implantable centrifugal devices, such as the Cleveland Clinic CorAide pump.[159,160] Nonetheless, if a patient cannot be weaned off support with the standard centrifugal pumps after one week, the system should be converted to a longer-term device. One report of 35 patients receiving the Sarns pump for postcardiotomy support found that more than 70% of patients could be weaned with a 52% hospital survival rate. Thus, even though these devices are not approved for this indication, they are very effective, with results competitive with the more sophisticated devices.[161]

b. Several devices use axial flow technology with a nonpulsatile rotary pump that withdraws blood from the left ventricle and pumps it into the aorta. These devices provide systemic flow and can also improve blood supply to ischemic zones and produce diastolic and systolic unloading. The original system, now known as the Medtronic hemopump, consists of a transthoracic catheter that is situated near the aortic valve that withdraws blood from the left ventricle and expels it into the ascending aorta. Three of the newer implantable devices include the DeBakey Micromed VAD and the Heartmate II LVAS, which have an inflow cannula inserted into the apex of the left ventricle with the pump sitting in an extracardiac position, and the implantable Jarvik 2000 device, which is placed directly into the left ventricle. Blood is then returned through an outflow graft to the ascending aorta. These devices have been used successfully as bridges to transplantation and might prove satisfactory when used for destination therapy.[162–165]

2. **Pulsatile pumps**

   a. The **Abiomed BVS® 5000** system is a pulsatile pneumatic device that is located at the patient's bedside (Figure 11.5). Specially designed catheters provide venous return to the pump, and a catheter with an integral graft is sewn to the outflow vessel. These catheters drain the right atrium and perfuse the pulmonary artery for RVAD support, or drain the left atrium/ventricle and return flow to the aorta for LVAD support. This system is indicated primarily for temporary support of patients with postinfarction or postbypass cardiogenic shock, and its use should generally be restricted to about 2 weeks. If continued VAD support is still required, the system should be converted to a longer-term device. The Abiomed system functions in series with the heart, with ejection occurring once the bladder has reached a designated volume. It requires anticoagulation with an ACT of 150–200 seconds. One of its drawbacks is the formation of fibrinous clot in the outflow chamber that may give rise to thromboembolism.[166]

   b. The **Abiomed AB5000™** ventricle became available in 2004 (Figure 11.6). This device resembles the Thoratec pneumatic VAD system (described below) in providing a pneumatically driven device that lies on the abdominal wall. The device includes an Angioflex membrane and proprietary trileaflet valves. This system avoids the extensive tubing and bedside arrangement of the BVS 5000 device and should be less susceptible to thrombus formation within the housings near the valves. It can be used for uni- or biventricular support.

   c. The **Thoratec VAD** is a pulsatile pneumatic paracorporeal device that lies on the abdominal wall. The patient is tethered only by the pneumatic driveline. Cannulation is similar to that of the Abiomed systems with specially designed catheters and grafts to provide drainage and blood return. These cannulas can be attached to one or two separate units to provide uni- or biventricular support. This device can provide long-term temporary support and can be used as a bridge to transplantation. It also requires full anticoagulation. Results in the Thoratec voluntary registry show that 38% of patients could be weaned from the device, of whom 59% survived to be discharged from the hospital. When placed as a bridge to transplantation, 40% died, but 60% were transplanted with an 86% survival.[167,168]

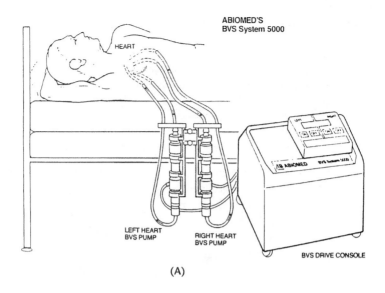

ABIOMED'S
BVS System 5000

HEART

LEFT HEART
BVS PUMP

RIGHT HEART
BVS PUMP

BVS DRIVE CONSOLE

(A)

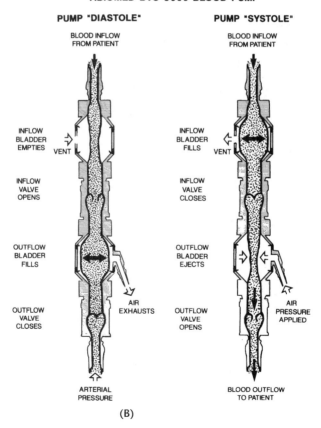

ABIOMED BVS 5000 BLOOD PUMP

PUMP "DIASTOLE"

BLOOD INFLOW
FROM PATIENT

INFLOW
BLADDER
EMPTIES

VENT

INFLOW
VALVE
OPENS

OUTFLOW
BLADDER
FILLS

OUTFLOW
VALVE
CLOSES

AIR
EXHAUSTS

ARTERIAL
PRESSURE

PUMP "SYSTOLE"

BLOOD INFLOW
FROM PATIENT

INFLOW
BLADDER
FILLS

VENT

INFLOW
VALVE
CLOSES

OUTFLOW
BLADDER
EJECTS

OUTFLOW
VALVE
OPENS

AIR
PRESSURE
APPLIED

BLOOD OUTFLOW
TO PATIENT

(B)

Figure 11.5 • The Abiomed BVS® 5000 System. (A) The devices are located at the patient's bedside and are connected to the drive console for pneumatic activation. (B) A cross-sectional view of the heart pumps during systole and diastole. *(Image courtesy of Abiomed, Inc.)*

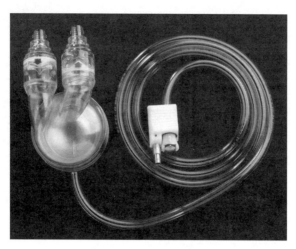

Figure 11.6 • The Abiomed AB5000™ ventricle attached to a pneumatic drive line. *(Image courtesy of Abiomed, Inc.)*

    d. The **Thoratec HeartMate VE** is an implantable, pulsatile, electric device that can provide only LV assist (Figure 11.7). Blood drains from the LV apex through a porcine valve into the device, which then ejects a stroke volume when the chamber is filled or at a fixed rate.

        i. This device has a unique textured surface that decreases the risk of thromboembolism. Most patients can be treated with aspirin alone.

        ii. This device is used primarily as a bridge to transplantation. Its low complication rate and efficacy in providing pulsatile flow allow for correction of preexisting organ system dysfunction prior to transplantation. Patients are fully ambulatory and can be discharged with a battery pack. The system requires a driveline that exits the lower abdominal wall and is often the site of infection. Nearly 70% of patients receiving the device are successfully transplanted.[136,169] If the patient is not a transplantation candidate, the device may be utilized for destination therapy, although the long-term results are somewhat discouraging.[129]

        iii. Degeneration of the porcine valve may occur in patients receiving long-term support. This should be suspected when the device output progressively rises, due to valvular regurgitation back into the left ventricle. This results in very rapid filling of the device with an increase in ejection rate. The device has been modified to address this problem.

        iv. If a patient receiving a HeartMate requires RVAD support, the Thoratec system is usually selected. If BiVAD support is required from the outset, usually two Thoratec pneumatic VAD or the Abiomed BV 5000 ventricles are used to support both ventricles.

    e. The **Novacor LVAS** (World Heart Corp, Oakland, CA) is an implantable, pulsatile, electrical device that can provide only LV assist. It functions like the HeartMate system, but has a higher incidence of thromboembolism

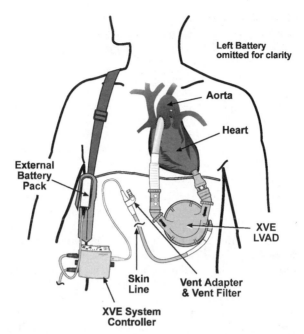

Figure 11.7 • The Thoratec HeartMate vented electric LVAD system. The device rests in a preperitoneal pocket in the left upper quadrant. Blood enters the device through an apical cannulation site and is pumped through a graft sewn to the ascending aorta. This device may run off battery power transmitted through a percutaneous driveline. *(Reprinted with permission from Thoratec Corporation.)*

despite anticoagulation. This device is used nearly exclusively as a bridge to transplantation. It has been reported to be associated with a 20–35% risk of neurologic complications, which are usually thromboembolic in nature.[170,171] However, recent advancements in perioperative management have reduced the incidence of this as well as other complications associated with this device, such as bleeding and infection. These advances include preperitoneal implantation, use of newer generation vascular grafts, extensive drainage of the insertion pockets, and a more restricted anticoagulation protocol.[172]

    f. A number of other devices are being investigated to provide destination therapy. These include LVADs, such as the wireless **Arrow LionHeart LVAS**, and total artificial hearts, such as the **AbioCor TAH** (Abiomed, Danvers MA).[173–175] The critical element in these devices is biocompatibility to reduce the risk of thromboembolism and blood element damage and improved transcutaneous energy transmission systems to reduce the risks of infection.

G. Complications. Continuing improvements in technology and perioperative care have reduced, but not eliminated, some of the complications associated with the long-term use of circulatory assist devices. These include the following:

1. **Mediastinal bleeding.** Use of aprotinin at the time of device implantation has been successful in reducing transfusion requirements. Nonetheless, upward of 50% of patients require reexploration for evacuation of mediastinal clot that can cause tamponade (manifested by inadequate drainage into the device).[176] Contributing factors include the large amount of dead space around the catheters in the mediastinum, coagulopathies present at the time of implantation, the requirement for anticoagulation for most devices, and the occurrence of fibrinolysis and platelet activation due to the extracorporeal circuit.[177] If aprotinin is used for LVAD insertion, the likelihood of an anaphylactic response upon reexposure to aprotinin at the time of LVAD removal and transplantation is increased and should always be kept in mind.[178]

2. **Mediastinitis and sepsis.** Nosocomial infections affect 40–50% of patients receiving VADs, many of which are device related, and some of which are not. They most commonly originate at the driveline exit site that is used for energy transmission. Because long-term antibiotic usage is commonplace, resistant organisms are often identified. In addition, many patients are debilitated and malnourished and have numerous intravascular and other invasive catheters that can become colonized. Although the infection risk is lowest with implantable devices with primary wound closure, bacteremia is still very common, being noted in almost 50% of patients in a study at the Cleveland Clinic.[179] The most common organisms are *Staphylococcus aureus* and coagulase-negative, *Candida*, and *Pseudomonas aeruginosa*. Infection is associated with a significantly increased mortality, especially so in the case of fungal endocarditis, which occurs in about 20% of patients. If this develops, antifungal therapy with either device removal and replacement or urgent transplantation may lead to a successful result.[179–181] In general, driveline site infections are controllable and do not influence the results of transplantation.[182]

3. **Thromboembolism** resulting in stroke has been noted in about 20% or more in patients receiving the Novacor device, but in only 3% of patients with the HeartMate device, even in the absence of anticoagulation. Clot formation within other devices occurs despite careful attention to anticoagulation. Very careful attention to anticoagulation protocols may reduce the incidence of stroke, which is related to device design and the thrombogenic potential of the blood-contacting surfaces.[170–172]

4. **Malignant ventricular arrhythmias** may develop as a result of myocardial ischemia, infarction, or the use of catecholamines. They may also originate from an arrhythmogenic focus in a dilated myopathic ventricle. BiVADs function during ventricular fibrillation, as can LVADs as long as the PVR is not high. If LVAD flow cannot be maintained, the patient may require placement of an RVAD. Fibrillation may foster thrombus formation in the ventricles and should be treated aggressively. Early cardioversion should be considered to reduce thrombus formation and prevent RV injury from prolonged fibrillation.[183]

5. **Renal failure** is less common with pulsatile devices and is usually caused by prolonged episodes of hypotension or low cardiac output prior to insertion of the devices. It generally returns to the patient's baseline after VAD implantation, except when there is evidence of other organ system failure (especially hepatic) or infection. Early aggressive treatment with CVVH should be considered. The mortality rate for patients with persistent renal failure on VAD support is very high.

6. **Respiratory failure** is usually attributable to a prolonged duration of CPB, sepsis, use of multiple blood products, and perhaps a long period of nonpulsatile flow with certain devices.

7. **Vasodilatory** shock due to inappropriately low levels of vasopressin is not uncommon in patients requiring placement of LVADs. In fact, vasopressin hypersensitivity may be noted. Use of arginine vasopressin 0.1 U/min effectively increases mean arterial pressure in these patients.[134]

8. Patients receiving LVADs become immunologically sensitized and have a reduced rate of transplantation due to crossmatch issues. Furthermore, they have a higher risk of rejection. However, after transplantation, survival appears to be similar to that in nonbridged recipients who are not sensitized. Immunomodulatory treatment with intravenous immunoglobulins and cyclophosphamide may be beneficial in offsetting the problems associated with sensitization.[184]

VI. Systemic Hypertension

A. General comments

1. Systemic hypertension is fairly common after open-heart surgery. In the immediate postoperative period, it usually results from vasoconstriction due to systemic hypothermia and from enhanced sympathetic nervous system activity associated with elevated levels of various hormones caused by the use of extracorporeal circulation. Hypertension is more common in patients with preserved ventricular function, preoperative hypertension, and those undergoing surgery for aortic valve disease.

2. Hypertension may result from elevated SVR or hyperdynamic myocardial performance, or both. Therefore, it is imperative that cardiac hemodynamics be assessed before therapeutic interventions are initiated. **One should never assume that hypertension is the result of hyperdynamic cardiac performance.** Withdrawal of inotropic support when hypertension is due to intense vasoconstriction may precipitate rapid hemodynamic deterioration if the cardiac output is marginal.

3. Treatment is indicated to maintain the systolic blood pressure below 140 mm Hg or the mean arterial pressure below 100 mm Hg. Aggressive treatment is warranted to minimize the potential adverse effects of hypertension. These include an increase in afterload, which can precipitate myocardial ischemia, dysrhythmias, or myocardial failure, mediastinal bleeding, suture line disruption, aortic dissection, and stroke.

B. Etiology

1. The hormonal milieu of CPB, including elevated levels of norepinephrine, renin-angiotensin, and vasopressin

2. Vasoconstriction from hypothermia, vasopressors, or a low cardiac output state

3. Fever, anxiety, pain, agitation and awakening when sedatives wear off

4. Abnormal arterial blood gases (ABGs) (hypoxia, hypercarbia, acidosis)

5. Pharyngeal manipulation (readjusting an endotracheal tube, placing a nasogastric tube or echo probe)

6. Hyperdynamic ventricles, especially those with LVH

7. Altered baroreceptor function: following combined CABG-carotid endarterectomy

8. Severe acute hypoglycemia

C. **Assessment**

1. Careful patient examination, especially for breath sounds and peripheral perfusion

2. Assessment of cardiac hemodynamics

3. Measurement of ABGs, serum potassium, hematocrit

4. Review of chest x-ray and 12-lead ECG

5. **Note:** Don't forget to check the chest drainage unit for the amount of mediastinal bleeding!

D. **Treatment**. Systolic pressure should be maintained between 100 and 140 mm Hg (mean arterial pressure around 90 mm Hg). The objective is to reduce the SVR sufficiently enough to reduce myocardial oxygen demand without compromising coronary perfusion pressure. A secondary benefit is frequently an improvement in myocardial function. Ideally, an antihypertensive agent should prevent myocardial ischemia without adversely affecting heart rate, AV conduction, or myocardial contractility.

1. Ensure satisfactory oxygenation and ventilation.

2. Use vasodilator medications if the cardiac output is satisfactory (see next section).

3. Provide inotropic support along with vasodilators if the cardiac output is marginal (cardiac index < 2.0–2.2 L/min/m²)

4. Sedate with propofol 25–50 (μg/kg/min (2–6 mg/kg/h), midazolam 2.5–5.0 mg IV, or morphine 2.5–5.0 mg IV. Sedation usually should be minimized to allow for early extubation unless hypertension is labile and difficult to control with antihypertensive medications. However, in the fully ventilated patient in whom delayed extubation is anticipated, sedation is an appropriate first step in the control of hypertension.

5. Control shivering with meperidine 25–50 mg IV or pharmacologic paralysis (**always** with sedation).

VII. Vasodilators and Antihypertensive Medications

A. General comments

1. A variety of medications can be used to control systemic hypertension (Table 11.5). Their hemodynamic effects depend on the patient's intravascular volume status and myocardial function, and the site at which they exert their antihypertensive action. Vasodilators may reduce blood pressure by increasing venous capacitance (reducing preload) or decreasing arterial resistance (which reduces afterload and usually preload as well). Other antihypertensive medications reduce blood pressure by inhibiting central adrenergic discharge or exerting a negative inotropic effect, a property also shared by several of the vasodilators. Thus, a careful cardiac assessment is required to ensure that the appropriate medication is selected.

2. Antihypertensive medications are most commonly used during the early phase of postoperative recovery when the patient is hypothermic, vasoconstricted,

Table 11.5 • Mixes and Dosage Ranges for Intravenous Antihypertensive Medications

Medication	Mix	Dosage Range
Nitroprusside	50 mg/250 mL	0.1–8 µg/kg/min
Nitroglycerin	50 mg/250 mL	0.1–10 µg/kg/min
Calcium channel blockers		
Nicardipine	50 mg/250 mL	2.5 mg over 5 min; repeat 4 times at 10-min intervals, then 2–4 mg/h
Diltiazem	250 mg/250 mL	0.25 mg/kg over 2 min, then 0.35 mg/kg over 2 min, then 5–15 mg/h
Verapamil	120 mg/250 mL	0.1 mg/kg bolus over 2 min, then 2–5 µg/kg/min
β-blockers		
Esmolol	2.5 g/250 mL	0.25–0.5 mg/kg/min bolus then 50–200 µg/kg/min
Labetalol	200 mg/200 mL	0.25 mg/kg over 2 min, then 0.5 mg every 15 min
		1–4 mg/min
Enalaprilat		0.625–1.25 mg IV over 30 min, then 0.2 mg/h
Fenoldopam	10 mg/250 mL	0.05–0.1 µg/kg/min initial infusion, up to 0.8 µg/kg/min

and hypertensive. They are tapered as the patient vasodilates in order to maintain a systolic blood pressure of 100–140 mm Hg. Vasodilators may also be used alone or in conjunction with inotropic medications to improve myocardial function by lowering SVR.

3. The most commonly used medication in the ICU is sodium nitroprusside (SNP), although other intravenous medications, such as NTG, calcium channel blockers (nicardipine or diltiazem), fenoldopam, enalaprilat, β-blockers (continuous infusion of esmolol or labetalol, or intermittent metoprolol) can also be considered in selected situations.

4. Most patients who were not hypertensive before surgery exhibit only transient hypertension after surgery and usually do not require further antihypertensive therapy. For those with a history of hypertension, oral medications must be initiated before transfer from the ICU. The appropriate choice depends on the patient's hemodynamic and renal function (see page 399).

B. Sodium nitroprusside (SNP)

  1. Hemodynamic effects

  a. SNP primarily relaxes arterial smooth muscle and reduces SVR and PVR. It has a lesser effect on venous capacitance, which also reduces preload. The overall effect is a reduction in systemic blood pressure and filling pressures, often resulting in an improvement in LV function. Maintenance or improvement in cardiac output usually requires a modest volume infusion to restore filling pressures to an optimal level. The theory is to "optimize preload → reduce afterload → restore preload." The development of a reflex tachycardia during SNP infusion usually reflects hypovolemia and may increase myocardial oxygen demand.

  b. SNP should theoretically be avoided in the ischemic heart. It dilates resistance vessels in the coronary circulation and can produce a coronary steal syndrome by shunting blood away from ischemic zones. In addition, if filling pressures do not decrease when systemic perfusion pressure falls, the diastolic transmyocardial gradient for coronary blood flow will be reduced, potentially producing myocardial ischemia.

  c. SNP is a very dangerous drug that always requires close monitoring with an indwelling arterial cannula. It has a very rapid onset of action (within seconds) and can lower the blood pressure precipitously. Fortunately, its effects dissipate within a few minutes.

  2. Indications

  a. To control systemic hypertension caused by an increase in SVR. SNP is the best antihypertensive drug to use if cardiac function is marginal, filling pressures are elevated, and SVR is high.

  b. To improve myocardial function when the SVR is elevated, whether systemic hypertension is present or not. The best results are often obtained with concomitant inotropic support.

  3. The usual **starting dose** is 0.1 µg/kg/min with a mix of 50 mg/250 mL. The bottle must be wrapped in aluminum foil to prevent metabolic breakdown from light. The dosage is gradually increased to a maximum of 8 µg/kg/min.

  4. Adverse effects

  a. Potentiation of myocardial ischemia from a reduction in diastolic perfusion pressure, shunting of blood from ischemic zones, or reflex tachycardia.

  b. Reflex increase in contractility and dp/dt that must be managed with β-blockers in a patient with an aortic dissection.

  c. Inhibition of hypoxic vasoconstriction, which produces ventilation-perfusion mismatch and hypoxia.

  d. Tachyphylaxis due to its vasodilating effects.

  e. Cyanide toxicity. SNP is metabolized to cyanide, which is then converted to thiocyanate in the liver. Cyanide toxicity, manifested by metabolic acidosis and an elevated mixed venous PO_2, may occur when large doses (> 8 µg/kg/min) are given for several days (cumulative dose > 1 mg/kg over 12–24 hours) or if hepatic dysfunction is present. Moderate cyanide toxicity is treated by converting the cyanide to thiocyanate for its excretion by the kidneys.

  i. Sodium bicarbonate for metabolic acidosis in doses of 1 mEq/kg.

    ii. Sodium thiosulfate 150 mg/kg IV (approximately 12.5 g in a 50-mL D5W solution given over 10 minutes)

   f. **Thiocyanate toxicity** (level > 5 mg/dL) may develop from chronic use of SNP, especially when there is impaired renal excretion of this metabolite. It is manifested by dyspnea, vomiting, and mental status changes with dizziness, headache, and loss of consciousness. **Management** of both severe cyanide and thiocyanate toxicity involves use of nitrite preparations to induce metHb formation. The metHb combines with cyanide to form cyanmethemoglobin, which is nontoxic.

    i. Amyl nitrite inhalation of 1 ampule over 15 seconds

    ii. Sodium nitrite 5 mg/kg IV slow push. This is usually given at a rate of 2.5 mL/min of a 3% solution to a total of 10–15 mL. One-half of this dose can be used subsequently if toxicity recurs.

    iii. Sodium thiosulfate in the dose noted above can then be administered to convert the cyanide that is gradually dissociated from cyanmethemoglobin into thiocyanate for excretion.

C. Nitroglycerin (NTG)

  1. Hemodynamic effects

   a. NTG is primarily a venodilator that lowers blood pressure by reducing preload, filling pressures, stroke volume, and cardiac output. If filling pressures are satisfactory, NTG will maintain aortic diastolic perfusion pressure, although at high doses some arterial vasodilatation does occur. In the presence of hypovolemia or a marginal cardiac output, NTG should be avoided because it lowers cardiac output further and produces a reflex tachycardia.

   b. NTG dilates coronary conductance vessels and improves blood flow to ischemic zones.[185]

  2. Indications

   a. **Hypertension** in association with myocardial ischemia or high filling pressures

   b. ECG changes of **myocardial ischemia**

   c. **Coronary spasm** or prevention of radial artery spasm

   d. **Pulmonary hypertension,** to reduce RV afterload and improve RV function

   e. **Preoperative ischemia.** NTG is useful before revascularization to reduce preload while phenylephrine is used to maintain coronary perfusion pressure.

  3. Starting dose is 0.1 μg/kg/min with a mix of 50 mg/250 mL. The dose can be titrated up to 10 μg/kg/min. It must be administered through nonpolyvinylchloride tubing because polyvinylchloride tubing absorbs up to 80% of the NTG.

  4. Adverse effects. NTG is metabolized by the liver to nitrites, which oxidize Hb to metHb. Methemoglobinemia and impaired oxygen transport can occur if the patient receives excessive doses of IV NTG (over 10 μg/kg/min for several days) or has renal or hepatic dysfunction. The diagnosis is suggested by the presence of chocolate-brown blood and a lower oxygen saturation measured by oximetry than one would expect from the Pao_2. It can be confirmed by an elevated metHb level (> 1% of total hemoglobin). Symptoms (cyanosis, progressive weakness, and acidosis) are usually not noted until the metHb level exceeds 15–20%. The treatment is intravenous methylene blue 1 mg/kg of a 1% solution.[186]

D. β-blockers

    1. Hemodynamic effects

        a. In contrast to the vasodilating drugs, β-blockers reduce blood pressure primarily by their negative inotropic and chronotropic effects. They reduce contractility, lowering the stroke volume and cardiac output, and also slow the heart rate by depressing the sinoatrial (SA) node. Their antihypertensive activity may also be attributable to a decrease in central sympathetic outflow and suppression of renin activity.

        b. β-blockers slow AV conduction and can precipitate heart block. Pacemaker backup should be available when IV β-blockers are given. This electrophysiologic effect is beneficial in reducing the ventricular rate response to atrial tachyarrhythmias.

    2. Indication. β-blockers can be used to control postoperative systolic hypertension associated with a satisfactory cardiac output. They are especially beneficial in the hyperdynamic, tachycardic heart that is often noted in patients with normal preoperative LV function and/or LVH. **Note:** Intravenous β-blockers should be avoided in hypertensive patients with compromised cardiac output.

    3. Esmolol is a cardioselective, ultrafast, short-acting β-blocker with an onset of action of 2 minutes, reaching a steady-state level in 5 minutes, and with reversal of effect in 10–20 minutes.[187] Because of its very short duration of action, esmolol is the β-blocker of choice in the ICU for transient hypertension control in the patient with a satisfactory cardiac output.

        a. Esmolol must be used with extreme caution when the patient is hypertensive but has a marginal cardiac output. Frequently, blood pressure and cardiac output are maintained by fast heart rates at low stroke volumes. Use of esmolol in this circumstance will often reduce blood pressure and cardiac output by a negative inotropic effect with little reduction in heart rate. Even in patients with an excellent cardiac output, the reduction is blood pressure is generally more pronounced than the decrease in heart rate.

        b. Esmolol can be used safely in the patient with a history of bronchospasm because of its cardioselectivity.

        c. The recommended initial dosage is a 0.25–0.5 mg/kg load over 1 minute, followed by 50 μg/kg/min over 4 minutes. Because patients tend to be very sensitive to esmolol in the immediate postoperative period, a smaller test dose should be considered to determine its effect on heart rate and blood pressure. If an adequate antihypertensive effect is not achieved, a repeat loading dose is given and a maintenance infusion of 100 μg/kg/min is given. Two more reloading doses can be given with additional 50 μg/kg/min increases in the maintenance infusion rate. Little additional effect is gained at doses over 200 μg/kg/min.

        d. The mix for continuous infusion is 2.5 g/250 mL.

    4. Labetalol has both α- and β-blocking properties as well as a direct vasodilatory effect. The ratio of β to α effects is 3:1 for the oral form and 7:1 for the intravenous form. In the postoperative cardiac surgical patient, IV labetalol reduces blood pressure primarily by its negative inotropic and chronotropic effects. The α-blocking effect prevents reflex vasoconstriction.[188]

    a. The onset of action for IV labetalol is rapid, with a maximal blood pressure response at 5 minutes for a bolus injection and 10–15 minutes for a continuous infusion. Since the approximate duration of action is 6 hours, labetalol is useful when a **longer-acting antihypertensive drug** is desired. It is a very useful medication for the patient with an **aortic dissection**, both pre- and postoperatively.

    b. Labetalol is given as a 0.25 mg/kg bolus over 2 minutes with subsequent doses of 0.5 mg/kg every 15 minutes until effect is achieved (to a total dose of 300 mg).

    c. Alternatively, a continuous IV infusion can be given at a rate of 1–4 mg/min, mixing 40 mL of the 5 mg/mL solution in 160 mL (200 mg/200 mL).

  5. **Metoprolol** is a cardioselective β-blocker that can be used for control of **hypertension** after surgery, but is usually given in oral form (25–50 mg PO bid) starting about 8 hours after surgery for AF prophylaxis. The primary indications for its intravenous use are control of **ischemia** and **slowing of the ventricular response to AF**. It is given in 5-mg increments every 5 minutes for up to three doses until effect is achieved. The onset of action is 2–3 minutes with a peak effect in 20 minutes, and a duration of action of up to 5 hours.

E. **Calcium channel blockers**

  1. **Hemodynamic effects**

    a. The calcium channel blockers are very effective for control of hypertension after surgery, primarily by relaxing vascular smooth muscle and producing peripheral vasodilatation. A variety of medications are available that have differing effects on cardiovascular hemodynamics and electrophysiology (Table 11.6). Use of these medications during the perioperative period has been shown to reduce the incidence of MI, ischemia, and supraventricular arrhythmias and may also improve survival.[189,190] However, they are usually used as adjuncts to other antihypertensive medications for selected indications.

    b. Other effects may include coronary vasodilatation, negative inotropy, a reduction in SA nodal automaticity (slowing the sinus mechanism), and slowing of AV nodal conduction (decreasing the ventricular rate response to atrial tachyarrhythmias).

  2. **Indications**

    a. Control of **hypertension when the cardiac output is satisfactory** or if there is evidence of myocardial ischemia. Nicardipine may be used if there is evidence of compromised ventricular function because it lacks a negative inotropic effect, but diltiazem and verapamil should be avoided in this situation because of their negative inotropic properties.

    b. **Coronary vasospasm**[191]

    c. **Slowing the ventricular response** to AF/atrial flutter (diltiazem, verapamil)

  3. **Nicardipine**

    a. Nicardipine reduces blood pressure by reducing the SVR. It lacks a negative inotropic effect, produces a minimal increase in heart rate, and has no effect on AV conduction.

Table 11.6 • Effects of Calcium Channel Blockers

	Nicardipine	Diltiazem	Verapamil	Nifedipine	Amlodipine
Inotropy	0	↓	↓↓	0↑	0
Heart rate	0↑	↓	↓	↑	0↑
AV conduction	0	↓↓	↓↓	0	0
Systemic resistance	↓↓	↓↓	↓↓	↓↓	↓↓
Coronary vascular resistance	↓↓	↓↓	↓↓	↓↓	↓↓

0, no effect.

   b. Indications
     i. It is very effective and safe in controlling postoperative hypertension and may provide more stable BP control than SNP.[192] An advantage over other calcium channel blockers is that it has no negative inotropic effect and has been shown to decrease the extent and duration of myocardial ischemia after CABG in comparison with NTG.[193]
     ii. Nicardipine has been used to prevent radial artery spasm in a dosage of 0.25 μg/kg/min.[194] However, one study of preexisting vasospasm in coronary artery conduits found that nicardipine added to NTG caused no more dilatation than NTG alone.[191]
   c. Advantages over SNP[195]
     i. Nicardipine improves cardiac output with less reduction in filling pressures than SNP (which also causes venodilatation), thus necessitating less volume infusion.
     ii. It avoids the reflex tachycardia and coronary steal that could lead to myocardial ischemia.
     iii. It is a potent coronary vasodilator that may improve the distribution of blood flow to ischemic zones.
   d. Disadvantages
     i. Nicardipine has a rapid onset of action (1–2 minutes) but a longer duration of action than SNP, with an elimination half-life of 40 minutes. Although it can be titrated for optimal control of hypertension, the longer half-life could be problematic in the hemodynamically unstable patient.
     ii. It increases ventilation/perfusion mismatch and can produce hypoxemia.
   e. The dose is 2.5 mg over 5 minutes, repeated every 10 minutes to a total dose of 12.5 mg. An infusion of 2–4 mg/h is then begun, using a 50 mg/250 mL mix.

4. **Diltiazem**

  a. Diltiazem reduces systemic blood pressure by lowering the SVR. However, it also depresses systolic function by exerting a negative inotropic effect and slows the heart rate. Thus, it should be avoided if the cardiac output is marginal. Nonetheless, the slowing of a tachycardia in a patient with a satisfactory cardiac output may be beneficial in improving myocardial oxygen metabolism.[196]

  b. Indications

   i. Slowing the ventricular response to AF. Diltiazem slows AV conduction and can produce heart block; therefore, pacemaker backup must be available when it is administered intravenously. **Note:** The patient's blood pressure and cardiac output are often marginal when AF develops, and there is often reluctance to use diltiazem for rate control. However, a reduction in ventricular response usually improves stroke volume and blood pressure. If the blood pressure is marginal, a pure α-agent may be given. If the blood pressure is unacceptably low, then cardioversion should be performed.

   ii. Prevention of **arterial graft spasm** (specifically, the radial artery)

   iii. Management of **coronary artery spasm** (diltiazem is a potent coronary vasodilator)

   iv. Systemic hypertension, especially if being used primarily to prevent spasm (radial artery conduits) or manage AF. It may be used as an adjunct to other antihypertensive medications if blood pressure remains elevated.

  c. IV dosage is a 0.25 mg/kg bolus over 2 minutes, which may be followed by a repeat bolus of 0.35 mg/kg 15 minutes later. A continuous infusion is then given at a rate of 5–15 mg/h with a 250 mg/250 mL mix.

5. **Verapamil**

  a. Verapamil reduces systemic blood pressure by lowering SVR, but it also has moderate negative inotropic, chronotropic, and dromotropic effects that depress contractility, slow the heart rate, and depress AV conduction. In the early postoperative period, indications for its use are similar to those of diltiazem.

  b. IV dosage is a 0.1 mg/kg IV bolus followed by 2–5 μg/kg/min continuous infusion of a 120 mg/250 mL mix.

6. **Nifedipine** is a potent arterial vasodilator that lowers blood pressure by reducing SVR. This is frequently accompanied by a baroreceptor-mediated reflex tachycardia and a slight reflex increase in cardiac inotropy and AV conduction. In comparison with SNP, an IV infusion of nifedipine produces a more significant increase in cardiac output and a greater decrease in SVR, and does not lower preload due to the absence of venodilator effects.[197] Nifedipine is also a potent coronary vasodilator and thus is beneficial in managing **coronary spasm**.[191] It also reduces PVR and PA pressures. Although there are a few reports of its use in intravenous form for control of postoperative hypertension, this is not a common practice. It is primarily given sublingually or orally in a dosage of 10–30 mg q4h.

7. **Amlodipine** reduces SVR and blood pressure and may improve cardiac output due to a decrease in afterload. It has no negative inotropic effects and no

effect on the SA node or AV nodal conduction. It produces a gradual decrease in blood pressure that persists for 24 hours after an oral dose. Thus, it is indicated for the long-term control of hypertension in the stable patient. It is given in doses of 2.5–10 mg qd.

F. Enalaprilat is an intravenous ACE inhibitor. It inhibits activation of the renin-angiotensin system and blunts the increase in other vasoactive substances that normally rise with CPB (catecholamines, endothelin, and atrial natriuretic peptide).[198,199]

1. **Enalaprilat** reduces blood pressure by producing balanced arterial and venous vasodilatation without a reflex increase in heart rate. It thus reduces preload and afterload and reduces myocardial oxygen demand. It also does not produce hypoxic vasoconstriction and has no effect on gas exchange and oxygen delivery. This drug can be considered in the hemodynamically stable patient with hypertension and depressed ventricular function who is unable to tolerate oral medications. It has been shown to improve cardiac and renal function in patients with LV dysfunction even when hypertension is not present. It can subsequently be converted to the oral form of enalapril 5 mg qd (half this dose if creatinine clearance is < 30 mL/min) or other oral ACE inhibitors.

2. **Dosage**: Enalaprilat is given in a bolus dose of 0.625–1.25 mg IV over 5 minutes q6h, which produces an initial clinical response in 15 minutes with a peak effect in 4 hours. Some studies have used higher bolus dosages (0.06 mg/kg) or a continuous infusion of 1 mg/h with a doubling of the dose every 30 minutes until effect is achieved (to a total dose of 10 mg).[198-200]

G. **Hydralazine**

1. Hydralazine is a direct arteriolar vasodilator that decreases SVR and systemic blood pressure. The reduction in afterload may improve myocardial function but is usually accompanied by a compensatory tachycardia.

2. **Indication**: Hydralazine is most commonly used as a substitute for potent IV antihypertensive medications if the patient is hemodynamically stable but remains **hypertensive several days after surgery.** It is beneficial when the patient **cannot take or absorb oral medications** or if toxicity from or resistance to other IV antihypertensive medications develops.

3. The usual dosage is 20–40 mg IM q4h or 5 mg IV q15 minutes until effect. The onset of action after IV injection is about 5–10 minutes with a peak effect at 20 minutes and a duration of action of 3–4 hours. Thus, it is difficult to titrate and should not be used if the patient is hemodynamically unstable. However, a continuous infusion of 1.5 μg/kg/min has been used in postoperative cardiac patients with excellent reduction in afterload.[201]

H. **Fenoldopam mesylate**

1. Fenoldopam is a dopamine (DA_1) receptor agonist that is a rapid-acting peripheral and renal vasodilator. Its antihypertensive effect is accompanied by a reflex tachycardia, an increase in stroke volume index, and an increase in cardiac index.[202] It also lowers PVR, with potential theoretical benefits in patients with preexisting RV dysfunction. Its beneficial effect on renal function occurs because it dilates renal afferent arterioles, resulting in an increase in renal blood flow. It also produces hypokalemia, either through a direct drug effect or enhanced K^+-Na^+ exchange.

2. **Indication: Severe hypertension** when rapid onset of effect is necessary (although the duration of action is longer than that of SNP).[203] Limited studies suggest that it is an effective drug for use in post–cardiac surgical hypertension.

3. **Dosage**: Fenoldopam is given as a continuous infusion starting at 0.05–0.1 μg/kg/min using a 10 mg/250 mL mix. The dose may be increased in 0.05–0.1 μg/kg/min increments every 15 minutes until effect is achieved to a maximum of 0.8 μg/kg/min. The dosage used to provide a renoprotective effect (0.1 μg/kg/min) generally does not produce systemic hypotension. If a patient is receiving fenoldopam during surgery for this reason, it could be used as the primary antihypertensive drug after surgery but is probably not cost-effective.

I. **Nesiritide** is a balanced arterial and venous vasodilator that is used primarily in patients with decompensated heart failure. In cardiac surgery patients, it may improve RV or LV function in patients with elevated PA pressures by virtue of its vasodilator effects. It is not primarily indicated for the treatment of systemic hypertension.

J. **Selection of the appropriate antihypertensive medication in the postoperative cardiac surgical patient**

1. When filling pressures are normal or slightly elevated and the cardiac output is marginal, an arterial vasodilator, such as **nitroprusside**, should be selected. It reduces preload and afterload by producing arterial (and some venous) dilatation and often improves cardiac output. Consideration should be given to using inotropic agents and vasodilators together to optimally augment cardiac function. **Nicardipine** reduces SVR without any negative inotropic or chronotropic effects and can be used effectively in this situation. Its longer duration of action may prove detrimental if used during a period of hemodynamic instability.

2. When filling pressures are high and the cardiac output is satisfactory, a venodilator, such as **nitroglycerin**, may be beneficial. This reduces venous return, filling pressures, stroke volume, cardiac output, and blood pressure. It may be beneficial if there is evidence of myocardial ischemia. However, NTG is best avoided when hypovolemia or a marginal cardiac output is present.

3. When the heart is hyperdynamic with adequate filling pressures, a high cardiac output, and frequently a tachycardia, medications with negative inotropic and chronotropic properties, such as **esmolol** or the calcium channel blockers (**diltiazem, verapamil**), should be selected. These medications are beneficial in improving myocardial oxygen metabolism, especially when there is evidence of ischemia.

4. Once the patient is able to tolerate oral medications, the IV medications should be tapered while the blood pressure is monitored for response to PO medications. It is most appropriate to restart the medications the patient was taking before surgery, but others should be considered under certain circumstances.

   a. β-blockers (metoprolol 25–75 mg PO bid) are initiated in virtually all patients to reduce the incidence of AF and to control blood pressure. Their use may be limited by slow heart rates.

   b. The next choice is usually an ACE inhibitor, such as lisinopril 5–10 mg PO qd. This should be considered for all patients with poor ventricular function (ejection fraction < 35%) but must be used cautiously in patients with renal dysfunction.

   c. The third choice is usually a calcium channel blocker, which is often used routinely for patients receiving radial artery grafts.

   d. In patients with bradycardia, clonidine or an angiotensin receptor blocker can be chosen.

   e. Long-acting nitrates are alternative coronary vasodilators that can be used in patients receiving radial artery grafts and may also provide an antihypertensive benefit.

VIII. Cardiac Arrest

A. Cardiac arrest is a serious and dreaded complication of any cardiac operation that occurs with an incidence of approximately 2%. It can occur unexpectedly at the conclusion of surgery, during transport from the operating room, in the ICU, or later during convalescence on the floor. It must be managed immediately by standard advanced cardiac life support (ACLS) protocols and, if not immediately successful, by open-chest massage. Prompt and aggressive cardiopulmonary resuscitation (CPR) is essential to restore satisfactory cardiac function and hopefully prevent severe neurologic sequelae from compromising the results of a successful CPR.[204] The mortality rate for patients sustaining a cardiac arrest after cardiac surgery is approximately 30%. Survival is most likely when an arrhythmia or bleeding is the predisposing cause; patients arresting from pump failure rarely survive.[205]

B. Basic and ACLS recommendations should be followed:

   A: Establish an **airway**

   B: Provide **breathing** with positive-pressure ventilation (15–20/min)

   C: Provide **circulation** by chest compressions (100/min); place intravenous lines if not present

   D: Defibrillate for VF/pulseless ventricular tachycardia (VT)

C. **Etiology and assessment** (Table 11.7). An evaluation to determine the possible cause of a cardiac arrest should be undertaken as the resuscitation is underway.

   1. Listen to the chest, check the ventilator function, ABGs, acid-base, and electrolyte status. If the patient is not intubated, secure an airway first, administer oxygen, and then intubate. Do **not** try to intubate before delivering oxygen by face mask because this may prolong the period of hypoxemia.

     • Severe ventilatory or oxygenation disturbance (hypoxia, hypercarbia from pneumothorax, endotracheal tube displacement, acute pulmonary embolism)

     • Severe acid-base and electrolyte disturbances (acidosis, hypo- or hyperkalemia)

   2. Check the chest tube drainage and review the chest x-ray.

     • Acute impairment of venous return (tension pneumothorax, cardiac tamponade, occasionally with sudden cessation of massive bleeding)

     • Acute hypovolemia (massive mediastinal bleeding)

   3. Assess whether inotropes, vasopressors, and vasodilators are being administered at the correct rate.

     • Inadvertent cessation of inotropic support

     • Profound vasodilatation from bolusing of nitroprusside

Table 11.7 • Most Common Causes of Postoperative Cardiac Arrest

Cause	Treatment
Hypovolemia	Volume infusions
Hypoxia	Hand ventilation with 100% O_2
Hydrogen ion acidosis	Sodium bicarbonate
Hyperkalemia	Calcium chloride, glucose/insulin/ bicarbonate drip
Hypokalemia	KCl infusion
Hypothermia	Warming blankets
Tamponade	Pericardiocentesis, subxiphoid exploration, or emergency sternotomy
Tension pneumothorax	Needle decompression, chest tube
Thrombosis (myocardial infarction)	IABP, emergency cardiac catheterization
Thrombosis (pulmonary embolism)	Anticoagulation, embolectomy, IVC umbrella

Tablets:
  Drug overdose
  Digoxin
  β-blockers, calcium
    channel blockers
	
	Gastric lavage, activated charcoal
	Digibind
	Inotropic support, pacing

4. Examine the cardiac monitor and ECG.
   - Third-degree heart block (may occur spontaneously or if AV pacing fails in a patient with complete heart block)
   - Acute ischemia (graft thrombosis, coronary spasm)
   - Ventricular tachyarrhythmias (VT or VF)

C. **Treatment**
   1. **Hand ventilate** with 100% oxygen at a rate of 15–20/min; listen for bilateral breath sounds. Intubate after establishing an adequate airway if the patient is no longer intubated.
   2. Assess current rhythm from monitor:
      a. **VT or VF** necessitates immediate defibrillation with 200 joules; if unsuccessful, increase to 300 and then 360 joules.
      b. **Asystole**: turn on the atrial and/or ventricular pacing wires.

Table 11.8 • Drug Doses Used During Cardiac Arrest

Vasopressin	40 units IV push × 1 dose
Epinephrine	1-mg IV push, repeat doses q3–5 min
Amiodarone	300-mg IV push; can give 150 mg q5 min to total 2.2 g/24 h
Lidocaine	1–1.5 mg/kg bolus, followed by 0.5–0.75 mg/kg boluses every 5–10 min to total dose of 3 mg/kg
Magnesium sulfate	1–2 g in 10 mL D5W
Procainamide	20 mg/min up to total dose of 17 mg/kg

3. **Initiate external cardiac massage** at a rate of 100/min if unable to defibrillate or establish pacing within 30 seconds. Efficient massage can provide about 25% of the normal cardiac output. Massage can result in disruption of the sternal closure, injury to bypass grafts, or damage to the ventricular myocardium from prosthetic valves. This potential damage can be minimized if compressions are **delayed for a very short time** to prepare and use the defibrillator or attach the pacing wires to a pacemaker.

4. **Ventricular fibrillation and pulseless ventricular tachycardia**

   a. **Defibrillation** is essential for VF or pulseless VT and should be repeated with increasing energy levels (200, 300, 360 joules, if necessary).

   b. Initial medications (Table 11.8)
      • **Vasopressin** 40 units IV as a single dose provides comparable or superior efficacy to epinephrine in promoting return of spontaneous circulation.[206]
      • **Epinephrine** 1 mg IV push (10 mL of 1:10,000 solution) should be given if VT/VF persists or recurs after three attempts at defibrillation. It may be repeated every 3–5 minutes.

   c. Antiarrhythmic drugs may improve the success of defibrillation and should be used for persistent/recurrent VT/VF or malignant ventricular ectopy. Defibrillation should be repeated after each dose of medication.
      • **Amiodarone** should be given first in a bolus dose of 300 mg; a dose of 150 mg may be repeated every 3–5 minutes to a maximum of 2.2 g IV/24 h. It is then given as an infusion of 1 mg/min for 6 hours, then 0.5 mg/min for 18 hours with conversion to oral dosing if necessary.[207]
      • **Lidocaine** may be given for refractory VT/VF as a 1–1.5 mg/kg bolus followed by 0.5–0.75 mg/kg boluses every 5–10 minutes to a total dose of 3 mg/kg.
      • **Magnesium sulfate** 1–2 g in 10 mL of D5W IV may be helpful for refractory VF or torsades de pointes, especially if hypomagnesemia is suspected.

- **Procainamide** may also be given for refractory VF. Give 20 mg/min IV until the arrhythmia is suppressed, hypotension occurs, the QRS complex widens to 50% of its original width, or a total dose of 17 mg/kg is given.

d. **Note:** If cardiac arrest occurs away from the ICU setting and intravenous access is not immediately available, lidocaine and epinephrine are very effective when given down an endotracheal tube. Two to 2.5 times the usual IV dose should be diluted in 10 mL of normal saline.[208]

5. **Asystole** that is unresponsive to epicardial pacing.

- Attempt **transcutaneous pacing.**
- **Epinephrine** bolus 1 mg IV (10 mL of a 1:10,000 solution) every 3–5 minutes; an infusion of 2–10 µg/min can be used for bradycardia.
- **Atropine** 1 mg IV with repeat doses of 1.0 mg every 3–5 minutes to a total dose of 0.04 mg/kg.

6. **Bradycardia** that is unresponsive to epicardial pacing

- **Atropine** 1 mg IV with repeat doses of 0.5–1.0 mg every 3–5 minutes to a total dose of 0.04 mg/kg
- Attempt **transcutaneous pacing.**
- **Dopamine** 5–20 µg/kg/min (200 mg/250 mL mix)
- **Epinephrine** 2–10 µg/min (1 mg/250 mL mix)
- **Isoproterenol** infusion 2–10 µg/min (2 µg = 30 drops/min of a 1 mg/250 mL mix)

7. **Pulseless electrical activity** refers to a variety of rhythms that are associated with no detectable blood pressure (including electromechanical dissociation). It is therefore important to palpate for a pulse and not to be deceived by pacing spikes or the patient's QRS complex on the monitor, which may represent isolated electrical activity without any effective myocardial contraction. **Epinephrine** 1 mg IV (10 mL of a 1:10,000 solution) should be given. Common contributing factors are listed in Table 11.7.

8. **Persistent hypotension.** Reestablishment of satisfactory myocardial blood flow is the most important element in a successful resuscitation. Because coronary perfusion occurs during compression "diastole" (i.e., when the aortic pressure exceeds the right atrial pressure), elevation of SVR and coronary perfusion pressure is critical. This is best achieved with medications that have predominantly α effects (epinephrine, norepinephrine) or strong vasoconstrictor properties (vasopressin).

9. **If the patient cannot be resuscitated within 5–10 minutes of cardiac arrest, open-chest massage should be strongly considered** (see pages 284–285). Internal cardiac massage is nearly twice as effective as closed-chest compressions in increasing forward blood flow.

10. **Controversial medications during cardiac arrest**

a. **Sodium bicarbonate** should not be given routinely for the attended arrest during which excellent ventilation and cardiac compressions are achieved. Administration of sodium bicarbonate can depress cerebral and myocardial function, reduce SVR, exacerbate central venous acidosis, inactivate catecholamines administered simultaneously, and impair oxygen release to tissues. Its use should be guided by the results of ABGs drawn every 10 minutes during the arrest. It is given in doses of 1 meq/kg, with half the dose readministered 10 minutes later if ABGs are not available.

b. **Calcium chloride** 2 mL of a 10% solution (about 2–4 mg/kg) can be given for hypocalcemia, hyperkalemia, or persistent calcium channel blockade. Calcium may otherwise contribute to intracellular damage during periods of ischemia, and it is not routinely recommended during a cardiac arrest.

IX. Perioperative Myocardial Infarction

A. Although the current surgical population is older, has more left main and diffuse multivessel coronary disease, and has more urgent indications for surgery, the risk of developing a perioperative myocardial infarction (PMI) is less than 5%. This can be attributed to improvements in myocardial protection, use of off-pump surgery, and refinements in surgical technique. Depending on its extent, a PMI may be of little consequence to the patient or it may result in a low output state or malignant arrhythmias. Generally, a hemodynamically significant infarction results in increased perioperative mortality and reduced long-term survival, whereas one that is diagnosed enzymatically does not.[209–212]

B. **Predisposing factors**[213]

1. Left main or diffuse three-vessel disease

2. Preoperative ischemia or infarction. This includes acute coronary syndromes, including a non–ST-segment MI diagnosed by positive troponin levels, or evidence of ongoing ischemia, often following a failed percutaneous coronary intervention.

3. Poor LV systolic and diastolic function (low ejection fraction, CHF, LVEDP > 15 mm Hg, LVH)

4. Reoperations, which predispose to atheroembolism of debris or to graft thrombosis

5. Coronary endarterectomy

6. Long aortic cross-clamp period

C. **Mechanisms**

1. Prolonged ischemia during anesthetic induction or before the establishment of coronary reperfusion. This is usually caused by tachycardia, hypertension/hypotension, or ventricular distention, but may occasionally result from acute thrombosis of a critically narrowed artery or stenotic vein graft at reoperation.

2. Ischemia/reperfusion injury following cardioplegic arrest or inadequate myocardial protection. Research into the biochemical mechanism of PMI suggests that this insult is caused by activation of the Na^+-H^+ exchanger that leads to intracellular calcium accumulation, cell contracture, and cell death. Prophylactic use of a Na^+-H^+ exchange inhibitor, such as cariporide, in the perioperative period has been shown to reduce the incidence of PMI.[214]

3. Incomplete revascularization, including graft flow problems from anastomotic stenosis or graft thrombosis

4. Coronary vasospasm

5. Coronary air or particulate embolization (usually from patent but atherosclerotic vein grafts during reoperations)

D. Diagnosis. The diagnosis of a PMI is usually entertained by the combination of new ECG changes (new Q waves or ST changes), evidence of new regional or global wall motion abnormalities by echocardiography, and elevation of cardiac specific markers. However, several factors must be considered before concluding that myocardial necrosis has occurred.

1. Severe postcardiotomy ventricular dysfunction may suggest the development of a PMI but often represents a prolonged period of reversible myocardial depression ("stunning") that can recover after several days of pharmacologic or mechanical support. However, the persistence of new regional wall motion abnormalities on serial evaluations is more consistent with the occurrence of a PMI.

2. New Q waves on the ECG are noted in about 5–8% of patients after surgery. Up to 25% of these may be false positives, representing areas of altered depolarization or unmasking of old infarcts. In these patients, the new Q wave is not associated with elevation in enzyme markers to levels consistent with myocardial necrosis and is not associated with an adverse outcome.[215] The presence of ST-segment depression, deep T wave inversions, ventricular tachyarrhythmias, or a new bundle-branch block that persists for over 48 hours suggests some degree of myocardial injury, but each is a nonspecific indicator of PMI. T wave inversions, in particular, are occasionally noted several weeks after surgery when there has been no other evidence of PMI.

3. Creatine kinase myocardial band (CK-MB) levels are elevated in more than 90% of patients undergoing CABG. They can be elevated by atriotomy or ventriculotomy incisions, myocardial trauma, reperfusion VF, reperfusion of severely ischemic zones, and, in fact, by autotransfusion of shed mediastinal blood.[216]

   a. A PMI is generally diagnosed by a CK-MB level that exceeds 10 times the upper limit of normal (ULN) or when it exceeds 5 times the ULN in association with new Q waves.[209,217] CK-MB isoforms (elevated CK-MB$_2$) and the MB$_2$/MB$_1$ ratio can also be used to provide an earlier and more precise diagnosis of PMI, but are not readily measured.[218]

   b. It should be noted that the 2004 STS database specifications define a PMI as a CK-MB that exceeds 5 times the ULN with or without new Q waves. It also defines a PMI occurring more than 24 hours postoperatively by at least one of the following criteria:
      i. Evolutionary ST-segment elevation
      ii. New Q waves in two or more contiguous leads
      iii. New left bundle-branch block (LBBB) on ECG
      iv. CK-MB greater than 3 times the ULN

4. Troponin I (TnI) is a myofibrillar protein that is a very sensitive and specific biochemical marker of myocardial cell injury. Levels in patients undergoing non-CABG open-heart surgery and those undergoing CABG without MI do not exceed 15 µg/L, peak at 12 hours, and return to normal after 5 days. However, TnI levels > 15–20 µg/L within 12 hours and > 35 µg/L at 24 hours are consistent with a PMI.[219–222] It should be noted that there is some increase in TnT levels after defibrillation of VF but minimal increase after cardioversion for AF.[223]

E. **Presentation and treatment**

1. **Intraoperative ischemia.** Identification of new regional wall motion abnormalities by TEE is a sensitive means of assessing intraoperative myocardial ischemia. These changes precede evidence of ischemia noted with Swan-Ganz monitoring (elevation of PA pressures) or the ECG (ST-segment elevation). Aggressive treatment to reduce myocardial oxygen demand and maintain perfusion pressure is essential to lower the risk of PMI. In patients undergoing reoperative surgery, avoiding manipulation of patent but diseased grafts is essential to prevent atheroembolism.

2. **Postcardiotomy low cardiac output syndrome with/without ECG evidence of ischemia.** Although the duration of aortic clamping correlates with the level of detected cardiac markers,[224] fastidious attention to myocardial protection should offset the adverse effects of prolonged cross-clamping. The occurrence of severe postcardiotomy ventricular dysfunction, whether caused by ischemia, "stunning," or an infarction, requires careful evaluation and management.

   a. If myocardial dysfunction or ischemia is noted in the operating room at the conclusion of CPB, the adequacy of the operative procedure should be assessed. Supplemental grafts or graft revision may be necessary. IABP or circulatory assist devices may be indicated.

   b. The incidence of asymptomatic postoperative ischemia has been reported to be as high as 50% and should draw attention to means for optimizing postoperative cardiac function while minimizing the increase in oxygen demand.[30]

   c. If ECG changes are detected upon arrival in the ICU, intravenous NTG or calcium channel blockers (if spasm is suspected) should be given. Placement of an IABP and emergency coronary angiography with possible percutaneous coronary intervention or surgical graft revision should be strongly considered.

   d. Management of a hemodynamically significant MI involves supportive care until arrhythmias and hemodynamic instability resolve. Cardiac output should be optimized in standard fashion, but care must be taken to avoid excessive volume infusions and tachycardia that may increase myocardial oxygen demand and worsen an ischemic insult. Use of inamrinone/milrinone or placement of an IABP will minimize oxygen consumption. It is difficult to manage the sinus tachycardia that is frequently present in low cardiac output states because it usually represents a compensatory mechanism to maintain cardiac output. Sinus tachycardia is frequently a sign of an "injured heart" and can perpetuate myocardial ischemia and damage.

3. **Good cardiac output but low SVR.** The patient sustaining a small PMI may have a normal cardiac output accompanied by systemic hypotension. This syndrome usually requires use of an α-agent for several days to maintain an adequate systemic blood pressure until SVR returns to normal.

4. **Persistent ventricular ectopy** may reflect ischemia, infarction, or reperfusion of previously ischemic muscle. It should be managed with lidocaine and standard oral antiarrhythmic medications. β-blockers are generally used for their antiarrhythmic effect in patients with preserved ventricular function. However, nonsustained or sustained VT occurring in patients with impaired ventricular

function often requires electrophysiologic testing, use of an antiarrhythmic (e.g., amiodarone), and placement of an implantable cardioverter-defibrillator (ICD).

5. Some patients have an infarction diagnosed by electrocardiographic, enzymatic, or functional criteria but have no clinical or hemodynamic sequelae. These patients do not require special treatment.

F. Prognosis

1. An uncomplicated infarction does not influence operative mortality or long-term survival. Despite a return of ventricular function to baseline, the heart may fail to demonstrate functional improvement during exercise.

2. In contrast, a hemodynamically significant MI (one presenting as a low cardiac output syndrome or malignant arrhythmias) increases operative mortality and decreases long-term survival.[209–212]

3. The prognosis following a perioperative infarction is determined primarily by the adequacy of revascularization and the residual ejection fraction. One study reported that the prognosis for patients sustaining an MI with an ejection fraction > 40% and with complete revascularization was comparable to patients not developing a perioperative infarction.[225]

X. Coronary Vasospasm

A. Vasospasm has become increasingly recognized as a cause of postoperative morbidity and mortality following coronary artery bypass grafting. It can affect normal coronary arteries, bypassed vessels, saphenous vein grafts, or arterial grafts (ITA, radial, gastroepiploic artery).[226,227]

B. **Etiology** is speculative, possibly related to increased α-adrenergic tone, release of platelet thromboxane A_2, hypothermia, hypomagnesemia, calcium infusions, or rebound from withdrawal of calcium channel blockers used preoperatively. It is more commonly noted in young women with small coronary arteries.

C. **Diagnosis** of spasm can be extremely difficult to make. It is generally manifested by:

1. ST elevation in multiple leads

2. Hemodynamic collapse (low cardiac output, hypotension)

3. Ventricular arrhythmias

4. Heart block

D. The differential diagnosis of the scenario of cardiovascular instability, arrhythmias, and ECG changes must include other potential problems, such as preexisting myocardial dysfunction or ventricular arrhythmias, myocardial ischemia or infarction, reperfusion injury, or graft stenosis or occlusion subsequent to an operation. Any of these is more likely to be present than vasospasm. Coronary angiography may be necessary to make the appropriate diagnosis if there is no response to therapy. Angiography will usually demonstrate sluggish flow through grafts, diffuse spasm, and poor flow into distal native vessels. Resolution of spasm with intracoronary NTG or a calcium channel blocker confirms the diagnosis. Differentiation from technical problems at the anastomosis can be difficult due to poor flow. If there is little response to pharmacologic manipulation, reexploration may be indicated.

E. **Treatment** involves hemodynamic support and initiation of medications that can reverse the vasospasm. If the patient does not improve and/or ECG changes persist, emergency cardiac catheterization is indicated to identify and often correct the problem.

1. Optimize oxygenation and correct acidosis.

2. Optimize hemodynamic parameters. If an inotrope is indicated, a PDE inhibitor is the best choice because it is a potent vasodilator of the ITA and perhaps of native vessels as well.[91,111]

3. Start **IV NTG** at 0.5 µg/kg/min and raise as tolerated.

4. Select a **calcium channel blocker:**

   a. Nifedipine 10 mg SL, then 30 mg per NG q6h.

   b. IV diltiazem drip: 0.25 mg/kg IV bolus over 2 minutes, followed by a repeat bolus of 0.35 mg/kg 15 minutes later. A continuous infusion is then given at a rate of 5–15 mg/h using a 250 mg/250 mL mix.

   c. IV verapamil drip: 0.1 mg/kg bolus, followed by a 2–5 µg/kg/min infusion of a 120 mg/250 mL mix.

   d. When taking PO: Imdur 30 mg qd, Isordil 20 mg q8h, nifedipine 30 mg q6h, or diltiazem CD 180 mg qd.

XI. Pacing Wires and Pacemakers

Two temporary right atrial and two right ventricular epicardial pacing wire electrodes are usually placed at the conclusion of all open-heart procedures. These pacing wires have both diagnostic and therapeutic utility.

A. **Diagnostic uses**. Atrial pacing wires can be used to record atrial activity in both unipolar and bipolar modes. With suitably equipped monitors, these recordings can be obtained simultaneously with standard limb leads to distinguish among atrial and junctional arrhythmias and differentiate them from more life-threatening ventricular arrhythmias. Simultaneous ECGs and atrial electrogram (AEG) tracings for each of the most commonly encountered postoperative arrhythmias are provided in the next section. The technique for obtaining atrial wire tracings is either of the following:

1. A multichannel recorder can be used to print simultaneous monitor ECGs and AEGs. Most current monitoring systems have cartridges with three leads for recording the AEG: two of them represent the arm leads and are connected with alligator clips to the atrial pacing wires; the third represents a left leg lead and is attached to an electrode pad over the patient's flank. When the monitor channel for the AEG is set on lead I, a bipolar AEG is obtained (Figure 11.8). This shows a large atrial complex and a very small or undetectable ventricular complex. When the AEG monitor channel is set on lead II or III, a unipolar AEG is obtained. This demonstrates a large atrial and slightly smaller ventricular complex.

2. When a standard ECG machine is used, the two arm leads are connected to the atrial wires with alligator clips, and the leg leads are attached to the right and left legs. A bipolar AEG will be recorded in lead I and a unipolar AEG in lead II or III. Alternatively, the atrial wires can be connected to the V leads. Bipolar AEGs give a better assessment of atrial activity than do unipolar AEGs and can distinguish between sinus tachycardia and atrial arrhythmias. However, because the AEG and standard ECG tracings are not obtained simultaneously, a unipolar tracing is required to differentiate sinus from junctional tachycardia

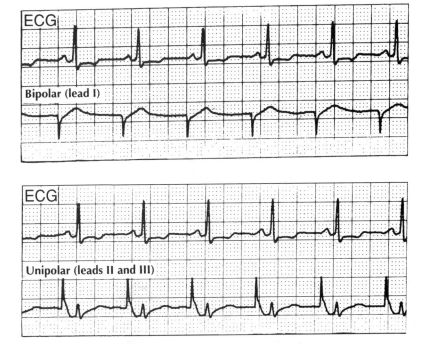

Figure 11.8 • Sinus rhythm in simultaneous monitor leads and AEGs. In the upper tracing, note that the bipolar AEG (lead I) produces predominantly an atrial complex with essentially no visible ventricular complex. In contrast, the unipolar tracing (leads II and III) on the bottom shows both a large atrial wave and a smaller ventricular complex.

because it can demonstrate the relationship between the larger atrial and smaller ventricular complexes.

B. Therapeutic uses

1. Optimal hemodynamics are achieved at a heart rate of around 90/min in the immediate postoperative period. Use of temporary pacing wires attached to an external pulse generator (Figure 11.9) to increase the heart rate is preferable to the use of positive chronotropic agents that have other effects on myocardial function. Atrial or AV pacing will nearly always demonstrate superior hemodynamics to ventricular pacing. Since AV delay is often prolonged after bypass, shortening it artificially using AV pacing can improve hemodynamics, especially in patients with impaired ventricular function.[228]

2. Reentrant rhythms can be terminated by rapid pacing. Rapid atrial pacing can terminate type I atrial flutter (flutter rate less than 350) and other paroxysmal supraventricular tachycardias. Rapid ventricular pacing can terminate VT.

C. Pacing nomenclature

1. The sophistication and reprogrammability of permanent pacemaker systems led to the establishment of a joint nomenclature by the North American Society of Pacing and Electrophysiology (NASPE) and the British Pacing

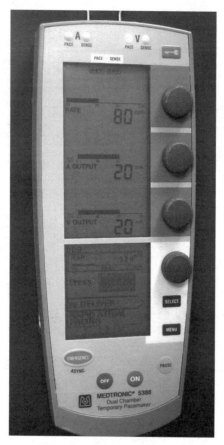

Figure 11.9 • The Medtronic model 5388 external pacemaker. This device can be used to provide pacing in a variety of modes, including AAI, DVI, DDD, and VVI pacing. It also has rapid atrial pacing capabilities. *(Image courtesy of Medtronic.)*

and Electrophysiology Group (BPEG). This nomenclature, referred to as the NBG code, classifies pacemakers by their exact mode of function (see Table 11.9).

2. Use of the first three letters is helpful in understanding the temporary pacemaker systems that are used after cardiac surgical procedures (Table 11.10). The most common modes are AOO (asynchronous atrial pacing), VVI (ventricular demand pacing), DVI (AV sequential pacing with ventricular demand), and DDD (AV sequential pacing with dual chamber sensing).

D. Atrial pacing

1. Atrial bipolar pacing is achieved by connecting both atrial electrodes to the pacemaker. This produces a smaller pacing stimulus artifact on a monitor than unipolar pacing and can often be difficult to detect even in multiple leads

Table 11.9 • NBG Pacemaker Identification Codes

| | Code Positions | | | |
I	II	III	IV	V
Chamber paced	Chamber sensed	Response to sensing	Programmable functions	Antitachyarrhythmia functions
V-ventricle	V-ventricle	T-triggers pacing	P-programmable rate and/or output	P-antitachyarrhythmia
A-atrium	A-atrium	I-inhibits pacing	M-multiprogrammable	S-shock
D-double	D-double	D-triggers and inhibits pacing	C-communicating functions (telemetry)	D-dual (pacer & shock)
0-none	0-none	0-none	R-rate modulation	0-none
S-single chamber	S-single chamber		0-none	

Table 11.10 • Temporary Pacing Modes Used After Heart Surgery

Code positions			Description
I	*II*	*III*	
A	O	O	Asynchronous atrial pacing
A	A	I	Atrial demand pacing
V	V	I	Ventricular demand pacing
D	V	I	AV sequential pacing (ventricular demand)
D	D	D	AV sequential pacing (both chambers sense)

A = atrium; V = ventricle; D = both chambers; O = does not apply

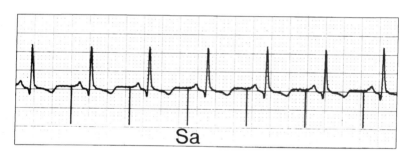

Figure 11.10 • Atrial pacing at a rate of 95/min. The atrial pacing stimulus artifact (Sa) is well seen in this tracing but is frequently difficult to identify on the monitor. The height of the atrial pacing spike may be increased on the monitor for better visualization, or it may be decreased to prevent problems with ECG interpretation or intraaortic balloon tracking.

(Figure 11.10). It does, however, prevent IABP consoles from misinterpreting large pacing spikes as QRS complexes.

2. Atrial pacing can also be achieved using transesophageal electrodes or a pacing catheter placed through "paceport" Swan-Ganz catheters. These are particularly beneficial during minimally invasive surgery.[229]

3. Pacing is usually accomplished in the AOO or AAI mode (Tables 11.9 and 11.10). The usual settings include a pulse amplitude of 10–20 mA in the asynchronous mode (insensitive to the ECG signal), set at a rate faster than the intrinsic heart rate. With the Medtronic Model 5388 external pacemaker, AAI demand pacing may be accomplished if atrial sensing is satisfactory.

4. **Indications**. Atrial pacing requires the ability to capture the atrium as well as normal conduction though the AV node. It is ineffective during AF/atrial flutter.

   a. Sinus bradycardia or desire to increase the sinus rate to a higher level

   b. Suppression of premature ventricular contractions: set at a rate slightly faster than the sinus mechanism

   c. Suppression of premature atrial complexes or prevention of AF (with dual-site atrial pacing)

   d. Slow junctional rhythm

   e. Overdriving supraventricular tachycardias (atrial flutter, paroxysmal atrial or AV junctional reentrant tachycardia). Rapid atrial pacing can interrupt a reentrant circuit and convert it to sinus rhythm or a nonsustained rhythm, such as AF, which may terminate spontaneously.

5. **Technique of overdrive pacing**

   a. Overdrive pacing is accomplished using pacemakers that can produce rates as high as 800 beats/min (see Figure 11.9). When attaching pacemaker wires to the generator, **be absolutely certain** that the atrial wires, not the ventricular wires, are being attached. Pacing initially 10–15 beats/min above the ventricular rate will confirm that the ventricle is not being paced, which can occur when atrial pacing wires are placed close to the ventricle.

   b. The patient must be attached to an ECG monitor during rapid atrial pacing. Bipolar pacing should be used to minimize distortion of the atrial complex. Pacing spikes are often best identified by evaluation of lead II.

   c. Turn the pacer to full current (20 mA) and to a rate about 10 beats faster than the tachycardia or flutter rate. When the atrium has been captured, increase the rate slowly until the morphology of the flutter waves changes (atrial complexes become positive). This is usually about 20–30% above the atrial flutter rate. Pacing for up to one minute may be required.

   d. The pacer should be turned off abruptly. Sinus rhythm, a pause followed by sinus rhythm, AF, or recurrent flutter may be noted (Figure 11.11). If severe bradycardia develops, the pacemaker may be turned on at a rate of around 60 until the sinus mechanism recovers.

E. **Atrioventricular pacing**

1. AV pacing is achieved by connecting both atrial wires to the atrial inlets and both ventricular wires to the ventricular inlets of an AV pacer (Figure 11.12). If two ventricular wires are not available or functioning, an atrial or skin lead can be used as a ground (the positive electrode) for ventricular pacing. The atrial and ventricular outputs are both set at 10–20 mA with a PR interval of 150 ms. Cardiac output can often be improved by increasing or decreasing the PR interval to alter ventricular filling time. The ECG will demonstrate both pacing spikes, although the atrial spike is often difficult to detect.

2. Current external pacemakers, such as the Medtronic model 5388, can pace in a variety of modes. The DDD mode senses atrial activity, following which the ventricle contracts at a preset time interval after the atrial contraction. This mode reduces the risk of triggering atrial, junctional, and pacemaker-induced arrhythmias. Careful monitoring is necessary in the event that the pacemaker tracks the atrial signal in AF/atrial flutter, resulting in a very fast ventricular response. However, setting an appropriate upper rate limit on these pacemakers

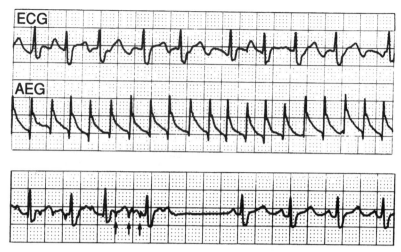

Figure 11.11 • Rapid atrial bipolar pacing of atrial flutter in sequential ECGs. The upper tracing confirms the rhythm as type I atrial flutter (rate 300/min) with variable AV block. In the lower tracing, rapid atrial pacing at a slightly faster rate entrains the atrium; the pacer is turned off and sinus rhythm resumes after a brief pause. The arrows indicate the atrial pacing stimulus artifact.

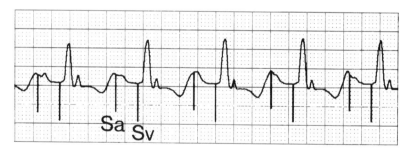

Figure 11.12 • Atrioventricular pacing at a rate of 100/min with a PR interval of about 160 ms. The P wave is often very poorly seen between the pacing stimulus artifacts. Sa = atrial; Sv = ventricular.

usually prevents this complication. Occasionally, a pacemaker-mediated tachycardia can develop from repetitive retrograde conduction from premature ventricular complexes (PVCs) that produces atrial deflections that are sensed and tracked.

3. If atrial activity is absent, either the DDD or DVI mode can be used. The DVI mode senses only the ventricle, so if a ventricular beat does not occur, both chambers are paced. This may lead to competitive atrial activity if the atrium is beating at a faster rate.

4. **Indications**
   a. Complete heart block
   b. Second-degree heart block to achieve 1:1 conduction
   c. First-degree heart block if 1:1 conduction cannot be achieved at a faster rate because of a long PR interval.

5. Additional comments
   a. Sequential AV pacing is ineffective during AF/atrial flutter.
   b. AV pacing is always preferable to ventricular pacing because of the atrial contribution to ventricular filling. This is especially important in noncompliant ventricles in which atrial contraction contributes up to 20–30% of the cardiac output.
   c. If sudden hemodynamic deterioration occurs during AV pacing, consider the possibility that AF has occurred with loss of atrial contraction. If AV conduction is slow, the ECG will demonstrate two pacing spikes with a QRS complex suggesting AV sequential pacing, although only ventricular pacing is occurring. This may be noted in the DDD mode with undersensing of AF or in the DVI mode in which the atrium is not sensed.

F. **Ventricular pacing**
   1. Ventricular pacing is achieved by connecting the two ventricular wires to the pulse generator for bipolar pacing or connecting one ventricular wire to the negative pole and an indifferent electrode (skin wire or an atrial wire) to the positive pole for unipolar pacing.
   2. The pacemaker is used in the VVI mode. The ventricular output is set at 10–20 mA in the synchronous (demand) mode. The rate selected depends on whether the pacemaker is being used for bradycardia backup, pacing at a therapeutic rate, or overdrive pacing (Figure 11.13). Ventricular pacing in the VOO or VVI mode with undersensing of native R waves may result in the delivery of an inappropriate spike on the T wave at a time when the ventricle is vulnerable, inducing ventricular tachyarrhythmias.
   3. **Indications**
      a. A slow ventricular response to AF or atrial flutter
      b. Failure of atrial pacing to maintain heart rate
      c. VT (overdrive pacing)

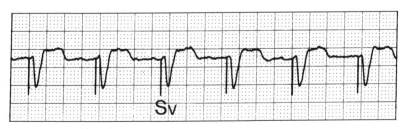

Figure 11.13 • Ventricular pacing at a rate of 80/min, demonstrating the wide ventricular complex. Since the patient's own mechanism is slower, the pacemaker produces all of the ventricular complexes. Sv = ventricular pacing stimulus artifact.

4. If a patient is dependent on AV or ventricular pacing, the pacing threshold must be tested. Gradually lower the **mA** until there is no capture. If the current necessary to generate electrical activity is rising or exceeds 10 mA, consideration should be given to placement of a transvenous pacing system (temporary or permanent).

5. If the pacemaker is in the demand mode, the sensing threshold should be checked. This determines the amplitude of the signal being measured in the chamber being sensed. Demand pacing relies on the native rhythm to determine when to pace. Undersensing results in inappropriate pacing, while oversensing inhibits pacing. To determine the sensing threshold, decrease the pacing rate to below the native rate and slowly decrease the sensitivity of the channel by increasing the sensing threshold (i.e., the amplitude below which the channel will not respond to a native signal). When an inappropriate pacing spike appears on the monitor or the "pacing" light begins to flash on the pacemaker when pacing should not be occurring, the sensing threshold will have been reached. **VT can be triggered by inappropriately sensing ventricular pacing wires.**

G. **Potential problems with epicardial pacing wires electrodes**

1. **Failure to function** may result from:

   a. Faulty connections of the connecting cord to the pacing wires or the pulse generator or a defective pacing cord

   b. Faulty pulse generator function (low battery)

   c. Undetected development of AF causing failure of atrial capture

   d. Electrodes located in areas of poor electrical contact and high threshold

   e. Undetected detachment of the wire electrode from the atrial or ventricular epicardium

2. **Options** to restore pacemaker function and reestablish a rhythm include:

   a. Checking all connections; changing the connecting cord

   b. Increasing the output of the pulse generator to maximal current (20 mA).

   c. Using a different wire electrode as the negative (conducting) electrode (reversing polarity)

   d. Unipolarizing the pacemaker by attaching the positive lead to a surface ECG electrode or skin pacing wire

   e. Converting to ventricular pacing if the atrial stimulus fails to produce capture

   f. Using a chronotrope (any of the catecholamines) to increase the intrinsic rate or possibly increase atrial sensitivity to the pacing stimulus

   g. Placing a transvenous pacing wire if the patient has heart block or severe bradycardia and is pacer-dependent

3. **Change in threshold**. The pacing threshold rises from the time of implantation because of edema, inflammation, or the formation of scar tissue near the electrodes. If an advanced degree of heart block persists for more than a few days, consideration should be given to the placement of a permanent transvenous pacemaker system.

4. **Oversensing problems**. If the atrial activity of AF/atrial flutter is sensed during DDD pacing, a very fast ventricular response will be noted. The upper rate limit should be programmed (i.e., lowered) to prevent this. If this is not

possible, the pacemaker should be converted to the VVI mode. Oversensing of T waves may lead to inhibition of VVI pacing.

5. **Competition with the patient's own rhythm**. When atrial or ventricular ectopy occurs during asynchronous pacing, suspect that the pacemaker is set at a rate similar to the patient's intrinsic mechanism. Turning off the pacemaker will eliminate the problem.

6. **Inadvertent triggering of VT or VF**. Use of ventricular pacing in the asynchronous mode can potentially trigger ventricular ectopy by competing with the patient's own mechanism. Appropriate sensing should always be confirmed if the pacemaker generator is left attached to the patient and is turned on. Ventricular pacing must always be accomplished in a demand mode (DVI, VVI, DDD). Pacing wires that are not being used should be electrically isolated to prevent stray AC or DC current near the wires from triggering VF. Wires should be placed in needle caps and left in accessible locations.

7. **Mediastinal bleeding** can occur if the pacing wires or the plastic carrier wire beyond the electrode (on Medtronic 6500 pacing wires) are placed close to bypass grafts, shearing them by intermittent contact during ventricular contractions. Bleeding from atrial or ventricular surfaces can occur if the wires are sewn too securely to the heart and excessive traction is applied for their removal. Pacing wires should generally be removed with the patient off heparin and before a therapeutic INR is achieved in patients receiving warfarin. The patient should be observed carefully for signs of tamponade for several hours after removal of epicardial wires.

8. **Inability to remove the wire electrodes from the heart**. The wire can be caught beneath a tight suture on the heart or, more likely, under a sternal wire or subcutaneous suture. Constant gentle traction, allowing the heart to "beat the wire loose" should be applied. A lateral chest x-ray may reveal where the wires are entrapped. If the wires cannot be removed, they should be pulled out as far as possible, cut off at the skin level, and allowed to retract. Infection can occur in pacing wire tracts, but it is unusual.

H. **Other temporary pacing modes**

1. Current defibrillator/monitors can provide transcutaneous pacing through gel pads attached to the patient's chest and back. This is most useful in emergency situations when epicardial pacing wires fail to function. This should not be relied on for more than a few hours because ventricular capture frequently deteriorates over time.

2. Placement of a 4–5F temporary transvenous ventricular pacing wire is indicated if the patient is pacemaker-dependent and the threshold of the epicardial wires is high or the wires fail to function. These wires are usually placed through an introducer in the internal jugular or subclavian vein. Several brands have balloon tips that assist in floating the pacing wire into the apex of the right ventricle, although fluoroscopy may occasionally be required.

3. Some Swan-Ganz catheters have extra channels that open into the right atrium and ventricle ("paceport catheters") through which pacing catheters can be placed. This is convenient during and following minimally invasive cardiac operations. It is also helpful in emergency situations since central venous access has already been

achieved. These pacing leads should not be relied on for chronic pacing in the pacemaker-dependent patient.

4. Transesophageal atrial pacing is valuable during minimally invasive procedures and can be used in the ICU on a temporary basis if AV conduction is preserved.[229]

I. Indications for permanent pacemakers

1. Although the temporary use of epicardial pacing is very common immediately after surgery, the vast majority of patients with preoperative normal sinus rhythm will achieve a satisfactory sinus rate within a few days. Permanent pacing is more likely in patients who are elderly, have preoperative bundle branch blocks, or undergo surgery requiring long durations of CPB or aortic cross-clamping, especially with suboptimal myocardial protection. It is more common following surgery during which there may be trauma to the conduction system such as valve operations, especially for endocarditis or reoperations, or ablative arrhythmia operations.[230,231]

2. If a permanent pacemaker is being strongly considered, oral anticoagulation, most commonly used for recurrent atrial fibrillation or a valve prosthesis, should be withheld. Intravenous heparin should be used for thromboembolism prophylaxis and stopped for several hours before and after the pacemaker has been implanted.

3. Patients in whom pacemaker placement is indicated following surgery include those with the following conditions:

   a. Complete heart block (usually following aortic valve surgery)

   b. Symptomatic or significant sinus node dysfunction, slow nodal mechanism, or slow ventricular response to atrial fibrillation (usually rates less than 50/min). The slow rate should be persistent after the discontinuation of medications, such as β-blockers, sotalol, calcium channel blockers, amiodarone, and digoxin, that are commonly used for either AF prophylaxis or treatment.

   c. Tachycardia-bradycardia syndrome (usually a fast response to paroxysmal atrial fibrillation but upon conversion to sinus rhythm with medications, a slow sinus mechanism)

   d. Advanced second-degree heart block with a slow ventricular response

4. The optional timing of the placement of a permanent pacemaker system has not been determined. In some patients, the indication may be transient and a delay in pacemaker implantation may obviate its need. However, this frequently prolongs the length of stay. Because of the low morbidity of pacemaker implantation, it may be more cost-effective to place the pacemaker after about 4–5 days to expedite the patient's discharge. A study from the Mayo Clinic showed that 40% of patients were not pacer-dependent at follow-up, although about 85% of patients requiring implantation for complete heart block became pacer-dependent.[230]

XII. Cardiac Arrhythmias

The development of cardiac arrhythmias following open-heart surgery is fairly common. A supraventricular arrhythmia, especially atrial fibrillation (AF), is noted in about 25% of patients. Ventricular arrhythmias are less common and usually reflect some degree of myocardial injury.

Whereas AF is usually benign, ventricular arrhythmias may warrant further evaluation and treatment because of their potentially life-threatening nature.

The mechanisms underlying the development of most arrhythmias are those of altered automaticity (impulse formation) and conductivity (impulse conduction). An understanding of these mechanisms and the electrophysiologic effects of the antiarrhythmic drugs has provided a rational basis for their use (see page 444). The management of arrhythmias commonly noted after open-heart surgery is summarized in Table 11.11.

A. **Etiology.** Although the factors that contribute to the development of various cardiac arrhythmias may differ, there are several common causes that should be considered.

1. Cardiac problems

    a. Underlying heart disease
    b. Preexisting arrhythmias
    c. Myocardial ischemia or infarction
    d. Poor intraoperative myocardial protection
    e. Pericardial inflammation

2. Respiratory problems

    a. Endotracheal tube irritation or misplacement
    b. Hypoxia, hypercarbia, acidosis
    c. Pneumothorax

3. Electrolyte imbalance (hypo- or hyperkalemia, hypomagnesemia)

4. Intracardiac monitoring lines (PA catheter)

5. Surgical trauma (atriotomy, ventriculotomy, dissection near the conduction system)

6. Drugs (digoxin, vasoactive medications, proarrhythmic effects of antiarrhythmic medications)

7. Hypothermia

8. Fever, anxiety, pain

9. Gastric dilatation

B. **Assessment**

1. Check the ABGs, ventilator function, position of the endotracheal tube, and chest x-ray for mechanical problems.

2. Check serum electrolytes (especially potassium).

3. Review a 12-lead ECG for ischemia and a more detailed examination of the arrhythmia. If the diagnosis is not clearcut, obtain an atrial electrogram (AEG). This is frequently beneficial in differentiating among some of the more common arrhythmias by providing an amplified tracing of atrial activity.

C. **Sinus bradycardia**

1. Sinus bradycardia is present when the sinus rate is less than 60/min. It is frequently caused by persistent β-blockade and the use of narcotics, and may result in atrial, junctional, or ventricular escape rhythms.

2. Because sinus bradycardia reduces cardiac output, the heart rate should be maintained around 90/min following the termination of CPB to optimize hemodynamics. An increase in heart rate can improve myocardial contractility and cardiac output.

Table 11.11 • Treatment of Common Arrhythmias

Arrhythmia	Treatment
Sinus bradycardia	Pacing: atrial or AV > ventricular Chronotropic medication
Third-degree heart block	Pacing: AV > ventricular Isoproterenol
Sinus tachycardia	Address cause β-blocker
Premature atrial complexes	No treatment Atrial pacing (preferably dual-site) Digoxin Procainamide β-blocker or sotalol Verapamil Magnesium sulfate

Atrial fibrillation	Cardioversion if hemodynamically compromised
	Rate control:
	  Diltiazem
	  β-blocker or sotalol
	  Digoxin
	Convert:
	  Amiodarone or procainamide
	  Sotalol
	  Propafenone/ibutilide
	  Electrical cardioversion
	V-pace if slow response

Atrial flutter	Cardioversion if compromised Rapid atrial pacing See atrial fibrillation
Slow junctional rhythm	Pacing (atrial > AV > ventricular) Chronotropic medication
Paroxysmal supraventricular tachycardias (PAT or AVNRT)	Atrial overdrive pacing Cardioversion Adenosine Verapamil/diltiazem β-blocker Digoxin

Nonparoxysmal AV junctional tachycardia	On digoxin: stop digoxin
	           potassium
	           phenytoin
	Not on digoxin: digoxin

Premature ventricular complexes	Treat hypokalemia Atrial overdrive pacing Lidocaine Procainamide
Ventricular tachycardia/fibrillation	Defibrillation Amiodarone Lidocaine Procainamide

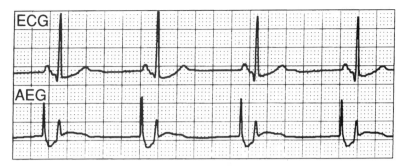

Figure 11.14 • Sinus bradycardia at a rate of 54/min recorded simultaneously in lead I and a unipolar AEG. The AEG demonstrates the larger atrial complex, a PR interval of 0.18 ms, and the smaller ventricular complex.

3. **Diagnosis.** See Figure 11.14.

4. **Treatment**

a. Atrial pacing should be used to take advantage of the 20–30% increase in stroke volume that results from the contribution of atrial filling. This is particularly important in the early postoperative period when reperfusion and myocardial edema impair ventricular compliance and cause diastolic dysfunction. Atrial contraction is especially important in patients with LVH, such as those with aortic valve disease or systemic hypertension.

b. AV pacing should be used if abnormal AV conduction is present with a slow ventricular rate (second- or third-degree AV block).

c. If pacing wires were not placed at the conclusion of surgery or if they fail to function, atropine 0.01 mg/kg IV (usually 0.5–1 mg IV) or one of the catecholamines can be used to stimulate the sinus mechanism. Either epinephrine 1–2 μg/min or isoproterenol 0.3–4 μg/min (starting at 5 microdrops/min of a 1 mg/250 mL mix) is often useful. However, these medications (as well as dopamine and dobutamine) not only increase the heart rate but have other hemodynamic effects as well.

d. Ventricular pacing can be used if the atrium fails to capture or there is little response to pharmacologic management. It will nearly always produce less effective hemodynamics than a supraventricular mechanism. If the ventricular pacing wires fail to function, the other pacing modes listed on page 417 can be considered.

e. Patients with known sick sinus or tachycardia-bradycardia syndrome often have problems with slow heart rates postoperatively and may require placement of a permanent pacemaker.

D. **Conduction abnormalities and heart block**

1. Transient disturbances of AV conduction are noted in about 25% of patients following coronary bypass surgery. They are more frequent when cold cardioplegic arrest is used for myocardial protection, especially when calcium channel blockers are used as additives.

a. Conduction abnormalities are more common in patients with compromised LV function, hypertension, severe coronary disease (especially involving the

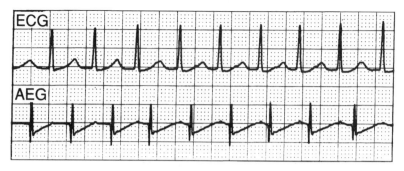

Figure 11.15 • First-degree AV block recorded simultaneously in lead II and a bipolar AEG. The PR interval is approximately 0.26 ms.

right coronary artery in a right-dominant system), long aortic cross-clamp periods, and extremely low myocardial temperatures. These findings suggest that ischemic or cold injury to the conduction system may be responsible for these problems. Although most resolve within 24–48 hours, the persistence of a new left bundle-branch block (LBBB) suggests the possible occurrence of a perioperative infarction.[232–234]

   b. Conduction abnormalities occurring after aortic valve replacement (AVR) may be caused by hemorrhage, edema, suturing, or debridement near the AV node and His bundle. Although persistent conduction abnormalities do not appear to influence the long-term prognosis after CABG,[234] LBBB is an ominous prognostic sign after AVR.[235]

   c. Exposure of the mitral valve by the biatrial transseptal approach involves division of the sinus node artery and anterior internodal pathways. Although some studies have not documented a higher incidence of postoperative rhythm disturbances, others have shown a high incidence of ectopic atrial rhythms, junctional rhythms, and varying degrees of heart block. Nearly 20% of patients may require a permanent pacer for bradycardia or complete heart block when this approach is used.[236,237]

2. **Diagnosis**. See Figures 11.15–11.19.

3. **Treatment**

   a. Use of both temporary atrial and ventricular pacing wires are invaluable in the management of heart block in the immediate postoperative period. Atrial wires alone would not be expected to be beneficial when AV conduction is impaired.

   b. **First-degree AV block** usually does not require treatment. If the PR interval is markedly prolonged, attempts to achieve faster atrial pacing will not achieve 1:1 conduction because the AV node will remain refractory when the next impulse arrives. This will produce functional second-degree heart block. AV pacing in the DDD or DVI mode can be used in this situation. Shortening a prolonged AV interval can significantly improve hemodynamics, especially in patients with impaired LV function.[228]

   c. **Second-degree AV block**

   i. Mobitz type I (Wenckebach) is characterized by progressive PR interval prolongation culminating in a nonconducted P wave (Figure 11.16).

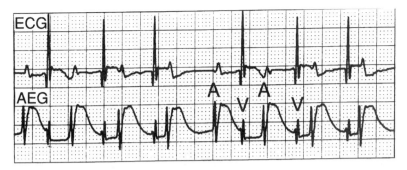

Figure 11.16 • Mobitz type I (Wenckebach) second-degree block. The unipolar AEG demonstrates a constant atrial rate of 120 with progressive lengthening of the A-V (PR) intervals until the ventricular complex is dropped. In the AEG, the atrial activity is represented by the larger of the two complexes. A = atrial complex; V = ventricular complex.

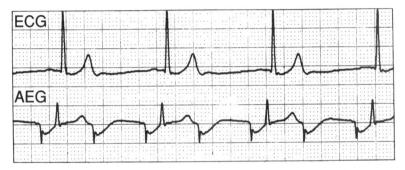

Figure 11.17 • High-grade second-degree block. Atrial activity is present at a rate of 100/min with 2:1 block, producing a ventricular rate of 50/min.

This usually does not require treatment unless the ventricular rate is slow. In this situation, it can be treated by AV pacing (DVI) at a slightly faster rate; if the atrial rate is too fast to overdrive, it can be treated by DDD pacing.

   ii. Mobitz type II is characterized by intermittent nonconducted P waves without progressive PR elongation. If the ventricular rate is too slow, AV pacing in the DVI or DDD mode should be used.

   iii. High-grade second-degree heart block is characterized by a constant PR interval with dropped QRS complexes in a mathematical relationship (2:1, 3:1) (Figure 1.17). It is treated in a similar fashion to Mobitz type II block.

  d. **Complete heart block** requires AV pacing in the DDD or DVI mode if there is atrial inactivity or a slow atrial rate (Figures 11.18 and 11.19). The DVI mode may increase the risk of developing AF if frequent PACs are present. The DDD mode is most beneficial in tracking a faster atrial rate and then providing a sequential ventricular contraction. Ventricular pacing

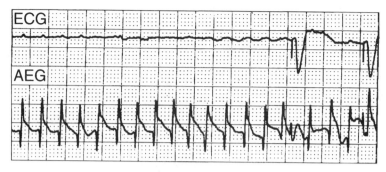

Figure 11.18 • Complete AV block. The AEG demonstrates type I atrial flutter, but the monitor ECG shows no ventricular complex until ventricular pacing is initiated.

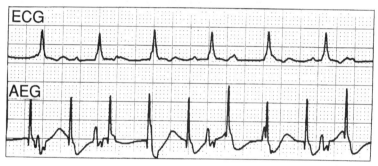

Figure 11.19 • Complete AV block with AV dissociation. The unipolar AEG demonstrates an atrial rate of 140 (large spikes) with no clear-cut relationship to the QRS complex, which represents a junctional mechanism at a rate of 100/min.

should be used if AF/atrial flutter is present. Pacing is usually not necessary when there is AV dissociation with an adequate junctional or idioventricular rate. However, it can be accomplished in the DDD mode if the atrial rate is not too fast.

e. If heart block persists, the patient's medications should be reviewed. β-blockers, calcium channel blockers, and digoxin should be withheld to assess the patent's intrinsic rate and conduction. If complete heart block persists for more than a few days with the patient off these medications, a permanent pacemaker system should be placed. Nonetheless, about 40% of patients in whom permanent pacemakers are placed are not dependent on their system at follow-up. The most significant predictor of pacemaker dependency is its insertion for complete heart block.[230]

E. **Sinus tachycardia**

1. Sinus tachycardia is present when the sinus rate exceeds 100 beats/min. It generally occurs at rates less than 130. A faster and regular ventricular rate

suggests the presence of paroxysmal supraventricular (atrial or junctional) tachycardia or atrial flutter with 2:1 block.

2. Fast heart rates are detrimental to myocardial metabolism. They can exacerbate myocardial ischemia by increasing oxygen demand and decreasing the time for diastolic coronary perfusion. They also reduce the time for ventricular filling and can reduce stroke volume, especially in patients with LVH and diastolic dysfunction.

3. **Etiology**

    a. Benign hyperdynamic reflex response related to sympathetic overactivity:
- Pain, anxiety, fever
- Adrenergic rebound (patient on β-blockers preoperatively)
- Drugs (catecholamines, pancuronium)
- Gastric dilatation
- Anemia
- Hypermetabolic states (sepsis)

    b. Compensatory response to myocardial injury or impaired cardiorespiratory status:
- Hypoxia, hypercarbia, acidosis
- Hypovolemia or low stroke volumes noted with small, stiff left ventricles with LVH and diastolic dysfunction
- Myocardial ischemia or infarction
- Cardiac tamponade
- Tension pneumothorax

4. **Diagnosis**. See Figure 11.20.

5. **Treatment**

    a. Correction of the underlying cause

    b. Sedation and analgesia

    c. β-blockers can be used if the heart is hyperdynamic with an excellent cardiac output. They must be used cautiously, however, when cardiac function is marginal. Tachycardia is a compensatory mechanism to maintain cardiac output when the stroke volume is low, and attempts to slow the

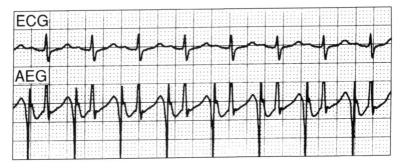

Figure 11.20 • Sinus tachycardia at a rate of 130/min on simultaneous recordings of monitor lead II and a unipolar AEG. Note the larger atrial and smaller ventricular complex in the unipolar AEG tracing, which demonstrates the 1:1 AV conduction.

heart rate may prove detrimental. Even when the cardiac output is satisfactory, β-blockers often lower the blood pressure significantly more than they reduce the heart rate.

   i. Esmolol 0.25–0.5 mg/kg IV over 1 minute followed by a continuous infusion of 50–200 μg/kg/min. A trial bolus of 0.125 mg/kg is frequently beneficial in determining whether the patient can tolerate esmolol.

   ii. Metoprolol 5 mg IV increments every 5 minutes for 3 doses

  d. Calcium channel blockers have mild negative chronotropic effects on the SA node, but they do not play a major role in the treatment of sinus tachycardia.

  e. Note: Both β-blockers and calcium channel blockers individually are safe to administer intravenously, but their simultaneous use should only be considered if functional pacing wires are present.

F. Premature atrial complexes

  1. Premature atrial complexes (PACs) are premature beats arising in the atrium that generally have a different configuration than the normal P wave and produce a PR interval that exceeds 120 ms. Although benign, they often herald the development of AF or atrial flutter, and this occurrence can be very difficult to prevent.

  2. Magnesium sulfate may be beneficial in reducing the incidence of PACs in the immediate postoperative period. The dose is 2 g in 100 mL solution.

  3. Diagnosis. See Figure 11.21.

  4. Treatment

   a. Patients with PACs generally do not need treatment, but because PACs frequently precede the development of AF, medications that can alter atrial automaticity and conduction or slow the ventricular response to AF can be considered. These include β-blockers, digoxin, and calcium channel blockers. Use of type IA antiarrhythmics (procainamide) slows atrial conduction but can accelerate AV conduction if atrial flutter develops.

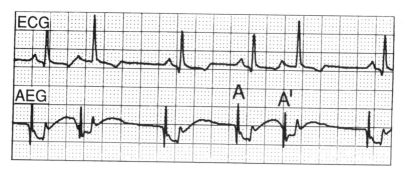

Figure 11.21 • Premature atrial complexes (PACs) in monitor lead II and a unipolar AEG. Note the slightly different morphology of the normal (A) and premature (A') atrial complexes and the slightly shorter PR interval following the PACs that indicates a focus different from the sinus node. The PR interval exceeds 120 ms, thus differentiating these beats from premature junctional complexes.

b. Digoxin is useful in decreasing the frequency of PACs and slows conduction through the AV node if AF does develop. However, by increasing conduction velocity in the atrium, digoxin can theoretically increase the risk of developing AF if PACs are present.

c. Temporary right atrial pacing at a faster rate ("overdrive pacing") may suppress PACs, but it may also trigger atrial arrhythmias and induce AF. This may occur even in the AAI mode when there is difficulty sensing atrial activity leading to inappropriate pacing. This problem generally does not occur with permanent dual-chamber pacemakers. If PACs occur during atrial pacing, one should suspect competition with the patient's own rhythm.[238] Dual-site atrial pacing may suppress PACs and also prevent AF.

G. **Atrial fibrillation or flutter**

1. Atrial fibrillation (atrial rate > 380) and atrial flutter (atrial rate generally < 380) are the most common arrhythmias noted after open-heart surgery. Despite various prophylactic measures to decrease their incidence, they still occur in about 25–30% of patients. The underlying mechanism is probably increased dispersion of repolarization, but predisposing factors have not been well identified. It has been proposed that there is a reversible trigger that causes AF in postoperative patients when there is an underlying electrophysiologic substrate for its development.[239]

2. The incidence of AF is greater in older patients, those with a history of atrial arrhythmias, lung disease (especially when requiring prolonged postoperative ventilation), right coronary artery stenosis, valve surgery, elevated preoperative BNP levels, increased P wave duration, and patients not receiving β-blockers after surgery. Technical considerations that may predispose to AF include venting through the right superior pulmonary vein, long cross-clamp times, more systemic hypothermia, division of the aortic anterior epicardial fat pad, and postoperative right atrial pacing.[240–243] The efficacy of off-pump coronary surgery in reducing the incidence of AF is controversial.[244,245]

3. The potential adverse effects of these rhythms are a compromise in cardiac hemodynamics and systemic thromboembolism from left atrial thrombus.[246] Because of the resources required to manage AF once it occurs, it has a substantial impact on hospital costs.

4. These arrhythmias occur most commonly on the second and third postoperative day. By that time, myocardial function has recovered to baseline and few adverse hemodynamic effects are noted. However, when atrial tachyarrhythmias occur during the first 24 hours, when the patient is hemodynamically unstable, or in patients with noncompliant hypertrophied ventricles, a rapid ventricular response can precipitate ischemia and lower cardiac output by eliminating the atrial contribution to ventricular filling.

5. After the initial 24 hours, AF is frequently an incidental finding on the ECG monitor. Symptoms such as palpitations, nausea, fatigue, or light-headedness may be noted, especially in patients with LVH or poor ventricular function.

6. **Etiology**

a. Enhanced sympathetic activity ("hyperadrenergic state") or adrenergic rebound in patients taking β-blockers preoperatively

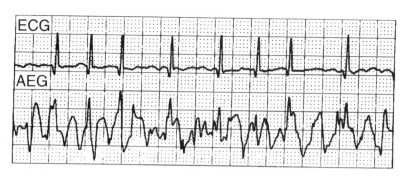

Figure 11.22 • Atrial fibrillation with a ventricular response of 130/min. The AEG demonstrates the chaotic atrial activity that is characteristic of atrial fibrillation.

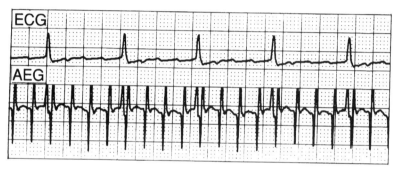

Figure 11.23 • Atrial flutter with 4:1 AV block. The unipolar AEG demonstrates an atrial rate of about 300 with a ventricular response of about 75/min.

      b. Atrial ischemia from poor myocardial preservation during aortic cross-clamping

      c. Atrial distention from fluid shifts

      d. Surgical trauma or pericardial inflammation

      e. Metabolic derangements (hypoxia, hypokalemia, hypomagnesemia)

7. Diagnosis. See Figures 11.22 and 11.23.

8. Prevention

      a. Initiation of low-dose β-**blockers** starting within 12–24 hours of surgery is effective in lowering the incidence of AF.[247–253] Metoprolol 25–50 mg bid or atenolol 25 mg qd is most commonly used. The addition of digoxin to one of the β-blockers may increase efficacy, although digoxin alone is not effective because early postoperative AF is usually caused by a hyperadrenergic state.[254] In fact, digoxin may render the atrium more susceptible to the development of AF because it increases atrial excitability and conduction velocity, reduces the atrial refractory period, and increases the number of fibrillatory wavelets.

      b. **Sotalol** is a β-blocker with class III antiarrhythmic properties that, at a dose of 80 mg bid, is more effective than standard β-blockers in preventing supraventricular tachyarrhythmias.[255,256] However, it is a negative inotrope and is not tolerated in about 20% of patients, in whom hypotension, bradycardia, or AV block may develop. Sotalol may also cause QT prolongation and polymorphic ventricular arrhythmias, including torsades de pointes. It is excreted by the kidneys and should probably be avoided in patients with renal dysfunction.

c. **Amiodarone** is a class III antiarrhythmic with some class I, II, and IV properties. It is effective in reducing the incidence of AF, either when given alone (if β-blockers are contraindicated) or in conjunction with β-blockers.[257–264] It is as effective as sotalol but more effective than propranolol.[257,258] The timing (pre-, intra-, or postoperative), route (IV vs. PO), and dosage of amiodarone that provide the best prophylaxis are unknown because different regimens have been used in virtually all studies. The most cost-effective approach is probably one that starts amiodarone the day of surgery and continues it for several days postoperatively. An acceptable dosing regimen for amiodarone is similar to that recommended for other indications: a 150-mg IV load over 15 minutes, followed by a 60 mg/h infusion × 8 hours, then 30 mg/h × 16 hours, then 400 mg po bid for 1 week. The drug is stopped at the time of hospital discharge if effective for prophylaxis. If the patient develops intermittent AF and converts, the drug may be continued for several weeks, with the dosage being weaned down to 200 mg qd, and stopped after 4–6 weeks. Amiodarone may be particularly beneficial in patients with COPD, in whom the incidence and morbidity of AF are greater.[265] However, the potential for acute amiodarone toxicity that can produce hypoxemia must be kept in mind.[266]

d. **Magnesium sulfate** (2 g in 100-mL doses) is arguably effective in decreasing the number of episodes of postoperative AF.[267–271] It appears to be most effective when given with a β-blocker, such as sotalol, and when the serum magnesium level is low.[271–273] Since its administration is benign and of potential benefit, it is worthwhile administering to all patients during surgery and on postoperative day 1 in addition to β-blockers.

e. Dual-site **atrial pacing** has been shown in numerous studies to reduce the incidence of AF.[274–276] In one study that showed no overall benefit, the incidence of AF was reduced in patients receiving concomitant β-blockers.[277] It is theorized that intraatrial conduction delays may contribute to AF. Dual-site pacing alters the atrial activation sequence and may achieve more uniform electrical activation of the atria. It may also overdrive suppress PACs, eliminate compensatory pauses after PACs, and reduce the dispersion of refractoriness that may contribute to AF.[239]

f. The efficacy of numerous other medications in preventing AF has been studied. Propafenone (300 mg bid) was found to be as effective as atenolol.[278] Procainamide was also found to be effective.[279] Triiodothyronine 0.8 μg/kg (about 50–80 μg) at the time of removal of the cross-clamp with a 6-hour infusion of 0.113 μg/kg/h (8–11 μg/h) has been shown to halve the rate of AF, but it is very expensive and rarely used.[105] Other medications, including digoxin alone, verapamil, and diltiazem have not been uniformly efficacious.[253]

9. **Management** of the unstable patient initially involves cardioversion, whereas for the stable patient, the plan involves rate control, anticoagulation if AF persists, and attempts to achieve conversion to sinus rhythm (Box 11.4). An attempt should be made to achieve conversion because most patients will subsequently remain in sinus rhythm and not require long-term use of medications. This is in contradistinction to patients not undergoing cardiac surgery in whom a rate-controlled strategy has similar survival results but potentially fewer adverse effects than attempts to achieve rhythm control.[280]

   a. **Electric cardioversion** with 50–100 joules can be used in a variety of circumstances.

      i. Cardioversion should always be considered first if there is evidence of significant hemodynamic compromise. This is more common in the early postoperative period when a very rapid ventricular response may be present and myocardial function is moderately depressed from surgery. It is also more likely to have adverse effects in patients with significant LVH. **Note:** There is an increased risk of precipitating malignant ventricular arrhythmias if cardioversion is attempted when the digoxin level is significantly elevated, especially if hypokalemia or hypercalcemia is also present.

      ii. If a patient fails to convert to normal sinus rhythm (NSR) with medications after 24–36 hours, cardioversion can be performed so that anticoagulation can be avoided. If more than 36 hours has elapsed and anticoagulation has not been given, preliminary TEE should be considered to rule out left atrial thrombus before performing cardioversion.[281–283] The decision to continue warfarin for one month after delayed cardioversion must be considered because de novo thrombus may form due to mechanical atrial inactivity after electrical cardioversion.[284]

      iii. If a patient cannot be converted pharmacologically or electrically, warfarin should be given for 3 weeks and then elective cardioversion attempted. If successful, warfarin should be continued for an additional 4 weeks.

   b. **Rapid atrial pacing** should be attempted to convert atrial flutter (see Figure 11.11 and page 413 for technique of rapid atrial pacing). It is usually successful in converting only type I flutter (atrial rate less than 350). A variety of type IA, IC, and III antiarrhythmics (procainamide, propafenone, and ibutilide) increase the efficacy of rapid atrial pacing by prolonging the atrial flutter cycle length.[285–287] The type IA drugs do not alter or may increase the duration of the excitable gap in the reentrant circuit, whereas the type III agents shorten the excitable gap. Although the latter may limit the ability of pacing to capture tissue in the reentrant circuit, equivalent efficacy has been noted.

   c. **Rate control** can be achieved most readily with one of the rapid-acting intravenous medications and more chronically with digoxin. Once the rate has been controlled, the IV medications can be converted to oral ones.

      i. **β-blockers** are very effective in achieving rate control and have the advantage of converting about 50% of patients to sinus rhythm. If an oral β-blocker has already been given, it can be supplemented by an

Box 11.4 • Management Protocols for Atrial Fibrillation/Flutter

1. Prophylaxis
   a. Magnesium sulfate 2 g IV after CPB and on first postoperative morning
   b. Metoprolol 25–50 mg PO (or per nasogastric tube) starting 8 hours after surgery
   c. Alternatives
      i. Dual-site atrial pacing
      ii. Sotalol 80 mg bid
      iii. Amiodarone started either PO preoperatively or IV the day of surgery
2. Treatment
   a. Cardioversion with 50–100 joules if unstable
   b. Rapid atrial pace if atrial flutter
   c. Increase prophylactic β-blocker dose if hemodynamically stable
   d. Rate control:
      * IV **diltiazem** 0.25 mg/kg IV over 2 minutes, followed 15 minutes later by 0.35 mg/kg over 2 minutes, followed by a continuous infusion of 10–15 mg/h, if necessary
      * IV **metoprolol** 5 mg IV q5 min × 3 doses
   e. Conversion to sinus rhythm and anticoagulation
      * Magnesium sulfate 2 g IV
      * Option #1: heparin/warfarin after 24–36 hours of AF; await spontaneous conversion on β-blockers and discharge home in either sinus rhythm or atrial fibrillation
      * Option #2: early cardioversion within 24–36 hours following use of one of the following:
         • β-blockers or calcium channel blockers
         • **Amiodarone** 150 mg over 30 minutes, followed by an infusion of 1 mg/min × 6 hours, then 0.5 mg/min × 12 hours
         • **Procainamide** given either IV (10 mg/kg) or after 4 doses of Procan SR 500 mg q6h
         If unsuccessful, heparinize and give warfarin; discharge home in AF off medications.
         If successful, continue PO Procan or amiodarone for 4 weeks
         If cardioversion is performed after 36–48 hours, preliminary TEE is essential to rule out left atrial thrombus
      * Option #3: pharmacologic management alone, with anticoagulation after 36 hours if AF persists:
         • **Amiodarone** in IV dose listed above, then an oral dose of 400 mg tid reduced to 200 mg PO qd over 4 weeks; discontinue at discharge if unsuccessful (except after Maze procedures) or after 4 weeks if converts to NSR
         • **Procan SR** 500–1000 mg q6h with same plan for continuation
         • **Sotalol** 80 mg q4h × 4 doses, then 80 mg bid and stop other β-blockers
         • **Propafenone** 1 mg/kg IV over 2 minutes, followed 10 minutes later by another 1 mg/kg dose; if IV not available, give one oral dose of 600 mg
         • **Ibutilide** 1 mg infusion over 10 minutes (0.01 mg/kg if < 60 kg) with a second infusion 10 minutes later
         • **Dofetilide** 500 μg PO bid

IV dose. If the patient has a relatively slow heart rate (whether already receiving a β-blocker or not) and then develops AF, diltiazem is a better selection to avoid the bradycardia that may occur after conversion.

• **Metoprolol** is the preferred β-blocker because it can be given in the ICU or on the postoperative floor. It is a negative inotrope, so it must be used cautiously in patients with significantly compromised LV function or hypotension. It is given in 5-mg IV increments every 5 minutes up to a total dose of 15 mg. The onset of action is 2–3 minutes with a peak effect noted at 20 minutes. The duration of action is approximately 5 hours.

• **Esmolol** can be used in the ICU setting with arterial line monitoring, but it is a very dangerous drug due to its tendency to produce hypotension. It has an onset of action of 2 minutes and a rapid reversal of effect in 10–20 minutes. Thus, it may prove safer than longer acting β-blockers if adverse effects develop, such as bronchospasm, conduction disturbances, excessive bradycardia, or LV dysfunction. However, if the patient does not convert to NSR, a continuous infusion may be needed until an oral β-blocker can be started. The dose is 0.125–0.5 mg/kg IV over 1 minute, followed by an infusion of 50–200 µg/kg/min.

ii. **Diltiazem** is preferred in patients with a slow sinus mechanism prior to the development of AF. Although it is effective in slowing the ventricular response, it is not as effective as the β-blockers in converting the patient to sinus rhythm.[288–290] It is given in a dose of 0.25 mg/kg IV over 2 minutes, followed 15 minutes later by 0.35 mg/kg over 2 minutes, followed by a continuous infusion of 10–15 mg/h, if necessary. Heart rate response is noted in about 3 minutes, with a peak effect within 7 minutes. The reduction in heart rate lasts 1–3 hours after a bolus dose. The median duration of action is 7 hours after a 24-hour continuous infusion. Diltiazem is more effective in slowing the ventricular response to AF than flutter.

• Because diltiazem is a vasodilator and a negative inotrope, hypotension is the most common side effect. Thus, it must be used cautiously in patients with compromised ventricular function. If the patient is hypotensive with a rapid ventricular rate, an α-agent can be used to support SVR during diltiazem dosing (unless cardioversion is felt to be indicated).

• **Note:** Extreme caution must be used when administering any IV calcium channel blocker concomitantly with an IV β-blocker because of the risk of inducing complete AV block. Availability of functional pacing wires is essential.

iii. Concomitant with the selection of one of the preceding medications, use of **digoxin** might also be considered because of its efficacy in chronically slowing the ventricular response. Digoxin alone is less effective than the β-blockers and calcium channel blockers in slowing the ventricular response to AF in the early postoperative period because its vagotonic effect on the AV node is offset by the increased sympathetic tone that contributes to the rapid ventricular response. However, one study comparing diltiazem and digoxin found that the conversion rate to NSR after 24 hours was slightly better with digoxin.[291] Furthermore, the combination of these medications has been shown to be more effective than diltiazem alone in achieving faster and more stable rate control.[292]

- The initial dose is 0.5 mg IV, followed by 0.25 mg IV q4–6h × 3 doses (up to a total dose of 1.25 mg within 24 hours; less in elderly patients), and then 0.125–0.25 mg qd. The serum potassium level should be > 4.0 mEq/L when digoxin is given because hypokalemia can precipitate digoxin-toxic rhythms.
- The onset of action of IV digoxin is about 30 minutes with a peak effect in 2–3 hours.

   iv. **Amiodarone** is effective in reducing the ventricular response to AF due to its multiple mechanisms of action (β-blockade, class III effects). It is especially useful in the patient with borderline hemodynamics. However, the rapidity and degree of slowing of the ventricular response is less than that of the β-blockers and calcium channel blockers, which may have to be given after an amiodarone load if a fast rate persists.[293]

  d. **Anticoagulation.** Heparinization should be considered for patients with recurrent or persistent AF to minimize the risk of stroke from embolization of left atrial thrombus. In one study, it was noted that 14% of patients developed thrombus and 39% had spontaneous echo contrast in the left atrium within 3 days of the development of AF.[294] Generally, heparin should be started within 24–36 hours of the development of AF to minimize the risk of thrombus formation while awaiting a beneficial response to medications. A strategy of early cardioversion may avert the need for anticoagulation. However, anticoagulation is essential before later cardioversion to reduce the risk of thromboembolism.

  e. **Conversion to sinus rhythm.** "Spontaneous" conversion to sinus rhythm is fairly common with the use of β-blockers or calcium channel blockers. One study found that 80% of patients converted to NSR within 24 hours without the use of class I or III medications, and conversion was more likely in patients receiving β-blockers postoperatively, especially in the absence of severe LV dysfunction and diabetes.[295] The conversion rate noted in this study seems quite high when compared with other studies that have evaluated the effectiveness of a variety of medications in converting AF to NSR. These studies have shown that most of the medications listed below have an approximate conversion rate of 50–60%.[296] If a patient cannot be converted pharmacologically, a strategy of anticoagulation, rate control, and subsequent cardioversion is a viable and cost-effective alternative strategy.

   i. **Magnesium sulfate** 2 g IV over 15 minutes is a benign and relatively effective means of converting patients back to sinus rhythm, with a conversion rate of 60% within 4 hours in one study.[297]

  ii. **β-blockers,** in addition to being used for prophylaxis, are effective for both rate control and conversion. The prophylactic dose can be increased if the patient's blood pressure and heart rate are acceptable. Substitution of sotalol (80 mg bid) for the selective β-blockers may be considered because it is slightly more successful in producing conversion.

Many patients cannot tolerate sotalol because of bradycardia or hypotension.

iii. **Amiodarone** has seen increasing usage for the treatment of AF and is considered by many to be the treatment of choice due to its efficacy and safety profile. Acute administration is associated with modest hypotension, more so than noted with the type IC drugs.[298] Although it does produce QT prolongation, this is not accompanied by a significant proarrhythmic effect. It is safer than procainamide in patients with renal or LV dysfunction. Conversion occurs with a similar frequency to the type IC drugs listed below but usually takes longer.[296] It may be given with the standard IV load (150 mg over 15 minutes, followed by a 60 mg/h infusion × 6 hours, then 30 mg/h × 18 hours) followed by an oral taper (400 mg bid for 1 week, 400 mg qd for 1 week, 200 mg qd for 2 weeks. Alternatively, it may be given as an oral load of 400 mg tid for 1 week, followed by the same wean. One study found that a load of 30 mg/kg PO was safe and effective in converting patients to NSR.[299]

iv. **Procainamide** is a type IA medication that has traditionally been the drug of choice for conversion. It is as effective as amiodarone, but it is more proarrhythmic, a mild negative inotrope, and is renally excreted, and thus must be used with caution in patients with renal dysfunction. It is also associated with more short-term side effects (GI upset, hallucinations). Because of its vagolytic effects, it can accelerate AV conduction in AF/atrial flutter, so it should be given only after the ventricular rate has been brought under control.

- One option is to administer a brief course of IV procainamide (10 mg/kg over 60 minutes, followed by a 2 mg/min infusion), with an attempt at electric cardioversion within 24 hours if conversion does not occur pharmacologically. Alternatively, oral dosing of 500–1000 mg Procan SR q6h with or without a 10 mg/kg IV load can be used prior to electric cardioversion.

- Another option is to use either regimen (more commonly the oral load) in an attempt to achieve pharmacologic conversion. If this does not occur after therapeutic levels are achieved, the drug is stopped and a rate-control/anticoagulation protocol is used. If conversion does occur, the procainamide is continued arbitrarily for 4 weeks.

v. The type IC and III antiarrhythmics have been successful in converting 50–70% of patients with recent-onset AF back to sinus rhythm. They generally cause less hypotension than drugs mentioned above and produce more rapid conversion.

- **Propafenone** (class IC) is effective in slowing the ventricular response and in rapidly converting patients to sinus rhythm within a few hours. The intravenous dose is 1–2 mg/kg IV over 15 minutes, followed 10 minutes later by another 1 mg/kg dose. The IV form of propafenone was not available in the United States in 2004, but one oral dose of 600 mg achieves a similar conversion rate, although it may take longer.[300–302] IV propafenone has been found to be equivalent to amiodarone but better than procainamide in achieving conversion, and it achieves conversion more rapidly.[303,304]

- **Ibutilide** (class III) is given as a 1-mg infusion over 10 minutes (0.01 mg/kg if < 60 kg) with a second infusion 10 minutes later, if necessary. It is more successful in converting atrial flutter than AF.[305] Mean time to conversion is about 30 minutes. Because of the proarrhythmic risk, the infusion should be stopped as soon as the arrhythmia has terminated, VT occurs, or there is marked prolongation of the QT interval. Ibutilide is particularly useful in patients with poor ventricular function or chronic lung disease. In comparative studies, ibutilide was found to be more effective than procainamide and sotalol, and just as effective as amiodarone, in converting AF/atrial flutter to sinus rhythm.[306,307]
- **Dofetilide** (class III) has no negative inotropic effects and is beneficial when there are contraindications to class I drugs (LV dysfunction) or β-blockers (bradycardia, chronic obstructive pulmonary disease). It is usually given in a dosage of 500 μg PO bid. One study using IV dofetilide (up to 8 μg/kg over 15 minutes) found that it was more successful in converting atrial flutter (70%) than fibrillation (30%) within 1 hour.[308] It also causes QT prolongation and is proarrhythmic. The dosage must be adjusted by creatinine clearance and the baseline QTc.

vi. **Low-energy internal cardioversion** using epicardial defibrillation wires sewn to the left and right atria at the time of surgery is 90% successful in restoring sinus rhythm.[309,310]

H. Other supraventricular tachycardias

1. This designation refers to a tachycardia of sudden onset that arises either in the atrium (paroxysmal atrial tachycardia, or PAT) or in the AV nodal region (atrioventricular nodal reentrant tachycardia, or AVNRT), or uses the AV node as an integral part of the reentrant circuit (AVRT). These rhythms usually occur at a rate of 150–250/min and are uncommon after cardiac surgery. PAT with AV block may be associated with ischemic heart disease and commonly results from digoxin toxicity. As with any arrhythmia causing a rapid ventricular response, immediate treatment is indicated because of potential adverse effects on myocardial metabolism and function.

2. **Diagnosis.** Differentiation among sinus tachycardia, PAT, AVNRT, AVRT, and atrial flutter with 2:1 block may require examination of an AEG (Figure 11.24). Carotid sinus massage is often recommended as a diagnostic modality to differentiate among various arrhythmias by slowing the ventricular response to atrial tachyarrhythmias. However, it must be used with caution in patients with coronary artery disease, not only because it may precipitate asystole but because it may produce an embolic stroke in patients with coexistent carotid artery disease.

3. **Treatment**
   a. Rapid atrial overdrive pacing may capture the atrium and cause reversion to sinus rhythm.
   b. Cardioversion should be considered if there is evidence of hemodynamic compromise.
   c. Vagal stimulation often breaks a reentrant rhythm involving the AV node. Carotid sinus massage must be used cautiously as noted above.

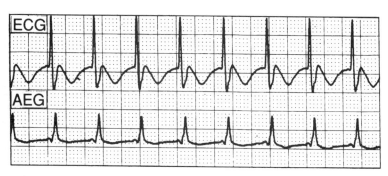

Figure 11.24 • AV junctional tachycardia at a rate of about 140/min recorded in simultaneous monitor and bipolar AEGs. Note the nearly simultaneous occurrence of retrograde atrial activation in the AEG and the antegrade ventricular activation in the monitor lead.

    d. Adenosine produces transient high-grade AV block and is successful in terminating supraventricular tachycardia caused by AVNRT.[311] It is given as a 6-mg rapid IV injection via a central line followed by a saline flush. A repeat dose of 12 mg may be given 2 minutes later. The half-life of adenosine is only 10 seconds. Adenosine can help distinguish AVRT and AVNRT (in which it terminates the circuit) from atrial flutter or fibrillation, in which it may produce transient slowing of the ventricular rate.

    e. Calcium channel blockers are effective in converting AVNRT to sinus rhythm in about 90% of patients.

        i. Diltiazem 0.25 mg/kg IV over 2 minutes, followed 15 minutes later by 0.35 mg/kg, if necessary.[312]

        ii. Verapamil 2.5–10 mg IV over 5–10 minutes

    f. Additional measures that can be used for AVNRT if the above fail include:

        i. Digoxin 0.5 mg IV in a patient not previously on digoxin

        ii. Metoprolol 5 mg q5 minutes to a total dose of 15 mg

        iii. Edrophonium 5-mg slow IV push, followed by a 10-mg dose

    g. PAT with block is usually associated with digoxin toxicity, and treatment should be provided accordingly:

        i. Digoxin should be withheld and a digoxin level obtained

        ii. Administration of potassium chloride

        iii. Digibind (digoxin immune Fab [ovine]) starting at a dose of 400 mg (10 vials) over 30 minutes if severe digoxin toxicity

        iv. Phenytoin (Dilantin) 250 mg IV over 5 minutes

I. AV junctional rhythm and nonparoxysmal AV junctional tachycardia

    1. An AV junctional rhythm occurs when junctional tissue has a faster intrinsic rate than the sinus node. When it occurs at a rate less than 60 beats/min, it is termed a junctional escape rhythm.

    2. Nonparoxysmal AV junctional tachycardia occurs at a rate of 70–130 beats/min. In the postoperative patient, this rhythm may reflect digitalis toxicity, pericarditis, or an inferior infarction. Its presence may be suggested by a regularized ventricular rate with underlying AF and can be confirmed with an AEG.

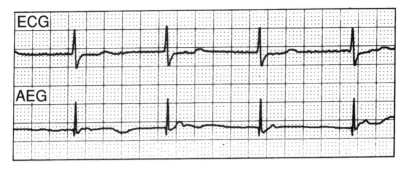

Figure 11.25 • Slow junctional rhythm at a rate of 54/min. Note the simultaneous occurrence of atrial and ventricular activation.

3. As with any nonatrial rhythm, cardiac output is diminished by lack of synchronous atrial and ventricular contractions.

4. **Diagnosis.** See Figures 11.24 and 11.25. The focus may be localized by the relationship of the P wave to the QRS on a surface ECG (short PR interval if high nodal, invisible P wave if midnodal, and P wave following the QRS if low nodal). The P-QRS relationship is more evident on an AEG.

5. **Treatment**

   a. Slow junctional rhythm

      i. Atrial pacing if AV conduction is normal.

      ii. AV pacing if AV conduction is depressed.

      iii. Use of a vasoactive drug with chronotropic β_1 action to stimulate the sinus mechanism; any drug the patient is receiving that might slow the sinus mechanism should be stopped.

   b. Nonparoxysmal junctional tachycardia

      i. If the patient is receiving digoxin, it should be stopped. Severe digoxin toxicity may be treated with digibind. Use of potassium, lidocaine, phenytoin, or a β-blocker may be helpful.

      ii. Overdrive pacing at a faster rate may establish AV synchrony.

      iii. If the patient is not on digoxin, it should be started. If the rhythm is not well tolerated, use of a β-blocker or calcium channel blocker can be considered to slow the junctional focus with use of atrial or AV pacing to establish AV synchrony.

J. **Premature ventricular complexes**

1. PVCs are fairly uncommon when complete revascularization has been accomplished with good myocardial protection. When they develop de novo, they may reflect transient perioperative phenomena, such as augmented sympathetic tone or increased levels of catecholamines (endogenous or exogenous), irritation from a Swan-Ganz catheter or endotracheal tube, abnormal acid-base status, hypoxemia, etc. Thus, most PVCs are self-limited, benign, and not predictive of more serious, life-threatening arrhythmias. Ventricular ectopy is also fairly common in patients following an MI and may persist after surgery, although ischemia-induced ectopy may be improved.

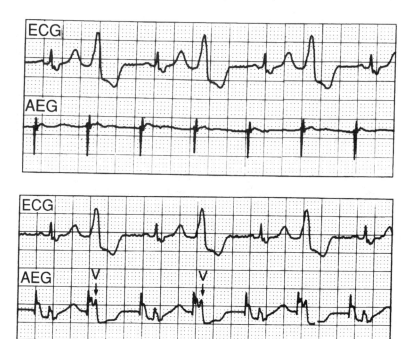

Figure 11.26 • Premature ventricular complexes (ventricular bigeminy) recorded simultaneously from monitor lead II and bipolar (upper) and unipolar (upper) AEGs. Note the wide QRS complex of unifocal morphology representing the PVC on the ECG. The bipolar AEG shows that the interval between atrial complexes is maintained despite the PVCs. The unipolar tracing shows that the PVC directly follows the sinus beat but leaves the ventricle refractory to the following beat, producing a full compensatory pause. V = premature ventricular complex.

2. Nonetheless, PVCs developing de novo may also reflect poor intraoperative myocardial protection, myocardial ischemia or infarction, and may herald malignant ventricular arrhythmias. Therefore, some surgical groups believe that even occasional PVCs should never be ignored in the early postoperative period. During the first 24 hours after surgery, when a multitude of cardiac and noncardiac precipitating factors may be present, it is of potential benefit and little risk to treat any ventricular ectopy. Persistent complex ventricular ectopy in patients with depressed LV function (ejection fraction < 40%) may require further evaluation and treatment.

3. **Diagnosis.** See Figure 11.26.

4. **Treatment**

   a. Correct the serum potassium with an intravenous KCl infusion at a rate up to 10–20 mEq/h through a central line. Some patients require potassium levels between 4.5 and 5.0 mEq/L to eliminate ventricular ectopy.

   b. Atrial pace at a rate exceeding the current sinus rate ("overdrive pacing") unless tachycardia is present.

c. Lidocaine 1 mg/kg with 1–2 repeat doses of 0.5 mg/kg 10 minutes apart. A continuous infusion of 1–2 mg/min of a 1 g/250 mL mix should be started. Do not exceed 4 mg/min to avoid seizure activity. Consider the patient's weight, hepatic function, and any underlying CHF when calculating a maximal dose.[313]

d. Magnesium sulfate (2 g in 100 mL IV) administered at the termination of bypass has been shown to reduce the incidence of ventricular ectopy.[314]

K. Ventricular tachycardia and ventricular fibrillation

1. Etiology

a. VT/VF occur postoperatively in about 1–3% of patients undergoing open-heart surgery and carry a mortality rate of 20–25%.[315, 316]

b. Ventricular tachyarrhythmias result from disorders of impulse formation or propagation. When they are present preoperatively on the basis of ischemia, resolution may be anticipated with revascularization of the ischemic zones. However, if they occur preoperatively as a consequence of a prior MI, they may be exacerbated by reperfusion.

c. Reperfusion of zones of ischemia or infarction can also trigger de novo malignant ventricular arrhythmias. They develop commonly in patients with prior infarction, unstable angina, an ejection fraction < 40%, NYHA class III–IV CHF, and when bypass grafts are placed to noncollateralized occluded vessels, especially the left anterior descending artery. Potential triggers include residual ischemia or development of a PMI secondary to incomplete revascularization, anastomotic problems, or acute graft closure.[315-319]

i. Nonsustained ventricular tachycardia (NSVT) (VT lasting less than 30 seconds) may be encountered for reasons similar to those of PVCs and may occur in patients with normal or abnormal ventricular function.

ii. Sustained monomorphic VT (VT lasting over 30 seconds) is usually noted in patients with a previous myocardial infarction and depressed LV function, often with formation of an LV aneurysm. The border zone between scar and viable tissue provides the electrophysiologic substrate for a reentry mechanism that passes through myocyte bands surviving within the infarct.

iii. Sustained polymorphic VT with a normal QT interval is usually caused by increased dispersion of repolarization in areas of reperfused ischemia or infarction. Triggered activity in the form of delayed afterdepolarizations and occasionally enhanced automaticity are the mechanisms involved. Polymorphic VT may be facilitated by perioperative phenomena such as ischemia, hemodynamic instability, use of catecholamines or intrinsic sympathetic activity, withdrawal of β-blockers, and other metabolic problems. Similarly, VF may be triggered by an acute ischemic insult.

iv. Polymorphic VT with QT prolongation is called **torsades de pointes.** The mechanism involves early afterdepolarizations, a form of triggered activity. It usually complicates the use of type IA and III antiarrhythmic medications, especially if hypokalemia is present. Other medications that can contribute to torsades de pointes are metoclopramide,

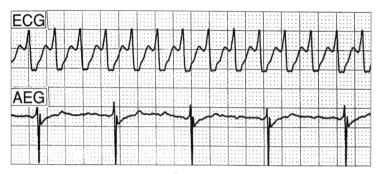

Figure 11.27 • Ventricular tachycardia recorded simultaneously in lead II and a bipolar AEG. There is dissociation between the sinus rhythm at a rate of 72/min noted in the AEG and the wide complex ventricular tachycardia occurring at a rate of 210/min noted in the monitor lead.

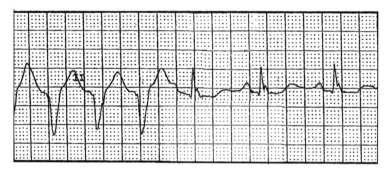

Figure 11.28 • Nonsustained ventricular tachycardia at a rate around 130/min that spontaneously reverted to a sinus mechanism at a rate of 75/min.

droperidol (for nausea), and high-dose haloperidol (> 35 mg/day) used for agitation in the ICU.[320]

   d. If the patient has a VVI or DDD pacemaker, the use of electrocautery during surgery can inactivate the sensing circuit, converting it to the VOO mode. This may result in bizarre-appearing arrhythmias and may trigger VF. These pacemakers must be evaluated upon arrival in the ICU and reprogrammed if necessary.[321]

2. Diagnosis. See Figures 11.27–11.30. A common arrhythmia commonly confused with VT is AF with a rate-dependent conduction block (aberrancy) that produces a wide QRS complex. This should be distinguished by its irregularity, although this may be difficult to detect at fast heart rates.

3. Evaluation and treatment depend on the status of LV function, the nature of the arrhythmia (nonsustained vs. sustained, monomorphic or polymorphic VT), and whether the VT is inducible.

   a. Any potential triggering factors should be identified and managed. These include acid-base and electrolyte abnormalities, intracardiac catheters, myocardial ischemia or infarction, CHF, and potentially proarrhythmic medications.

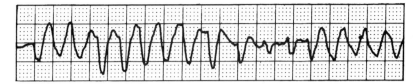

Figure 11.29 • Ventricular fibrillation on monitor lead.

b. The prognosis of symptomatic **PVCs or NSVT with preserved LV function** is favorable. Lidocaine and magnesium may be used perioperatively to decrease the incidence of NSVT, and β-blockers and perhaps amiodarone should be utilized subsequently.[313,322] One follow-up study of patients who developed postoperative VT/VF, 85% of whom had an ejection fraction greater than 30%, reported an equivalent prognosis of patients who survived 30 days after surgery with use of medications alone to that of control patients who did not develop VT/VF.[316]

c. **NSVT in patients with depressed LV function** may be associated with a poor prognosis without treatment. Extrapolating from the MADIT I and MUSTT trials (see p. 41), an electrophysiologic study and ICD placement should be considered if NSVT develops after surgery in these patients.[323]

d. Any patient developing **VF or sustained VT that is pulseless or associated with hemodynamic instability** requires immediate defibrillation per ACLS protocol.[204] If unsuccessful, emergency thoracotomy and open-chest massage are indicated.

e. **Sustained VT** occurring **without hemodynamic compromise** can be managed by:

    i. Ventricular overdrive pacing to terminate the reentry circuit.

    ii. Cardioversion if VT persists or hemodynamic compromise develops.

    iii. Amiodarone 150 mg over 15 minutes, then 1 mg/min (60 mg/h) for 6 hours, then 0.5 mg/min (30 mg/h) for 18 hours.

f. Electrophysiologic testing is essential for patients with sustained VT and impaired ventricular function in whom the prognosis is not favorable.

    i. **Monomorphic VT** is inducible in 80% of patients with spontaneous VT and is usually associated with a remote infarct and an arrhythmogenic substrate causing a reentry mechanism. This usually requires antiarrhythmic therapy (usually amiodarone) and virtually always requires the placement of an ICD.[323]

    ii. **Polymorphic VT** is usually associated with myocardial infarction, ischemia, or reperfusion, and should prompt further evaluation for ongoing ischemia. This may involve coronary arteriography to identify potential graft occlusion or an anastomotic stenosis, which may be a correctable problem. It is often transient, and therapy must be individualized.

g. **Torsades de pointes**[324]

    i. Cardiovert immediately for hemodynamic compromise or prolonged episodes (usually because VF is suspected).

    ii. Administer potassium chloride, unless hyperkalemia is present, to shorten the QT interval.

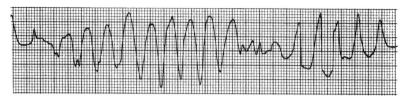

Figure 11.30 • Torsades de pointes on monitor lead. Note how the QRS complex appears to "twist" around the isoelectric baseline. Torsades usually has a pause-dependent onset initiated by a premature ventricular complex discharging at the end of a T wave, usually associated with a long QT interval.

    iii. Ventricular pace at 90–100/min or start an isoproterenol infusion at 1–4 µg/min.[325] This will shorten the action potential to prevent early afterdepolarization.

    iv. Magnesium 1–2 g and β-blockers may eliminate triggered activity to prevent recurrence but do not shorten the QT interval.

XIII. Antiarrhythmic Medications

A variety of medications are available for the control of supraventricular and ventricular arrhythmias (Table 11.12). A basic understanding of their mechanism of action is critical to the appropriate selection of these drugs for the management of various arrhythmias as noted in the preceding sections.[326–328] In this section, a more detailed discussion of drugs most commonly used in patients undergoing cardiac surgery will be presented.

    A. Vaughn-Williams classification of antiarrhythmic medications

        Class I   **Sodium channel blockers**
                Class IA Quinidine
                           Procainamide
                           Disopyramide
                Class IB Lidocaine
                           Mexiletine
                           Phenytoin
                Class IC Propafenone
        Class II   **β-adrenergic blockers**
        Class III **Potassium channel blockers**
                Amiodarone
                Sotalol
                Ibutilide
                Dofetilide
        Class IV **Calcium channel blockers**

    B. Table 11.13 shows the effects of the various classes of antiarrhythmic drugs on automaticity, conduction velocity, and the effective refractory period (ERP). The appropriate class of antiarrhythmic drug that can be selected for the management of the common arrhythmias is as follows:

Table 11.12 • Doses and Therapeutic Levels of Common Antiarrhythmic Drugs

Drug	IV	PO	Therapeutic Levels
IA			
Procainamide	Load: 10 mg/kg Drip: 1–4 mg/min	Procan SR 500–1000 mg q6h	Procan: 4–10 μg/mL NAPA: 2–8 μg/mL
IB			
Lidocaine	Load: 1 mg/kg → 0.5 mg/kg, 1–2 times 10 min apart Drip: 2–4 mg/min (1 g/250 mL)		1–5 μg/mL
IC			
Propafenone	1 mg/kg IV over 2 min, followed 10 min later by another 1 mg/kg dose	600 mg PO load, then 150–300 mg q8h	0.2–3.0 μg/mL
III			
Amiodarone	150 mg over 15 min, then 1 mg/min × 6h, 0.5 mg/min × 18 hours, then convert to PO	400 mg tid, reduced weekly to 200 mg qd	1–2.5 μg/mL
Sotalol		80–160 mg bid	
Ibutilide	1 mg infusion over 10 min (0.01 mg/kg if < 60 kg) with a second infusion 10 min later		
Dofetilide		500 μg PO bid	

1. Alterations in automaticity
   a. Sinus tachycardia (sinus node): class II, IV
   b. Ventricular ectopy (Purkinje and ventricular fibers): class IA, IB, IC, II, III
   c. Digoxin-toxic ectopy (delayed afterdepolarizations: IB (phenytoin)

Table 11.13 • Electrophysiologic Properties of Antiarrhythmic Drugs

Property		Class IA	Class IB	Class IC	Class II	Class III	Class IV
Automaticity							
SA node		—	—	—	↓	—	↓
Vent ectopic foci (Purkinje)		↓	↓	↓	↓	—	—
Delayed afterdepolarizations[a]		—	↓	↓	↓	—	↓
Conduction							
Atria	CV	↓	—	↓	—	—	—
	ERP	↑	—	↑	—	—	—
AV node	CV	—	—	↓	↓	—	↓
	ERP	—	—	↑	↑	—	↑
His-Purkinje	CV	↓	↓	↓	—	—	—
	ERP	↓	↑	↑	↑	—	—
Ventricle	CV	↓	↓	↓	—	—	—
	ERP	↑	↓	↑	—	↑	—

[a] Mechanism of digoxin-induced ventricular ectopy.
CV = conduction velocity; ERP = effective refractory period.

    2. Alterations in conduction velocity and ERP
       a. Conversion of AF (atrium): class IA, IC, II, III
       b. To slow the response to AF (AV node): class II, III, IV, digoxin
       c. Conversion of AVNRT or AVRT: class II, IV, digoxin
       d. VT (interrupt reentrant circuits in His-Purkinje fibers or ventricle): class IA, IB, III
  C. **Note:** The clinical indications listed below for each of the antiarrhythmic medications are those for which there is documented efficacy. FDA approval has not necessarily been provided for each of these indications.
  D. **Procainamide**
    1. Clinical indications
       a. Prevention/conversion of AF
       b. Suppression of premature supraventricular and ventricular complexes and sustained ventricular tachyarrhythmias

   c. Wolff-Parkinson-White (WPW) syndrome (slows conduction over accessory pathways)

2. Dosage

   a. IV: 100 mg q5 min up to 1000 mg (never more than 50 mg/min), then a 2–4 mg/min drip (1 g/250 mL mix).

   b. PO: 500–1000 mg load, then Procan SR 500–1000 mg q6h or Procanbid 1–2.5 g q12h = 50 mg/kg/day.

   c. Conversion of IV to PO: Give one-fourth of the total daily IV dose as Procan SR q6h or one-half as Procanbid; stop the IV infusion immediately after the first oral dose.

3. Metabolism: hepatic to active metabolite *N*-acetylprocainamide (NAPA) and then excreted by the kidneys

4. Therapeutic level: 4–10 µg/mL of procainamide and 2–8 µg/mL of NAPA

5. Hemodynamic effects: decreases SVR, negative inotrope in high doses

6. Special electrophysiologic concerns

   a. Slowing of the atrial rate in atrial flutter and vagolytic effects on AV conduction may increase the ventricular response to AF/atrial flutter. Medications that prevent accelerated AV conduction must be given first.

   b. Evidence of toxicity:

      i. QT prolongation and polymorphic VT

      ii. Myocardial depression

      iii. NAPA has different electrophysiologic properties than procainamide. It may accumulate in patients with CHF and renal failure. It has a longer half-life than procainamide (7 hours vs. 4 hours) and can lead to cardiac toxicity, including early afterdepolarizations, triggered activity, and ventricular arrhythmias, including torsades de pointes, especially in the ischemic heart.

7. Noncardiac side effects: GI (nausea, anorexia), CNS (insomnia, hallucinations, psychosis, depression), rash, drug fever, agranulocytosis, lupus-like syndrome with long-term use

E. Disopyramide (Norpace)

1. Clinical indications

   a. Suppression of ventricular and supraventricular arrhythmias

   b. Termination and prevention of recurrence of AVNRT

   c. Prevention/conversion of AF

   d. WPW syndrome (slows conduction over accessory pathways)

2. Dosage: 100–200 mg PO q6h

3. Metabolism: 65% renal, 35% hepatic

4. Hemodynamic effects: strong negative inotrope (thus useful in patients with hypertrophic obstructive cardiomyopathy)

5. Therapeutic level: 2–5 µg/mL

6. Special electrophysiologic concerns

   a. Slowing of the atrial rate in atrial flutter and vagolytic effects on AV conduction require prior use of medications (digoxin) to prevent accelerated AV conduction.

b. May cause torsades de pointes or other ventricular tachyarrhythmias associated with QT prolongation.

7. Noncardiac side effects: anticholinergic (urinary retention, constipation, blurred vision), nausea, dizziness, insomnia

F. Lidocaine

1. Clinical indications: PVCs and ventricular tachyarrhythmias
2. Dosage
   a. 1 mg/kg IV followed by a continuous infusion of 2–4 mg/min (1 g/250 mL mix); a dose of 0.5 mg/kg may be given 20 minutes later to achieve a stable plasma concentration.
   b. A rebolus of 0.5 mg/kg should be given to increase plasma levels if the infusion rate is increased.
3. Metabolism: hepatic; half-life is 15 minutes after one dose and 2 hours with constant infusion (often longer with hepatic impairment)
4. Therapeutic level: 1–5 µg/mL
5. Hemodynamic effects: none in the absence of severe LV dysfunction
6. Noncardiac side effects: CNS (dizziness, delirium, tremors, seizures), GI (nausea)

G. Propafenone

1. Clinical indication: conversion of AF
2. Dosage
   a. PO: 600 mg load, then 150–300 mg q8h
   b. IV: 1 mg/kg IV over 2 minutes, followed 10 minutes later by another 1 mg/kg dose (used for conversion of AF) (not available in United States)
3. Metabolism: hepatic
4. Therapeutic level: 0.2–3.0 µg/mL
5. Hemodynamic effects: negative inotrope in patients with compromised ventricular function
6. Special electrophysiologic concerns
   a. Proarrhythmic effects are noted in 5% of patients.
   b. Has some β-blocker activity and can produce AV block and sinus node depression.
   c. It doubles the digoxin level.
7. Noncardiac side effects are noted in 15% of patients: CNS (dizziness, diplopia), GI upset

H. β-adrenergic blockers

1. Clinical indications
   a. Prevention/treatment of postoperative AF/atrial flutter
   b. Sinus tachycardia
   c. Ventricular arrhythmias associated with digoxin toxicity, myocardial ischemia, or QT prolongation
   d. AVNRT and reciprocating tachycardias in WPW syndrome
2. Dosages
   a. Metoprolol (relative potency is 2.5:1 for IV/PO)

     i. IV: 5 mg q5 minutes for 3 doses

     ii. PO: 25–100 mg q12h

   b. Atenolol: 25–50 mg PO qd

   c. Esmolol: IV: 500 µg/kg load, then 50–200 µg/kg/min drip

3. Metabolism: hepatic (metoprolol), renal (atenolol), blood (esmolol)

4. Hemodynamic and electrophysiologic effects: negative inotropes; can produce hypotension, bradycardia, and heart block

5. Noncardiac side effects: bronchospasm (less with the cardioselective β-blockers atenolol and metoprolol), diarrhea, impotence, depression, intermittent claudication

I. Amiodarone

1. Clinical indications

   a. Prevention/conversion of postoperative AF

   b. Pulseless VT/VF (first choice)

   c. Sustained ventricular tachyarrhythmias

2. Dosage

   a. PO: 400 mg tid, tapered to 200 mg qd over several weeks

   b. IV: 150 mg over 15 min, then 1 mg/min × 6 h, 0.5 mg/min × 18 hours, then 1 g/day

3. Metabolism: hepatic (half-life of 50 days)

4. Therapeutic level: 1.0–2.5 µg/mL

5. Hemodynamic effects: β-blocker; coronary and peripheral vasodilator (α-adrenergic effect)

6. Special electrophysiologic concerns

   a. May produce bradycardia and heart block.

   b. Prolongs the QT interval but rarely causes ventricular arrhythmias.

   c. Reduces clearance (and therefore increases serum levels) of drugs metabolized by the liver. These include **digoxin, warfarin,** and procainamide. **Doses of these medications should be reduced by about one-half.**

7. Noncardiac side effects are noted in more than 50% of patients, especially during chronic therapy. These include pulmonary toxicity, hepatic dysfunction, corneal microdeposits (in nearly all patients), photosensitivity, GI upset, CNS symptoms (tremor, ataxia, paresthesias), and neuropathy. Acute pulmonary toxicity has been reported but is rare.[266]

J. Sotalol

1. Clinical indications

   a. Prevention/treatment of postoperative AF

   b. Suppression of ventricular tachyarrhythmias

2. Dosage: 80–160 mg PO bid

3. Metabolism: excreted unchanged in the urine

4. Hemodynamic effects: causes a decrease in heart rate with some negative inotropic effect, hypotension

5. Special electrophysiologic effects

    a. Exhibits β-blocker and class III effects.

    b. Produces torsades de pointes or proarrhythmic effects in about 4% of patients. Torsades de pointes is dose-related and predictable from the QT interval.

  6. Side effects: fatigue, dyspnea, dizziness, heart failure, nausea and vomiting

K. Ibutilide

  1. Clinical indication: conversion of recent-onset AF and atrial flutter

  2. Dosage: 1 mg IV over 10 minutes (0.01 mg/kg if less than 60 kg) with a second dose if no response

  3. Metabolism: hepatic

  4. Therapeutic level: unknown

  5. Hemodynamic effects: no significant hemodynamic effects

  6. Special electrophysiologic concerns

    a. Dose-related prolongation of the QT interval (avoid if the QT interval exceeds 440 ms). QT prolongation may contribute to torsades de pointes, but sustained polymorphic VT may occur even in the absence of a prolonged QT interval.

    b. Monomorphic or polymorphic VT (sustained or nonsustained) is noted in about 10% of patients; careful monitoring in the ICU is essential for 4 hours after an administered dose (half-life is 6 hours) or until the QT interval has returned to baseline.

  7. Noncardiac side effects: headache, nausea

L. Dofetilide

  1. Clinical indication: conversion of AF/atrial flutter

  2. Dosage: 500 μg PO bid (based on renal function and QT prolongation)

  3. Metabolism: renal

  4. Therapeutic level: unknown

  5. Hemodynamic effects: no negative inotropic effects

  6. Special electrophysiologic concerns:

    a. Slightly decreases the sinus rate but has no effect on AV conduction

    b. Proarrhythmic effect from QT prolongation, so contraindicated if QTc > 440 ms (or if creatinine clearance is < 20 mL/min)

    c. Has drug interaction with verapamil, which contraindicates its use

    d. All class I or III antiarrhythmic medications should be stopped for 3 half-lives before dofetilide is given.

    e. Amiodarone must be stopped for 3 months (or a level < 0.3 mg/L) before dofetilide is given.

M. Calcium channel blockers (verapamil and diltiazem)

  1. Clinical indications

    a. Control rapid ventricular response to AF/atrial flutter

    b. Prevent AVNRT and reciprocating tachycardias of WPW syndrome (AVRT); contraindicated for AF in WPW syndrome

    c. Ischemic ventricular ectopy

2. Dosages

    a. Diltiazem

        i. IV: 0.25 mg/kg IV bolus over 2 minutes, with a repeat bolus of 0.35 mg/kg 15 minutes later; then a continuous infusion of 10–15 mg/h (250 mg/250 mL mix).

        ii. PO: 30–90 mg q8h (or 180–360 mg qd of long-acting preparation)

    b. Verapamil

        i. IV: 2.5–10 mg bolus over 1 minute with repeat dose in 30 minutes; then a continuous infusion of 2–5 µg/kg/min (120 mg/250 mL mix).

        ii. PO: 80–160 mg q8h

3. Metabolism: hepatic

4. Therapeutic level: 0.1–0.15 µg/mL (verapamil)

5. Hemodynamic effects: mild negative inotropes, hypotension from decreased SVR

6. Special electrophysiologic effects

    a. Can precipitate asystole, bradycardia, or heart block when used concomitantly with IV β-blockers.

    b. Verapamil reduces clearance of digoxin and increases the digoxin level by about 35%.

    c. Noncardiac side effects: GI (constipation, nausea), headache, dizziness, elevation in liver function tests.

N. Adenosine

1. Clinical indication: paroxysmal supraventricular tachycardias with AV nodal reentry (AVNRT or AVRT).

2. Dosage: 6 mg rapid IV injection through a central line followed by a saline flush; a second dose of 12 mg may be given 2 minutes later if necessary.

3. Metabolism: rapidly degraded in blood, with a half-life of less than 10 seconds.

4. Electrophysiologic effects: produces transient high-grade AV block that can be used to unmask atrial activity and differentiate the causes of narrow- and wide-complex tachycardias.

5. Side effects: flushing, dyspnea, or chest pressure of very brief duration

O. Digoxin

1. Clinical indications

    a. Rapid ventricular response to AF/atrial flutter (less effective than calcium channel blockers or β-blockers due to the mechanism of early postoperative AF)

    b. Recurrent paroxysmal supraventricular tachycardia

2. Dosage

    a. IV: 0.5 mg, then 0.25 mg q4–6h to total dose of 1.0–1.25 mg, then 0.125 mg qd

    b. PO: 0.5 mg, then 0.25 mg q4–6h to total dose of 1.25 mg, then 0.25 mg qd

        i. Maintenance dose depends on serum level and therapeutic effect

        ii. Dose is 0.125 mg qod for patients in renal failure

        iii. IV dose is two-thirds of the PO dose

3. Metabolism: renal
4. Therapeutic level: 1–2 ng/mL (drawn not less than 6 hours after an oral dose or 4 hours after an intravenous dose)

   a. Serum levels are increased by medications that reduce its clearance or volume of distribution; thus, digoxin dosing should be reduced accordingly.
   b. **Levels are increased by amiodarone** (by 70–100%) and verapamil (by 35%). Thus, dose of digoxin should be halved.
5. Hemodynamic effects: slight inotropic effect, peripheral vasodilatation
6. Special electrophysiologic concerns: see comments below on digoxin toxicity
7. Noncardiac side effects: GI (anorexia, nausea, vomiting), CNS (headache, fatigue, confusion, seizures), visual symptoms

P. **Comments on digoxin toxicity**[329]

1. Digoxin is used primarily to slow the ventricular response to AF/atrial flutter by virtue of its vagotonic effect (at low dose) and its direct effect (at high dose) on the AV node. It is less effective than other medications in slowing the ventricular response to AF in the early postoperative period when a high adrenergic state is present. Thus, it is not the drug of choice for acute rate control. However, it can provide additional rate control, especially when AF is persistent.

2. Aggressive digitalization for rapid AF is usually not successful in achieving rate control and can lead to digoxin toxicity for a number of reasons in the early postoperative period.

   a. There is increased sensitivity to digoxin related to augmented sympathetic tone, myocardial ischemia, electrolyte imbalance (hyper- or hypokalemia, hypercalcemia, hypomagnesemia), acid-base imbalance, or use of vasoactive or antiarrhythmic drugs (quinidine or verapamil).
   b. Large doses need to be given to achieve effect because digoxin's vagotonic effects are offset by increased sympathetic tone. IV doses are usually given to provide 1.25 mg within the first 24 hours but subsequent IV doses should be two-thirds of the oral doses to avoid toxicity.
   c. The volume of distribution is lower in many elderly patients with decreased lean body mass.
   d. Hypokalemia from postoperative diuresis and hypomagnesemia predispose to digoxin toxicity.
   e. Renal excretion may be impaired in patients with chronic renal insufficiency. Elderly patients have reduced glomerular filtration rates and excrete digoxin less efficiently.

3. Digoxin toxicity should be considered in any patient receiving digoxin who develops a change in rhythm. These include, in decreasing order of frequency:

   a. PVCs (multiform and bigeminy)
   b. Nonparoxysmal AV junctional tachycardia
   c. AV block: first-degree or Wenckebach second-degree block
   d. Paroxysmal atrial tachycardia with 2:1 block
   e. VT (especially bidirectional VT at a rate of 140–180/min)
   f. Sinus bradycardia or SA block

3. Digoxin toxicity in a patient with AF is usually manifested by:
   a. Slow ventricular response (< 50/min)
   b. AV dissociation with AV junctional escape or accelerated junctional rhythm. Regularization of the ventricular rate in the presence of AF should always raise concern about the development of complete heart block with a junctional escape rhythm.
4. Treatment
   a. Bradyarrhythmias are treated by atrial, AV, or ventricular pacing, depending on the underlying atrial rhythm and the status of AV conduction. Atropine can be used, but isoproterenol should be avoided because it may induce malignant ventricular arrhythmias.
   b. Tachyarrhythmias
      i. Potassium chloride, except in the presence of high-grade AV block because hyperkalemia can potentiate the depressant effect of digoxin on AV conduction.
      ii. Lidocaine at usual doses
      iii. Phenytoin (Dilantin), 100 mg IV every 5 min to a maximum of 1 g, then 100–200 mg PO q8h
   c. Digibind (digoxin immune Fab [Ovine]) 400 mg (10 vials) IV, which may be repeated in several hours, can be used for life-threatening digoxin toxicity.
5. Special concerns
   a. Digoxin toxicity decreases the threshold for postcardioversion malignant arrhythmias. This may be exacerbated when hypokalemia or hypercalcemia is present. Use of lidocaine, phenytoin, or lower energy levels should be considered.
   b. Dialysis is ineffective in removing digoxin. Its half-life is 36–48 hours.

References

1. Douglas PS, Edmunds LH, Sutton MSJ, Geer R, Harken AH, Reichek N. Unreliability of hemodynamic indexes of left ventricular size during cardiac surgery. Ann Thorac Surg 1987;44: 31–4.

2. Hansen RM, Viquerat CE, Matthay MA, et al. Poor correlation between pulmonary arterial wedge pressure and left ventricular end-diastolic volume after coronary artery bypass surgery. Anesthesiology 1986;64:764–70.

3. Stewart RD, Psyhojos T, Lahey SJ, Levitsky S, Campos CT. Central venous catheter use in low-risk coronary artery bypass grafting. Ann Thorac Surg 1998;66:1306–11.

4. Schwann TA, Zacharias A, Riordan CJ, Durham SJ, Engoren M, Habib RH. Safe, highly selective use of pulmonary artery catheters in coronary artery bypass grafting: an objective patient selection method. Ann Thorac Surg 2002;73:1394–1402.

5. Eichhorn EJ, Diehl JT, Konstam MA, Payne DD, Salem DN, Cleveland RJ. Left ventricular inotropic effect of atrial pacing after coronary artery bypass grafting. Am J Cardiol 1989;63: 687–92.

6. Mielck F, Buhre W, Hanekop G, Tirilomis T, Hilgers R, Sonntag H. Comparison of continuous cardiac output measurements in patients after cardiac surgery. J Cardiothorac Vasc Anesth 2003;17:211–6.

7. Bein B, Worthmann F, Tonner PH, et al. Comparison of esophageal Doppler, pulse contour analysis, and real-time pulmonary artery thermodilution for the continuous measurement of cardiac output. J Cardiothorac Vasc Anesth 2004;18:185–9.

8. Su NY, Huang CJ, Tsai P, Hsu YW, Hung YC, Cheng CR. Cardiac output measurement during cardiac surgery: esophageal Doppler versus pulmonary artery catheter. Acta Anaesthesiol Sin 2002;40:127–33.

9. Gan GJ. The esophageal Doppler as an alternative to the pulmonary artery catheter. Current Opin Crit Care 2000;6:214–21.

10. Poeze M, Ramsay G, Greve JW, Singer M. Prediction of postoperative cardiac surgical morbidity and organ failure within 4 hours of intensive care unit admission using esophageal Doppler ultrasonography. Crit Care Med 1999;27:1288–94.

11. Cotter G, Moshkovitz Y, Kaluski et al. Accurate, noninvasive continuous monitoring of cardiac output by whole-body electrical bioimpedance. Chest 2004;125:1431–40.

12. Felbinger TW, Reuter DA, Eltzschig HK, Moerstedt K, Goedje O, Goetz AE. Comparison of pulmonary arterial thermodilution and arterial pulse contour analysis: evaluation of a new algorithm. J Clin Anesth 2002;14:296–301.

13. Hamilton TT, Huber LM, Jessen ME. Pulse CO: a less-invasive method to monitor cardiac output from arterial pressure after cardiac surgery. Ann Thorac Surg 2002;74:S1408–12.

14. Johnson RG, Thurer RL, Kruskall MS, et al. Comparison of two transfusion strategies after elective operations for myocardial revascularization. J Thorac Cardiovasc Surg 1992;104: 307–14.

15. Doak GJ, Hall RI. Does hemoglobin concentration affect perioperative myocardial lactate flux in patients undergoing coronary artery bypass surgery? Anesth Analg 1995;80:910–6.

16. Baron JG. Which lower value of haematocrit or haemoglobin concentration should guide the transfusion of red blood cell concentrates during and after extracorporeal circulation? Ann Fr Anesth Réanim 1995;14(suppl):21–7.

17. Spiess BD, Ley C, Body SC, et al. Hematocrit value on intensive care unit entry influences the frequency of Q-wave myocardial infarction after coronary artery bypass grafting. J Thorac Cardiovasc Surg 1998;116:460–7.

18. Vamvakas EC, Carven JH. Transfusion and postoperative pneumonia in coronary artery bypass grafting surgery: effect of the length of storage of transfused cells. Transfusion 1999;39:701–10.

19. Fransen E, Maessen J, Dentener M, Senden N, Buurman W. Impact of blood transfusions on inflammatory mediator release in patients undergoing cardiac surgery. Chest 1999;116:1233–9.

20. Chelemer SB, Prato BS, Cox PM Jr, O'Connor GT, Morton JR. Association of bacterial infection and red blood cell transfusion after coronary artery bypass surgery. Ann Thorac Surg 2002;73: 138–42.

21. Sommers MS, Stevenson JS, Hamlin RL, Ivey TD, Russell AC. Mixed venous oxygen saturation and oxygen partial pressure as predictors of cardiac index after coronary artery bypass grafting. Heart Lung 1993;22:112–20.

22. Magilligan DJ Jr, Teasdall R, Eisinminger R, Peterson E. Mixed venous oxygen saturation as a predictor of cardiac output in the postoperative cardiac surgical patient. Ann Thorac Surg 1987;44:260–2.

23. Balik K, Pachl J, Hendl J, Martin B, Jan P, Jan H. Effect of the degree of tricuspid regurgitation on cardiac output measurements by thermodilution. Intensive Care Med 2002;28:1117–21.

24. Ardehali A, Ports TA. Myocardial oxygen supply and demand. Chest 1990;98:699–705.

25. Griffin MJ, Hines RL. Management of perioperative ventricular dysfunction. J Cardiothorac Vasc Anesth 2001;15:90–106.

26. Royster RL, Butterworth JF IV, Prough DS, et al. Preoperative and intraoperative predictors of inotropic support and long-term outcome in patients having coronary artery bypass grafting. Anesth Analg 1991;72:729–36.

27. Bernard F, Denault A, Babin D, et al. Diastolic dysfunction is predictive of difficult weaning from cardiopulmonary bypass. Anesth Analg 2001;92:291–8.

28. Rao V, Ivanov J, Weisel RD, Cohen G, Borger MA, Mickle DA. Lactate release during reperfusion predicts low cardiac output syndrome after coronary bypass surgery. Ann Thorac Surg 2001;71:1925–30.

29. Breisblatt WM, Stein KL, Wolfe CJ, et al. Acute myocardial dysfunction and recovery: a common occurrence after coronary bypass surgery. J Am Coll Cardiol 1990;15:1261–9.

30. Smith RC, Leung JM, Mangano DT. Postoperative myocardial ischemia in patients undergoing coronary artery bypass surgery. Anesthesiology 1991;74:464–73.

31. Casthely PA, Shah C, Mekhjian H, et al. Left ventricular diastolic function after coronary artery bypass grafting: a correlative study with three different myocardial protection techniques. J Thorac Cardiovasc Sug 1997;114:254–60.

32. Schmidlin D, Schuepbach R, Bernard E, Ecknauer E, Jenni R, Schmid ER. Indications and impact of postoperative transesophageal echocardiography in cardiac surgical patients. Crit Care Med 2001;29:2143–8.

33. Weisel RD, Burns RJ, Baird RJ, et al. A comparison of volume loading and atrial pacing following aortocoronary bypass. Ann Thorac Surg 1983;36:332–44.

34. Richer M, Robert S, Lebel M. Renal hemodynamics during norepinephrine and low-dose dopamine infusions in man. Crit Care Med 1996;24:1150–6.

35. Morimatsu H, Uchino S, Chung J, Bellomo R, Raman J, Buxton B. Norepinephrine for hypotensive vasodilatation after cardiac surgery: impact on renal function. Intensive Care Med 2003;29:1106–12.

36. Argenziano M, Choudhri AF, Moazami N, et al. Vasodilatory hypotension after cardiopulmonary bypass: risk factors and potential mechanisms. Circulation 1997;96(suppl I):I–680.

37. Argenziano M, Chen JM, Choudhri AF, et al. Management of vasodilatory shock after cardiac surgery: identification of predisposing factors and use of a novel pressor agent. J Thorac Cardiovasc Surg 1998;116:973–80.

38. Dunser MW, Mayr AJ, Ulmer H, et al. Arginine vasopressin in advanced vasodilatory shock: a prospective, randomized, controlled trial. Circulation 2003;107:2313–9.

39. Morales DLS, Garrido MJ, Madigan JD, et al. A double-blind randomized trial: prophylactic vasopressin reduces hypotension after cardiopulmonary bypass. Ann Thorac Surg 2003;75:926–30.

40. Levin RL, Degrange MA, Bruno GF, et al. Methylene blue reduces mortality and morbidity in vasoplegic patients after cardiac surgery. Ann Thorac Surg 2004;77:496–9.

41. Leyh RG, Kofidis T, Struber M, et al. Methylene blue: the drug of choice for catecholamine-refractory vasoplegia after cardiopulmonary bypass? J Thorac Cardiovasc Surg 2003;125:1426–31.

42. Martikainen TJ, Tenhunen JJ, Uusaro A, Ruokonen E. The effects of vasopressin on systemic and splanchnic hemodynamics and metabolism in endotoxin shock. Anesth Analg 2003;97:1756–63.

43. Davila-Roman VG, Waggoner AD, Hopkins WE, Barzilai B. Right ventricular dysfunction in low output syndrome after cardiac operations: assessment by transesophageal echocardiography. Ann Thorac Surg 1995;60:1081–6.

44. Perings SM, Perings C, Kelm M, Strauer BE. Comparative evaluation of thermodilution and gated blood pool method for determination of right ventricular ejection fraction at rest and during exercise. Cardiology 2001;95:161–3.

45. Gordon G, Rastegar H, Khabbaz K, Schumann R, England M. Perioperative use of nesiritide in adult cardiac surgery. Anesth Analg 2004;98:SCA1–134.

46. Moazami N, Damiano RJ, Bailey MS, et al. Nesiritide (BNP) in the management of postoperative cardiac patients. Ann Thorac Surg 2003;75:1974–6.

47. Ichinose F, Robert JD Jr, Zapol WM. Inhaled nitric oside. A selective pulmonary vasodilator. Current uses and therapeutic potential. Circulation 2004;109:3106–11.

48. Solina AR, Ginsberg SH, Papp D, et al. Dose response to nitric oxide in adult cardiac surgery patients. J Clin Anesth 2001;13:281–6.

49. Maxey TS, Smith CD, Kern JA, et al. Beneficial effects of inhaled nitric oxide in adult cardiac surgical patients. Ann Thorac Surg 2002;73:529–32.

50. Frostell CG, Blomqvist H, Nedenstierna G, Lundberg J, Zapol WM. Inhaled nitric oxide selectively reverses human hypoxic pulmonary vasoconstriction without causing systemic vasodilation. Anesthesiology 1995;78:427–35.

51. Solina AR, Ginsberg SH, Papp D, et al. Response to nitric oxide during adult cardiac surgery. J Invest Surg 2002;15:5–14.

52. Fullerton DA, Jaggers J, Wollmering MM, Piedalue F, Grover FL, McIntyre RC Jr. Variable response to inhaled nitric oxide after cardiac surgery. Ann Thorac Surg 1997;63:1251–6.

53. Fullerton DA, Jaggers J, Piedalue F, Grover FL, McIntyre RC Jr. Effective control of refractory pulmonary hypertension after cardiac operations. J Thorac Cardiovasc Surg 1997;113:363–70.

54. Ivy DD, Kinsella JP, Ziegler JW, Abman SH. Dipyridamole attenuates rebound pulmonary hypertension after inhaled nitric oxide withdrawal in postoperative congenital heart disease. J Thorac Cardiovasc Surg 1998;115:875–82.

55. Pearl JM, Nelson DP, Raake JL, et al. Inhaled nitric oxide increases endothelin-1 levels: a potential cause of rebound pulmonary hypertension. Crit Care Med 2002;30:89–93.

56. Solina A, Papp D, Ginsberg S, et al. A comparison of inhaled nitric oxide and milrinone for the treatment of pulmonary hypertension in adult cardiac surgery patients. J Cardiothorac Vasc Anesth 2000;14:12–7.

57. Camara ML, Aris A, Alvarez J, Padro JM, Caralps JM. Hemodynamic effects of prostaglandin E_1 and isoproterenol early after cardiac operations for mitral stenosis. J Thorac Cardiovasc Surg 1992;103:1177–85.

58. Tritapepe L, Voci P, Cogliati AA, Pasotti E, Papalia U, Menichetti A. Successful weaning from cardiopulmonary bypass with central venous prostaglandin E1 and left atrial epinephrine infusion in patients with acute pulmonary hypertension. Crit Care Med 1999;27:2180–3.

59. Haché M, Denault A, Bélisle S, et al. Inhaled epoprostenol (prostacyclin) and pulmonary hypertension before surgery. J Thorac Cardiovasc Surg 2003;125:642–9.

60. Lowson SM, Doctor A, Walsh BK, Doorley PA. Inhaled prostacyclin for the treatment of pulmonary hypertension after cardiac surgery. Crit Care Med 2002;30:2762–4.

61. De Wet CJ, Affleck DG, Jacobsohn E, et al. Inhaled prostacyclin is safe, effective, and affordable in patients with pulmonary hypertension, right heart dysfunction, and refractory hypoxemia after cardiothoracic surgery. J Thorac Cardiovasc Surg 2004;127:1058–67.

62. Sablotzki A, Czeslick E, Schubert S, et al. Iloprost improves hemodynamics in patients with severe chronic cardiac failure and secondary pulmonary hypertension. Can J Anaesth 2002;49:1076–80.

63. Rex S, Busch T, Vettelschoss M, de Rossi L, Rossaint R, Buhre W. Intraoperative management of severe pulmonary hypertension during cardiac surgery with inhaled iloprost. Anesthesiology 2003;99:745–7.

64. Kieler-Jensen N, Houltz E, Milocco I, Ricksten SE. Central hemodynamics and right ventricular function after coronary artery bypass surgery. A comparison of prostacyclin, sodium nitroprusside, and nitroglycerin for treatment of postcardiac surgical hypertension. J Cardiothorac Vasc Anesth 1993;7:555–9.

65. Schmid ER, Burki C, Engel MH, Schmidlin D, Tornic M, Seifert B. Inhaled nitric oxide versus intravenous vasodilators in severe pulmonary hypertension after cardiac surgery. Anesth Analg 1999;89:1108–15.

66. Fullerton DA, Jones SD, Grover FL, McIntyre RC Jr. Adenosine effectively controls pulmonary hypertension after cardiac operations. Ann Thorac Surg 1996;61:1118–24.

67. Brutsaert DL, Sys SU, Gillebert TC. Diastolic dysfunction in post-cardiac surgical management. J Cardiothorac Vasc Anesth 1993;7(suppl 1):18–20.

68. Aral A, Oguz M, Ozberrak H, et al. Hemodynamic advantages of left atrial epinephrine administration in open heart surgery. Ann Thorac Surg 1997;64:1046–9.

69. Butterworth JF IV, Prielipp RC, Royster RL, et al. Dobutamine increases heart rate more than epinephrine in patients recovering from aortocoronary bypass surgery. J Cardiothorac Vasc Anesth 1992;6:535–41.

70. Bailey JM. Dopamine: one size doesn't not fit all. Anesthesiology 2000;92:303–5.

71. Esson ML, Schrier RW. Diagnosis and treatment of acute tubular necrosis. Ann Intern Med 2002;137:744–52.

72. Gelfman DM, Ornato JP, Gonzalez ER. Dopamine-induced increase in atrioventricular conduction in atrial fibrillation-flutter. Clin Cardiol 1987;10:671–3.

73. Lassnigg A, Donner E, Grubhofer G, Presterl E, Druml W, Hiesmayr M. Lack of renoprotective effects of dopamine and furosemide during cardiac surgery. J Am Soc Nephrol 2000;11: 97–104.

74. Woo EB, Tang AT, el-Gamel A, et al. Dopamine therapy for patients at risk of renal dysfunction following cardiac surgery: fact or fiction? Eur J Cardiothorac Surg 2002;22:106–11.

75. Romson JL, Leung JM, Bellows WH, et al. Effects of dobutamine on hemodynamics and left ventricular performance after cardiopulmonary bypass in cardiac surgical patients. Anesthesiology 1999;91:1318–28.

76. Fowler MB, Alderman EL, Oesterle SN, et al. Dobutamine and dopamine after cardiac surgery: greater augmentation of myocardial blood flow with dobutamine. Circulation 1984;70(suppl I): I-103–11.

77. Van Trigt P, Spray TL, Pasque MK, Peyton RB, Pellom GL, Wechsler AS. The comparative effects of dopamine and dobutamine on ventricular mechanics after coronary artery bypass grafting: a pressure–dimension analysis. Circulation 1984;70(suppl I):I-112–7.

78. DiSesa VJ, Brown E, Mudge GH Jr, Collins JJ Jr, Cohn LH. Hemodynamic comparison of dopamine and dobutamine in the postoperative volume-loaded, pressure-loaded, and normal ventricle. J Thorac Cardiovasc Surg 1982;83:256–63.

79. Dupuis JY, Bondy R, Cattran C, Nathan JH, Wynands JE. Amrinone and dobutamine as primary treatment of low cardiac output syndrome following coronary artery surgery: a comparison of their effects on hemodynamics and outcome. J Cardiothorac Vasc Anesth 1992;6:542–53.

80. Feneck RO, Sherry KM, Withington PS, Oduro-Dominah A, and the European Milrinone Multicenter Trial Group. Comparison of the hemodynamic effects of milrinone with dobutamine in patients after cardiac surgery. J Cardiothorac Vasc Anesth 2001;15:306–15.

81. Levy JH, Bailey JM, Deeb GM. Intravenous milrinone in cardiac surgery. Ann Thorac Surg 2002; 73:325–30.

82. Royster RL, Butterworth JF IV, Prielipp RC, Robertie PG, Kon ND. A randomized, blinded trial of amrinone, epinephrine, and amrinone/epinephrine after cardiopulmonary bypass (CPB). Anesthesiology 1991;75:A148.

83. Olsen KH, Kluger J, Fieldman A. Combination high dose amrinone and dopamine in the management of moribund cardiogenic shock after open heart surgery. Chest 1988;94:503–6.

84. Royster RL, Butterworth JF IV, Prielipp RC, et al. Combined inotropic effects of amrinone and epinephrine after cardiopulmonary bypass in humans. Anesth Anal 1993;77:662–72.

85. Rathmell JP, Prielipp RC, Butterworth JF, et al. A multicenter, randomized, blind comparison of amrinone with milrinone after elective cardiac surgery. Anesth Analg 1998;86:683–90.

86. Ko W, Zelano JA, Fahey AL, et al. The effects of amrinone versus dobutamine on myocardial mechanics after hypothermic global ischemia. J Thorac Cardiovasc Surg 1993;105:1015–24.

87. Alhashemi JA, Hooper J. Treatment of milrinone-associated tachycardia with beta-blockers. Can J Anaesth 1998;45:67–70.
88. Kikura M, Sato S. The efficacy of preemptive milrinone or amrinone therapy in patients undergoing coronary artery bypass grafting. Anesth Anal 2002;94:22–30.
89. Kikura M, Lee MK, Safon RA, Bailey JM, Levy JH. The effects of milrinone on platelets in patients undergoing cardiac surgery. Anesth Analg 1995;81:44–8.
90. Liu JJ, Doolan LA, Xie B, Chen JR, Buxton BF. Direct vasodilator effect of milrinone, an inotropic drug, on arterial coronary bypass grafts. J Thorac Cardiovasc Surg 1997;113:108–113.
91. Lobato EB, Janelle GM, Urdaneta F, Martin TD. Comparison of milrinone versus nitroglycerin, alone and in combination, on grafted internal mammary artery flow after cardiopulmonary bypass: effects on α-adrenergic stimulation. J Cardiothorac Vasc Anesth 2001;15:723–7.
92. Kikura M, Levy JH, Bailey JM, Shanewise JS, Michelsen LG, Sadel SM. A bolus dose of 1.5 mg/kg amrinone effectively improves low cardiac output states following separation from cardiopulmonary bypass in cardiac surgical patients. Acta Anaesthesiol Scand 1998;42:825–33.
93. Kirsh MM, Bove E, Detmer M, Hill A, Knight P. The use of levarterenol and phentolamine in patients with low cardiac output following open-heart surgery. Ann Thorac Surg 1980;29:26–31.
94. DeHert SG, Ten Broecke PW, De Mulder PA, et al. The effects of calcium on left ventricular function early after cardiopulmonary bypass. J Cardiothorac Vasc Anesth 1997;11:864–9.
95. Drop LJ, Scheidegger D. Plasma ionized concentration: important determinant of the hemodynamic response to calcium infusion. J Thorac Cardiovasc Surg 1980;79:425–31.
96. Royster RL, Butterworth JF IV, Prielipp RC, et al. A randomized, blinded, placebo-controlled evaluation of calcium chloride and epinephrine for inotropic support after emergence from cardiopulmonary bypass. Anesth Analg 1992;74:3–13.
97. Butterworth JF, Zaloga GP, Prielipp RC, Tucker WY Jr, Royster RL. Calcium inhibits the cardiac stimulating properties of dobutamine but not of amrinone. Chest 1992;101:174–80.
98. Reinhardt W, Mocker K, Jockenhovel F, et al. Influence of coronary artery bypass surgery on thyroid hormone parameters. Horm Res 1997;47:1–8.
99. Sabatino L, Cerillo AG, Ripoli A, Pilo A, Glauber M, Iervasi G. Is the low tri-iodothyronine state a crucial factor in determining the outcome of coronary artery bypass patients? Evidence from a clinical pilot study. J Endocrinol 2002;175:577–86.
100. Klemperer JD, Klein I, Gomez M, et al. Thyroid hormone treatment after coronary-artery bypass surgery. N Engl J Med 1995;333:1522–7.
101. Bennett-Guerrero E, Jimenez JL, White WD, D'Amico EB, Baldwin BI, Schwinn DA. Cardiovascular effects of intravenous triiodothyronine in patients undergoing coronary artery bypass surgery. A randomized, double-blind, placebo-controlled trial. Duke T₃ study group. JAMA 1996;275:687–92.
102. Mullis-Jansson S, Argenziano M, Corwin S, et al. A randomized double-blind study of the effect of triiodothyronine on cardiac function and morbidity after coronary bypass surgery. J Thorac Cardiovasc Surg 1999;117:1128–35.
103. Klemperer JD. Thyroid hormone and cardiac surgery. Thyroid 2002;12:517–21.
104. Klemperer JD, Zelano J, Helm RE et al. Triiodothyronine improves left ventricular function without oxygen wasting effects after global hypothermic ischemia. J Thorac Cardiovasc Surg 1995;109:457–65.
105. Klemperer JD, Klein IL, Ojamaa K, et al. Triiodothyronine therapy lowers the incidence of atrial fibrillation after cardiac operations. Ann Thorac Surg 1996;61:1323–9.
106. Fonarow GC. Nesiritide: practical guide to its safe and effective use. Rev Cardiovasc Med 2001;2(suppl2):532–5.
107. Ramanathan T, Shirota K, Morita S, Nishimura T, Huang Y, Hunyor SN. Glucose-insulin-potassium solution improves left ventricular mechanics in diabetics. Ann Thorac Surg 2002;73:582–7.
108. MacGregor DA, Butterworth JF 4th, Zaloga CP, Prielipp RC, James R, Royster RL. Hemodynamic and renal effects of dopexamine and dobutamine in patients with reduced cardiac output following coronary artery bypass grafting. Chest 1994;106:835–41.
109. Boldt J, Kling D, Zickmann B, Dapper F, Hempelmann G. Efficacy of the phosphodiesterase inhibitor enoximone in complicated cardiac surgery. Chest 1990;98:53–8.

110. Labriola C, Siro-Brigiani M, Carrata F, Santangelo F, Amantea B. Hemodynamic effects of levosimendan in patients with low-output failure after cardiac surgery. Int J Clin Pharmacol Ther 2004;42:204–11.

111. Dzimiri N, Chester AH, Allen SP, Duran C, Yacoub MH. Vascular reactivity of arterial coronary artery bypass grafts: implications for their performance. Clin Cardiol 1996;19:165–71.

112. Maccioli GA, Lucas WJ, Norfleet EA. The intra-aortic balloon pump: a review. J Cardiothorac Anesth 1988;2:365–73.

113. Baskett RJF, Ghali WA, Maitland A, Hirsch GM. The intraaortic balloon pump in cardiac surgery. Ann Thorac Surg 2002;74:1276–87.

114. Kang N, Edwards M, Larbalestier R. Preoperative intraaortic balloon pumps in high-risk patients undergoing open heart surgery. Ann Thorac Surg 2001;72:54–7.

115. Craver JM, Murrah CP. Elective intraaortic balloon counterpulsation for high-risk off-pump coronary artery bypass operations. Ann Thorac Surg 2001;71:1220–3.

116. Kim KB, Lim C, Ahn H, Yang JK. Intraaortic balloon pump therapy facilitates posterior off-pump coronary artery bypass grafting in high-risk patients. Ann Thorac Surg 2001;71:1964–8.

117. Khir AW, Price S, Heinein MY, Parker KH, Pepper JR. Intra-aortic balloon pumping: effects on left ventricular diastolic function. Eur J Cardiothorac Surg 2003;24:277–82.

118. Meyns BP, Nishimura Y, Jashari R, Racz R, Leunens VH, Flameng WJ. Ascending versus descending aortic balloon pumping: organ and myocardial perfusion during ischemia. Ann Thorac Surg 2000;70:1264–9.

119. Arafa OE, Pedersen TH, Svennevig JL, Fosse E, Geiran OR. Vascular complications of the intraaortic balloon pump in patients undergoing open heart operations: a 15-year experience. Ann Thorac Surg 1999;67:645–51.

120. Boffa DJ, Tak V, Jansson SL, Ko W, Krishnasastry KV. Atheroemboli to superior mesenteric artery following cardiopulmonary bypass. Ann Vasc Surg 2002;16:228–30.

121. Venkateswaran RV, Charman SC, Goddard M, Large SR. Lethal mesenteric ischemia after cardiopulmonary bypass: a common complication? Eur J Cardiothorac Surg 2002;22:534–8.

122. Ho AC, Hong CL, Yang MW, Lu PP, Lin PJ. Stroke after intraaortic balloon counterpulsation associated with mobile atheroma in thoracic aorta diagnosed using transesophageal echocardiography. Chang Gung Med J 2002;25:612–6.

123. Swartz MT, Sakamoto T, Arai H, et al. Effects of intraaortic balloon position on renal artery blood flow. Ann Thorac Surg 1992;53:604–10.

124. Shimamoto H, Kawazoe K, Kito H, Fujita T, Shimamoto Y. Does juxtamesenteric placement of intra-aortic balloon interrupt superior mesenteric flow? Clin Cardiol 1992;15:285–90.

125. Christensen JT, Cohen M, Ferguson JJ III. Trends in intraaortic ballon counterpulsation complications and outcomes in cardiac surgery. Ann Thorac Surg 2002;74:1086–91.

126. Davies AR, Bellomo R, Raman JS, Gutteridge GA, Buxton BF. High lactate predicts the failure of intraaortic balloon pumping after cardiac surgery. Ann Thorac Surg 2001;71:1415–20.

127. Matsuda H, Matsumiya G. Current status of left ventricular assist devices: the role of bridging to heart transplantation and future perspectives. J Artif Organs 2003;6:157–61.

128. Wheeldon DR. Mechanical circulatory support: state of the art and future perspectives. Perfusion 2003;18:233–43.

129. Rose EA, Gelijns AC, Moskowitz AJ, for the REMATCH Study Group. Long-term use of a left ventricular assist device for end-stage heart failure. N Engl J Med 2001;345:1435–43.

130. Klotz S, Deng MC, Stypmann J, et al. Left ventricular pressure and volume unloading during pulsatile versus nonpulsatile left ventricular assist devices support. Ann Thorac Surg 2004;77:143–9.

131. Aaronson KD, Patel H, Pagani FD. Patient selection for left ventricular assist device therapy. Ann Thorac Surg 2003;75:S29–35.

132. Rao V, Oz MC, Flannery MA, Catanese KA, Argenziano M, Naka Y. Revised screening scale to predict survival after insertion of a left ventricular assist device. J Thorac Cardiovasc Surg 2003;125:855–62.

133. Williams MR, Oz MC. Indications and patient selection for mechanical ventricular assistance. Ann Thorac Surg 2001;71:S86–91.

134. Morales DLS, Gregg D, Helman DN, et al. Arginine vasopressin in the treatment of 50 patients with postcardiotomy vasodilatory shock. Ann Thorac Surg 2000;69:102–6.

135. Barbone A, Rao V, Oz MC, Naka Y. LVAD support in patients with bioprosthetic valves. Ann Thorac Surg 2002;74:232–4.

136. Schmid C, Welp H, Klotz S, Baba HA, Wilhelm MJ, Scheld HH. Outcome of patients surviving to heart transplantation after being mechanically bridged for more than 100 days. J Heart Lung Transplant 2003;22:1054–8.

137. Schmid C, Radovancevic B. When should we consider right ventricular support? Thorac Cardiovasc Surg 2002;50:204–7.

138. Radovancevic B, Gregoric ID, Tamez F, et al. Biventricular support with the Jarvik 2000 axial flow pump: a feasibility study. ASAIO J 2003;49:604–7.

139. Wagner F, Dandel M, Gunther G, et al. Nitric oxide inhalation in the treatment of right ventricular dysfunction following left ventricular assist device implantation. Circulation 1997;96(suppl II): II-291–6.

140. Chen JM, Levin HR, Rose EA, et al. Experience with right ventricular assist devices for perioperative right-sided circulatory failure. Ann Thorac Surg 1996;61:305–10.

141. Fukamachi K, McCarthy PM, Smedira NG, Vargo RL, Starling RC, Young JB. Preoperative risk factors for right ventricular failure after implantable left venricular assist device insertion. Ann Thorac Surg 1999;68:2181–4.

142. Ochiai Y, McCarthy PM, Smedira NG, et al. Predictors of severe right ventricular failure after implantable left ventricular assist device insertion: analysis of 245 patients. Circulation 2002;106(suppl I):I-198–202.

143. Nakatani S, Thomas JD, Savage RM, Vargo RL, Smedira NG, McCarthy PM. Prediction of right ventricular dysfunction after left ventricular assist device implantation. Circulation 1996;94 (suppl II):II-216–21.

144. Kavarana MN, Pessin-Minsley MS, Urtecho J, et al. Right ventricular dysfunction and organ failure in left ventricular assist device recipients: a continuing problem. Ann Thorac Surg 2002;73: 745–50.

145. Magliato KE, Kleisli T, Soukiasian HJ, et al. Biventricular support in patients with profound cardiogenic shock: a single center experience. ASAIO J 2003;49:475–9.

146. Muehrcke DD, McCarthy PM, Stewart RW et al. Extracorporeal membrane oxygenation for postcardiotomy cardiogenic shock. Ann Thorac Surg 1996;61:684–91.

147. Pagani FD, Aaronson KD, Swaniker F, Bartlett RH. The use of extracorporeal life support in adult patients with primary cardiac failure as a bridge to implantable left ventricular assist device. Ann Thorac Surg 2001;71:S77–81.

148. Smedira NG, Blackstone EH. Postcardiotomy mechanical support: risk factors and outcomes. Ann Thorac Surg 2001;71(suppl):S60–6.

149. Smedira NG, Moazami N, Golding CM, et al. Clinical experience with 202 adult patients receiving extracorporeal membrane oxygenation for cardiac failure: survival at five years. J Thorac Cardiovasc Surg 2001;122:92–102.

150. Wang SS, Ko WJ, Chen YS, Hsu RB, Chou NK, Chu SH. Mechanical bridge with extracorporeal oxygenation and ventricular assist to heart transplantation. Artif Organs 2001;25:599–602.

151. Chen YS, Chao A, Yu HY, et al. Analysis and results of prolonged resuscitation in cardiac arrest patients by extracorporeal membrane oxygenation. J Am Coll Cardiol 2003;41:197–203.

152. Bartlett RH. Extracorporeal life support in the management for severe respiratory failure. Clin Chest Med 2000;21:555–61.

153. Pego-Fernandes PM, Stolf NAG, Moreira LFP, et al. Influence of Biopump with and without intraaortic balloon on the coronary and carotid flow. Ann Thorac Surg 2000;69:536–40.

154. Smith C, Bellomo R, Raman JS, et al. An extracorporeal membrane oxygenation-based approach to cardiogenic shock in an older population. Ann Thorac Surg 2001;71:1421–7.

155. Fiser SM, Tribble CG, Kaza AK, et al. When to discontinue extracorporeal membrane oxygenation for postcardiotomy support. Ann Thorac Surg 2001;71:210–4.

156. Yap HJ, Chen YC, Fang JT, Huang CC. Combination of continuous renal replacement therapies (CRRT) and extracorporeal membrane oxygenation (ECMO) for advanced cardiac patients. Ren Fail 2003;25:183–93.

157. Ko WJ, Lin CY, Chen RJ, Wang SS, Lin FY, Chen YS. Extracorporeal membrane oxygenation support for adult postcardiotomy cardiogenic shock. Ann Thorac Surg 2002;73:538–45.

158. Doll N, Kiaii B, Borger M, et al. Five-year results of 219 consecutive patients treated with extracorporeal membrane oxygenation for refractory postoperative cardiogenic shock. Ann Thorac Surg 2004;77:151–7.

159. Saito S, Westaby S, Piggot D, et al. End-organ function during chronic nonpulsatile circulation. Ann Thorac Surg 2002;74:1080–5.

160. Ochiai Y, Golding LA, Massiello AL et al. Cleveland Clinic CorAide blood pump circulatory support without anticoagulation. ASAIO J 2002;48:249–52.

161. Curtis JJ, McKenney-Knox CA, Wagner-Mann CC. Postcardiotomy centrifugal assist: a single surgeon's experience. Artif Organs 2002;26:994–7.

162. Meyns B, Sergeant P, Wouters P, et al. Mechanical support with microaxial blood pumps for postcardiotomy left ventricular failure: can outcome be predicted? J Thorac Cardiovasc Surg 2000; 120:393–400.

163. Vitali E, Lanfranconi M, Ribera E, et al. Successful experience in bridging patients to heart transplantation with the MicroMed DeBakey ventricular assist device. Ann Thorac Surg 2003;75:1200–4.

164. Frazier OH, Delgado RM III, Kar B, Patel V, Gregoric ID, Myers TJ. First clinical use of the redesigned HeartMate II left ventricular assist system in the United States. A case report. Tex Heart Inst J 2004;31:157–9.

165. Frazier OH, Myers TJ, Westaby S, Gregoric ID. Clinical experience with an implantable, intracardiac, continuous flow circulatory support device: physiologic implications and their relationship to patient selection. Ann Thorac Surg 2004;77:133–42.

166. Samuels LE, Holmes EC, Thomas MP, et al. Management of acute cardiac failure with mechanical assist: experience with the Abiomed BVS 5000. Ann Thorac Surg 2001;71(suppl):S67–72.

167. Korfer R, El-Banayosy A, Arusoglu L, et al. Single-center experience with the Thoratec ventricular assist device. J Thorac Cardiovasc Surg 2000;119:596–600.

168. Farrar DJ. The Thoratec ventricular assist device: a paracorporeal pump for treating acute and chronic heart failure. Semin Thorac Cardiovasc Surg 2000;12:243–50.

169. Morgan JA, John R, Rao V, et al. Bridging to transplant with the HeartMate left ventricular assist device: the Columbia Presbyterian 12-year experience. J Thorac Cardiovasc Surg 2004;127: 1309–16.

170. Thomas CE, Jichici D, Petrucci R, Urrutia VC, Schwartzman RJ. Neurologic complications of the Novacor left ventricular assist device. Ann Thorac Surg 2001;72:1311–5.

171. El-Banayosy A, Arusoglu L, Kizner L, et al. Novacor left ventricular assist system versus HeartMate vented electric left ventricular assist system as a long-term mechanical circulatory support device in bridging patients: a prospective study. J Thorac Cardiovasc Surg 2000;119:581–7.

172. Strauch JT, Speilvogel D, Haldenwang PL, et al. Recent improvements in outcome with the Novacor left ventricular assist device. J Heart Lung Transplant 2003;22:674–80.

173. El-Banayosy A, Aarusoglu L, Kizner L, et al. Preliminary experience with the LionHeart left ventricular assist device in patients with end–stage heart failure. Ann Thorac Surg 2003;75:1469–75.

174. Myers TJ, Robertson K, Pool T, Shah N, Gregoric I, Frazier OH. Continuous flow pumps and total artificial hearts: management issues. Ann Thorac Surg 2003;75(suppl):S79–85.

175. Dowling RD, Gray LA JR, Etoch SW, et al. Initial experience with the AbioCor implantable replacement heart system. J Thorac Cardiovasc Surg 2004;127:131–41.

176. Goldstein DJ, Beauford RB. Left ventricular assist devices and bleeding: adding insult to injury. Ann Thorac Surg 2003;75(suppl):S42–7.

177. Spanier T, Oz M, Levin H, et al. Activation of coagulation and fibrinolytic pathways in patients with left ventricular assist devices. J Thorac Cardiovasc Surg 1996;112:1090–7.

178. Milano CA, Patel VS, Smith PK, Smith MS. Risk of anaphylaxis from aprotinin re-exposure during LVAD removal and heart transplantation. J Heart Lung Transplant 2002;21:1127–30.

179. Malani PN, Dyke DB, Pagani FD, Chenoweth CE. Nosocomial infections in left ventricular assist device recipients. Clin Infect Dis 2002;34:1295–300.

180. Gordon SM, Schmitt SK, Jacobs M, et al. Nosocomial blood stream infections in patients with implantable left ventricular assist devices. Ann Thorac Surg 2001;72:725–30.

181. Nurozler F, Argenziano M, Oz MC, Naka Y. Fungal left ventricular assist device endocarditis. Ann Thorac Surg 2001;71:614–8.

182. Morgan JA, Park Y, Oz MC, Naka Y. Device related infections while on left ventricular assist device support do not adversely impact bridging to transplant or transplant survival. ASAIO J 2003;49:748–50.

183. Oz MC, Rose EA, Slater J, Kuiper JJ, Catanese KA, Levin HR. Malignant ventricular arrhythmias are well tolerated in patients receiving long-term left ventricular assist devices. J Am Coll Cardiol 1994;24:1688–91.

184. John R, Lietz K, Schuster M, et al. Immunologic sensitization in recipients of left ventricular assist devices. J Thorac Cardiovasc Surg 2003;125:578–91.

185. Fremes SE, Weisel RD, Mickle DAG, et al. A comparison of nitroglycerin and nitroprusside: I. Treatment of postoperative hypertension. Ann Thorac Surg 1985;39:53–60.

186. Bojar RM, Rastegar H, Payne DD, et al. Methemoglobinemia from intravenous nitroglycerin: a word of caution. Ann Thorac Surg 1987;43:332–4.

187. Kataria B, Dubois M, Lea D, et al. Evaluation of intravenous esmolol for treatment of postoperative hypertension. J Cardiothorac Anesth 1990;4:13–6.

188. Sladen RN, Klamerus KJ, Swafford MWG, et al. Labetalol for the control of elevated blood pressure following coronary artery bypass grafting. J Cardiothorac Anesth 1990;4:210–21.

189. Wijeysundera DN, Beattie WS, Rao V, Karski J. Calcium antagonists reduce cardiovascular complications after cardiac surgery: a meta-analysis. J Am Coll Cardiol 2003;41:1496–505.

190. Wijeysundera DN, Beattie WS, Rao V, Ivanov J, Karkouti K. Calcium antagonists are associated with reduced mortality after cardiac surgery: a propensity analysis. J Thorac Cardiovasc Surg 2004;127:755–62.

191. Chanda J, Canver CC. Reversal of preexisting vasospasm in coronary artery conduits. Ann Thorac Surg 2001;72:476–80.

192. Vincent JL, Berlot G, Preiser JC, Engelman E, Dereume JP, Khan RJ. Intravenous nicardipine in the treatment of postoperative arterial hypertension. J Cardiothorac Vasc Anesth 1997;11:160–4.

193. Apostolidou I, Skubas NJ, Bakola A, et al. Effects of nicardipine and nitroglycerin on perioperative myocardial ischemia in patients undergoing coronary artery bypass surgery. Semin Thorac Cardiovasc Surg 1999;11:77–83.

194. Grigore AM, Castro JL, Swistel D, Thys DM. Nicardipine infusion for the prevention of radial artery spasm during myocardial revascularization. J Cardiothorac Vasc Anesth 1998;12:556–7.

195. David D, Dubois C, Loria Y. Comparison of nicardipine and sodium nitroprusside in the treatment of paroxysmal hypertension following aortocoronary bypass surgery. J Cardiothorac Vasc Anesth 1991;5:357–61.

196. Mullen JC, Miller DR, Weisel RD, et al. Postoperative hypertension: a comparison of diltiazem, nifedipine, and nitroprusside. J Thorac Cardiovasc Surg 1988;96:122–32.

197. Bertolissi M, De Monte A, Giodano F. Comparison of intravenous nifedipine and sodium nitroprusside for treatment of acute hypertension after cardiac surgery. Minerva Anestesiol 1998;64:321–8.

198. Tohmo H, Karanko M, Klossner J, et al. Enalaprilat decreases plasma endothelin and atrial natriuretic peptide levels and preload in patients with left ventricular dysfunction after cardiac surgery. J Cardiothorac Vasc Anesth 1997;11:585–90.

199. Boldt J, Schindler E, Harter K, Gorlach G, Hampelmann G. Influence of intravenous administration of angiotensin-converting enzyme inhibitor enalaprilat on cardiovascular mediators in cardiac surgery patients. Anesth Analg 1995;80:480–5.

200. Wagner F, Yeter R, Bisson S, Siniawski H, Hetzer R. Beneficial hemodynamic and renal effects of intravenous enalaprilat following coronary artery bypass surgery complicated by left ventricular dysfunction. Crit Care Med 2003;31:1421–8.

201. Swartz MT, Kaiser GC, Willman VL, Codd JE, Tyras DH, Barner HB. Continuous hydralazine infusion for afterload reduction. Ann Thorac Surg 1981;32:188–92.

202. Gombotz H, Plaza J, Mahla E, Berger J, Metzler H. DA1-receptor stimulation by fenoldopam in the treatment of postcardiac surgical hypertension. Acta Anaesthesiol Scand 1998;42:834–40.

203. Yakazu Y, Iwasawa K, Narita H, Kindscher JD, Benson KT, Goto H. Hemodynamic and sympathetic effects of fenoldopam and sodium nitroprusside. Acta Anaesthesiol Scan 2001;45:1176–80.

204. Guidelines 2000 for cardiopulmonary resuscitation and emergency cardiovascular care. Circulation 2000:102:I-1–228.

205. El-Banayosy A, Brehm C, Kizner L, et al. Cardiopulmonary resuscitation after cardiac surgery: a two-year study. J Cardiothorac Vasc Anesth 1998;12:390–2.

206. Wenzel V, Krismer AC Artnz HR, et al. A comparison of vasopressin and epinephrine for out-of-hospital cardiopulmonary resuscitation. N Engl J Med 2004;350:105–13.

207. Dorian P, Cass D, Schwartz B, Cooper R, Geleznikas R, Barr A. Amiodarone as compared with lidocaine for shock-resistant ventricular fibrillation. N Engl J Med 2002;346:884–90.

208. Prengel AW, Lindner KH, Hahnel J, Ahnefeld FW. Endotracheal and endobronchial lidocaine administration: effects on plasma lidocaine concentration and blood gases. Crit Care Med 1991;19:911–5.

209. Gavard JA, Chaitman BR, Sakai S, et al. Prognostic significance of elevated creatine kinase MB after coronary bypass surgery and after an acute coronary syndrome: results from the GUARDIAN trial. J Thorac Cardiovasc Surg 2003;126:807–13.

210. Brener SJ, Lytle BW, Schneider JP, Ellis SG, Topol EJ. Association between CK-MB elevation after percutaneous and surgical revascularization and three-year mortality. J Am Coll Cardiol 2002;40:1961–7.

211. Costa MA, Carere RG, Lichtenstein SV, et al. Incidence, predictors, and significance of abnormal cardiac enzyme rise in patients treated with bypass surgery in the Arterial Revascularization Therapies Study (ARTS). Circulation 2001;104:2689–93.

212. Steuer J, Horte LG, Lindahl B, Stahle E. Impact of perioperative myocardial injury on early and long-term outcome after coronary artery bypass grafting. Eur Heart J 2002;23:1219–27.

213. Jain U. Myocardial infarction during coronary artery bypass surgery. J Cardiothorac Vasc Anesth 1992;6:612–23.

214. Boyce SW, Bartels C, Bolli R, et al. Impact of sodium-hydrogen exchange inhibition by cariporide on death or myocardial infarction in high-risk CABG surgery patients: results of the CABG surgery cohort of the GUARDIAN trial. J Thorac Cardiovasc Surg 2003;126:420–7.

215. Svedjeholm R, Dahlin LG, Lundberg G, et al. Are electrocardiographic Q-wave criteria reliable for diagnosis of perioperative myocardial infarction after coronary surgery? Eur J Cardiothorac Surg 1998;13:655–61.

216. Schmidt H, Mortensen PE, Folsgaard SL, Jensen EA. Cardiac enzymes and autotransfusion of shed mediastinal blood after myocardial revascularization. Ann Thorac Surg 1997;63:1288–92.

217. Ryan TJ, Anderson JL, Antman EM, et al. ACC/AHA guidelines for the management of patients with acute myocardial infarction: a report of the American College of Cardiology/American Heart Association task force on practice guidelines (Committee on management of acute myocardial infarction). J Am Coll Cardiol 1996;28:1328–1428.

218. Birdi I, Angelini GD, Bryan AJ. Biochemical markers of myocardial injury during cardiac operations. Ann Thorac Surg 1997;63:879–84.

219. Alyanakian MA, Dehoux M, Chatel D, et al. Cardiac troponin I in diagnosis of perioperative myocardial infarction after cardiac surgery. J Cardiothorac Vasc Anesth 1998;12:288–94.

220. Vermes E, Mesguich M, Houel R, et al. Cardiac troponin I release after open heart surgery: a marker of myocardial protection? Ann Thorac Surg 2000;70:2087–90.

221. Gensini GF, Fusi C, Conti AA, et al. Cardiac troponin I and Q wave perioperative myocardial infarction after coronary artery bypass surgery. Crit Care Med 1998;26:2066–70.

222. Sadony V, Korber M, Albes G, et al. Cardiac troponin I levels for diagnosis and quantitation of perioperative myocardial damage in patients undergoing coronary artery bypass surgery. Eur J Cardiothorac Surg 1998;13:57–65.

223. Runsiö M, Kallner A, Kallner G, Rosenqvist M, Bergfeldt L. Myocardial injury after electrical therapy for cardiac arrhythmias assessed by troponin-T release. Am J Cardiol 1997;79:1241–5.

224. Etievent JP, Chocron S, Toubin G, et al. Use of cardiac troponin I as a marker of perioperative myocardial ischemia. Ann Thorac Surg 1995;59:1192–4.

225. Force T, Hibberd P, Weeks G, et al. Perioperative myocardial infarction after coronary artery bypass surgery. Clinical significance and approach to risk stratification. Circulation 1990;82:903–12.

226. Lemmer JH Jr, Kirsh MM. Coronary artery spasm following coronary artery surgery. Ann Thorac Surg 1988;46:108–15.

227. Paterson HS, Jones MW, Baird DK, Hughes CF. Lethal postoperative coronary artery spasm. Ann Thorac Surg 1998;65:1571–3.

228. Broka SM, Ducart AR, Collard EL, et al. Hemodynamic benefit of optimizing atrioventricular delay after cardiopulmonary bypass. J Cardiothorac Vasc Anesth 1997;11:723–8.

229. Atlee JL III, Pattison CZ, Mathews EL, Hedman AG. Transesophageal atrial pacing for intraoperative sinus bradycardia or AV junctional rhythm: feasibility as prophylaxis in 200 anesthetized adults and hemodynamic effects of treatment. J Cardiothorac Vasc Anesth 1993;7:436–41.

230. Glikson M, Dearani JA, Hyberger LK, Schaff HV, Hammill SC, Hayes DL. Indications, effectiveness, and long-term dependency in permanent pacing after cardiac surgery. Am J Cardiol 1997;80:1309–13.

231. Gordon RS, Ivanov J, Cohen G, Ralph-Edwards AL. Permanent cardiac pacing after a cardiac operation: predicting the use of permanent pacemakers. Ann Thorac Surg 1998;66:1698–704.

232. Hippelainen M, Mustonen P, Manninen H, Rehnberg S. Predictors of conduction disturbances after coronary bypass grafting. Ann Thorac Surg 1994;57:1284–8.

233. Mustonen P, Poyhonen M, Rehnberg S, et al. Conduction defects after coronary artery bypass grafting—a disappearing problem? Ann Chir Gynaecol 2000;89:33–9.

234. Mustonen P, Hippelainen M, Vanninen E, Rehnberg S, Tenhunen-Eskelinen M, Hartikainen J. Significance of coronary artery bypass grafting–associated conduction defects. Am J Cardiol 1998;81:558–63.

235. Thomas JL, Dickstein RA, Parker FB, et al. Prognostic significance of the development of left bundle conduction defects following aortic valve replacement. J Thorac Cardiovasc Surg 1982;84:382–6.

236. Gaudino M, Alessandrini F, Glieca F, et al. Conventional left atrial versus superior septal approach for mitral valve replacement. Ann Thorac Surg 1997;63:1123–7.

237. Garcia-Villarreal OA, Gonzalez-Oviedo R, Rodriguez-Gonzalez H, Martinez-Chapa HD. Superior septal approach for mitral valve surgery: a word of caution. Eur J Cardiothorac Surg 2003;24:862–7.

238. Chung MK, Augostini RS, Asher CR, et al. Ineffectiveness and potential proarrhythmia of atrial pacing for atrial fibrillation prevention after coronary artery bypass grafting. Ann Thorac Surg 2000;69:1057–63.

239. Fan K, Lee K, Lau CP. Mechanisms of biatrial pacing for prevention of postoperative atrial fibrillation: insights from a clinical trial. Card Electrophysiol Rev 2003;7:147–53.

240. Hogue CW Jr, Hyder ML. Atrial fibrillation after cardiac operation: risks, mechanisms, and treatment. Ann Thorac Surg 2000;69:300–6.

241. Hill LL, Kattapuram M, Hogue CW Jr. Management of atrial fibrillation after cardiac surgery, Part I: Pathophysiology and risks. J Cardiothorac Vasc Anesth 2002;16:483–94.

242. Cummings JE, Gill I, Akhrass R, Dery M, Biblo LA, Quan KJ. Preservation of the anterior fat pad paradoxically decreases the incidence of postoperative atrial fibrillation in humans. J Am Coll Cardiol 2004;43:994–1000.

243. Wazni OM, Martin DO, Marrouche NF, et al. Plasma B-type natriuretic peptide levels predict postoperative atrial fibrillation in patients undergoing cardiac surgery. Circulation 2004;119:124–7.

244. Athanasiou T, Aziz O, Mangoush O, et al. Do off-pump techniques reduce the incidence of postoperative atrial fibrillation in elderly patients undergoing coronary artery bypass grafting? Ann Thorac Surg 2004;77:1567–74.

245. Salamon T, Michler RE, Knott KM, Brown DA. Off-pump coronary artery bypass grafting does not decrease the incidence of atrial fibrillation. Ann Thorac Surg 2003;75:505–7.

246. Lahtinen J, Biancari F, Salmela E, et al. Postoperative atrial fibrillation is a major cause of stroke after on-pump coronary artery bypass surgery. Ann Thorac Surg 2004;77:1241–4.

247. Chung MK. Cardiac surgery: postoperative arrhythmias. Crit Care Med 2000;28(suppl):N136–44.

248. Hill LL, De Wet C, Hogue CW Jr. Management of atrial fibrillation after cardiac surgery, Part II: Prevention and treatment. J Cardiothorac Vasc Anesth 2002;16:626–37.

249. Crystal E, Connolly SJ, Sleik K, Ginger TJ, Yusuf S. Interventions on prevention of postoperative atrial fibrillation in patients undergoing heart surgery. A meta-analysis. Circulation 2002; 106:75–80.

250. Balser JR. Pro: all patients should receive pharmacologic prophylaxis for atrial fibrillation after cardiac surgery. J Cardiothorac Vasc Anesth 1999;13:98–100.

251. Rajagopal A, Cheng DCH. Pro: atrial arrhythmias prophylaxis is required for cardiac surgery. J Cardiothorac Vasc Anesth 2002;16:114–7.

252. Solomon AJ. Pharmacological approach for the prevention of atrial fibrillation after cardiovascular surgery. Card Electrophys Rev 2003;7:172–7.

253. Kowey PR, Taylor JE, Rials SJ, Marinchak RA. Meta-analysis of the effectiveness of prophylactic drug therapy in preventing supraventricular arrhythmia early after coronary artery bypass grafting. Am J Cardiol 1992;69:963–5.

254. Roffman JA, Fieldman A. Digoxin and propranolol in the prophylaxis of supraventricular tachydysrhythmias after coronary artery bypass surgery. Ann Thorac Surg 1981;31:496–500.

255. Sanjuan R, Blasco M, Carbonell N, et al. Preoperative use of sotalol versus atenolol for atrial fibrillation after cardiac surgery. Ann Thorac Surg 2004;77:838–43.

256. Parikka H, Toivonen L, Heikkila L, Virtanen K, Jarvinen A. Comparison of sotalol and metoprolol in the prevention of atrial fibrillation after coronary artery bypass surgery. J Cardiovasc Pharmacol 1998;31:67–73.

257. Wurdeman RL, Mooss AN, Mohiuddin SM, Lenz TL. Amiodarone vs. sotalol as prophylaxis against atrial fibrillation/flutter after heart surgery. A meta-analysis. Chest 2002;121:1203–10.

258. Solomon AJ, Greenberg MD, Kilborn MJ et al. Amiodarone vs. a beta-blocker to prevent atrial fibrillation after cardiovascular surgery. Am Heart J 2001;142:811–5.

259. Haan CK, Geraci SA. Role of amiodarone in reducing atrial fibrillation after cardiac surgery in adults. Ann Thorac Surg 2002;73:1665–9.

260. White CM, Giri S, Tsikouris JP, et al. A comparison of two individual amiodarone regimens to placebo in open heart surgery patients. Ann Thorac Surg 2002;74:69–74.

261. Katariya K, DeMarchena E, Bolooki H. Oral amiodarone reduces incidence of postoperative atrial fibrillation. Ann Thorac Surg 1999;68:1599–604.

262. Daoud EG, Strickberger SA, Man KC, et al. Preoperative oral amiodarone as prophylaxis against atrial fibrillation after heart surgery. N Engl J Med 1997;337:1785–91.

263. Yazigi A, Rahbani P, Zeid HA, Madi-Jebara S, Haddad F, Hayek G. Postoperative oral amiodarone as prophylaxis against atrial fibrillation after coronary artery surgery. J Cardiothorac Vasc Anesth 2002;16:603–6.

264. Yagdi T, Nalbantgil S, Ayik F, et al. Amiodarone reduces the incidence of atrial fibrillation after coronary artery bypass grafting. J Thorac Cardiovasc Surg 2003;125:1420–5.

265. Kuralay E, Cingoz F, Kilic S, et al. Supraventricular tachyarrhythmias prophylaxis after coronary artery surgery in chronic obstructive pulmonary disease patients (early amiodarone prophylaxis trial). Eur J Cardiothorac Surg 2004;25:224–30.

266. Kaushik S, Hussain A, Clarke P, Lazar HL. Acute pulmonary toxicity after low-dose amiodarone therapy. Ann Thorac Surg 2001;72:1760–1.

267. Boyd WC, Thomas SJ. Pro: magnesium should be administered to all coronary artery bypass graft surgery patients undergoing cardiopulmonary bypass. J Cardiothorac Vasc Anesth 2000;14: 339–43.

268. Speziale G, Ruvolo G, Fattouch K, et al. Arrhythmia prophylaxis after coronary artery bypass grafting: regimens of magnesium sulfate administration. Thorac Cardiovasc Surg 2000;48:22–6.

269. Hazelrigg SR, Boley TM, Cetindag IB, et al. The efficacy of supplemental magnesium in reducing atrial fibrillation after coronary artery bypass grafting. Ann Thorac Surg 2004;77:824–30.

270. Kaplan M, Kut MS, Icer UA, Dermirtas MM. Intravenous magnesium sulfate prophylaxis for atrial fibrillation after coronary artery bypass surgery. J Thorac Cardiovasc Surg 2003;125: 344–52.

271. Maslow AD, Regan MM, Heindle S, Panzica P, Cohn WE, Johnson RG. Postoperative atrial tachyarrhythmias in patients undergoing coronary artery bypass graft surgery without cardiopulmonary bypass: a role for intraoperative magnesium supplementation. J Cardiothorac Vasc Anesth 2000;14: 524–30.

272. Forlani S, De Paulis R, de Notaris S, et al. Combination of sotalol and magnesium prevents atrial fibrillation after coronary artery bypass grafting. Ann Thorac Surg 2002;74:720–6.

273. Kiziltepe U, Eyileten ZB, Sirlak M, et al. Antiarrhythmic effect of magnesium sulfate after open heart surgery: effect of blood levels. Int J Cardiol 2003;89:153–8.

274. Archbold RA, Schilling RJ. Atrial pacing for the prevention of atrial fibrillation after coronary artery bypass graft surgery: a review of the literature. Heart 2004;90:129–33.

275. Debrunner M, Naegeli B, Genoni M, Turina M, Bertel O. Prevention of atrial fibrillation after cardiac valvular surgery by epicardial, biatrial synchronous pacing. Eur J Cardiothorac Surg 2004; 25:16–20.

276. Cooper JM, Katcher MS, Orlov MV. Implantable devices for the treatment of atrial fibrillation. N Engl J Med 2002;346:2062–8.

277. Gerstenfeld EP, Hill MRS, French SN, et al. Evaluation of right atrial and biatrial temporary pacing for the prevention of atrial fibrillation after coronary artery bypass surgery. J Am Coll Cardiol 1999;33:1981–8.

278. Merrick AF, Odom NJ, Keenan DJR, Grotte GJ. Comparison of propafenone to atenolol for the prophylaxis of postcardiotomy supraventricular tachyarrhythmias: a prospective trial. Eur J Cardiothorac Surg 1995;9:146–9.

279. Laub GW, Janiera L, Muralidharan S, et al. Prophylactic procainamide for prevention of atrial fibrillation after coronary artery bypass grafting: a prospective, double-blind, randomized, placebo-controlled study. Crit Care Med 1993;21:1474–8.

280. The atrial fibrillation follow-up investigation of rhythm management (AFFIRM) investigators. A comparison of rate control and rhythm control in patients with atrial fibrillation. N Engl J Med 2003;347:1825–33.

281. Klein AL, Grimm RA, Murray RD, et al. Use of transesophageal echocardiography to guide cardioversion in patients with atrial fibrillation. N Engl J Med 2001;344:1411–20.

282. Klein AL, Murray RD, Grimm RA. Role of transesophageal echocardiography-guided cardioversion of patients with atrial fibrillation. J Am Coll Cardiol 2001;37:691–704.

283. Black IW, Fatkin D, Sagar KB, et al. Exclusion of atrial thrombus by transesophageal echocardiography does not preclude embolism after cardioversion of atrial fibrillation. A multicenter study. Circulation 1994;89:2509–13.

284. Harjai KJ, Mobarek SK, Cheirif J, Boulos LM, Murgo JP, Abi-Samra F. Clinical variables affecting recovery of left atrial mechanical function after cardioversion from atrial fibrillation. J Am Coll Cardiol 1997;30:481–6.

285. Stambler BS, Wood MA, Ellenbogen KA. Comparative efficacy of intravenous ibutilide versus procainamide for enhancing termination of atrial flutter by atrial overdrive pacing. Am J Cardiol 1996;77:960–6.

286. Oral H, Souza JJ, Michaud GF, et al. Facilitating transthoracic cardioversion of atrial fibrillation with ibutilide pretreatment. N Engl J Med 1999;340:1849–54.

287. D'Este D, Bertaglia E, Mantovan R, Zanocco Z, Franceschi M, Pascotto P. Efficacy of intravenous propafenone in termination of atrial flutter by overdrive transesophageal pacing previously ineffective. Am J Cardiol 1997;79:500–2.

288. Ellenbogan KA, Dias VC, Cardello FP, et al. Safety and efficacy of intravenous diltiazem in atrial fibrillation or atrial flutter. Am J Cardiol 1995;75:45–9.

289. Mooss AN, Wurdeman RL, Mahiuddin SM, et al. Esmolol versus diltiazem in the treatment of postoperative atrial fibrillation/atrial flutter after open heart surgery. Am Heart J 2000;140: 176–80.

290. Hilleman DE, Reyes AP, Mooss AN, Packard KA. Esmolol versus diltiazem in atrial fibrillation following coronary artery bypass graft surgery. Curr Med Res Opin 2003;19:376–82.

291. Tisdale JE, Padhi ID, Goldberg AD, et al. A randomized, double-blind comparison of intravenous diltiazem and digoxin for atrial fibrillation after coronary artery bypass surgery. Am Heart J 1989;135:739–47.

292. Wattanasuwan N, Khan IA, Mehta NJ, et al. Acute ventricular rate control in atrial fibrillation. IV combination of diltiazem and digoxin vs IV diltiazem alone. Chest 2001;119:502–6.

293. Karth GD, Geppert A, Neunteufl T, et al. Amiodarone versus diltiazem for rate control in critically ill patients with atrial tachyarrhythmias. Crit Care Med 2001;29:1149–53.

294. Stoddard MF, Dawkins PR, Prince CR, Ammash NM. Left atrial appendage thrombus is not uncommon in patients with acute atrial fibrillation and a recent embolic event: a transesophageal echocardiographic study. J Am Coll Cardiol 1995;25:452–9.

295. Soucier RJ, Mirza S, Abordo MG, et al. Predictors of conversion of atrial fibrillation after cardiac operations in the absence of class I or III antiarrhythmic medications. Ann Thorac Surg 2001;72:694–8.

296. Chevalier P, Durand-Dubief A, Burri H, Cucherat M, Kirkorian G, Touboul P. Amiodarone versus placebo and class Ic drugs for cardioversion of recent-onset atrial fibrillation: a meta-analysis. J Am Coll Cardiol 2003;41:255–62.

297. Gullestad L, Birkeland K, Molstad P, Hoyer MM, Vanberg P, Kjekshus J. The effect of magnesium versus verapamil on supraventricular arrhythmias. Clin Cardiol 1993;16:429–34.

298. Cheung AT, Weiss SJ, Savino JS. Acute circulatory actions of intravenous amiodarone loading in cardiac surgical patients. Ann Thorac Surg 2003;76:535–41.

299. Peuhkurinen K, Niemala M, Ylitalo A, Linnaluoto M, Lilja M, Juvonen J. Effectiveness of amiodarone as a single oral dose for recent-onset atrial fibrillation. Am J Cardiol 2000;85:462–5.

300. Boriani G, Capucci A, Lenzi T, Sanguinetti M, Bagnani B. Propafenone for conversion of recent-onset atrial fibrillation. A controlled comparison between oral loading dose and intravenous administration. Chest 1995;108:355–8.

301. Khan IA. Single oral loading dose of propafenone for pharmacological cardioversion of recent-onset atrial fibrillation. J Am Coll Cardiol 2001;37:542–7.

302. Boriani G, Martignani C, Biffi M, Capucci A, Branzi A. Oral loading with propafenone for conversion of recent-onset atrial fibrillation: a review on in-hospital treatment. Drugs 2002;62: 415–23.

303. Geelen P, O'Hara GE, Roy N, et al. Comparison of propafenone versus procainamide for the acute treatment of atrial fibrillation after cardiac surgery. Am J Cardiol 1999;84:345–7.

304. Blanc JJ, Voinov C, Maarek M. Comparison of oral loading dose of propafenone and amiodarone for converting recent-onset atrial fibrillation. Am J Cardiol 1999;84:1029–32.

305. VanderLugt KT, Mattiani T, Denker S, et al. for the Ibutilide investigators. Efficacy and safety of ibutilide fumarate for the conversion of atrial arrhythmias after cardiac surgery. Circulation 1999;100:369–75.

306. Volgman AS, Carberry PA, Stambler B, et al. Conversion efficacy and safety of intravenous ibutilide compared with intravenous procainamide in patients with atrial flutter or fibrillation. J Am Coll Cardiol 1998;31:1414–9.

307. Bernard EO, Schmid ER, Schmidlin D, Scharf C, Candinas R, Germann R. Ibutilide versus amiodarone in atrial fibrillation: a double-blinded, randomized study. Crit Care Med 2003;31:1031–4.

308. Lindeboom JE, Kingma JH, Crijns HJGM, Dunselman PHJM. Efficacy and safety of intravenous dofetilide for rapid termination of atrial fibrillation and flutter. Am J Cardiol 2000;85:1031–3.

309. Patel AN, Hamman BL, Patel AN, et al. Epicardial atrial defibrillation: successful treatment of postoperative atrial fibrillation. Ann Thorac Surg 2004;77:831–7.

310. Bechtel JFM, Christiansen JF, Sievers HH, Bartels C. Low-energy cardioversion versus medical treatment for the termination of atrial fibrillation after CABG. Ann Thorac Surg 2003;75:1185–8.

311. Wilbur SL, Marchlinski FE. Adenosine as an antiarrhythmic agent. Am J Cardiol 1997;79:30–7.

312. Dougherty AH, Jackman WM, Naccarelli GV, Friday KJ, Dias VC, for the IV Diltiazem Study group. Acute conversion of paroxysmal supraventricular tachycardia with intravenous diltiazem. Am J Cardiol 1992;70:587–92.

313. Johnson RG, Goldberger AL, Thurer RL, Schwartz M, Sirois C, Weintraub RM. Lidocaine prophylaxis in coronary revascularization patients: a randomized, prospective trial. Ann Thorac Surg 1993;55:1180–4.

314. England MR, Gordon G, Salem M, Chernow B. Magnesium administration and dysrhythmias after cardiac surgery. JAMA 1992;268:2395–402.

315. Steinberg JS, Gaur A, Sciacca R, Tan E. New-onset sustained ventricular tachycardia after cardiac surgery. Circulation 1999;99:903–8.

316. Ascione R, Reeves BC, Santo K, Khan N, Angelini GD. Predictors of new malignant ventricular arrhythmias after coronary surgery. A case-control study. J Am Coll Cardiol 2004;43:1630–8.

317. Topol EJ, Lerman BB, Baughman KL, Platia EV, Griffith LSC. De novo refractory ventricular tachyarrhythmias after coronary revascularization. Am J Cardiol 1986;57:57–9.

318. Azar RR, Berns E, Seecharran B, Veronneau J, Lippman N, Kluger J. De novo monomorphic and polymorphic ventricular tachycardia following coronary artery bypass grafting. Am J Cardiol 1997;80:76–8.

319. Saxon LA, Wiener I, Natterson PD, Laks H, Drinkwater D, Stevenson WG. Monomorphic versus polymorphic ventricular tachycardia after coronary artery bypass grafting. Am J Cardiol 1995;75:403–5.

320. Sharma ND, Rosman HS, Padhi ID, Tisdale JE. Torsades de pointes associated with intravenous haloperidol in critically ill patients. Am J Cardiol 1998;81:238–40.

321. Lamas GA, Antman EM, Gold JP, Braunwald NS, Collins JJ. Pacemaker backup-mode reversion and injury during cardiac surgery. Ann Thorac Surg 1986;41:155–7.

322. Pinto RP, Romerill DB, Nasser WK, Schier JJ, Surawicz B. Prognosis of patients with frequent premature ventricular complexes and nonsustained ventricular tachycardia after coronary artery bypass surgery. Clin Cardiol 1996;19:321–4.

323. Gollob MH, Seger JJ. Current status of the implantable cardioverter-defibrillator. Chest 2001;119:1210–21.

324. Roden DM. A practical approach to torsade de pointes. Clin Cardiol 1997;20:285–90.

325. Laub GW, Muralidharan S, Janeira L, et al. Refractory postoperative torsades de pointes syndrome successfully treated with isoproterenol. J Cardiothorac Vasc Anesth 1993;7:210–2.

326. Miller JH, Zipes DP. Management of the patient with a cardiac arrhythmia: pharmacological, electrical, and surgical techniques. In: Braunwald E, Zipes DP, Libby P, eds. Heart Disease. A textbook of cardiovascular medicine, 6th ed. Philadelphia: W.B. Saunders, 2001:700–66.

327. Olgin JF, Zipes DP. Specific arrhythmias: diagnosis and treatment. In: Braunwald E, Zipes DP, Libby P, eds. Heart Disease. A textbook of cardiovascular medicine, 6th ed. Philadelphia: W.B. Saunders, 2001:815–89.

328. Weng JT, Smith DE, Moulder PV. Antiarrhythmic drugs: electrophysiological basis of their clinical usage. Ann Thorac Surg 1986;41:106–12.

329. Bhatia SJS, Smith TW. Digitalis toxicity: mechanisms, diagnosis, and management. J Cardiac Surg 1987;2:453–65.

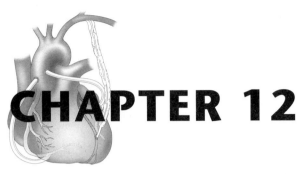

CHAPTER 12

Fluid Management, Renal and Metabolic Problems

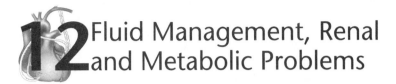

Fluid Management, Renal and Metabolic Problems

Judicious fluid management and maintenance of satisfactory renal function are two important elements in the perioperative care of the cardiac surgical patient. Careful attention to these issues is essential to optimize hemodynamic performance, minimize respiratory morbidity, avert electrolyte abnormalities, and avoid drug toxicity. Because renal function has such a significant impact on the function of other organ systems, it is understandable that renal insufficiency is one of the most significant risk factors for a poor surgical outcome.[1-6]

A basic understanding of body water distribution, awareness of the factors that influence renal function, steps that can be taken to optimize renal perfusion, and early identification and treatment of incipient or established renal dysfunction are essential to optimize the surgical result.

I. Body Water Distribution

Approximately 60% of the body weight (50% in women) is water with two-thirds of this residing in the intracellular space and one-third in the extracellular space. In the latter, two-thirds is in the interstitial space (the so-called "third space"), and one-third constitutes the intravascular volume.

    A. Water moves freely among all three compartments and shifts so as to normalize serum osmolarity (which generally reflects the serum sodium concentration).

    B. Sodium moves freely between the intravascular and interstitial spaces but does not move passively into cells. Therefore, if a patient receives a hypotonic sodium load (e.g., 0.45% saline), which would lower the serum osmolarity and sodium concentration, water will move from the extracellular space to the intracellular space to normalize these values. The presence of **a low serum sodium concentration in the postoperative patient usually indicates total body water overload.**

    C. Protein remains within the intravascular space and is the primary determinant of plasma oncotic pressure. If colloid or protein is administered, plasma oncotic pressure will increase and fluid will be drawn to the intravascular space from the interstitial space. Conversely, if the serum albumin is low, fluid will tend to shift to the interstitial space, contributing to tissue edema.

    D. Starling's law governs the influence of hydrostatic and oncotic pressures on fluid shifts. For example, elevated hydrostatic pressure (e.g., increased pulmonary capillary wedge pressure, PCWP) or lower intravascular colloid oncotic pressure (e.g., low serum albumin) will shift fluid into the lung interstitium. Conversely, raising the intravascular oncotic pressure with colloid (e.g., 25% albumin) will tend to draw fluid from the lung interstitium back to the intravascular space.

    E. Starling's law describes fluid shifts in the absence of abnormalities in membrane integrity. However, open-heart surgery using cardiopulmonary bypass (CPB) is associated with a systemic inflammatory response marked by increased membrane permeability and a transient capillary leak. When this leak is present, administered fluid will shift more readily into the interstitial space than if the capillary leak is absent. Clinically, this is most evident as increased extravascular lung water that impairs oxygenation and can lead to noncardiogenic pulmonary edema. However, expansion of the interstitial space may also contribute to cerebral edema (mental obtundation), hepatic congestion (jaundice), splanchnic congestion (ileus), and impaired renal perfusion.

II. Effects of Cardiopulmonary Bypass and Off-Pump Surgery on Renal Function

A. The performance of open-heart surgery may be associated with subtle or overt effects on renal function. Clinical assessment is commonly based only on urine output and measurement of the serum creatinine level. Thus, if urine output is adequate with minimal change in the serum creatinine (Cr), renal function is considered to be unaffected by surgery. However, even in a patient with normal preoperative renal function and stable hemodynamics, a subclinical degree of renal dysfunction with tubular damage is invariably present. There are a number of sensitive and sophisticated markers of renal dysfunction that can be used to assess whether renal damage is occurring and whether interventions are beneficial in preserving renal function. These include tests of:

1. Glomerular function: creatinine clearance
2. Glomerular damage: microalbuminuria
3. Proximal tubular function: fractional excretion of sodium (FE_{Na}), retinol-binding protein
4. Proximal tubular damage: increased levels of N-acetyl-β-D-glucosaminidase (NAG), α_1-microglobulin, neutral endopeptidase, glutathione transferase-α
5. Distal tubular function: free water clearance
6. Distal tubular damage: glutathione transferase-π

B. Extracorporeal circulation for open-heart surgery produces a variety of effects on renal blood flow (RBF), as well as on glomerular and tubular function. Low-flow, hypothermic, nonpulsatile perfusion with hemodilution increases effective RBF, marginally decreases the glomerular filtration rate (GFR), decreases filtration fraction, and decreases renal vascular resistance.[7] Bypass is associated with an increase in the FE_{Na} and free water clearance, but also with an increase in virtually all kidney-specific proteins that are markers for tubular damage.[8,9]

C. Numerous aspects of CPB can influence renal function.[10,11]

1. Elevated levels of hormones include the following with their specific effects noted:
   a. Renin and aldosterone (sodium retention and potassium excretion)
   b. Angiotensin II (renal vasoconstriction and sodium retention)
   c. Vasopressin (increases renal vascular resistance)
   d. Atrial natriuretic factor (ANF) and urodilan (increase natriuresis and diuresis after bypass)[12]
   e. Epinephrine and norepinephrine (increase systemic resistance)
   f. Plasma free cortisol after CPB (sodium retention and potassium excretion)

2. Other vasoactive substances released during CPB include complement, kallikrein, and bradykinin, which alter vascular tone and contribute to the generalized inflammatory response that increases capillary permeability.

3. **Hypothermia** decreases renal cortical blood flow by producing vasoconstriction. It also decreases GFR slightly, decreases renal tubular function, and reduces free water and osmolar clearance. These effects are offset to some degree by hemodilution during CPB. During the phase of rewarming, vasodilatation and hyperemia of tissue beds result in "third spacing" of fluid. Hypothermia may also cause hypokalemia due to a transcellular shift.

4. **Hemodilution** with a crystalloid prime reduces plasma oncotic pressure, promoting movement of fluid from the vascular space to the interstitial space. A reduction in viscosity increases outer renal cortical blood flow, leading to an increase in urine output, free water clearance, and sodium and potassium excretion.

5. **Medications.** Preoperative medications (amiodarone, angiotensin-converting enzyme [ACE] inhibitors, angiotensin receptor blockers, and calcium channel blockers), as well as drugs used during surgery (nitroglycerin, nitroprusside, inhalational anesthetics, narcotics, and anxiolytics), can produce significant vasodilatation that increases fluid requirements.

6. **Ischemic/reperfusion injury** associated with the use of cardioplegia for myocardial protection can produce myocardial edema, a reduction in diastolic compliance, and impairment of myocardial function. This may alter the relationship between the left-sided filling pressures and left ventricular (LV) end-diastolic volume.

D. Off-pump coronary bypass surgery (OPCAB) has been proposed as a means of minimizing many of the alterations caused by CPB to reduce the risk of postoperative renal insufficiency.[13] Avoidance of the pump may result in better preservation of glomerular and tubular function with less evidence of damage.[14,15] However, off-pump surgery is associated with significant fluid administration, use of comparable anesthetic and vasoactive medications, cytokine release that can damage proximal tubules, and alterations in perfusion pressure that can adversely affect renal function. Although OPCAB may reduce the incidence of acute renal failure (ARF) requiring dialysis in patients with non–dialysis-dependent renal insufficiency, its benefits are not as well defined in patients at low risk.[16–19] Furthermore, postoperative renal dysfunction is invariably related to preexisting renal disease or significant hemodynamic alterations in the perioperative period, independent of whether CPB is used, unless the duration of CPB is exceedingly long.[9] Thus, particular attention to fluid management and renal function remains paramount no matter which technique of surgery is used.

III. Routine Fluid Management in the Early Postoperative Period

A. As a result of hemodilution on CPB, most patients are in a state of total body sodium and water overload at the conclusion of surgery, commonly being about 5% above their preoperative weight (estimated at 800 mL/m^2/h, but quite variable in amount).[20] Cardiac filling pressures may not reflect this state of fluid overload because several factors that accompany CPB, including a capillary leak, decreased plasma colloid osmotic pressure, and vasodilatation, may suggest that the patient is hypovolemic or euvolemic. Thus, filling pressures may be low or require ongoing fluid administration to be maintained despite excessive body water.

B. This fluid requirement occurs at a time when urine output may be high or marginal (<1 mL/kg/h). During the first 4–6 hours after surgery, cardiac output is often depressed, and the achievement of satisfactory hemodynamics is dependent on both preload and inotropic support. Thus, fluid must invariably be administered to maintain intravascular volume and cardiac hemodynamics at the expense of expansion of the interstitial space. It should be noted that early extubation is helpful in reducing fluid requirements because it eliminates the adverse effects of positive-pressure ventilation on venous return and ventricular function.

C. It can be difficult to decide which fluid to administer to maintain filling pressures. Clearly, any fluid infused during a period of altered capillary membrane integrity will expand the interstitial space, but fluids that can more effectively expand the intravascular space while minimizing expansion of the interstitial space are preferable.[21]

1. Blood and colloids are superior to hypotonic or even isotonic crystalloid solutions in expanding the intravascular volume. Although a rapid infusion of crystalloid is effective in increasing intravascular volume acutely (630 mL expansion at the end of a 5-minute infusion of 1 L of lactated Ringer's solution [LR]), this benefit is transient. LR rapidly redistributes into the interstitial space, retaining barely 20% of the infused volume within the intravascular compartment after an hour.[22] Similarly, only 250 mL of a liter of infused normal saline (NS) is retained in the intravascular compartment after 1 hour.[23] In contrast, after a 5-minute infusion of 1 L of 6% hetastarch, the intravascular volume expands by 1123 mL with more long-lasting effects.[22]

2. In general, it is reasonable to initially administer a moderate amount of inexpensive crystalloid (up to 1 L) if the patient is oxygenating well.[24] Infusing greater amounts may contribute to tissue edema, commonly impairing oxygenation. Interestingly, use of LR exclusively may create a hypercoagulable state.[25]

3. Colloids should be selected if additional volume is required. The selection of colloid should be based on the patient's pulmonary and renal function and the extent of mediastinal bleeding. Colloid solutions have become relatively inexpensive, so cost should not be an issue.

   a. **Albumin (5%)** provides excellent volume expansion (approximately 800 mL retained per liter administered) and has primarily dilutional effects on clotting parameters. It also has oxygen free-radical scavenging and antiinflammatory properties. Albumin has a half-life of 16 hours and leaves the bloodstream at about 5–8 g/h.[26]

   b. **Hespan** (6% hetastarch in saline or HES) and **Hextend** (6% hetastarch in balanced electrolyte solution) are both high-molecular-weight hydroxyethyl starch compounds that provide excellent volume expansion that decreases gradually over the ensuing 24–36 hours. Both may be retained in the intravascular space better than 5% albumin in conditions of endothelial capillary leakage.

      i. HES demonstrates significant adverse hemostatic effects that are not seen with Hextend.[27,28] These include decreased levels of factors I, VIII:C, and von Willebrand factor, platelet dysfunction, and fibrinolysis. Multiple studies have shown that patients who receive HES during surgery (often in the pump prime) have a much greater risk of perioperative bleeding.[29] When given postoperatively, the risk of bleeding can be minimized if the dose is restricted to 20 mL/kg.[30] However, if a patient is bleeding and requires volume, Hespan is best avoided. Lower molecular weight compounds (such as 10% pentastarch, not available in the United States) have less effect on coagulation, but provide effective plasma expansion for a shorter period of time.[31]

ii. The high-molecular-weight hetastarch preparations are excreted in the urine, whereas the lower molecular weight hetastarches undergo glomerular filtration. Nonetheless, Hespan and Hextend should probably be used cautiously in the patient with preexisting renal dysfunction.[32]

iii. There is concern that saline-based solutions (such as 5% albumin and Hespan) can induce renal dysfunction. They provide a chloride load that can produce progressive renal vasoconstriction, a decrease in glomerular filtration rate, and a hyperchloremic metabolic acidosis. Furthermore, patients receiving normal saline have been noted to develop central nervous system changes and abdominal discomfort.[33] Thus, use of a balanced electrolyte vehicle may provide better acid-base and electrolyte balance and better organ perfusion.

c. Hypertonic solutions are effective in augmenting intravascular volume by extracting fluid from the interstitial and intracellular spaces. They may reduce the amount of fluid required to maintain intravascular volume when there is total body fluid overload. **25% albumin** can increase the intravascular volume by 450 mL for every 100 mL administered. **Hypertonic saline (3%)** can also be used. Studies from Europe have shown that **hypertonic saline (7.5%)** can produce renal vasodilatation, increase GFR, and produce an intense diuresis.[34,35] It should be noted that use of these hypertonic solutions can produce hyperoncotic renal failure if the patient is dehydrated because glomerular filtration of hyperoncotic colloid molecules may cause stasis of tubular flow.[32]

D. It cannot be overemphasized that the purpose of postoperative fluid administration is to maintain **adequate** intravascular volume to ensure **satisfactory** cardiac output and tissue perfusion. Administration of excessive volume to maintain high filling pressures and the highest possible cardiac output will increase tissue edema, primarily manifest as increased extravascular lung water. This can be detrimental to pulmonary function and will often delay extubation. In addition, intravascular volume expansion may decrease the hematocrit and also reduce the level of clotting factors, possibly necessitating homologous blood or plasma transfusions.

E. When cardiac function is satisfactory but there is an ongoing volume requirement to maintain filling pressures or blood pressure, often from a combination of the capillary leak, vasodilatation, or excellent urine output, "flooding" the patient with volume should be resisted. After 1.5–2 L of fluid is given, an α-agent, such as phenylephrine or norepinephrine, should be used. If both cardiac output and urine output remain marginal after fluid administration, inotropic support should be considered first, with α-agents used only if systemic resistance remains low. Use of α-agents at substantial doses is always of concern because they may produce renal vasoconstriction and compromise renal function. One study showed that norepinephrine reduced RBF without any change in GFR or urine output, and that this decrease in RBF could be offset by dopamine.[36] However, another study showed that use of norepinephrine in the vasodilated patient did not have adverse effects on renal function.[37]

F. Generally, diuretics are best avoided in the first 6 hours after surgery unless inexplicable oliguria, pulmonary edema, or borderline oxygenation is present. When the patient has achieved a stable core temperature and the capillary leak has ceased, usually after the first 6–12 hours, filling pressures stabilize or rise with little fluid administration. By this time, myocardial function has usually recovered, inotropic support can be gradually withdrawn, and the patient can be extubated. Diuresis should then be initiated to excrete the excess salt and water administered during CPB and the early postoperative period. Patients who have undergone operations that require long periods of bypass (usually > 3 hours) or who have persistent low-output syndromes may experience a longer period of "capillary leak" that requires further fluid administration to maintain filling pressures.

G. Diuresis can be augmented most efficiently by the use of loop diuretics.

1. Most patients with preserved renal function respond to furosemide (Lasix) 10–20 mg IV. In the absence of renal insufficiency, furosemide has a half-life of 1.5–2 hours, and thus it can be administered every 4 hours, if necessary.[38] Not infrequently, the diuresis persists after one dose.

2. A gentle continuous diuresis may be obtained in patients with significant fluid overload and hemodynamic instability using a bolus dose of 40 mg followed by a continuous infusion of 0.1–0.5 mg/kg/h (usually 10–20 mg/h) of furosemide.[39] This may decrease the total dosage requirements and usually improves the diuretic response, especially in patients who are diuretic "tolerant." The addition of a thiazide (chlorothiazide 500 mg IV) is beneficial in overcoming this problem of tolerance, which may be caused by compensatory hypertrophy of the distal nephron segments in response to increased exposure to solute from long-term use of loop diuretics.

3. Diuretics are continued in IV or oral form until the patient has achieved his or her preoperative weight. Despite the nearly universal use of routine diuretics to achieve an earlier diuresis, one study showed no clinical benefit to this practice in low-risk patients with normal renal function.[40]

4. Guidelines for the hemodynamic and fluid management of typical postoperative scenarios are presented in Chapter 8.

IV. Prevention of Renal Dysfunction

A. The risk of renal dysfunction is very low when a patient with normal renal function undergoes an uneventful operation without hemodynamic compromise. In contrast, the presence of any degree of preoperative renal dysfunction increases the risk of postoperative renal dysfunction and mortality.[41]

1. It has been estimated that the risk of renal dysfunction increases by 4.8-fold for each 1 mg/dL increment in serum creatinine.[42]

2. One study found that the risk of dialysis exceeded 30% if the preoperative creatinine was > 2.5 mg/dL.[43]

3. Both the preoperative creatinine and the degree of perioperative rise in creatinine correlate with operative mortality.[44] The overall mortality risk for patients with a preoperative creatinine > 1.5 mg/dL ranges from 5–30%.[44–48] The mortality risk has been estimated at about 5% for patients with a creatinine of 1.5–2.5 mg/dL, 15–30% in non–dialysis-dependent patients with a creatinine > 2.5 mg/dL, and 15% for those on long-term dialysis.[46,49–51]

4. These alarming statistics emphasize the crucial importance of taking any steps possible to preserve renal function in the perioperative period, especially in patients at increased risk.

B. The definition of preoperative renal insufficiency is commonly based on an elevated serum creatinine (usually > 1.5 mg/dL or > 130 μmols/L (1 mg/dL = 88 μmols/L). Starting in 2004, the STS database defined it as a creatinine ≥ 2.0 mg/dL. However, the serum creatinine may be normal with a greater than 50% reduction in renal function. A more sensitive estimate of renal function can be obtained using the creatinine clearance (C_{CR}). This approximates the GFR and provides an estimate of the number of functioning nephrons. Because it is more indicative of renal reserve and the ability to the kidneys to tolerate surgical stress, the C_{CR} correlates best with postoperative renal dysfunction and mortality.[52,53] A C_{CR} less than 55 mL/min has been found to provide the best threshold below which surgical risk increases.[53] The C_{CR} is estimated from the Cockcroft and Gault equation as follows:

$$C_{CR} = \frac{(140 - age) \times wt(kg)}{72 \times Cr} \times 0.8 \text{ (for females)}$$

This can be calculated more precisely using a 24-hour or 2-hour urine specimen using the equation:

$$C_{CR} = (U_{CR}/P_{CR}) \times (volume/1440 \text{ min, or } 120 \text{ min})$$

where U_{CR} and P_{CR} are the urinary and plasma creatinine concentrations.

C. The presence of any degree of preoperative renal insufficiency should lead to a search for potentially treatable causes that might lower the risk of progressive dysfunction postoperatively. Identifying and correcting these contributing factors before surgery and using prophylactic measures during and after surgery to optimize renal perfusion and tubular function may ameliorate the complications associated with the development of oliguric renal failure. These may include electrolyte abnormalities, pulmonary and cardiac dysfunction, bleeding, infection, and delayed return of gastrointestinal (GI) function affecting nutrition, let alone the possibility of requiring dialysis and its attendant complications.

D. **Risk factors** for the development of postoperative renal dysfunction have been elucidated in a number of studies.[41,44,54–62]

1. Preoperative factors
   a. Preexisting renal dysfunction as defined above
   b. Radiocontrast administration < 48 hours prior to surgery
   c. Increasing age: 2.5-fold increase in risk for each 10-year age increment[42]
   d. LV dysfunction, especially with symptoms of congestive heart failure (CHF)
   e. Emergency operations
   f. Comorbidities: diabetes mellitus, especially in combination with hypertension and peripheral vascular disease
   g. Acute endocarditis
2. Intraoperative factors
   a. Reoperations
   b. Concomitant coronary artery bypass grafting (CABG)–valve operations
   c. Isolated valve operations (mitral more than aortic)[60]
   d. Use of deep hypothermic circulatory arrest
   e. Long durations of bypass (generally over 2–2.5 hours) but unrelated to normothermic or moderately hypothermic bypass[9,41,61]
   f. Ascending aortic atherosclerosis[62]

Table 12.1 • Factors Contributing to Pre- and Postoperative Renal Insufficiency

Preoperative factors	Low cardiac output states/hypotension (cardiogenic shock from acute MI, mechanical complications of MI) Medications that interfere with renal autoregulation (ACE inhibitors, NSAIDs) Nephrotoxins (contrast-induced ATN, especially in diabetic vasculopaths); medications (metformin, aminoglycosides) Renal atheroembolism (catheterization, IABP) Interstitial nephritis (antibiotics, NSAIDs, furosemide) Glomerulonephritis (endocarditis)
Intraoperative factors	Cardiopulmonary bypass (nonpulsatile, low flow, low-pressure perfusion) Low cardiac output syndrome/hypotension after CPB Hemolysis and hemoglobinuria from prolonged duration of CPB
Postoperative factors	Low cardiac output states (decreased contractility, hypovolemia, absent AV synchrony in hypertrophied hearts) Hypotension Intense vasoconstriction (low-flow states, α-agents) Atheroembolism (IABP) Sepsis Medications (cephalosporins, aminoglycosides, ACE inhibitors)

    g. Postcardiotomy hemodynamic dysfunction
    h. Low urine output on bypass
  3. Postoperative factors
    a. Hemodynamic instability with hypotension and low cardiac output, including right ventricular failure and systemic venous hypertension
    b. Postoperative bleeding
    c. Respiratory failure with hypoxemia
 E. A number of etiologic mechanisms may contribute to perioperative acute renal insufficiency (Table 12.1). They may be categorized as prerenal (reduced renal perfusion), renal (intrinsic renal insults), or postrenal (obstructive uropathy). When the kidneys have sustained an acute preoperative insult, they seem to be particularly sensitive to the nonpulsatile flow of CPB and to tenuous postcardiotomy hemodynamics. This may be due to endothelial injury with the first insult that limits vasodilatation with subsequent ischemic insults. The BUN and creatinine should therefore be allowed to return to baseline before proceeding with surgery.
 F. Patients with chronic renal failure (CRF) have increased susceptibility to fluid overload, hyponatremia, hyperkalemia, and metabolic acidosis in the perioperative period. Patients on chronic dialysis should be dialyzed within the 24 hours before and after surgery. Intraoperative hemofiltration should also be performed to reduce the positive fluid balance. The overall mortality rate for patients on chronic dialysis

---

Box 12.1 • Preoperative and Intraoperative Measures to Reduce the Incidence of Renal Dysfunction

A. Preoperative Measures

1. Use hydration during cardiac catheterization.
2. Use acetylcysteine or fenoldopam during catheterization.
3. Optimize hemodynamic status.
4. Withhold medications that adversely affect renal function (ACE inhibitors, NSAIDs) or can cause lactic acidosis when an ionic dye is used (metformin).
5. Repeat serum creatinine if preoperative renal dysfunction, especially in diabetics, and defer surgery, if possible, until creatinine has returned to baseline.
6. Correct all acid-base and metabolic problems.

B. Intraoperative Measures

1. Perform off-pump surgery if possible.
2. Use antifibrinolytics cautiously if renal dysfunction (aprotinin is safe if on dialysis).
3. Maintain a high perfusion pressure (75–80 mm Hg) on bypass.
4. Use fenoldopam during bypass (0.1 µg/kg/min).
5. Add mannitol to the pump.
6. Use a heparin-coated circuit, if available.
7. Consider using leukocyte-reducing filters on pump.
8. Use hemofiltration to remove excess fluid.
9. Optimize post-bypass hemodynamics.

---

undergoing open-heart surgery is approximately 15% but is most significantly increased in those with advanced NYHA class and those undergoing urgent or emergent surgery.[50,51]

G. **Preoperative measures (Box 12.1)**

1. Minimize nephrotoxicity of contrast studies by using nonionic contrast media. Adequate hydration (0.45% D5/NS at 75 mL/h) should be provided before, during, and after the study for up to 12 hours. Medications that are commonly prescribed to attenuate the nephrotoxic effects of contrast media in patients at increased risk of renal dysfunction include:

   a. **Acetylcysteine** is usually given in an oral dose of 600 mg bid beginning 12 hours before the procedure and continuing q12h for a total of 4 doses. Alternatively, it may be given IV as 150 mg/kg in 500 mL NS over 30 minutes prior to contrast exposure followed by 50 mg/kg in 500 mL NS over the subsequent 4 hours.[63,64]

   b. **Fenoldopam** given in a dose of 0.1 µg/kg/min has shown in some studies to be useful in reducing the incidence of contrast-induced nephropathy, especially in diabetics and patients with moderate renal failure.[65,66] However, a comparative study of n-acetylcysteine and fenoldopam found the former to be more effective in preventing nephrotoxicity.[67]

   c. **Note:** Furosemide should be avoided in these patients because it increases the risk of ARF. Dopamine provides no advantage over hydration alone.[68]

2. Repeat the serum creatinine 12 hours after contrast studies and defer surgery, if possible, until the creatinine has returned to baseline.

3. Identify and eliminate any medications with adverse effects on renal function (especially nonsteroidal antiinflammatory drugs [NSAIDs], ACE inhibitors, and metformin).

4. Optimize hemodynamic status. Occasionally, emergency surgery is indicated in patients with marginal hemodynamic function on inotropes and an intraaortic balloon, in which case one often has to accept the inevitable but frequently transient deterioration in postoperative renal function.

5. Correct acid-base or metabolic abnormalities associated with renal insufficiency, such as hyponatremia, hyper- or hypokalemia, hypomagnesemia, hyperphosphatemia, metabolic acidosis (from CRF), or alkalosis (from use of diuretics).

H. **Intraoperative measures** should be taken in an attempt to augment renal reserve by improving RBF, enhancing the GFR, and preventing tubular damage in patients with known renal dysfunction or risk factors for its development.

1. Perform off-pump coronary surgery if possible.

2. Maintain optimal hemodynamic performance before and after CPB.

3. Maintain a higher mean perfusion pressure (around 80 mm Hg) on bypass. This can be achieved by increasing the systemic flow rate or using vasopressors. Norepinephrine may be preferable to phenylephrine since it is less likely to be associated with renal damage. Vasopressin is an alternative in patients whose condition is refractory to norepinephrine; in fact, it has been shown to improve renal perfusion in patients with vasodilatory shock.[69]

4. The "pump run" should be kept as short as possible. Generally, the longer the duration of CPB, the greater the incidence of renal failure.[9,41,61] A very prolonged bypass run (>4 hours) may cause hemoglobinuria, which can impair tubular function.

5. Avoid extreme hemodilution (hematocrits <20%) on CPB. One study documented an inverse correlation between the lowest hematocrit on pump with the rise in postoperative creatinine, especially in obese patients.[70]

6. Use heparin-coated circuits, if available.[71]

7. Leukodepletion on pump using leukocyte-reducing filters may attenuate glomerular and tubular injury. This has been shown to lower the levels of microalbumin and retinol-binding protein indexed to creatinine.[72]

8. **Fenoldopam** should be considered in patients with a serum creatinine > 1.4 mg/dL, initiating an infusion of 0.03–0.1 µg/kg/min before CPB and continuing in the ICU for about 12 hours.

   a. This medication is a selective agonist of the dopamine-1 (DA1) receptor that has beneficial effects on renal function at this dose range without causing systemic vasodilatation.

   b. Fenoldopam produces a dose-dependent increase in renal plasma flow with a decrease in renal vascular resistance and maintenance of GFR. It increases blood flow to both the renal cortex and medulla and inhibits tubular reabsorption of sodium. Thus it produces diuresis, natriuresis, and kaliuresis.[73–75] Studies have shown preservation of renal function as well as some improvement in serum creatinine and C_{CR} after CPB in patients with an elevated creatinine.[75]

9. **Nesiritide** (B-type natriuretic peptide) may provide a renoprotective benefit when used during surgery, although this has not been well studied. It dilates the renal afferent arterioles and, to a lesser extent, the efferent arterioles leading to augmented glomerular filtration. It also has a direct tubular effect on sodium and water handling. Thus it exhibits strong natriuretic and diuretic properties. During periods of neurohormonal activation, such as cardiopulmonary bypass, it also inhibits the renin-angiotensin-aldosterone axis.[76] It is given in a bolus dose of 2 µg/kg over one minute followed by an infusion of 0.01–0.03 µg/kg/min.

10. Use of "renal-dose" **dopamine** (2–3 µg/kg/min) has been a common practice to optimize urine output and preserve renal function in patients at risk. However, numerous studies have failed to demonstrate any renoprotective effect of dopamine during surgery, both in patients with normal and abnormal renal function. Although dopamine may increase urine output, it has been shown to produce early renal tubular damage equal to or worse than that noted in control patients.[77-79]

11. **Diltiazem** has been evaluated as a means of preserving renal function, but its benefits are controversial.[80-83] Studies have provided conflicting evidence on whether there is preservation of glomerular and tubular integrity or any early improvement in renal function. One study did find that it caused a late deterioration in renal function.[42] It may produce an increase in urine output but no difference in creatinine clearance.

    a. Diltiazem reduces renal vascular resistance by dilating afferent arterioles, resulting in an increase in RBF and GFR. It increases sodium excretion and creatinine and free water clearance by a direct effect on tubular reabsorption. Diltiazem may also minimize the increase in calcium influx into renal tubular cells that could cause renal dysfunction.

    b. The use of diltiazem has been limited by its vasodilatory effects, and deterioration of renal function could be related to hypotension on pump.

12. Although neither dopamine nor diltiazem can be recommended individually to provide any renal protection, one study of an infusion of dopamine (2 µg/kg/min) + diltiazem (2 µg/kg/min) did demonstrate that this combination increased creatinine clearance, osmotic clearance, and free water clearance with no increase in markers of tubular damage.[84]

13. **Furosemide** is often given during surgery to augment urine output and is beneficial in patients with significant volume overload, severe oliguria, or hyperkalemia. However, its use may be associated with an increased, rather than a decreased, risk of renal impairment, even in patients with normal preoperative function.[79] Thus, it is not renoprotective and should be used only for the indications listed.

14. **Mannitol** may be added to the pump to increase tubular flow and produce a diuresis. It increases oncotic pressure, reduces tissue edema, and may reduce cell swelling after cardioplegic arrest. Usually 25–50 g is added to the pump prime.[85]

15. **Hemofiltration** can be performed to remove free water prior to terminating bypass. This is beneficial in removing excess fluid from patients with preoperative CHF, especially when the urine output is poor. It may improve hemodynamics, hemostasis, and pulmonary function in higher risk patients, although it has no direct beneficial effect on renal function.[86]

16. Use of antifibrinolytic drugs should be considered to minimize the bleeding diathesis that commonly accompanies renal dysfunction (uremic platelet

dysfunction). However, both ε-aminocaproic acid (Amicar) and aprotinin may affect renal function, so they must be used with caution.

a. ε-aminocaproic acid is associated with some degree of renal tubular dysfunction (elevated urine β_2-microglobulin levels) but generally does not alter creatinine clearance. It is probably the safest antifibrinolytic drug to use in patients with non–dialysis-dependent renal dysfunction.[87,88]

b. Aprotinin is actively absorbed by the renal tubular system where it remains for 5–6 days and produces a reversible overload of tubular reabsorption mechanisms. Patients with normal preoperative renal function usually compensate for this abnormality with little increase in creatinine, but those with altered tubular function may sustain additional tubular injury.[89–91] Studies have shown that 20% of patients develop an increase in serum creatinine over 0.5 mg/dL and 4% have a greater than 2 mg/dL increase, both of which are greater than in patients not receiving aprotinin.[92] Although guidelines for dosing in patients with moderate renal dysfunction are not available, lower doses should probably be used. It should be safe to use aprotinin in patients with CRF on dialysis.

V. Postoperative Oliguria and Renal Insufficiency

A. The use of hemodilution during CPB expands the extracellular volume and usually produces an excellent urine output in the immediate postoperative period. Oliguria is considered to be present in the postoperative cardiac surgical patient when the urine output is **less than 0.5 mL/kg/h.** Transient oliguria is commonly noted in the first 12 hours after surgery and may respond to a volume infusion or low-dose inotropic support. However, the persistence of oliguria is usually a manifestation of an acute renal insult caused by prolonged hypotension or a low cardiac output state. The serum creatinine will frequently be lower immediately after bypass due to hemodilution but will rise soon after if renal function is compromised.

B. The incidence of postoperative renal dysfunction depends on its definition. Most studies have defined it as an increase in serum creatinine of 50% or a 0.5 mg/dL (44 μmols/L) increase above the preoperative level; alternatively, it may be defined as a decrease in creatinine clearance >15 mL/min to less than 40 mL/min.[55] This extent of dysfunction affects about 10% of patients undergoing cardiac surgery. The 2004 STS database specifications defined it as an increase in serum creatinine to ≥2.0 mg/dL *and* to twice the preoperative level. According to this definition, it occurs in less than 5% of patients. Several studies have used a more liberal definition of renal failure and have found a higher incidence. For example, the incidence was reported to be 17% for a 30% change in serum creatinine and 42% for a 25% increase in two studies.[44,54]

1. **Nonoliguric renal failure,** defined as a rise in creatinine with a urine output >400 mL/day, is more common and may occur after an uneventful operation in a patient with preexisting renal dysfunction or risk factors for its development. This usually reflects less renal damage and is associated with a mortality rate of about 10%. Most patients can be managed by judicious fluid administration and high-dose diuretics to optimize urine output while awaiting spontaneous recovery of renal function.

2. **Oliguric renal failure,** defined as urine output <400 mL/day, occurs in only about 1–2% of patients, but often requires dialysis, which is associated with a mortality rate approaching 50%. This mortality rate has not changed over the past 10–15 years despite the early institution of various forms of dialysis and general improvements in postoperative care. This reflects the higher risk population undergoing

surgery and the morbidity of conditions frequently associated with renal failure, such as low cardiac output states, respiratory failure, infection, and stroke. In one study, the occurrence of three of these factors before or during the first 48 hours after initiation of hemodialysis was associated with a 90% mortality in contrast to only 15% when none was present.[93]

C. **Etiology of postoperative renal insufficiency (see Table 12.1)**

1. Despite the complex effects of low-flow, low-pressure, nonpulsatile perfusion with hemodilution and hypothermia on renal function, ischemic acute tubular necrosis (ATN) is most commonly the result of a **low cardiac output state.** A common contributing factor is intense peripheral vasoconstriction, often related to use of α-agents. The primary impact of oliguria is noted during the first few 12–24 hours after surgery when fluid overload and hyperkalemia can lead to pulmonary and myocardial complications and impair recovery from surgery.

2. The kidneys have a tremendous capacity to autoregulate and maintain RBF, GFR, filtration fraction, and tubular reabsorption in the face of reduced renal perfusion pressure. Intrinsic renal mechanisms that maintain autoregulation include a reduction in afferent arteriolar resistance and an increase in efferent arteriolar resistance. When a low cardiac output state or hypotension persists or potent vasopressor medications are used, the filtration reserve is exceeded, resulting in intense renal vasoconstriction and a fall in GFR. The development of renal failure often represents a continuum in which these compensatory mechanisms for prerenal problems are exhausted and ischemic ATN develops.[94] Patients with compromised renal reserve preoperatively are particularly sensitive to these insults.

D. Thus the management of both prerenal azotemia and ATN consists of measures to optimize renal perfusion. With the initial insult of impaired perfusion, the picture of prerenal azotemia will be present (Table 12.2) with values indicating preserved

Table 12.2 • Evaluation of the Etiology of Oliguria

	Prerenal	Renal
BUN/Cr	>20:1	<10:1
U/P creatinine	>40	<20
U_{osm}	>500	<400
U/P osmolality	>1.3	<1.1
Urine specific gravity	>1.020	1.010
U_{Na} (mEq/L)	<20	>40
FE_{Na}	<1%	>2%
Urinary sediment	Hyaline casts	Tubular epithelial cells Granular casts

tubular function. If this is recognized, the prerenal insult can often be corrected and ATN averted. If the prerenal insults are prolonged, ATN will develop with clinical and laboratory evidence of tubular dysfunction.[95]

E. Three patterns of ARF were described following open-heart surgery nearly 20 years ago and in principle still hold true today (Figure 12.1).[96] In the first, termed **"abbreviated ARF,"** a transient intraoperative insult occurs that causes renal ischemia. The serum creatinine peaks on the fourth postoperative day and then returns to normal. In the second pattern, termed **"overt ARF,"** the acute insult is followed by a more prolonged period of cardiac dysfunction. The creatinine usually rises to a higher level and returns toward baseline gradually over the course of 1–2 weeks once hemodynamics improve. The third pattern (**"protracted ARF"**) is characterized by an initial insult followed by a period of cardiac dysfunction that resolves. Just as the creatinine begins to fall, another insult occurs, often as a result of sepsis or a hypotensive event, that triggers a progressive, often irreversible rise in creatinine. Oliguria accompanying the rise in creatinine may adversely affect pulmonary function, but the early institution of dialysis may remove fluid and minimize pulmonary edema.

F. **Assessment** (see Table 12.2)[95,97]

1. Assess cardiac hemodynamics (filling pressures, cardiac output).

2. Identify any drugs being prescribed with adverse effects on renal function.

3. Obtain a serum BUN, creatinine, electrolytes, and osmolarity. **Note:** An elevation in creatinine with minimal or parallel rise in BUN is frequently noted with ATN. In contrast, a disproportionate rise in BUN with little rise in creatinine may reflect a prerenal process or increased protein intake, total parenteral nutrition (TPN), GI bleeding, hypercatabolism, or steroid administration, which increase urea production.

4. Examine the urinary sediment. Tubular epithelial or granular ("muddy brown") casts are indicative of tubular injury, whereas hyaline casts are seen in low perfusion states. The sediment is important to examine because test results regarding tubular function, such as the urine sodium and osmolality, may be inaccurate with use of diuretics.

5. Measure the urine sodium (U_{Na}) and creatinine (U_{Cr}) concentrations and the urine osmolarity (U_{osm}). These tests can differentiate prerenal from renal causes, but again, their interpretation will be influenced by the use of diuretics. $U_{Na} < 20$ mEq/L and $U_{osm} > 500$ mOsm/kg are strongly suggestive of prerenal disease. However, in oliguric patients, the U_{Na} will rise as the urine volume falls, leading to a higher U_{Na}, even in prerenal states.

   a. In this situation, calculation of the fractional excretion of sodium (FE_{Na}) is helpful:

$$FE_{Na} = \frac{U_{Na} \times P_{cr}}{P_{Na} \times U_{cr}} \times 100$$

   where U and P are the urinary and plasma concentrations of sodium and creatinine, respectively.

   b. In the oliguric patient, an FE_{Na} above 1–2% is noted in patients who develop ATN, whereas an $FE_{Na} < 1\%$ reflects retained tubular function with absorption of sodium and water, suggesting a prerenal problem. With an improvement in

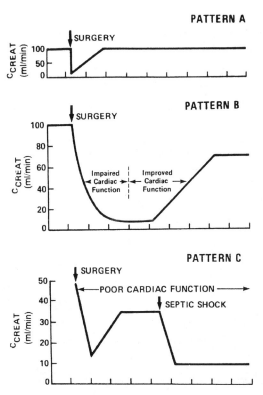

Figure 12.1 • Patterns of acute renal failure (ARF) observed after open-heart surgery. (A) Abbreviated ARF. (B) Overt ARF. (C) Protracted ARF. The reduction in creatinine clearance (C_{cr}) noted here is paralleled by a rise in serum creatinine. *(Reproduced with permission from Myers BD, Moran SM. Hemodynamically mediated acute renal failure. N Engl J Med 1986;314: 97–105. Copyright © 1986 Massachusetts Medical Society. All rights reserved.)*

hemodynamics, a rise in FE_{Na} may be noted during recovery of renal function due to sodium mobilization. However, a low FE_{Na} may be noted in patients with ATN associated with contrast nephrotoxicity or hepatorenal syndrome.

6. Monitor other electrolytes, blood glucose, and acid-base balance frequently.

7. Obtain a renal ultrasound to assess kidney size and rule out obstruction. A renal scan may be performed if a renal embolus is suspected.

G. **Management of oliguria** (Box 12.2). Interventions are beneficial at the first sign of renal dysfunction and may prevent frank ATN.[95,97] However, once ATN has occurred, very little can be done to promote recovery of renal function except to prevent additional insults. Generally, attention should be directed towards maintaining urine output to reduce tissue edema. If significant electrolyte or metabolic problems arise, they must be handled by additional means or by dialysis.

1. Ensure that the Foley catheter is in the bladder and is patent (this may rule out an obstructive uropathy). Irrigate with saline if necessary or consider changing the catheter empirically.

Box 12.2 • Management of Low Urine Output

1. Ensure that Foley catheter is in the bladder and is patent
2. Optimize cardiac function:
   - Treat hypovolemia
   - Control arrhythmias
   - Improve contractility
   - Reduce elevated afterload, but allow BP to drift up to 150 mm Hg
3. Administer diuretics or other medications:
   - Give increasing doses of furosemide (up to 500 mg IV) or a continuous infusion of 10–60 mg/h
   - Add chlorothiazide 500 mg IV to the loop diuretic
   - Consider bumetanide 4–10 mg or a 1 mg bolus, then 0.5–2 mg/h infusion
   - Cocktail of furosemide, dopamine ± mannitol
   - Nesiritide 2 µg/kg over 1 minute followed by an infusion of 0.01–0.03 µg/kg/min
   - Dopamine 2–3 µg/kg/min
4. If above fail:
   - Limit fluid to insensible losses
   - Readjust drug doses
   - Avoid potassium supplements
   - Nutrition: Essential amino acid diet
               High-nitrogen tube feeds if on dialysis
               TPN with 4.25% amino acid/35% dextrose
5. Consider early ultrafiltration or dialysis

---

2. Avoid nephrotoxins (NSAIDs, nephrotoxic antibiotics).
3. Optimize hemodynamics. Any additional insult that causes hypotension and a further decrease in renal perfusion will contribute to a state of protracted ARF. These insults include hypovolemia (often GI bleeding), arrhythmias (ventricular tachycardia, rapid atrial fibrillation), antihypertensive medications, or sepsis.
   a. Optimize preload without being overzealous; in a state of capillary leak, often seen in sepsis, excessive fluid administration may produce noncardiogenic pulmonary edema.
   b. Optimize heart rate and treat arrhythmias.
   c. Improve contractility with inotropes.
   d. Reduce afterload with vasodilators and try to eliminate drugs that can cause renal vasoconstriction; avoid ACE inhibitors[98] and angiotensin receptor blockers (ARBs).
      i. Do not be overly aggressive in the reduction of systemic blood pressure because patients with preexisting hypertension and chronic renal insufficiency often

have renal artery stenosis and require a higher blood pressure (130–150 mm Hg systolic) to maintain renal perfusion.

   ii. If inotropic drugs with vasodilator properties are used, such as inamrinone, milrinone, or dobutamine, an α-agent may be necessary to maintain systemic blood pressure. In this situation, norepinephrine is the preferred drug because it may have less effect on renal function.[37] Nonetheless, it probably does produce some degree of renal vasoconstriction and is more likely to compromise kidneys with preexisting dysfunction.

   e. If cardiac output remains marginal despite the use of multiple inotropes, consider placing an intraaortic balloon pump. This may result in an abrupt and dramatic increase in urine output.

4. If oliguria persists despite optimization of hemodynamics, the next step is selection of a **diuretic.** Diuretics do not have a direct effect on renal functional recovery or the natural history of ATN, and in fact may increase operative mortality and delay recovery of renal function.[69,95,99–101] However, they can often convert oliguric to nonoliguric renal failure if administered early after the onset of renal failure and may minimize the adverse impact of fluid retention on pulmonary function. An improvement in urine output suggests that the extent of renal injury is less severe in patients with "diuretic-responsive" ATN.

   a. A loop diuretic is chosen first to improve urine output. Loop diuretics inhibit sodium reabsorption in the ascending limb of the loop of Henle and increase solute (sodium) presentation to the distal tubules. By inhibiting tubular water reabsorption, they increase solute and free water clearance and prevent tubular obstruction. To a lesser extent, they may also act as renal vasodilators, increasing RBF and GFR, and they may improve medullary oxygenation.

   b. **Furosemide** is given in incremental doses starting at 10 mg IV. However, once acute renal failure is established, a dose of 100 mg IV is commonly required and should be given over 20–30 minutes to minimize ototoxicity. If urine output fails to increase within a few hours, the following steps can be taken:

      i. Increase the dose of furosemide up to 200 mg IV (limiting the cumulative daily dose to 1 g).

      ii. Use a **continuous infusion** of IV furosemide.[38,39,102] Give a loading dose of 40–100 mg, and then initiate an infusion of 10–40 mg/h. Rebolus before an increase in the infusion rate.

      iii. Alternatively, bumetanide can be given either as a bolus dose of 4–10 mg IV or as a 1 mg load followed by a continuous infusion of 0.5–2 mg/h depending on the estimated creatinine clearance.[38] There is little evidence, however, that one loop diuretic is better than any other.

5. Various **combinations** of medications may be effective in improving diuresis.

   a. Add a **thiazide** diuretic to the loop diuretic. These include chlorothiazide 500 mg IV, metolazone (Zaroxolyn) 5–10 mg PO or via an nasogastric tube, or hydrochlorothiazide 50–200 mg PO qd. Thiazides block distal nephron sites and act synergistically with the loop diuretics, which increase exposure of the distal tubules to solute. This combination is particularly effective in patients who tend to be diuretic-resistant and may have a low U_{Na} despite a loop diuretic.[38,103]

   b. The combination of dopamine and furosemide may be synergistic because the renal vasodilatation and improved RBF produced by dopamine improve the delivery of furosemide to the loop and increase solute diuresis.[104]

   c. The combination of mannitol (500 mL of 20% Osmitrol), furosemide (1 g), and dopamine (2–3 µg/kg/min) started within the first 6 hours of oliguria has been shown to produce a significant diuresis and early restoration of renal function.[105]

6. **Nesiritide** is very effective in producing a diuresis and lowering pulmonary artery pressures in patients with heart failure and other states of neurohormonal activation (such as use of CPB). It acts primarily by dilating afferent arterioles, and to a lesser extent, efferent arterioles, and improves RBF. It can improve the delivery of diuretics to the tubules, thus producing a synergistic effect with the loop diuretics. Therefore it may be of benefit in patients who are diuretic-resistant. It is given in a bolus dose of 2 µg/kg over 1 minute followed by an infusion of 0.01–0.03 µg/kg/min.[76,106]

7. One trial of **fenoldopam** initiated postoperatively in patients with a 50% rise in serum creatinine or a 25% rise for a creatinine > 1.5 mg/dL showed that a 72-hour infusion of 0.05–0.2 µg/kg/min significantly reduced the requirement for dialysis with an insignificant reduction in mortality.[107]

8. Despite the common use of **"renal-dose" dopamine** (2–3 µg/kg/min) for oliguric renal failure, numerous studies have shown that dopamine does not prevent ATN and has no impact on the duration of ATN, the need for dialysis, or on survival once ATN has developed.[95,108–115]

   a. Dopamine acts on DA1, α, and DA2 receptors. In normal subjects or those with CHF, dopamine has been shown to increase RBF and GFR, resulting in diuresis and natriuresis. However, it is more likely that diuresis is related to dopamine's positive inotropic effects or influence on tubular function. Studies have also shown that its renal effects and plasma levels cannot be predicted based on dosing alone.[108]

   b. Despite a lack of benefit on renal function per se, dopamine usually increases urine output (which is beneficial in improving pulmonary function) and may convert oliguric ATN to nonoliguric ATN. Patients in whom this can be accomplished generally have lesser degrees of ATN and are considered to have "diuretic-responsive ATN."

   c. A comprehensive review of dopamine use in critically ill ICU patients has suggested that dopamine may actually be deleterious to recovery. It was shown to worsen splanchnic oxygenation, impair GI function, impair endocrine and immunologic systems, and blunt the respiratory drive.[111]

   d. The influence and benefits of dopamine and dobutamine on renal function have been evaluated in several studies. One study showed that renal-dose dopamine increased urine output without improving creatinine clearance, whereas dobutamine did just the opposite.[116] Other studies have shown that dopamine can produce diuresis and improve creatinine clearance unrelated to any hemodynamic effects, whereas dobutamine has no effect on any renal variable.[117,118]

9. **Note: Mannitol** is an osmotic diuretic that is frequently used during surgery to increase serum osmolality during hemodilution to minimize tissue edema. It improves renal tubular flow, reduces tubular cell swelling, and improves urine output.[85,119] Nonetheless, it is best avoided in the postoperative period because its oncotic effect mobilizes fluid into the intravascular space. This could theoretically

lead to pulmonary edema if fluid overload is present and urine output does not improve. In fact, a significant increase in serum osmolality can cause renal vasoconstriction and induce renal failure.

H. Management of established renal failure

1. Once renal failure is established, treatment should be directed towards optimizing hemodynamics while minimizing excessive fluid administration, providing appropriate nutrition, and initiating early dialysis to hopefully reduce morbidity and improve survival. The blood pressure should be maintained at a higher level than usual in hypertensive patients whose kidneys may require higher perfusion pressures.

2. Restrict fluids with mL/mL of fluid replacement (i.e., input = output) plus 500 mL D5/0.2% NS/day (about 200 mL/m^2/day). Daily weights are helpful in assessing changes in day-to-day fluid status but must also take into consideration the influence of nutritional status on body mass.

3. Monitor electrolytes and blood glucose
   a. Avoid potassium supplements and medications that increase potassium levels (β-blockers, ACE inhibitors). Correct hyperkalemia as described on page 492.
   b. Hyponatremia should be treated with fluid restriction.
   c. Metabolic acidosis should be corrected if serum bicarbonate falls below 15 mEq/L.
   d. Correct hyperglycemia and abnormalities of calcium, phosphate, or magnesium metabolism.

4. Medications
   a. Eliminate drugs that impair renal function (aminoglycosides, NSAIDs, ACE inhibitors, ARBs).[98]
   b. Avoid or adjust doses of medications that are excreted or metabolized by the kidneys (particularly digoxin, procainamide, and antibiotics) (see Appendices 7 and 8).
   c. Give antacid medications (proton pump inhibitors) to minimize the risk of GI bleeding.

5. Remove the Foley catheter and catheterize daily or PRN depending on urine output. Culture the urine.

6. Improve the patient's nutritional state with enteral nutrition if possible.
   a. If the patient is able to eat, an essential amino acid diet should be used. Protein should not be restricted if the patient is on hemodialysis, which can result in the loss of 3–5 g/h of protein. Patients on dialysis should receive approximately 1.5 g/kg/day of protein.
   b. If the patient is unable to eat but has a functional GI tract, a high-nitrogen tube feeding can be used if the patient is on dialysis. For most patients with acute renal insufficiency, there is no need to alter the amount of protein, and standard tube feedings can be used unless hyperkalemia is present. In patients with chronic renal insufficiency that does not require dialysis, a low-protein supplement can be used to provide 0.5–0.8 g/kg/day of protein.
   c. If the patient is unable to tolerate enteral feedings, TPN using a 4.25% amino acid/35% dextrose solution that contains no potassium, magnesium, or phosphate is recommended.
   d. Consider the prompt initiation of dialysis or ultrafiltration.

Table 12.3 • Techniques of Hemofiltration and Dialysis				
If the patient has:	**HD**	**SCUF**	**CVVH**	**CVVHD**
Unstable hemodynamics	–	+++	+++	+++
Contraindication to heparin	++	+	+	+
Vascular access problems	+++	+++	+++	+++
Volume overload	++	+++	+++	+++
Hyperkalemia	+++	0	++	+++
Severe uremia	+++	0	+	++
Respiratory compromise	++	+++	+++	+++

HD = hemodialysis; SCUF = slow continuous ultrafiltration; CVVH = continuous venovenous hemofiltration; CVVHD = continuous venovenous hemodialysis with filtration.
– = avoid; 0 = minimal effect; + = useful; ++ = better; +++ = even better.

VI. Hemofiltration and Dialysis (Table 12.3)[120,121]

A. Hemofiltration or hemodialysis can be used to remove excessive fluid and solute to improve electrolyte balance, and they may also reduce the risk of bleeding and infection associated with uremia. Thus, the general **indications** for their use are hypervolemia, hyperkalemia, and metabolic acidosis. However, the important and sometimes difficult decision is whether these modalities should be initiated at the first sign of oliguric ATN or a rising creatinine. One study of "prophylactic" preoperative dialysis for patients with a preoperative creatinine greater than 2.5 mg/dL showed a dramatic increase in survival compared with patients on whom dialysis was performed only if the creatinine increased to 50% above baseline.[122] Another study reported that early initiation of CVVH (averaging less than 2.5 days after surgery) increased survival.[123] Another showed that early and aggressive dialysis was beneficial in improving survival.[124] Thus, there is accumulating evidence that early intervention before the BUN and creatinine are markedly elevated may be beneficial in improving outcomes. This should be especially true in the early postoperative cardiac surgical patient who is already in a state of total body water overload.

B. Whether hemofiltration or dialysis should be selected depends primarily on the indication for its use and the hemodynamic stability of the patient. Devices that provide continuous hemofiltration using only venous access have abrogated concern in unstable patients or those with limited arterial access.

C. Intermittent hemodialysis (HD)

1. **Principle.** Solute passes by diffusion down a concentration gradient from the blood, across a hollow-fiber semipermeable membrane, and into a dialysate bath. Some solute is also transported by convection resulting from a difference in hydrostatic pressure (ultrafiltration).

2. **Indications.** HD is indicated for the management of hyperkalemia, acid-base imbalances, fluid overload, or a hypercatabolic state in the hemodynamically stable patient. It is the most efficient means of removing solute (urea, creatinine) and correcting severe acid-base abnormalities. It does not obligatorily remove fluid but can be combined with ultrafiltration to achieve this goal.

3. **Access.** Standard intermittent HD is performed using a single 12F double-lumen catheter (such as the Niagara Slim-Cath, Bard Access Systems, Inc., Salt Lake City, UT) placed in the internal jugular or subclavian vein, although the latter is more likely to be associated with venous thrombosis. Placement in the femoral vein may lead to lower extremity venous thrombosis but can be used for very short-term dialysis. To reduce the infection risk in patients requiring more extended periods of dialysis, a double-lumen Permcath (Quinton Instrument Co., Seattle, WA) or HemoGlide or HemoSplit long-term hemodialysis catheter (Bard Access Systems) can be placed in the internal jugular vein and brought through a subcutaneous tunnel. Subsequently, a fistula can be created for permanent dialysis. When recovery appears unlikely and a fistula is being considered, the arm vessels on one side should be protected as much as possible.

4. **Technique.** Intermittent HD is performed over a 3–4 hour period. The blood is pumped into the dialysis cartridge at a rate of 300–500 mL/min, while the dialysate solution is infused at a rate of 500 mL/min in a direction countercurrent to blood flow. Although heparin is commonly used, heparin-free HD is possible in patients with bleeding problems or heparin-induced thrombocytopenia.

5. **Limitations**

   a. Use of biocompatible membranes, bicarbonate baths, initial high dialysate sodium, cool temperatures, and volumetric control during dialysis have attenuated some of the circulatory instability noted during the procedure.[95] However, hypovolemia or blunted sympathetic reflexes commonly occur during intermittent HD, especially if there is an attempt to remove a large volume of fluid in a short period of time. Colloid or blood transfusions and hemodynamic support (usually with α-agents or PO midodrine) are frequently necessary. Therefore, HD is best avoided in the hemodynamically unstable patient.

   b. Dialysis machines are complex, costly, and require special expertise.

D. Continuous venovenous systems can be used in a variety of ways, including slow continuous ultrafiltration (SCUF), continuous venovenous hemofiltration (CVVH), and continuous venovenous hemodiafiltration (CVVHD).[121]

1. **Principle.** An occlusive pump is included in a circuit that actively withdraws blood from the venous system, pumps it through a diafilter, and returns it to the venous system. For CVVHD, dialysis fluid runs countercurrent to the direction of blood flow within the diafilter. Solute then passes by diffusion down a concentration gradient across a hemofilter into the dialysate solution.

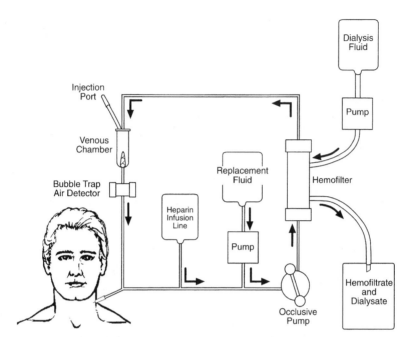

Figure 12.2 • Continuous venovenous hemofiltration (CVVH) and dialysis (CVVHD) setup. An occlusive pump withdraws blood from the venous circuit, pumps it through a diafilter, and returns it to the venous system through a double-lumen catheter placed in the internal jugular vein. Dialysis is accomplished by infusing a dialysate solution into the diafilter in a direction countercurrent to blood flow.

2. **Indications:** These systems are indicated for the management of fluid overload, especially in the hemodynamically unstable or hypotensive patient. Slow correction of electrolyte imbalance can be achieved with CVVH using a crystalloid solution of different composition as replacement fluid. Severe electrolyte imbalance or hypercatabolic states are better managed with CVVHD.

3. **Access** is obtained using a 12F double-lumen catheter (12 gauge for each lumen) placed in the internal jugular, subclavian, or femoral vein.

4. **Technique** (Figure 12.2)

   a. A high-efficiency biocompatible hemodialysis cartridge is attached downstream to an occlusive pump and heparin is infused into the inflow portion of the circuit to maintain a dialyzer output (venous) PTT of 45–60 seconds.

   b. For SCUF, the ultrafiltrate rate is set at the desired amount to achieve net negative fluid balance and no replacement fluid is given. The system is more prone to clotting because the hematocrit is higher at the return end of the hemofilter after plasma has been removed by ultrafiltration.

   c. For CVVH, the pump is usually set to deliver blood at a rate of 100 mL/min and the ultrafiltrate rate is usually set at a preselected rate (usually 999 mL/h). The blood then passes through a bubble trap air detector and is returned to the patient. A citrate replacement solution (which obviates the need for heparin) or a bicarbonate solution (if hepatic dysfunction is present) is infused into the inflow circuit or into the venous chamber. The amount of fluid administered is dictated by the desired negative fluid balance per hour. This can achieve a moderate amount of solute removal. If citrate is used, a continuous infusion of calcium gluconate is given if ionized calcium is less than 1.0 mmol/L.

  d. For CVVHD, dialysis fluid (Dianeal 1.5% with 4 mL of 23% NaCl per 2 L bag) is infused into the dialysis cartridge at a rate of 999 mL/h.

5. Limitations

  a. Heparinization within the circuit is required to prevent clotting.

  b. The pump adds some complexity and cost to the system compared with arteriovenous hemofiltration.

E. Continuous arteriovenous hemofiltration (CAVH). This technique of ultrafiltration is commonly used during surgery to remove excessive fluid before terminating CPB. It is beneficial in improving hemodynamics, hemostasis, and pulmonary function in higher risk patients.[86] Postoperatively, its use is limited by the need for arterial access, heparinization to minimize clotting of the hemofilter, and satisfactory arterial pressure to provide the hydrostatic pressure to achieve hemofiltration. Because of these drawbacks, CAVH has been replaced by CVVH in most units.

F. Peritoneal dialysis is rarely used in cardiac surgical patients because it produces abdominal distention and glucose absorption that can compromise the patient's respiratory status, and it carries the risk of peritonitis. Its use is usually limited to patients on long-term peritoneal dialysis.

VII. Hyperkalemia

A. Etiology

  1. High-volume, high-potassium cardioplegia solutions used in the operating room. The potassium load is usually eliminated promptly by normally functioning kidneys, but hyperkalemia can be problematic in patients with intrinsic renal dysfunction or oliguria from other causes.

  2. Low cardiac output states associated with oliguria. Potassium levels may rise with alarming and life-threatening rapidity.

  3. Severe tissue ischemia, whether peripheral (from severe peripheral vascular disease or complication of an intraaortic balloon pump) or intraabdominal (mesenteric ischemia). Hyperkalemia is often the first clue to the existence of these problems.

  4. Acute and chronic renal insufficiency.

  5. Medications that impair potassium excretion or increase potassium levels (ACE inhibitors, potassium-sparing diuretics, NSAIDs, ARBs, β-blockers).

Note: Remember that hyperkalemia is exacerbated by acidosis, which often accompanies low output or ischemic syndromes. A 0.2 unit change in pH produces about a 1 mEq/L change in serum potassium concentration. However, in conditions of organic acidosis, the potassium is more likely to rise due to tissue breakdown and release of potassium from cells (lactic acidosis) or from insulin deficiency and hyperglycemia (ketoacidosis), rather than from a change in pH.

  B. Manifestations are predominantly electrocardiographic. An asystolic arrest may occur when the potassium rises rapidly to a level exceeding 6.5 mEq/L. The ECG changes of hyperkalemia do not always develop in classic progressive fashion and are more related to the rate of rise of serum potassium than to the absolute level. These changes include:

1. Peaked T waves
2. ST depression
3. Smaller R waves
4. Prolonged PR interval
5. Loss of P waves
6. QRS widening, bradycardia, asystole, ventricular fibrillation
7. When the heart is being paced, hyperkalemia may result in failure to respond to the pacemaker stimulus.

C. **Treatment** entails stabilizing the cell membrane, shifting potassium into cells, and increasing its excretion from the body.

1. Optimize cardiac function.
2. If evidence of advanced cardiac toxicity (K^+ > 6.0 mEq/L), administer calcium gluconate 5–10 mL of a 10% solution (0.5–1 g) IV over 15 minutes to stabilize the cell membranes.
3. Identify and remove any potential source of potassium intake or medication that may increase the potassium level (as above).
4. Shift potassium into cells:
   a. Regular insulin 10 units/25 g of 50% dextrose IV.
   b. $NaHCO_3$ (1 ampule = 50 mEq/L) to correct metabolic acidosis and raise the pH to 7.40–7.50.
   c. Aerosolized β-agonists by nebulizer. They may improve potassium uptake into cells.
5. Enhance potassium excretion:
   a. Furosemide 10–200 mg IV
   b. Kayexalate enema 50 g in 50 mL sorbitol as retention enema or 50 g PO with 50 mL of sorbitol q6h
   c. 9α-fluorohydrocortisone acetate (Florinef) may be helpful in patients with low renin or aldosterone levels. It may transfer K^+ into cells or increase GI excretion.

VIII. Hypokalemia[125]

A. **Etiology**

1. Profound diuresis without adequate potassium replacement. Potassium excretion parallels the urine output after bypass, which tends to be copious because of hemodilution. The use of potent diuretics may produce a significant diuresis and kaliuresis in the early postoperative period.
2. Insulin to manage hyperglycemia
3. Alkalosis (metabolic or respiratory)
4. Significant nasogastric tube drainage

B. **Manifestations.** Hypokalemia promotes atrial, junctional, or ventricular ectopy, and enhances digoxin-induced arrhythmias. The ECG may demonstrate flattened ST segments, decreased T wave amplitude, and the presence of "u" waves.

C. Treatment. Potassium replacement may resolve ectopic beats by several mechanisms that alter automaticity and conduction.

1. It is essential that renal function and urine output be evaluated before a KCl drip is started, because acute hyperkalemia can develop very rapidly when oliguria or renal dysfunction is present. A slower infusion rate is advisable in this situation, with frequent rechecking of the serum potassium level.

2. In the ICU setting, KCl is administered through a central line at a rate of 10–20 mEq/h (mix of 80 mEq/250 mL). The serum potassium rises approximately 0.1 mEq/L for each 2 mEq of KCl administered.

3. When a central line is not present, a concentrated potassium drip cannot be administered peripherally because it scleroses veins. The maximum concentration of KCl that can be administered peripherally is 60 mEq/L. Oral potassium (usually 10–20 mEq tablets) is somewhat unpalatable, but coated preparations are available.

IX. Hypocalcemia

A. Calcium plays a complex role in myocardial reperfusion damage and myocardial energetics. Ionized calcium (normal = 1.1–1.3 mmol/L) should be measured because total calcium levels, which are affected by protein binding, usually decrease during surgery because of hemodilution, hypothermia, shifts in pH, and the use of citrated blood. Hypocalcemia is usually associated with prolongation of the QT interval on the ECG tracing.

B. Treatment

1. It is common practice to empirically administer a 500 mg bolus of calcium chloride at the termination of bypass to support systemic vascular resistance and possibly increase myocardial contractility.[126] It is also commonly mixed with protamine to offset the vasodilatory effects associated with the intravenous administration of protamine.

2. It is questionable whether treatment of hypocalcemia identified in the ICU is of any value in improving cardiovascular function. In fact, calcium salts may attenuate the cardiotonic effects of catecholamines, such as dobutamine or epinephrine, although they have little effect on the efficacy of inamrinone or milrinone.[127] Nonetheless, if the ionized calcium level is measured and found to be < 1 mmol/L, calcium gluconate (10 mL of 10% solution) may be given, although there is no clear benefit to doing so. Calcium chloride is best avoided for "asymptomatic" hypocalcemia to minimize any acute hemodynamic effects.

3. Calcium chloride (0.5–1 g IV) may be given in emergency situations to provide temporary circulatory support when a low cardiac output syndrome or acute hypotension develops suddenly. The transient improvement in hemodynamics allows time for analysis of causative factors and the institution of other pharmacologic support. $CaCl_2$ should not be given routinely during a cardiac arrest.

X. Hypomagnesemia

A. Magnesium plays a role in energy metabolism and cardiac impulse generation. Low levels have been associated with coronary spasm, low cardiac output syndromes, prolonged ventilatory support, a higher incidence of postoperative atrial and ventricular arrhythmias, perioperative infarction, and a higher mortality rate.[128,129]

B. Magnesium levels (normal = 1.5–2 mEq/L) are usually not measured during surgery, but they are reduced in more than 70% of patients studied.[130] This may be the result of diuresis usage or simple hemodilution.

C. Administration of magnesium sulfate (2 g in 100 mL solution) to raise the serum level to 2 mEq/L has been shown in many studies to reduce the incidence of postoperative atrial and ventricular dysrhythmias.[131–134] This benefit may also be seen during and after off-pump surgery.[135] In addition, magnesium has been found to inhibit the vasoconstrictive response to epinephrine but not its cardiotonic effects.[136] Administering 2 g of $MgSO_4$ at the conclusion of bypass and on the first postoperative morning can be recommended.

XI. Metabolic Acidosis

A. Etiology

1. A low cardiac output state, often with peripheral vasoconstriction or poor peripheral perfusion, is the primary cause of metabolic acidosis. This scenario is often noted in the immediate postoperative period when the patient not only has marginal myocardial function but is also vasoconstricted from hypothermia. The use of α-agents commonly impairs tissue perfusion perpetuating the metabolic acidosis.

2. Low-dose epinephrine occasionally causes a metabolic acidosis out of proportion to its α effects when the cardiac output is satisfactory. This may reflect a metabolic type B lactic acidosis (not associated with tissue hypoxia) caused by metabolic factors that increase lactic acid production, such as hyperglycemia and lipolysis.[137]

3. Intraabdominal catastrophes, such as mesenteric ischemia from a low-flow state, should always be considered when progressive metabolic acidosis occurs.

4. Sepsis

5. High doses of sodium nitroprusside

6. Renal failure

7. Acute hepatic dysfunction

8. Diabetic ketoacidosis

B. Effects

1. Adverse effects from metabolic acidemia usually do not occur until the pH is less than 7.20.[138] A pure metabolic acidosis (low serum bicarbonate with acidemic pH) may be noted in the heavily sedated patient in whom there is no respiratory compensation. However, compensatory hyperventilation will usually occur during intermittent mandatory ventilation or spontaneous ventilation to decrease the PCO_2 and partially neutralize the pH to minimize these effects. Nonetheless, some of the deleterious effects of metabolic acidemia may be related to the metabolic products associated with the acidemia, rather than the absolute level of pH, although they may be reversed by administration of sodium bicarbonate.

2. The presence of a progressive or significant metabolic acidosis (as assessed by the serum bicarbonate level) is more likely than not an indication of a serious ongoing problem that must be corrected before adverse consequences occur. These include:

    a. Cardiovascular effects
- Decreased contractility and cardiac output; reduction in hepatic and renal blood flow
- Attenuation of the positive inotropic effects of catecholamines[139]
- Venoconstriction and arteriolar dilatation, which increase filling pressures and decrease systemic pressures
- Increased pulmonary vascular resistance
- Sensitization to reentrant arrhythmias and reduction in the threshold for ventricular fibrillation

    b. Respiratory effects
- Dyspnea and tachypnea
- Decreased respiratory muscle strength

    c. Metabolic changes
- Increased metabolic demands
- Hyperglycemia caused by tissue insulin resistance and inhibition of anaerobic glycolysis
- Decreased hepatic update and increased hepatic production of lactate
- Hyperkalemia
- Increased protein catabolism

    d. Cerebral function
- Inhibition of brain metabolism and cell volume regulation
- Obtundation and coma

3. Type A lactic acidosis reflects impaired tissue oxygenation and anaerobic metabolism resulting from circulatory failure. The acidosis is self-perpetuating in that excess lactate is produced at a time when there is suppression of hepatic lactate utilization. The lactate ion, probably more than the acidemia, contributes to potential cardiovascular dysfunction. Elevated lactate levels (>3 mmol/L) are not uncommon after open-heart surgery but should raise suspicion of a low cardiac output state with severe tissue ischemia. This is noted more often in patients with long bypass runs, lower mean arterial pressures on pump, and use of vasopressors. To some degree, this may be related to splanchnic ischemia during surgery as well as a low cardiac output syndrome postpump. A lactate level > 3 mmol/L upon arrival in the ICU has been associated with a worse outcome.[137]

4. Type B lactic acidosis occurs in the absence of tissue hypoxia. It may be a catecholamine-induced metabolic effect (especially with epinephrine) caused by hyperglycemia and alterations in fatty acid metabolism that cause pyruvate accumulation and elevated levels of lactic acid. Acute hepatic failure may also present with severe lactic acidosis due to failure to clear lactic acid.[137,140,141]

C. Treatment should be directed primarily to reversal of the underlying cause. Whether correction of a primary metabolic acidosis (not one that compensates for a primary respiratory alkalosis) should be considered when the serum bicarbonate is less than 15 mEq/L (base deficit greater than 8–10 mmol/L) is controversial.

    1. Proponents of bicarbonate administration suggest that severe metabolic acidosis has significant deleterious effects on cardiovascular function that can be corrected with a more normal pH. Furthermore, more responsiveness to catecholamines does seem to occur with a higher pH. Thus, correction of the acidosis may be very important when the etiologic mechanism for the acidosis is unclear or not imminently remediable.[138,142]

2. However, others argue that the use of bicarbonate may correct only the blood pH, not the intracellular pH. They argue that no controlled studies have demonstrated improved hemodynamics attributable to use of sodium bicarbonate. In addition, sodium bicarbonate may have numerous deleterious effects such as hypernatremia and hyperosmolarity, increased affinity of hemoglobin for oxygen (and thus less tissue release), increased lactate levels, and reduced ionized calcium, which may reduce cardiac contractility.[143]

3. If one elects to correct the pH, there are several compounds that can be used:

   a. **Sodium bicarbonate** is administered in a dose calculated from the following equation:

   $$0.5 \times \text{body weight (kg)} \times \text{base deficit} = \text{mEq NaHCO}_3$$

   This should be administered over several hours in the patient with severe metabolic acidemia with careful monitoring of the serum sodium concentration.

   b. **Carbicarb** (available in Canada) is an equimolar solution of sodium bicarbonate and sodium carbonate.[144] One of its advantages over standard $NaHCO_3$ is that it does not undergo significant breakdown into CO_2 and H_2O; it also raises intracellular pH more consistently. The recommended dose is:

   $$0.2 \times \text{kg} \times \text{base deficit} = \text{mEq sodium}$$

   c. **Tromethamine** 0.3 M (THAM or Tris buffer) can be used if the patient has developed hypernatremia from multiple doses of $NaHCO_3$. It also limits CO_2 generation. It is usually given as a continuous infusion but is contraindicated in renal failure.

   $$\text{kg} \times \text{base deficit} = \text{mL of 0.3 M THAM}$$

XII. Metabolic Alkalosis[145]

A. Etiology

1. Excessive diuresis, especially from the loop diuretics
2. Nasogastric drainage with inadequate electrolyte replacement by IV solutions
3. TPN with inappropriate solute composition
4. Secondary as compensation for respiratory acidosis

B. Adverse effects

1. Lowers the serum potassium level, potentially leading to atrial and ventricular arrhythmias (especially digoxin-induced arrhythmias) and to neuromuscular weakness.
2. Has an adverse effect on the cardiovascular response to catecholamines that is comparable to that of acidosis.[139]
3. Shifts the oxygen-hemoglobin dissociation curve to the left, impairing oxygen delivery to the tissues. This effect is offset in chronic metabolic alkalosis by an increase in 2,3-diphosphoglycerate in red cells.
4. Produces arteriolar constriction, which can compromise cerebral and coronary perfusion. Neurologic abnormalities including headache, seizures, tetany, and

lethargy may occur, probably because of the associated hypocalcemia induced by alkalosis. These effects are usually seen with a pH > 7.60.

5. Decreases the central respiratory drive, leading to hypoventilation, CO_2 retention, and, potentially, hypoxemia.

C. **Treatment**

1. Metabolic alkalosis is sustained by hypovolemia ("contraction alkalosis"), hypokalemia, and hypochloremia. Thus, therapy should be directed towards correction of these factors.

2. Potential contributors to alkalosis should be assessed.

   a. Reduce doses of loop diuretics or thiazides. Use **acetazolamide** (Diamox) 250–500 mg IV in conjunction with a loop diuretic. This has a fairly weak diuretic effect when used alone. If hypokalemia is present, one of the potassium-sparing diuretics (spironolactone 25 mg PO qd or amiloride 5 mg PO qd) can be used. Eplerenone 50 mg PO qd, a new aldosterone antagonist, may be useful.

   b. Loss of gastric acid through a nasogastric tube can be reduced using H_2 blockers or a proton pump inhibitor.

   c. Avoid lactate (LR) and acetate (common in parenteral nutrition solutions) that are metabolized to bicarbonate.

3. The administration of chloride, usually as KCl or NaCl, is the primary treatment for metabolic alkalosis. The selection of the appropriate solute depends on the patient's serum potassium and volume status. The rate of administration of IV KCl is usually limited to 20 mEq/h, but can be slightly faster if the patient has significant hypokalemia and an ongoing profound diuresis.

4. Hydrochloric acid 0.1 N (100 mEq/L) may be administered through a central line at a rate of 10–20 mEq/h. It is rarely required in cardiac surgical patients. The total dose can be calculated based on a bicarbonate space of 50% body weight from either of the following methods:

   a. Chloride deficit:

   $$\text{mEq HCl} = 0.5 \times \text{kg} \times (103\text{-measured chloride})$$

   b. Base-excess method:

   $$\text{mEq HCl} = 0.5 \times \text{kg} \times \text{base excess}$$

   If a profound alkalosis is present, these doses should be given over 12 hours with intermittent reevaluation.

XIII. Hyperglycemia

A. **Etiology**

1. Preexisting diabetes mellitus exacerbated by the hormonal stress response to surgery

2. Impaired insulin production and peripheral insulin resistance during bypass resulting from elevated levels of the counterregulatory hormones, including cortisol, epinephrine, and growth hormone (even in nondiabetics).

3. TPN with inadequate insulin response

4. Sepsis (often the first manifestation of an occult sternal wound infection or an intraabdominal process)

B. Manifestations. Hyperglycemia contributes to excessive urine output from an osmotic diuresis, impairs wound healing, increases the risk of infection, and may impair blood pressure regulation. Although hypotonic fluid losses from the osmotic diuresis can cause hypernatremia, the glucose-induced shift of water from cells into the extracellular fluid compartment may cause hyponatremia. In this situation, the plasma osmolarity is elevated despite the low serum sodium, a condition treated by fluid administration rather than restriction.

C. Treatment

1. Strict blood glucose control in the ICU has been shown to reduce the risk of wound infection and mortality in diabetic patients.[146,147] Therefore, a hyperglycemia protocol should be followed with careful monitoring of blood sugars (Appendix 6). Excessively stringent control (keeping blood sugar <120 mg/dL) is potentially dangerous and probably not necessary. An intravenous bolus of insulin is rapidly cleared from the blood and may lower the potassium level without affecting the blood glucose. Therefore, a bolus followed by an infusion (using 100 units regular insulin/100 mL NS mix) is recommended.

2. All diabetic patients should have fingerstick blood sugars drawn before meals and at bedtime once they are started on an oral diet. The glucose level may be higher than suspected from the patient's oral intake because of the residual elevation of counterregulatory hormones from the operation. On the other hand, the blood sugar may remain acceptable without medications in some patients with poor oral intake.

3. Patients with type 1 diabetes mellitus should have their insulin doses gradually increased to preoperative levels depending on blood glucose levels and early postoperative insulin requirements. It is preferable to use a lower dose of intermediate-acting insulin initially (usually one-half of the usual dose) and supplement it with regular insulin as necessary. Insulin doses may be increased when the patient becomes more active and has an improved caloric intake.

4. In patients with type 2 diabetes, oral hypoglycemic medications should be restarted once the patient is taking a normal diet, with frequent checking of fingersticks to assess the adequacy of blood sugar control.

D. Hyperosmolar, hyperglycemic, nonketotic coma has been reported in patients with type 2 diabetes following surgery. It usually develops 4–7 days after surgery and is manifested by polyuria in association with a rising BUN or serum sodium. The resultant dehydration, often exacerbated by GI bleeding or use of high-nitrogen, hyperosmolar tube feedings, results in the hyperosmolar state.[148] Gradual correction of hypovolemia, hyperglycemia, hypokalemia, and hypernatremia is indicated.

E. Diabetic ketoacidosis is rarely seen following cardiac surgery but may be noted in persons with type 1 diabetes. Standard management with saline infusions, an insulin drip, and correction of potassium and acid-base abnormalities should be followed.

F. **Note: Hypoglycemia** is extremely uncommon after open-heart surgery unless excessive doses of insulin are administered. However, it may occur in patients with a severe hepatic insult with impaired glucose production.

XIV. Hypothyroidism

A. Hypothyroidism is difficult to manage preoperatively in the patient with ischemic heart disease because thyroid replacement may precipitate ischemic symptoms. It may be present more often than realized, however, in patients taking thyroid hormone replacement. One study showed a significantly greater operative mortality in patients taking thyroxine (T_4) preoperatively, perhaps for this reason.[149]

B. Serum total and free triiodothyronine (T_3 and free T_3) are significantly reduced after CPB and remain low for up to 6 days, whereas T_4 is low immediately after surgery, but returns to normal within 24 hours. This suggests that the conversion of T_4 to T_3 is delayed in some patients and this may account for the slower recovery of some patients after surgery.[150]

C. **Manifestations** include decreased myocardial contractility, bradycardia, high peripheral resistance, diastolic hypertension, and low cardiac output. Cardiac surgery is well tolerated in most patients with mild to moderate hypothyroidism. Ventricular dysfunction is rarely noted upon weaning from bypass.

D. Treatment
1. Should postcardiotomy ventricular dysfunction occur, 0.05–0.8 µg/kg of T_3 can be given in conjunction with an inotrope, such as inamrinone or milrinone, which does not depend on β-receptors for its action. The benefit of T_3 in improving hemodynamics and reducing the incidence of arrhythmias may occur because the T_3 level is lower after CPB.[151]
2. For the hypothyroid patient who has tolerated surgery uneventfully, treatment is initiated postoperatively with T_4 (Synthroid) 0.05 mg PO qd and subsequently increased depending on TSH and T_4 levels. If the patient is unable to take oral medications, one-half of the oral dose can be given intravenously.
3. If the patient is severely hypothyroid, consultation with an endocrinologist is imperative. Doses of T_4 that have been recommended include an initial IV dose of 0.4 mg, followed by 3 days of 0.1–0.2 mg IV daily, and then a maintenance dose of 0.05 PO qd.

XV. Adrenal Insufficiency

A. Adrenal insufficiency is a rare complication of cardiac surgery that may result from adrenal hemorrhage associated with heparinization (or other anticoagulation) and stress in an elderly patient.[152]

B. **Manifestations** include flank pain, nonspecific GI complaints (anorexia, nausea, vomiting, ileus, abdominal pain or distention), fever, and delirium. Late signs include hyperkalemia, hyponatremia, and hypotension with poor response to vasopressors. The clinical scenario can be confused with sepsis.

C. **Diagnosis** is confirmed by a low serum cortisol level and failure of cortisol levels to rise 1 hour after a 0.25 mg IV dose of cosyntropin (a synthetic ACTH analog). The level should rise fourfold or to a level greater than 20 µg/mL.[153]

    D. Treatment is with 100 mg of hydrocortisone IV every 8 hours as well as administration of glucose and NS. If additional mineralocorticoid is needed, fludrocortisone 0.05–0.2 mg qd can be given.

XVI. Pituitary Abnormalities

    A. **Pituitary apoplexy**[154]

        1. **Etiology**

            a. Ischemia, edema, or hemorrhage of an undetected pituitary tumor.

            b. CPB with heparinization and low cerebral blood flow may be contributory.

        2. **Presentation.** Compression of the optic chiasm and parasellar structures results in ophthalmoplegia, third-nerve palsy, visual loss, and headache.[155]

        3. **Treatment**

            a. Decrease intracerebral edema with hyperventilation, mannitol, and steroids (dexamethasone 10 mg q6h).

            b. Urgent hypophysectomy if no improvement.

    B. **Diabetes insipidus.** This is a rare complication of cardiac surgery caused by diminished production of antidiuretic hormone (ADH). The presence of polyuria, a urine osmolarity of 50–100 mOsm/L, and hypernatremia should raise suspicion of the diagnosis. Treatment involves use of DDAVP, administered either intranasally (1 or 2 sprays = 10–20 µg at bedtime), 1–2 µg IV/SC bid, or 0.05–0.4 mg PO bid.

References

1. Bernstein AD, Parsonnet V. Bedside estimation of risk as an aid for decision-making in cardiac surgery. Ann Thorac Surg 2000;69:823–8.
2. Higgins TL, Estafanous FG, Loop FD, et al. ICU admission score for predicting morbidity and mortality risks after coronary artery bypass grafting. Ann Thorac Surg 1997;64:1050–8.
3. Shroyer ALW, Coombs LP, Peterson ED, et al. The Society of Thoracic Surgeons: 30-day mortality and morbidity risk models. Ann Thorac Surg 2003;75:1856–64.
4. Edwards FH, Grover FL, Shroyer ALW, Schwartz M, Bero J. The Society of Thoracic Surgeons national cardiac surgery database: current risk assessment. Ann Thorac Surg 1997;63:903–8.
5. Mozes B, Olmer L, Galai N, Simchen E, for the ISCAB Consortium. A national study of postoperative mortality associated with coronary artery bypass grafting in Israel. Ann Thorac Surg 1998;66:1254–63.
6. Mangano CM, Diamondstone LS, Ramsay JG, Aggarwal A, Herskowitz A, Mangano DT. Renal dysfunction after myocardial revascularization: risk factors, adverse outcomes, and hospital resource utilization. The Multicenter Study of Perioperative Ischemia Research Group. Ann Intern Med 1998;128:194–203.
7. Lema G, Meneses G, Urzua J, et al. Effects of extracorporeal circulation on renal function in coronary surgical patients. Anesth Analg 1995;81:446–51.
8. Blaikley J, Sutton P, Walter M, et al. Tubular proteinuria and enzymuria following open heart surgery. Intensive Care Med 2003;29:1364–7.
9. Boldt J, Brenner T, Lehmann A, Suttner SW, Kumle B, Isgro F. Is kidney function altered by the duration of cardiopulmonary bypass? Ann Thorac Surg 2003;75:906–12.
10. Butterworth JF, Prielipp RC. Endocrine, metabolic, and electrolyte responses. In: Gravlee GP, Davis RF, Kurusz M, Utley JR, eds. Cardiopulmonary Bypass. Principles and Practice, 2nd ed. Philadelphia: Lippincott Williams & Wilkins, 2000:342–66.
11. Abraham VS, Swain JA. Cardiopulmonary bypass and the kidney. In: Gravlee GP, Davis RF, Kurusz M, Utley JR, eds. Cardiopulmonary Bypass. Principles and Practice, 2nd ed. Philadelphia: Lippincott Williams & Wilkins, 2000:382–90.
12. Sehested J, Wacker B, Forssmann WG, Schmitzer E. Natriuresis after cardiopulmonary bypass: relationship to urodilatin, atrial natriuretic factor, antidiuretic hormone, and aldosterone. J Thorac Cardiovasc Surg 1997;114:666–71.
13. Stallword MI, Grayson AD, Mills K, Scawn ND. Acute renal failure in coronary artery bypass surgery: independent effect of cardiopulmonary bypass. Ann Thorac Surg 2004;77:968–72.
14. Ascione R, Lloyd CT, Underwood MJ, Gomes WJ, Angelini GD. On-pump versus off-pump coronary revascularization: evaluation of renal function. Ann Thorac Surg 1999;68:493–8.
15. Ascione R, Nason G, Al-Ruzzeh S, Ko C, Ciulli F, Angelini GD. Coronary revascularization with or without cardiopulmonary bypass in patients with preoperative nondialysis-dependent renal insufficiency. Ann Thorac Surg 2001;72:2020–5.
16. Bucerius J, Gummert JF, Walther T, et al. On-pump versus off-pump coronary artery bypass grafting: impact on postoperative renal failure requiring renal replacement therapy. Ann Thorac Surg 2004;77:1250–6.
17. Loef BG, Epema AH, Navis G, Ebels T, van Oeveren W, Henning RH. Off-pump coronary revascularization attenuates transient renal damage compared with on-pump coronary revascularization. Chest 2002;121:1190–4.
18. Hayashida N, Teshima H, Chihara S, et al. Does off-pump coronary artery bypass really preserve renal function? Circ J 2002;66:921–5.
19. Gamoso MG, Phillips-Bute B, Landolfo KP, Newman MF, Stafford-Smith M. Off-pump versus on-pump coronary artery bypass surgery and postoperative renal dysfunction. Anesth Analg 2000;91:1080–4.
20. Utley JR, Stephens, DB. Fluid balance during cardiopulmonary bypass. In: Utley JR, ed. Pathophysiology and Techniques of Cardiopulmonary Bypass. Baltimore: Williams & Wilkins, 1982:26.
21. London MJ. Plasma volume expansion in cardiovascular surgery: practical realities, theoretical concerns. J Cardiothorac Anesth 1988;2:39–49.

22. McIlroy DR, Kharasch ED. Acute intravascular volume expansion with rapidly administered crystalloid or colloid in the setting of moderate hypovolemia. Anesth Analg 2003;96:1572–7.

23. Hauser CJ, Shoemaker WC, Turpin I, Goldberg SJ. Oxygen transport responses to colloids and crystalloids in critically ill surgical patients. Surg Gynecol Obstet 1980;150:811–6.

24. Gallagher JD, Moore RA, Kerns D, et al. Effects of colloid or crystalloid administration on pulmonary extravascular water in the postoperative period after coronary artery bypass grafting. Anesth Analg 1985;64:753–8.

25. Martin G, Bennett-Guerrero E, Wakeling H, et al. A prospective, randomized comparison of thromboelastographic coagulation profile in patients receiving lactated Ringer's solution, 6% hetastarch in balanced-saline vehicle, or 6% hetastarch in saline during major surgery. J Cardiothorac Vasc Anesth 2002;16:441–6.

26. Schwartzkopff W, Schwartzkopff B, Wurm W, Fresius H. Physiological aspects of the role of human albumin in the treatment of chronic and acute blood loss. Dev Biol Stand 1980;48:7–30.

27. Gan TJ, Bennett-Guerreo E, Phillips-Bute B, et al. Hextend, a physiologically balanced plasma expander for large volume use in major surgery: a randomized phase III clinical trial. Hextend study group. Anesth Analg 1999;88:992–8.

28. Wilkes NJ, Woolf RL, Powanda MC, et al. Hydroxyethyl starch in balanced electrolyte solution (Hextend): pharmacokinetic and pharmacodynamic profiles in healthy volunteers. Anesth Analg 2002;94:538–44.

29. Wilkes MM, Navickis RJ, Sibbald WJ. Albumin versus hydroxyethylstarch in cardiopulmonary bypass surgery: a meta-analysis of postoperative bleeding. Ann Thorac Surg 2001;72:527–33.

30. Avorn J, Patel M, Levin R, Winkelmayer WC. Hetastarch and bleeding complications after coronary artery surgery. Chest 2003;124:1437–42.

31. London MJ, Ho HS, Triedman JK, et al. A randomized clinical trial of 10% pentastarch (low molecular weight hydroxyethylstarch) versus 5% albumin for plasma volume expansion after cardiac operations. J Thorac Cardiovasc Surg 1989;97:785–87.

32. Boldt J, Preiebe HJ. Intravascular volume replacement therapy with synthetic colloids: is there an influence on renal function? Anesth Analg 2003;96:376–82.

33. Williams EL, Hildebrand KL, McCormick SA, Bedel MJ. The effect of lactated Ringer's solution versus 0.9% sodium chloride solution on serum osmolarity in human volunteers. Anesth Analg 1999;88:999–1003.

34. Jarvela K, Kaukinen S. Hypertonic saline (7.5%) decreases perioperative weight gain following cardiac surgery. J Cardiothorac Vasc Anesth 2002;16:43–6.

35. Jarvela K, Koskinen M, Kaukinen S, Koobi T. Effects of hypertonic saline (7.5%) on extracellular fluid volumes compared with normal saline (0.9%) and 6% hydroxyethylstarch after aortocoronary bypass graft surgery. J Cardiothorac Vasc Anesth 2001;15:210–5.

36. Richer M, Robert S, Lebel M. Renal hemodynamics during norepinephrine and low-dose dopamine infusions in man. Crit Care Med 1996;24:1150–6.

37. Morimatsu H, Uchino S, Chung J, Bellomo R, Raman J, Buxton B. Norepinephrine for hypotensive vasodilatation after cardiac surgery: impact on renal function. Intensive Care Med 2003;29:1106–12.

38. Brater DG. Diuretic therapy. N Engl J Med 1998;339:387–95.

39. Yelton SL, Gaylor MA, Murray KM. The role of continuous infusion loop diuretics. Ann Pharmacother 1995;29:1010–4.

40. Lim E, Ali ZA, Attaran R, Cooper G. Evaluating routine diuretics after coronary surgery: a prospective randomized controlled trial. Ann Thorac Surg 2002;73:153–5.

41. Antunes PE, Prieto D, de Oliveira JF, Antunes MJ. Renal dysfunction after myocardial revascularization. Eur J Cardiothorac Surg 2004;25:597–604.

42. Young EW, Diab A, Kirsh MM. Intravenous diltiazem and acute renal failure after cardiac operations. Ann Thorac Surg 1998;65:1316–9.

43. Durmaz I, Buket S, Atay Y, et al. Cardiac surgery with cardiopulmonary bypass in patients with chronic renal failure. J Thorac Cardiovasc Surg 1999;118:306–15.

44. Provenchere S, Plantefeve G, Hufnagel G, et al. Renal dysfunction after cardiac surgery with normothermic cardiopulmonary bypass: incidence, risk factors, and effect on clinical outcome. Anesth Analg 2003;96:1258–64.

45. Weerasinghe A, Nornick P, Smith P, Taylor K, Ratnatunga C. Coronary artery bypass grafting in non-dialysis-dependent mild-to-moderate renal dysfunction. J Thorac Cardiovasc Surg 2001; 121:1083–9.

46. Penta de Peppo A, Nardi P, De Paulis R, et al. Cardiac surgery in moderate to end-stage renal failure: analysis of risk factors. Ann Thorac Surg 2002;74:378–83.

47. Gibbs ER, Christian KG, Drinkwater DC Jr, Pierson RN III, Bender HW Jr, Merrill WH. Cardiac surgery in patients with moderate renal impairment. South Med J 2002;95:321–3.

48. Hirose H, Amano A, Takahashi A, Nagano N. Coronary artery bypass grafting for patients with non-dialysis-dependent renal dysfunction (serum creatinine greater than or equal to 2.0 mg/dL). Eur J Cardiothorac Surg 2001;20:565–72.

49. Christiansen S, Claus M, Philipp T, Reidemeister JC. Cardiac surgery in patients with end-stage renal failure. Clin Nephrol 1997;48:246–52.

50. Ko W, Kreiger KH, Isom OW. Cardiopulmonary bypass procedures in dialysis patients. Ann Thorac Surg 1993;55:677–84.

51. Horst M, Mehlhorn U, Hoerstrup SP, Suedkamp M, de Vivie ER. Cardiac surgery in patients with end-stage renal disease: a 10-year experience. Ann Thorac Surg 2000;69:96–101.

52. Wang F, Dupuis JY, Nathan H, Williams K. An analysis of the association between preoperative renal dysfunction and outcome in cardiac surgery: estimated creatinine clearance or plasma creatinine level as measures of renal function. Chest 2003;124:1852–62.

53. Walter J, Mortasawi A, Arnrich B, et al. Creatinine clearance versus serum creatinine as a risk factor in cardiac surgery. BMC Surg 2003;3:4.

54. Tuttle KR, Worral NK, Dahlstrom LR, Nandagopal R, Kausz AT, David CL. Predictors of ARF after cardiac surgical procedures. Am J Kidney Dis 2003;41:76–83.

55. Abrahamov D, Tamariz M, Fremes S, et al. Renal dysfunction after cardiac surgery. Can J Cardiol 2001;17:565–70.

56. Andersson LG, Ekroth R, Bratteby LE, Hallhagen S, Wesslen O. Acute renal failure after coronary surgery: a study of incidence and risk factors in 2009 consecutive patients. Thorac Cardiovasc Surg 1993;41:237–41.

57. Hayashida N, Chihara S, Tayama E, et al. Coronary artery bypass grafting in patients with mild renal insufficiency. Jpn Circ J 2001;65:28–32.

58. Ryckwaert F, Boccara G, Frappier JM, Colson PH. Incidence, risk factors, and prognosis of a moderate increase in plasma creatinine early after cardiac surgery. Crit Care Med 2002;30:1495–8.

59. Suen WS, Mok CK, Chiu SW, et al. Risk factors for development of acute renal failure (ARF) requiring dialysis in patients undergoing cardiac surgery. Angiology 1998;49:789–800.

60. Grayson AD, Khater M, Jackson M, Fox MA. Valvular heart operation is an independent risk factor for acute renal failure. Ann Thorac Surg 2003;75:1829–35.

61. Swaminathan M, East C, Phillips-Bute B, et al. Report of a substudy on warm versus cold cardiopulmonary bypass: changes in creatinine clearance. Ann Thorac Surg 2001;72:1603–9.

62. Davila-Roman VG, Kouchoukos NT, Schechtman KB, Barzilai B. Atherosclerosis of the ascending aorta is a predictor of renal dysfunction after cardiac operations. J Thorac Cardiovasc Surg 1999;117:111–6.

63. Baker CSR, Wragg A, Kumar S, De Palma R, Baker LRI, Knight CJ. A rapid protocol for the prevention of contrast-induced renal dysfunction: the RAPPID study. J Am Coll Cardiol 2003;41:2114–8.

64. Kay J, Chow WH, Chan TM, et al. Acetylcysteine for prevention of acute deterioration of renal function following elective coronary angiography and intervention. A randomized controlled trial. JAMA 2003;289:553–8.

65. Madyoon H. Clinical experience with the use of fenoldopam for prevention of radiocontrast nephropathy in high-risk patients. Rev Cardiovasc Med 2001;2 (suppl I):S26–30.

66. Kini AA, Sharma SK. Managing the high-risk patient: experience with fenoldopam, a selective dopamine receptor agonist, in prevention of radiocontrast nephropathy during percutaneous coronary intervention. Rev Cardiovasc Med 2001;2(suppl 1):S19–25.

67. Briguori C, Colombo A, Airoldi F, et al. N-acetylcysteine versus fenoldopam mesylate to prevent contrast agent-associated nephrotoxicity. J Am Coll Cardiol 2004;44:762–5.

68. Gare M, Haviv YS, Ben-Yehuda A, et al. The renal effect of low-dose dopamine in high-risk patients undergoing coronary angiography. J Am Coll Cardiol 1999;34:1682–8.

69. Lameire NH, De Vriese AS, Vanholder R. Prevention and nondialytic treatment of acute renal failure. Curr Opin Crit Care 2003;9:481–90.

70. Swaminathan M, Phillips-Bute BG, Conlon PJ, Smith PK, Newman MF, Stafford-Smith. The association of lowest hematocrit during cardiopulmonary bypass with acute renal injury after coronary artery bypass surgery. Ann Thorac Surg 2003;76:784–92.

71. Suehiro S, Shibata T, Sasaki Y, et al. Heparin-coated circuits prevent renal dysfunction after open heart surgery. Osaka City Med J 1999;45:149–57.

72. Tang ATM, Alexiou C, Hsu J, Sheppard SV, Haw MP, Ohri SK. Leukodepletion reduces renal injury in coronary revascularization: a prospective randomized study. Ann Thorac Surg 2002;74:372–7.

73. Ranucci M, Soro G, Barzaghi N, et al. Fenoldopam prophylaxis of postoperative acute renal failure in high-risk cardiac surgery patients. Ann Thorac Surg 2004;78:1332–8.

74. Garwood S, Swamidoss CP, Davis EA, Samson L, Hines RL. A case series of low-dose fenoldopam in seventy cardiac surgical patients at increased risk of renal dysfunction. J Cardiothorac Vasc Anesth 2003;17:17–21.

75. Caimmi PP, Pagani L, Micalizzi E, et al. Fenoldopam for renal protection in patients undergoing cardiopulmonary bypass. J Cardiothorac Vasc Anesth 2003;17:491–4.

76. Gordon G, Rastegar H, Khabbaz K, Schumann R, England M. Perioperative use of nesiritide in adult cardiac surgery. Anesth Analg 2004;98:SCA1–134.

77. Woo EB, Tang AT, el-Gamel A, et al. Dopamine therapy for patients at risk of renal dysfunction following cardiac surgery: fact or fiction? Eur J Cardiothorac Surg 2002;22:106–11.

78. Tang AT, El-Gamel A, Keevil B, Yonan N, Deiraniya AK. The effect of "renal-dose" dopamine on renal tubular function following cardiac surgery: assessed by measuring retinol binding protein (RBP). Eur J Cardiothorac Surg 1999;15:717–21.

79. Lassnigg A, Donner E, Grubhofer G, Presterl E, Druml W, Hiesmayr M. Lack of renoprotective effects of dopamine and furosemide during cardiac surgery. J Am Soc Nephrol 2000;11:97–104.

80. Amano A, Suzuki A, Sunamori M, Tofukuji M. Effect of calcium antagonist diltiazem on renal function in open heart surgery. Chest 1995;107:1260–5.

81. Zanardo G, Michielon P, Rosi P, et al. Effects of a continuous diltiazem infusion on renal function during cardiac surgery. J Cardiothorac Vasc Anesth 1993;7:711–6.

82. Bergman AS, Odar-Cederlof I, Westman L, Bjellerup P, Hoglund P, Ohqvist G. Diltiazem infusion for renal protection in cardiac surgical patients with preexisting renal dysfunction. J Cardiothorac Vasc Anesth 2002;16:294–9.

83. Piper SN, Kumle B, Maleck WH, et al. Diltiazem may preserve renal tubular integrity after cardiac surgery. Can J Anaesth 2003;50:285–92.

84. Yavuz S, Ayabakan N, Goncu MT, Ozdemir IA. Effect of combined dopamine and diltiazem on renal function after cardiac surgery. Med Sci Monit 2002;8:PI45–50.

85. Poullis M. Mannitol and cardiac surgery. Thorac Cardiovasc Surg 1999;47:58–62.

86. Kiziltepe U, Uysalel A, Corapcioglu T, Dalva K, Akan H, Akalin H. Effects of combined conventional and modified ultrafiltration in adult patients. Ann Thorac Surg 2001;71:684–93.

87. Butterworth J, James RL, Lin Y, Prielipp RC, Hudspeth AS. Pharmacokinetics of epsilon-aminocaproic acid in patients undergoing aortocoronary bypass surgery. Anesthesiology 1999;90:1624–35.

88. Stafford-Smith M, Phillips-Bute B, Reddan DN, Black J, Newman MF. The association of epsilon-aminocaproic acid with postoperative decrease in creatinine clearance in 1502 coronary bypass patients. Anesth Analg 2000;91:1085–90.

89. Schweizer A, Hohn L, Morel DR, Kalangos A, Licker M. Aprotinin does not impair renal haemodynamics and function after cardiac surgery. Br J Anaesth 2000;84:3–5.

90. Feindt PR, Walcher S, Volkmer I, et al. Effects of high-dose aprotinin on renal function in aortocoronary bypass grafting. Ann Thorac Surg 1995;60:1076–80.

91. O'Connor CJ, Brown DV, Avramov M, Barnes S, O'Connor HN, Tuman KJ. The impact of renal dysfunction on aprotinin. Pharmacokinetics during cardiopulmonary bypass. Anesth Analg 1999;89:1101–7.

92. Smith PK. Overview of aprotinin. Innovative strategies to improve open-heart surgery outcomes. Presented at symposium, Washington, DC, May 2002.

93. Lange HW, Aeppli DM, Brown DC. Survival of patients with acute renal failure requiring dialysis after open heart surgery: early prognostic indicators. Am Heart J 1987;113:1138–43.

94. Badr KF, Ichikawa I. Prerenal failure: a deleterious shift from renal compensation to decompensation. N Engl J Med 1988;319:623–9.

95. Esson ML, Schrier RW. Diagnosis and treatment of acute tubular necrosis. Ann Intern Med 2002;137:744–52.

96. Myers BD, Moran SM. Hemodynamically mediated acute renal failure. N Engl J Med 1986;314:97–105.

97. Klahr S, Miller SB. Acute oliguria. N Engl J Med 1998;338:671–5.

98. Manche A, Galea J, Busuttil W. Tolerance to ACE inhibitors after cardiac surgery. Eur J Cardiothorac Surg 1999;15:55–60.

99. Mehta RL, Pascual MT, Soroko S, Chertow GM for the PICARD study group. Diuretics, mortality, and nonrecovery of renal function in acute renal failure. JAMA 2002;288:2547–53.

100. Andreucci M, Russo D, Fuiano G, Minutolo R, Andreucci VE. Diuretics in renal failure. Miner Electrolyte Metab 1999;25:32–8.

101. Ventataram R, Kellum JA. The role of diuretic agents in the management of acute renal failure. Contrib Nephrol 2001;132:158–70.

102. Krasna MJ, Scott GE, Scholz PM, Spotnitz AJ, Mackenzie JW, Penn F. Postoperative enhancement of urinary output in patients with acute renal failure using continuous furosemide therapy. Chest 1986;89:294–5.

103. Vanky F, Broquist M, Svedjeholm R. Addition of a thiazide: an effective remedy for furosemide resistance after cardiac operations. Ann Thorac Surg 1997;63:993–7.

104. Lindner A. Synergism of dopamine and furosemide in diuretic-resistant, oliguric acute renal failure. Nephron 1983;33:121–6.

105. Sirivella S, Gielchinsky I, Parsonnet V. Mannitol, furosemide, and dopamine infusion in postoperative renal failure complicating cardiac surgery. Ann Thorac Surg 2000;69:501–6.

106. Rayburn BK, Bourge RC. Nesiritide: a unique therapeutic cardiac peptide. Rev Cardiovasc Med 2001;2(suppl 2):S25–31.

107. Tumlin J, Thourani VH, Guyton RA, Shaw A, Finkle K, Murray P. Fenoldopam mesylate reduces the incidence of dialysis in patients developing acute tubular necrosis following open heart surgery: results of a randomized, double-blind, placebo-controlled trial. Presented at the 40th Annual Meeting of the Society of Thoracic Surgeons, San Antonio, TX, January 2004.

108. Bailey JM. Dopamine: one size doesn't not fit all. Anesthesiology 2000;92:303–5.

109. Bellomo R, Chapman M, Finfer S, Hickling K, Myburg J. Low-dose dopamine in patients with early renal dysfunction: a placebo-controlled randomized trial. Australian and New Zealand Intensive Care Society (ANZICS) Clinical Trials Group. Lancet 2000;356:2139–43.

110. Kellum JA, Decker JM. Use of dopamine in acute renal failure: a meta-analysis. Crit Care Med 2001;29:1526–31.

111. Holmes CL, Walley KR. Bad medicine: low-dose dopamine in the ICU. Chest 2003;123:1266–75.

112. Burton CJ, Tomson CR. Can the use of low-dose dopamine for treatment of acute renal failure be justified? Postgrad Med J 1999;75:269–74.

113. Dishart MK, Kellum JA. An evaluation of pharmacological strategies for the prevention and treatment of acute renal failure. Drugs 2000;59:79–91.

114. Kellum JA. The use of diuretics and dopamine in acute renal failure: a systematic review of the evidence. Crit Care (Lond) 1997;1:53–9.

115. Gambaro G, Bertaglia G, Puma G, D'Angelo A. Diuretics and dopamine for the prevention and treatment of acute renal failure: a critical reappraisal. J Nephrol 2002;15:213–9.

116. Duke GJ, Briedis JH, Weaver RA. Renal support in critically ill patients: low-dose dopamine or low-dose dobutamine? Crit Care Med 1994;22:1919–25.
117. Ichai C, Passeron C, Carles M, Bouregba M, Grimaud D. Prolonged low-dose dopamine infusion induces a transient improvement in renal function in hemodynamically stable, critically ill patients: a single-blind, prospective, controlled study. Crit Care Med 2000;28:1329–35.
118. Ichai C, Soubielle J, Carles M, Giunti C, Grimaud D. Comparison of the renal effects of low to high doses of dopamine and dobutamine in critically ill patients: a single-blind randomized study. Crit Care Med 2000;28:921–8.
119. Better OS, Rubinstein I, Winaver JM, Knochel JP. Mannitol therapy revisited (1940–1997). Kidney Int 1997;51:886–94.
120. Pastan S, Bailey J. Dialysis therapy. N Engl J Med 1998;338:1428–37.
121. Forni LG, Hilton PJ. Continuous hemofiltration in the treatment of acute renal failure. N Engl J Med 1997;336:1303–9.
122. Durmaz I, Yagdi T, Calkavur T, et al. Prophylactic dialysis in patients with renal dysfunction undergoing on-pump coronary artery bypass surgery. Ann Thorac Surg 2003;75:859–64.
123. Bent P, Tan HK, Bellomo R, et al. Early and intensive continuous hemofiltration for severe renal failure after cardiac surgery. Ann Thorac Surg 2001;71:832–7.
124. Schiffl H, Lang SM, Fischer R. Daily hemodialysis and the outcome of acute renal failure. N Engl J Med 2002;346:305–10.
125. Genneri FJ. Hypokalemia. N Engl J Med 1998;339:451–8.
126. DiNardo JA. Pro: calcium is routinely indicated during separation from cardiopulmonary bypass. J Cardiothorac Vasc Anesth 1997;11:905–7.
127. Butterworth JF, Zaloga GP, Prielipp RC, Tucker WY Jr, Royster RL. Calcium inhibits the cardiac stimulating properties of dobutamine but not of amrinone. Chest 1992;101:174–80.
128. Parra L, Fita G, Gomar C, Rovira I, Marin JL. Plasma magnesium in patients submitted to cardiac surgery and its influence on perioperative morbidity. J Cardiovasc Surg (Torino) 2001;42:37–42.
129. Booth JV, Phillips-Bute B, McCants CB, et al. Low serum magnesium level predicts adverse cardiac events after coronary artery bypass graft surgery. Am Heart J 2003;145:1108–13.
130. Aglio LS, Stanford GG, Maddi R, Boyd JL III, Nussbaum S, Chernow B. Hypomagnesemia is common following cardiac surgery. J Cardiothorac Vasc Anesth 1991;5:201–8.
131. Kiziltepe U, Eyileten ZB, Sirlak M, et al. Antiarrhythmic effect of magnesium sulfate after open heart surgery: effect on blood levels. Int J Cardiol 2003;89:153–8.
132. Toraman F, Karabulut EH, Alhan HC, Dagdelen S, Tarcan S. Magnesium infusion dramatically decreases the incidence of atrial fibrillation after coronary artery bypass grafting. Ann Thorac Surg 2001;72:1256–61.
133. England MR, Gordon G, Salem M, Chernow B. Magnesium administration and dysrhythmias after cardiac surgery. A placebo-controlled, double-blind, randomized trial. JAMA 1992;268:2395–2402.
134. Boyd WC, Thomas SJ. Pro: magnesium should be administered to all coronary artery bypass graft surgery patients undergoing cardiopulmonary bypass. J Cardiothorac Vasc Anesth 2000;14:339–43.
135. Maslow AD, Regan MM, Heindle S, Panzica P, Cohn WF, Johnson RG. Postoperative atrial tachyarrhythmias in patients undergoing coronary artery bypass graft surgery without cardiopulmonary bypass: a role for intraoperative magnesium supplementation. J Cardiothorac Vasc Anesth 2000;14:524–30.
136. Prielipp RC, Zaloga GP, Butterworth JF IV, et al. Magnesium inhibits the hypertensive but not the cardiotonic actions of low-dose epinephrine. Anesthesiology 1991;74:973–9.
137. Maillet JM, Le Besnerais P, Cantoni M, et al. Frequency, risk factors, and outcome of hyperlactatemia after cardiac surgery. Chest 2003;123:1361–6.
138. Adrogué HJ, Madias NE. Management of life-threatening acid-base disorders. First of two parts. N Engl J Med 1998;338:26–34.
139. Kaplan JA, Guffin AV, Yin A. The effects of metabolic acidosis and alkalosis on the response to sympathomimetic drugs in dogs. J Cardiothorac Vasc Anesth 1988;2:481–7.

140. Raper R, Cameron G, Walker D, Bowley CJ. Type B lactic acidosis following cardiopulmonary bypass. Crit Care Med 1997;25:46–51.

141. Boldt J, Piper S, Murray P, Lehmann A. Severe lactic acidosis after cardiac surgery: sign of perfusions deficits? J Cardiothorac Vasc Anesth 1999;13:220–4.

142. Forsythe SM, Schmidt GA. Sodium bicarbonate for the treatment of lactic acidosis. Chest 2000;117:260–7.

143. Levraut J, Grimaud D. Treatment of metabolic acidosis. Curr Opin Crit Care 2003;9:260–5.

144. Leung JM, Landow L, Franks M, et al. Safety and efficacy of intravenous Carbicarb® in patients undergoing surgery: comparison with sodium bicarbonate in the treatment of mild metabolic acidosis. Crit Care Med 1994;22:1540–9.

145. Adrogué HJ, Madias NE. Management of life-threatening acid-base disorders. Second of two parts. N Engl J Med 1998;338:107–11.

146. Furnary AP, Gao G, Grunkemeier GL, et al. Continuous insulin infusion reduces mortality in patients with diabetes undergoing coronary artery bypass grafting. J Thorac Cardiovasc Surg 2003;125:1007–21.

147. Zerr KJ, Furnary AP, Grunkemeier GL, Bookin S, Kanhere V, Starr A. Glucose control lowers the risk of wound infection in diabetics after open heart operations. Ann Thorac Surg 1997;63:356–61.

148. Seki S. Clinical features of hyperosmolar hyperglycemic nonketotic diabetic coma associated with cardiac operations. J Thorac Cardiovasc Surg 1986;91:867–73.

149. Zindrou D, Taylor KM, Bagger JP. Excess coronary artery bypass graft mortality among women with hypothyroidism. Ann Thorac Surg 2002;74:2121–5.

150. Sabatino L, Cerillo AG, Ripoli A, Pilo A, Glauber M, Iervasi G. Is the low tri-iodothyronine state a crucial factor in determining the outcome of coronary artery bypass patients? Evidence from a clinical pilot study. J Endocrinol 2002;175:577–86.

151. Klemperer JD. Thyroid hormone and cardiac surgery. Thyroid 2002;12:517–21.

152. Sutherland FWH, Naik SK. Acute adrenal insufficiency after coronary artery bypass grafting. Ann Thorac Surg 1996;62:1516–7.

153. Tordjman K, Jaffe A, Trostanetsky Y, Greenman Y, Limor R, Stern N. Low-dose (1 microgram) adrenocorticotrophin (ACTH) stimulation as a screening test for impaired hypothalamo-pituitary-adrenal axis function: sensitivity, specificity, and accuracy in comparison with the high-dose (250 microgram) test. Clin Endocrinol 2000;52:633–40.

154. Cooper DM, Bazaral MG, Furlan AJ, et al. Pituitary apoplexy: a complication of cardiac surgery. Ann Thorac Surg 1986;41:547–50.

155. Kontorinis N, Holthouse DJ, Carroll WM, Newman M. Third nerve palsy after coronary artery bypass surgery. J Thorac Cardiovasc Surg 2001;122:400–1.

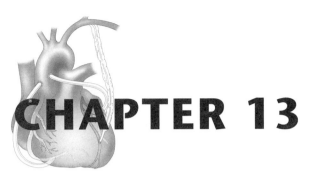

CHAPTER 13

Post-ICU Care and Other Complications

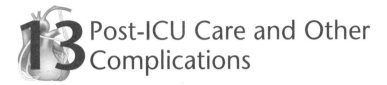

13 Post-ICU Care and Other Complications

I. General Comments

A. Following a brief stay in the ICU, most patients undergoing cardiac surgical procedures follow a routine pattern of recovery. The use of fast-track protocols and critical pathways ensures that the health care team and the patient have a clear understanding of what to expect at different junctures during recovery. Critical pathways are designed to standardize care and identify variances from the expected. However, they are not a substitute for careful patient examination that may identify problems that might otherwise be ignored by rigid adherence to protocols.

B. Most patients are transferred to an intermediate care unit or the postoperative cardiac surgical floor on the first postoperative day (POD). Invasive monitoring is no longer utilized, although bedside telemetry should be considered for several days to identify arrhythmias. It should be remembered that patients are still in an early phase of recovery from surgery with many physiologic derangements still present. Restoring the patient to a normal physiologic state requires careful attention to the prevention, identification, and management of complications that may develop at any time during the hospital stay. A detailed daily examination of the patient must be performed with particular attention paid to each organ system. Orders must be thought out carefully and written on an individualized basis to ensure the best possible postoperative care.

C. Although postoperative complications are more common in elderly patients and those with comorbidities, they may still develop unpredictably in low-risk, healthy patients despite an uneventful surgical procedure and early postoperative course. Problems such as atrial arrhythmias are very common and quite benign, with little influence on the patient's hospital course or long-term prognosis. In contrast, less common complications, such as stroke, mediastinitis, tamponade, renal failure, or an acute abdomen, may be devastating, resulting in early death or prolonged hospitalization with multisystem organ failure.

II. Transfer from the ICU and Postoperative Routines

The patient undergoing a routine recovery from surgery is usually extubated within 6–12 hours and off all inotropic support by the first postoperative morning. The following interventions are standardized and can be followed on a delayed basis for patients requiring a few additional days of care in the ICU. An example of the critical pathway for patients undergoing coronary artery bypass grafting (CABG) is noted in Table 13.1. Typical orders for transfer to the postoperative floor are noted in Box 13.1 and Appendix 3.

A. Postoperative day and night

    1. Wean vasoactive medications

    2. Wean patient from ventilator and extubate

Table 13.1 • Critical Pathway for Coronary Artery Bypass Grafting

	Preop Day or Office Visit	Day of Surgery	POD #1	POD #2–3	POD #4–5
Cardiovascular	Bilateral BP Height and weight	Monitor and treat: bleeding shivering arrhythmias hemodynamics Meds (start 8 h postop): ASA Metoprolol	VS q2h Telemetry D/C neck and arterial lines Meds: 2 g $MgSO_4$	VS q4-8h Telemetry	VS before D/C Remove pacing wires
Respiratory	RA O_2 saturation RA ABGs if COPD	Wean to extubate within 8–12 hours IS W/A q1h	40% face mask or nasal cannula IS W/A q1h Splinted cough	Nasal cannula at 2–4 L/min for O_2 sat <95% IS W/A q1h Splinted cough	Room air
Fluids and electrolytes		I & O q1h Keep u/o > 1 mL/kg/h	Weight I&O q2h Furosemide IV	Weight I&O qshift Furosemide IV	Weight Furosemide IV/PO until at preop weight
Wounds and drains	Hibiclens shower	OR dressing × 12 h Monitor/manage CT drainage	DSD with povidone-iodine wipe to wounds (unless covered with Dermabond) and pacing wire sites D/C CT when total drainage <100 mL/ last 8 h CT dressing intact × 48 h	DSD with povidone-iodine wipe to wounds and pacing wire sites	Wounds open to air; DSD with povidone-iodine wipe to pacing wires sites Remove staples early AM before D/C

Pain control		Continuous IV MS	IV → PCA MS IV ketorolac	Oxycodone or Tylenol no. 3	Oxycodone or Tylenol no. 3
Nutrition/GI	NPO after MN	NPO NGT to low suction	D/C NG tube Clear liquids	Advance to hi cal, hi prot, NAS diet ADA for diabetics Metamucil/Colace	Progress on diet
Activity	Ambulatory	OOB to chair × 1 after extubation	OOB to chair q8h	Ambulate × 3 in room with assist, then in hallway × 4	Ambulate × 6 in hallway; stair climb 12 stairs × 1
Test and labs	CXR, ECG, PT, PTT, plts, CBC, LBC, LFTs, U/A	On arrival: CXR, ECG, CBC, K+, ABG If bleeding: PT, PTT, plts, repeat HCT Obtain K+ q4h × 3	CXR after CT removal LBC, CBC PT (on warfarin)	K+ if on furosemide PT (on warfarin) PTT (on heparin)	CXR, ECG, CBC, LBC day before discharge Echo for valve pts
Anticoagulation	D/C warfarin 4 days before surgery		Warfarin (valve pts)	Warfarin (valve pts)	Start heparin POD #4 if subtherapeutic INR (mechanical valves)
Discharge planning	Home assessment			D/C planning status discussed by care team with discharge planners	Final review of meds; VNA follow-up, clinic or RMD follow-up
Teaching	Videos, critical pathway, NPO, shower instructions, incentive spirometry				Pt and family attend discharge class or view discharge video Nutrition instructions Medication instructions

---

Box 13.1 • Transfer Orders from the ICU

ALLERGIES:

1. Transfer to _____
2. Procedure: _____
3. Condition: _____
4. Vital signs q4h × 2 days, then qshift
5. ECG telemetry
6. I&O q8h
7. Daily weights
8. Foley catheter to gravity drainage; D/C at _____ ; due to void in 8 h
9. Spo$_2$ q8h and 1 time before and after ambulation
10. Chest tubes to –20 cm H$_2$O suction
11. Diet
    - □ NPO
    - □ Clear liquids/no added salt (NAS)
    - □ Full liquids/NAS
    - □ NAS, low fat, low cholesterol diet
    - □ Fluid restriction ___ mL per 24 hours (IV + PO)
    - □ _____ cal ADA, NAS low cholesterol diet, if diabetic
12. Activity
    - □ Bed rest
    - □ OOB and ambulate with assistance per protocol
13. Elastic antiembolism (TEDs) stockings
14. Dry sterile dressing changes qd until POD #4
15. Temporary pacemaker settings:
    - □ Pacemaker on: Mode: □ Atrial □ VVI □ DVI □ DDD
      Atrial output ____ mA   Ventricular output ____ mA
      Rate ___ /min   AV interval: ____ msecs
    - □ Pacer attached but off
    - □ Detach pacer but keep at bedside
16. Respiratory care
    - □ Oxygen via nasal prongs at 2–6 L/min to keep Spo$_2$ >92%
    - □ Incentive spirometer q1h when awake
17. Wire and wound care per protocol
18. Laboratory studies
    - □ Chest x-ray after chest tube removal
    - □ Daily PT, PTT if on heparin/warfarin
    - □ Daily platelet count if on heparin
    - □ Glucose via fingerstick/glucometer AC and qHS in diabetics
    - □ Chest x-ray, ECG, CBC, electrolytes, BUN, creatinine day prior to discharge

(continued)

Box 13.1 • (Continued)

MEDICATIONS:

1. Antibiotics
   - ☐ Cefazolin 1 g IV q8h for ____ more doses (6 doses total)
   - ☐ Vancomycin 1 g IV q12h for ___ more doses (4 doses total)
2. Cardiac medications
   - ☐ Metoprolol __ mg PO q12h. Hold for HR <60 and SBP <100
   - ☐ Digoxin 0.25 mg PO qd. Hold for HR <60
   - ☐ Antihypertensives:
   - ☐ Diltiazem 100 mg/100 mL NS @ ___ mg/h × 24 h, then 30 mg PO qid (radial artery grafts)
3. Anticoagulants/antiplatelet agents
   - ☐ Enteric-coated aspirin 325 mg PO qd (coronary bypass patients); hold for platelet count <75,000
   - ☐ Enteric-coated aspirin 81 mg (if on warfarin)
   - ☐ Heparin 25,000 U/500 mL D5W at _____ U/h starting on _____ (per protocol)
   - ☐ Coumadin ___ mg PO qd starting on ____ ; daily dose check with HO
4. Pain medications
   - ☐ Morphine sulfate via PCA pump or 10 mg IM q3h prn severe pain
   - ☐ Ketorolac 15–30 mg IV q6h prn pain, D/C after 72 hours
   - ☐ Acetaminophen with oxycodone (Percocet) 1 tab PO q4h prn pain
   - ☐ Acetaminophen with codeine (Tylenol #3) 1–2 tabs PO q4h prn pain
5. GI medications
   - ☐ Pantoprazole (Protonix) 40 mg PO qd
   - ☐ For nausea:
     - ☐ Metoclopramide 10 mg IV/PO q6h prn
     - ☐ Prochlorperazine 10 mg PO/IM q6h prn
   - ☐ Milk of magnesia 30 mL PO qhs prn
   - ☐ Metamucil 12 g in H_2O qd prn constipation
   - ☐ Docusate (Colace) 100 mg PO bid
   - ☐ Dulcolax suppository PR qd prn constipation
6. Diabetic patients
   - ☐ Oral hypoglycemic: _____
   - ☐ ___ units regular Humulin insulin SC ___ qAM ___ qPM
   - ☐ ___ units NPH Humulin insulin SC ___ qAM ___ qPM
   - ☐ Sliding scale: treat fingerstick/glucometer BS according the following scale at 06:00, 11:00, 15:00, and 20:00
     161–200, give ___ units regular Humulin insulin SC
     201–250, give ___ units regular Humulin insulin SC
     251–300, give ___ units regular Humulin insulin SC
     >300, call house officer

(continued)

Box 13.1 • (Continued)

---

7. Other medications
   ☐ Acetaminophen 650 mg PO q3h prn temp > 38.5°C
   ☐ Chloral hydrate 0.5–1.0 g PO qhs prn sleep
   ☐ Furosemide ____ mg IV/PO q __ h
   ☐ Potassium chloride ____ mEq PO bid (while on furosemide)
   ☐ Albuterol 2.5 mg/2.5 mL NS via nebulizer q6h prn
   ☐ Other medications:
8. Saline lock, flush q8h and prn

---

    3. Remove nasogastric tube

    4. Remove Swan-Ganz and arterial lines

    5. Get patient out of bed and into a chair

    6. Initiate β-blocker therapy and aspirin

B. POD #1

    1. Remove chest tubes

    2. Transfer patient to floor; place on telemetry and pulse oximetry × 72 hours

    3. Get patient out of bed and ambulating

    4. Advance diet

    5. Remove Foley catheter

    6. Start warfarin for valve patients

C. POD #2–3

    1. Stop antibiotics (after 36–48 hours)

    2. Advance diet to achieve satisfactory nutrition

    3. Increase activity level

    4. Continue diuresis to preoperative weight

    5. Commence planning for home services or rehabilitation

D. POD #3–4

    1. Obtain predischarge laboratory data (hematocrit [HCT], electrolytes, BUN, creatinine, chest x-ray, electrocardiogram [ECG])

    2. Remove pacing wires

    3. Do discharge teaching

E. POD #4–5

    1. Consider heparin for patients receiving mechanical valves

    2. Remove skin sutures or clips and place steristrips; leave sutures if there is an anticipated problem with wound healing (steroids)

    3. Discharge home

III. Differential Diagnosis of Common Postoperative Symptoms

The development of chest pain, shortness of breath, fever, or just feeling "plain lousy" with a poor appetite and fatigue during the early convalescent period is not unusual, especially in elderly patients. Although the cause of these signs and symptoms may be benign, they should not be taken lightly because they may indicate the presence of potentially serious problems that warrant investigation. Careful questioning and examination of the patient can prioritize diagnoses, direct the evaluation, and lead to prompt and appropriate treatment.

A. Chest pain

1. **Differential diagnosis.** The development of chest pain following cardiac surgery often raises the suspicion of myocardial ischemia, but the differential diagnosis must include several other potential causes. The greatest fear to a patient is that the recurrence of chest pain indicates a failed operation; the surgeon meanwhile may purposely try to provide alternative explanations. Although musculoskeletal pain is the most common cause of chest discomfort, significant problems that must be considered include:

   a. Myocardial ischemia
   b. Arrhythmias
   c. Sternal wound infection
   d. Pericarditis
   e. Pneumothorax
   f. Pneumonia
   g. Pulmonary embolism
   h. Gastroesophageal reflux

2. **Evaluation.** Careful physical examination (breath sounds, pericardial rub, sternal wound), a chest x-ray, and 12-lead ECG will usually provide the appropriate diagnosis and direct additional testing. Differentiation of ST-segment elevation related to ischemia as opposed to pericarditis is important. Consultation with the cardiology service is essential in managing patients with a suspected cardiac origin to their chest pain. Stress imaging or even coronary angiography may be warranted. Other diagnostic modalities include echocardiography, spiral computed tomography (CT) to rule out pulmonary embolism, standard chest CT, and sternal wound aspiration.

B. Shortness of breath

1. **Differential diagnosis.** Shortness of breath is usually caused by splinting from chest wall discomfort and is not uncommon in the anemic patient with underlying lung disease. However, significant shortness of breath, its acute onset, or deterioration in pulmonary status should raise awareness of a significant problem. The source may be of a primary pulmonary nature, but it may also be the consequence of cardiac or renal dysfunction. Diagnoses to be considered include:

   a. Pleuropulmonary problems
   • Atelectasis and hypoxia from mucus plugging or poor inspiratory effort
   • Pneumothorax
   • Pneumonia (aspiration)
   • Bronchospasm
   • An enlarging pleural effusion
   • Pulmonary embolism

   b. Cardiopulmonary problems: low cardiac output states or acute pulmonary edema caused by:
- Acute myocardial ischemia or infarction
- Cardiac tamponade
- Residual or new-onset mitral regurgitation (ischemic, systemic hypertension) or a recurrent ventricular septal defect
- Fluid overload (often with associated oliguric renal failure)
- Severe diastolic dysfunction
- Atrial or ventricular tachyarrhythmias

   c. Compensatory response to metabolic acidosis (low cardiac output state)

   d. Sepsis

  2. Evaluation. Careful lung examination may reveal absent breath sounds or diffuse rales/rhonchi suggesting a parenchymal process or pulmonary edema. Clinical evidence of cardiac tamponade (muffled heart sounds, pulsus paradoxus) should be sought. An arterial blood gas, chest x-ray, and ECG should be obtained. An echocardiogram gives an assessment of ventricular function, detects valve dysfunction or recurrent shunting, and may also identify a large pleural or pericardial effusion or tamponade. Spiral CT should be performed if a pulmonary embolism is suspected.

C. Fever

  1. Differential diagnosis. Fever is very common during the first 48–72 hours and is usually caused by atelectasis from poor inspiratory effort. Thorough evaluation of recurrent fevers is warranted after the first 72 hours. Potential causes of postoperative fever include:

   a. Atelectasis or pneumonia

   b. Urinary tract infection (UTI)

   c. Wound infections: sternum or leg

   d. Drug fever

   e. Sinusitis (usually in the patient with an indwelling endotracheal or nasogastric tube)

   f. An intraabdominal process

   g. Catheter sepsis

   h. Endocarditis (especially on a prosthetic valve)

   i. Decubitus ulcer

   j. Deep venous thrombosis (DVT) and pulmonary embolism

   k. Postpericardiotomy syndrome (PPS)

  2. Evaluation. The lungs, chest, and leg incisions should be examined carefully. A CBC with differential, chest x-ray, urinalysis, and appropriate cultures should be obtained. Indwelling central and arterial lines should be cultured and removed if in place for more than 5 days or if cultures return positive.[1] If the WBC is normal, a drug fever may be present. Occult sternal infections may be investigated with a chest CT scan, but needle aspiration should be performed if suspicion is high. Head CT scans can identify sinusitis. Transesophageal echocardiography (TEE) can be done to identify vegetations present on heart valves (native or prosthetic), consistent with endocarditis.

  3. Treatment. It is best to defer antibiotic therapy until an organism has been identified. However, a broad-spectrum antibiotic may be initiated based on the presumed source and organisms involved. This is especially important in patients who have received prosthetic material (valves, grafts). A narrower-spectrum antibiotic may be substituted subsequently. Occasionally a patient will have a fever and elevated WBC with no evident source, but will respond to a brief course of antibiotics. Additional comments on nosocomial infections and sepsis are found on pages 534–536.

IV. Respiratory Care and Complications

A. Respiratory function is still impaired when the patient is transferred to the postoperative floor, with many patients exhibiting shortness of breath with some splinting from chest wall discomfort. Arterial desaturation is not uncommon, and all patients should have an arterial saturation measured daily by pulse oximetry until the SaO_2 remains above 90%. Most patients have some degree of fluid overload and require diuresis, and steps must be taken to overcome a poor inspiratory effort and atelectasis. Potential complications, such as pneumonia, bronchospasm, pleural effusions, or pneumothorax, can be identified by examination and a chest x-ray. Standard orders should include:

1. Supplemental oxygen via nasal cannula at 2–6 L/min

2. Frequent use of incentive spirometry to encourage deep breathing

3. Progressive mobilization

4. Provision of adequate but not excessive analgesia. Patient-controlled analgesia (usually morphine) is particularly beneficial for one or two days following surgery, and may be supplemented with other pain medications, such as ketorolac (Toradol) 15–30 mg IV q6h for a few days. Most patients obtain adequate analgesia with oral medications 2–3 days after surgery and seem to do better with regular, rather than PRN, pain medications.

5. Chest physical therapy and bronchodilators administered via nebulizer should be used if copious secretions or bronchospasm are present, respectively.

6. Measures to reduce the risk of DVT (antiembolism stockings, pneumatic compression devices, SC heparin) should be considered depending on the patient's mobility and risk.

B. Significant decompensation of respiratory function is uncommon in the absence of preexisting lung disease or a history of heavy smoking. Potential pleuropulmonary contributory factors were noted above in section III.B. However, arterial desaturation may be a sign of cardiac disease (myocardial ischemia or mitral regurgitation), cardiac tamponade, or an early manifestation of renal dysfunction with progressive oliguria.

C. The management of respiratory insufficiency, pneumothorax, pleural effusions, and bronchospasm was discussed in Chapter 10. Less common complications, including diaphragmatic dysfunction from phrenic nerve paresis and pulmonary embolism, are discussed below.

D. **Diaphragmatic dysfunction** from phrenic nerve injury has been noted in 10–20% of patients, despite recognition of risk factors for its development.[2–4]

1. **Etiology**

a. Cold injury to the phrenic nerve from use of iced saline slush in the pericardial well is the primary cause of this problem. Avoidance of iced slush has been shown to reduce the incidence of phrenic nerve paresis. Systemic hypothermia has also been associated with abnormal diaphragmatic function.[4,5]

b. The phrenic nerve may be injured directly during proximal dissection of the internal thoracic artery (ITA) in the upper mediastinum, especially on the right side.[2,6,7] It may also be damaged when making a V incision in the pericardium to allow for better lie of the ITA pedicle. Phrenic nerve devascularization with ligation of the pericardiophrenic artery at the upper extent of the dissection may also be contributory, especially in diabetics.[8,9] Nonetheless, not all studies have identified ITA harvesting as a causative factor.[3]

2. Presentation

a. Most patients with unilateral phrenic nerve paresis have few respiratory symptoms and are extubated uneventfully. Difficulty weaning, shortness of breath, and the requirement for reintubation may be noted in patients with severe chronic obstructive pulmonary disease (COPD).

b. Bilateral phrenic nerve palsy usually produces tachypnea, paradoxical abdominal breathing, and CO_2 retention during attempts to wean from mechanical ventilation.

c. Note: Consideration should always be given to the possibility of an elevated left hemidiaphragm when a left pleural effusion is present. The position of the gastric bubble should identify the position of the diaphragm. A decubitus film may identify the size of the effusion. The location of the diaphragm must be given careful thought before a thoracentesis or tube thoracostomy is performed.

3. Evaluation

a. Chest x-ray will demonstrate an elevated hemidiaphragm at end-expiration during spontaneous ventilation, most commonly on the left side. This will not be evident during mechanical ventilation. An elevated hemidiaphragm may be difficult to appreciate if basilar atelectasis or a pleural effusion is present.

b. Diaphragmatic fluoroscopy ("sniff test") will demonstrate paradoxical upward motion of the diaphragm during spontaneous inspiration if unilateral paralysis is present (Kienböck's sign).

c. Ultrasonography will show a hypokinetic, immobile, or paradoxically moving diaphragm during respiration.

d. Transcutaneous phrenic nerve stimulation in the neck with recording of diaphragmatic potential over the 7th and 8th intercostal spaces can measure phrenic nerve conduction velocities and latency times.[10] This is helpful in assessing whether phrenic nerve dysfunction may be a contributing factor to a patient's respiratory problems.

e. Transdiaphragmatic pressure measurements can be used to make the diagnosis in patients with bilateral phrenic nerve palsies.[8]

4. Treatment is supportive until phrenic nerve function recovers, which may take up to 2 years. One study of patients with COPD found that nearly 25% of patients had persistent pulmonary problems with a decreased quality of life at midterm follow-up.[11] Diaphragmatic plication can provide significant symptomatic and objective improvement in patients with marked dyspnea from unilateral paralysis. This can performed via a thoracotomy or laparoscopically.[12] Ventilatory support is usually necessary for patients with bilateral involvement. Some patients can be treated at home with a cuirass respirator or a rocking bed.

E. **Pulmonary embolism** is very uncommon in patients undergoing open-heart surgery, with an incidence of about 1–2%.[13] The risk is quite low because of systemic heparinization and hemodilution during surgery and the presence of thrombocytopenia and platelet dysfunction in the early postoperative period. There have been concerns that off-pump surgery is associated with a prothrombotic state that may predispose to pulmonary embolism, but this has not been well studied.[14]

1. **Risk factors** for pulmonary embolism are generally those associated with an increased risk of DVT of the lower extremities.

   a. Prolonged bed rest before and after surgery

   b. Recent groin catheterization

   c. Hyperlipidemia, which is associated with a hypercoagulable state and platelet activation

   d. Postoperative congestive heart failure (CHF)

2. **Prevention.** Elastic graded compression stockings (TEDs stockings) should be placed after the initial leg dressing and ace wraps are removed. Few, if any, studies have examined any benefits of these stockings compared with placebo in cardiac surgery patients. However, it has been reported that there is no additional benefit of adding sequential compression devices (Venodyne) to these stockings, with an incidence of DVT of nearly 20% in both groups.[13,15] Another study showed that the incidence of pulmonary embolism was reduced by 60% (from 4% to 1.5%) by adding these devices to use of subcutaneous heparin.[16] Thus, it is not unreasonable to use compression devices and SC heparin in the high-risk patient who is poorly mobilized after surgery.

3. **Manifestations.** Pleuritic chest pain and shortness of breath are usually present. The acute onset of these symptoms distinguishes them from typical postoperative respiratory symptoms. The new onset of atrial fibrillation (AF), sinus tachycardia, or fever of unknown origin may be clues to the diagnosis.

4. **Assessment.** Arterial blood gases, chest x-ray, ECG, and spiral CT scanning should be obtained.[17] The presence of a low arterial oxygen saturation is nonspecific but may be compared with values obtained early in the postoperative course. A positive venous noninvasive study of the lower extremities in association with respiratory symptoms and hypoxia is suggestive evidence of a pulmonary embolism and should prompt further evaluation.

5. **Treatment** entails bed rest and anticoagulation with IV heparin for one week, followed by warfarin for 6 months. Thrombolytic therapy is contraindicated because of the recent sternotomy incision. A vena cava filter is recommended because of the high risk of recurrence despite anticoagulation and should be performed if anticoagulation is contraindicated. Interventional methods, including suction embolectomy and fragmentation therapy, or even emergency surgery may be necessary in the rare patient suffering a massive pulmonary embolism with refractory cardiogenic shock.[18]

V. Cardiac Care and Complications

A. Upon transfer to the postoperative floor, the patient should be attached to a telemetry system to continuously monitor the heart rate and rhythm for several days. Vital signs are obtained every shift if the patient is stable but more frequently if the patient's heart rate, rhythm, or blood pressure is abnormal or marginal.

B. The evaluation and management of complications noted most frequently in the ICU are presented in Chapter 11. These include low cardiac output states, perioperative infarction, cardiac arrest, coronary spasm, hypertension, and arrhythmias. This section will discuss several cardiac problems commonly noted during subsequent convalescence.

C. Arrhythmias and conduction problems

1. **Atrial arrhythmias** are the most common complication of open-heart surgery, occurring with a peak incidence on the second or third postoperative day. Although some patients become symptomatic with light-headedness, fatigue, or palpitations, most have no symptoms and are noted to be in AF or atrial flutter on the ECG monitor. Treatment entails rate control, attempted conversion to sinus rhythm, and anticoagulation if AF persists or recurs. Management protocols are discussed in detail on pages 427–435 and in Box 11.4 on page 431.

2. **Ventricular arrhythmias** are always of concern because they may be attributable to myocardial ischemia or infarction and may herald cardiac arrest. Low-grade ectopy or nonsustained ventricular tachycardia with normal ventricular function does not require aggressive therapy. In contrast, ventricular tachycardia with impaired left ventricular (LV) function requires further evaluation and probable implantable cardioverter-defibrillator placement. These issues are discussed on pages 439–441.

3. Temporary pacemaker wires are routinely removed on POD #3 but may be required for persistent complete heart block, sinus bradycardia, lengthy sinus pauses, or a slow ventricular response to AF. Patients undergoing valve surgery are more prone to conduction disturbances and more frequently require implantation of a permanent pacemaker.[19] Patients with sick sinus or tachybrady syndrome may have a rapid ventricular response to AF intermixed with a slow sinus mechanism that limits use of β-blockers. A permanent pacemaker system should be considered if these problems persist beyond 3 days. However, studies have shown that pacemaker dependence often resolves within a few months in patients in whom pacemakers are placed unless the indication was complete heart block.[19,20]

D. Hypertension. Blood pressure tends to return to its preoperative level several days after surgery once myocardial function has returned to baseline and the patient has been mobilized. A decrease in systolic blood pressure from preoperative levels may be noted in patients experiencing a perioperative infarction. In contrast, patients with aortic stenosis may develop significant systolic hypertension following aortic valve replacement. Oral medications must be substituted for the potent intravenous drugs used in the ICU. If blood pressure was well-controlled before surgery, the same medications should usually be restarted. Other considerations when selecting an antihypertensive medication include:

1. Poor ventricular function: use one of the angiotensin-converting enzyme (ACE) inhibitors (see Appendix 8).

2. Sinus tachycardia with good LV function, evidence of residual myocardial ischemia: use a β-blocker.

3. Coronary spasm or use of a radial artery graft: use a nitrate or calcium channel blocker (diltiazem, verapamil, nicardipine). These are excellent first-line medications to use in patients without significant ventricular dysfunction.

E. Hypotension may develop after transfer to the floor and should be evaluated using the differential diagnosis of shock or a low cardiac output state (see Chapter 11). Specific considerations several days after surgery include:

1. Hypovolemia: usually from aggressive diuresis, especially when profound anemia is present.
2. β-blockers used prophylactically to prevent AF.
3. Arrhythmias, especially AF/atrial flutter, and the medications used to manage them that can also lower the blood pressure (β-blockers, calcium channel blockers).
4. Aggressive use of antihypertensive medications: often from restarting the patient on their preoperative dose of antihypertensive medication, but occasionally in a patient who receives medications for hypertension associated with pain and sympathetic overactivity that then resolve.
5. Myocardial ischemia/infarction.
6. **Always** consider the possibility of delayed cardiac tamponade, especially, but not exclusively, in patients on anticoagulation (see section G below).

F. Recurrent myocardial ischemia. The development of recurrent angina or new ischemic ECG changes postoperatively always requires careful evaluation and treatment. Manifestations may include a low-output state, CHF and pulmonary edema, myocardial infarction, ventricular arrhythmias, or cardiac arrest.

1. **Etiology**
   a. Acute graft occlusion
   b. Hypoperfusion from anastomotic narrowing or inadequate flow (replacing a moderately diseased vein graft with a small ITA at reoperation)
   c. Unbypassed, diseased coronary arteries (incomplete revascularization)
   d. Coronary vasospasm

2. **Evaluation**
   a. Empiric use of a nitrate and/or calcium channel blocker may be helpful for ischemia or spasm and can be diagnostic.
   b. Urgent coronary arteriography should be considered when there are significant ECG changes. It may identify a technical problem with a graft or confirm the diagnosis of spasm.
   c. A stress imaging study can be performed to identify the presence of myocardial ischemia and differentiate between ischemic and nonischemic causes of chest pain.

3. **Treatment**
   a. Intensification of a medical regimen with nitrates and β-blockers is indicated.
   b. If a technical problem with a graft is identified, percutaneous coronary intervention is often the best course. If this is not feasible, but a major area of myocardium is in jeopardy, and the patient has not suffered a significant MI, reoperation can be considered. Not uncommonly, however, the coronary vessels supplying the ischemic zone are small and diffusely diseased, leaving small areas of the heart potentially ischemic. These vessels may not have been considered bypassable, or the graft flow was limited by small vessel size and runoff.
   c. The long-term results of coronary bypass surgery are influenced by the development of atherosclerotic disease in bypass conduits, unbypassed native arteries, or native arteries beyond the bypass sites. Factors that can improve these

results include use of the ITA, abstinence from smoking, control of hypercholesterolemia, and indefinite use of aspirin (use for 1 year will improve vein graft patency).[21] The late development of ischemia has also been attributed on rare occasion to a coronary steal syndrome, either from a coronary-subclavian steal or an ITA–pulmonary artery fistula.[22]

G. **Delayed tamponade.** Pericardial effusions are noted in nearly 50% of patients following surgery but usually resolve completely. A small percentage of patients have effusions that gradually increase in size and produce a low cardiac output state and tamponade.[23,24] This may be noted within the first week of surgery or several weeks later. Suspicion of this problem must remain high because symptoms often develop insidiously and are frequently difficult to differentiate from those noted in patients recovering slowly from surgery. **This is one of the most serious yet most potentially correctable of all postoperative problems.**

1. **Etiology**

   a. Use of antiplatelet agents (aspirin, clopidogrel) or anticoagulant drugs (heparin, warfarin) can cause slow intrapericardial bleeding from any source (soft tissues, raw pericardium, sutures lines).[25] This may occur even if the patient had minimal bleeding in the immediate postoperative period.

   b. Acute hemorrhage occurring after the chest tubes have been removed may occur from a right ventricular or atrial tear during removal of pacing wires. Rarely, a patient may develop a delayed rupture of an infarct zone or LV rupture from a mitral valve prosthesis.

   c. Late serous or serosanguineous effusions may develop from postpericardiotomy syndrome. Use of a nonsteroidal antiinflammatory drug (NSAID), such as diclofenac, may reduce the inflammatory response and lower the incidence of pericardial effusions.[26]

2. **Presentation.** Acute hemorrhage will present with refractory hypotension and often the clinical picture of acute cardiac tamponade. The classic picture of delayed tamponade is a low-output state manifested by malaise, shortness of breath, chest discomfort, anorexia, nausea, or a low-grade fever. These symptoms are frequently ascribed to medications or simply a slow recovery from surgery. Jugular venous distention, a pericardial rub, progressive orthostatic hypotension, tachycardia (often masked by use of β-blockers), and a pulsus paradoxus are often noted. Occasionally, the first sign is a decrease in urine output with rise in BUN and creatinine caused by progressive renal dysfunction from the low-output state.

3. **Evaluation.** A chest x-ray may reveal enlargement of the cardiac silhouette; however, frequently the chest x-ray is normal, depending on the site and rapidity of blood accumulation. Two-dimensional echocardiography can identify the pericardial effusion, confirm tamponade physiology (which may produce compression of individual cardiac chambers),[27] and assess the status of ventricular function (Figure 13.1). A surface echo often has limitations in obtaining certain acoustic windows that may be related to the patient's body habitus. Thus, it will occasionally not identify an effusion. If clinical suspicion remains high and the transthoracic image is suboptimal, TEE should be strongly considered.

4. **Treatment**

   a. Mediastinal exploration is indicated for active bleeding.

   b. Pericardiocentesis is the least invasive means of draining a large effusion that has produced cardiac tamponade. This is usually performed in the cardiac

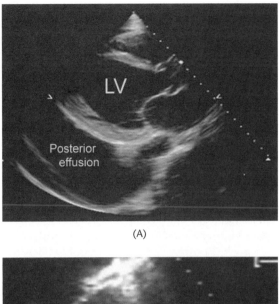

(A)

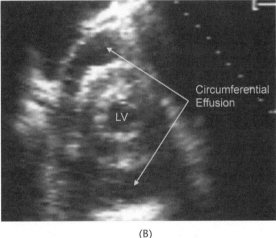

(B)

Figure 13.1 • Two-dimensional echocardiograms of significant postoperative pericardial effusions. (A) Transthoracic study in the parasternal long-axis view demonstrating a significant posterior effusion. (B) A transesophageal study in the transgastric short-axis view. Note the circumferential pericardial effusion that prevents adequate ventricular filling. Evidence of diastolic collapse will confirm the hemodynamic significance of the effusion. *(Image courtesy of Dr. Jeffrey T. Kuvin, Division of Cardiology, Tufts-New England Medical Center.)*

catheterization laboratory under ECG or two-dimensional echocardiographic guidance.[28]

   c. Subxiphoid exploration should be considered when the echocardiogram suggests that the fluid collection cannot be successfully approached percutaneously (usually a posterior collection) or when it is loculated. If this approach is ineffective in draining the effusion, the entire sternal incision may need to be opened.

    d. A pericardial "window" or limited pericardiectomy through a left thoracotomy approach should be considered for loculated posterior effusions or recurrent effusions several weeks after surgery.

    e. Antiinflammatory medications or steroids can be used for large effusions attributable to PPS that have not produced hemodynamic compromise.

H. Postpericardiotomy syndrome has been reported in 15–20% of patients following open-heart surgery and is considered to represent an autoimmune inflammatory response.[29-31] It may occur within the first week of surgery or several weeks to months later. PPS is more common in younger patients and those with a history of pericarditis or steroid usage. It must be aggressively managed because it may contribute to cardiac tamponade, early vein graft closure, or constrictive pericarditis. Use of prophylactic NSAIDs or colchicine (1.5 g/day) after surgery may reduce the incidence of PPS.[26,32]

  1. Presentation. Fever, malaise, precordial chest pain, arthralgias, and a pericardial rub are the diagnostic criteria. A pleural or pericardial effusion is usually present.

  2. Evaluation. Lymphocytosis, eosinophilia, and an elevated ESR are noted, but a fever workup is negative. Effusions are usually demonstrable by chest x-ray and echocardiography. In one study, the presence of cardiac muscle antibody correlated with PPS, but results of another study suggested that anti-heart antibodies may reflect an immune response to pericardial or myocardial injury, rather than being causally related.[31,32]

  3. Treatment

    a. Diuretics and aspirin should be used as the initial treatment. If there is minimal symptomatic relief, a 1-week course of an NSAID, such as ibuprofen 400 mg qid, is 90% effective. Aspirin should be stopped if this is used to minimize gastric irritation. Prednisone can be used if symptoms persist. It should be noted that regular use of NSAIDs (especially ibuprofen) may inhibit the cardioprotective antiplatelet effect of aspirin.[33]

    b. Pericardiocentesis may be necessary to drain a large symptomatic pericardial effusion.

    c. Pericardiectomy is recommended for recurrent large effusions.

I. Constrictive pericarditis is a late complication of cardiac surgery that is rare despite the development of dense adhesions that form in the mediastinum following surgery. It has been noted in patients with undrained early postoperative hemopericardium, use of warfarin, early PPS, and previous mediastinal radiation.[34]

  1. Presentation. The patient will note the insidious onset of dyspnea on exertion, chest pain, and fatigue. Peripheral edema and jugular venous distention are common, but pulsus paradoxus is uncommon.

  2. Evaluation

    a. Chest x-ray is frequently normal in the absence of a pericardial effusion.

    b. Two-dimensional echocardiography will demonstrate pericardial thickening and occasionally a small pericardial effusion.

    c. A CT scan usually documents a thick pericardium and the presence of pericardial fluid.

    d. Right heart catheterization provides the most definitive information. It documents the equilibration of diastolic pressures and demonstrates a diastolic dip-plateau pattern ("square root" sign) in the right ventricular pressure tracing (see Figure 1.20). On occasion, significant fluid overload produces hemodynamics consistent with constriction, when in fact there is no pathoanatomic evidence of epicarditis or thick pericardium other than the standard postoperative scarring.

3. **Treatment.** Pericardiectomy is indicated for clinically significant constriction. It is best performed through a sternotomy incision, which allows for adequate decortication of the right atrium and ventricle and much of the left ventricle. It also allows for the institution of cardiopulmonary bypass (CPB) in the event of a difficult or bloody operation. Relief of epicardial constriction is difficult and may result in surgical damage to bypass grafts or significant bleeding. A "waffle" or "turtle shell" procedure is performed with criss-crossing incisions made in the epicardial scar to relieve the constriction.

VI. Renal, Metabolic, and Fluid Management and Complications

A. Routine Care

1. Most patients are still substantially above their preoperative weight when transferred to the postoperative floor. Comparison of the patient's preoperative weight with daily weights obtained postoperatively is a guide to the use of diuretics to eliminate excess fluid. Achievement of dry body weight may require more aggressive diuresis if CHF was present before surgery. In the chronically ill patient, preoperative weight may be achieved despite fluid overload due to poor nutrition.

2. Dietary restriction (sodium and water) need not be overly strict in most cases. With the availability of potent diuretics to achieve negative fluid balance and the common problem of a poor appetite after surgery, it is more important to provide palatable food without restriction to improve the patient's caloric intake.

3. If a patient required diuretics before surgery (especially valve patients and those with poor myocardial function), it is advisable to continue them upon discharge from the hospital even if preoperative weight has been attained.

B. Transient renal failure (see also Chapter 12).

Patients with some element of preoperative renal dysfunction, severe hypertension, postoperative low cardiac output syndromes, or those requiring substantial doses of vasopressors may show evidence of gradual, progressive renal dysfunction. Diuretics are useful in reducing the immediate postoperative fluid overload and preventing the development of oliguric renal failure. However, postoperative management can be very difficult on the postoperative floor when methods of monitoring intravascular volume are limited. While diuretics are given to create a negative fluid balance, adequate intravascular volume must be maintained to prevent prerenal azotemia without producing pulmonary edema.

1. A common scenario is gradual elevation in the BUN and creatinine with low serum sodium, reflective of persistent total body water and salt overload. Medications must be adjusted to allow the hypertensive patient's blood pressure to rise to higher levels than normal. ACE inhibitors should be withheld, and diuretics must be used gently, if at all, to maintain adequate intravascular volume. If the patient was aggressively diuresed and has a poor appetite, additional hydration may be necessary. In most patients, the renal dysfunction is transient as long as the cardiac output remains satisfactory.

2. If fluid retention persists, contributing to respiratory compromise, and the BUN continues to rise, further evaluation and treatment are indicated. On occasion, medications (such as Bactrim) or an obstructive uropathy may be the cause of an unexplained rise in creatinine. **However, a rising BUN and creatinine of unclear cause, especially when associated with new-onset oliguria, should always raise the suspicion of delayed tamponade.** An echocardiogram should be obtained to assess myocardial function and rule out tamponade. The patient may require return to the ICU for intravenous inotropic support, ultrafiltration, or dialysis.

C. **Hyperkalemia** usually occurs in association with renal dysfunction. Its manifestations and treatment are discussed on pages 491–492. Particular attention should be directed to stopping any exogenous potassium intake or ACE inhibitors and reevaluating renal function.

D. **Hyperglycemia** in diabetics is a common postoperative problem. The blood glucose level may be elevated due to residual elevation of the counterregulatory hormones (glucagon, cortisol) after surgery. Stringent control of blood sugar during the early postoperative period not only reduces the incidence of wound infection but also reduces operative mortality (Appendix 6).[35–37] Once the patient is transferred to the floor, frequent fingersticks should be obtained (usually before meals and at bedtime) to assess the adequacy of blood sugar control.

1. Insulin resistance is commonly noted during the early postoperative period. Patients with type 1 diabetes mellitus should have their insulin doses gradually increased back to preoperative levels depending on oral intake and blood glucose levels. It is preferable to use a lower dose of intermediate-acting insulin initially and supplement it with regular insulin as necessary.

2. Oral hypoglycemics can be restarted once the patient has an adequate oral intake, usually starting at half the preoperative dose, and increasing the dose depending on oral intake and blood sugars.

E. Other electrolyte and endocrine complications are fairly unusual once the patient has been transferred to the postoperative floor. Chapter 12 discusses the evaluation and management of some of these problems.

VII. Hematologic Complications and Anticoagulation Regimens

A. Anemia

1. Despite the obligatory hemodilution associated with CPB, use of effective blood conservation strategies has reduced the requirements for perioperative blood transfusions. Furthermore, off-pump surgery is associated with a reduced transfusion requirement. Generally, the HCT should be maintained around 20% during CPB and then at least 22–24% postoperatively. However, transfusion to a higher HCT should be considered for elderly patients, those who feel significantly weak and fatigued, and those with ECG changes, hypotension, or significant tachycardia.

2. Although the HCT may rise gradually with postoperative diuresis, it frequently will not increase because of the shortened red cell life span caused by extracorporeal circulation and the loss of 30% of transfused red cells within 24 hours of transfusion.

3. Any patient with an HCT below 30% should be placed on iron therapy (ferrous sulfate or gluconate 300 mg tid for 1 month) at the time of discharge. Exogenous iron may not be necessary, however, if the patient has received multiple transfusions because of the storage of iron from hemolyzed cells.

4. Consideration may also be given to use of recombinant erythropoietin (Epogen) to stimulate red cell production (50–100 U/kg SC tiw).

B. **Thrombocytopenia** is caused by platelet destruction and hemodilution during extracorporeal circulation, but platelet counts gradually return to normal within several days. Impaired hemostasis noted in the early postoperative period is caused more commonly by platelet dysfunction induced by CPB, although it is attenuated somewhat by the use of the antifibrinolytic drugs.

1. **Etiology**
   a. Platelet activation or dilution during CPB
   b. Excessive bleeding without platelet replacement therapy
   c. Use of the intraaortic balloon pump (IABP)
   d. Medications that may reduce the platelet count, such as heparin or inamrinone

2. **Treatment.** Platelet transfusions are indicated:
   a. When the platelet count is less than 20,000–30,000/μL
   b. For ongoing bleeding when the platelet count is < 100,000/μL. Platelet administration may be considered when the platelet count is higher if platelet dysfunction is suspected.
   c. For a planned surgical procedure (such as a percutaneous IABP removal) when the platelet count is < 60,000/μL.

3. **Note:** Platelet counts must be monitored on a daily basis in any patient receiving heparin. A falling platelet count or heparin resistance may be an indication for in vitro aggregation testing to identify heparin-induced thrombocytopenia.

C. **Heparin-induced thrombocytopenia (HIT)** is a very serious complication of heparin therapy that may result in profound thrombocytopenia and widespread arterial and venous thrombosis. It carries a 20–30% mortality.[38]

1. **Classification**
   a. Type 1 HIT is a common entity that is not immune-mediated. Mild thrombocytopenia usually develops within 48 hours of initiating heparin. For a patient with a normal platelet count, the count rarely falls below 100,000 and heparin can usually be continued. However, in the postcardiac surgical patient with a reduced platelet count, the platelet count will generally fall to lower levels. The timing of onset of the thrombocytopenia and its pattern should be taken into consideration when deciding if this problem is benign or more consistent with type 2 HIT. Generally, if the postoperative platelet count continues to fall, especially to levels less than 70,000 (in a nonbleeding patient), type 2 HIT should be considered and all heparin should be stopped.
   b. Type 2 HIT is an immune-mediated phenomenon that is caused by the formation of IgG antibodies that bind to the heparin–platelet factor 4 (PF4) complex, producing platelet activation. This results in release of procoagulant microparticles that lead to thrombin generation. It also causes release of PF4, promoting more platelet activation. Antibody binding to glycosaminoglycans

on the surface of endothelial cells leads to endothelial cell damage and tissue factor expression. This procoagulant milieu promotes arterial and venous thrombosis in about 30% of patients, including stroke, myocardial infarction, mesenteric thrombosis, and DVT. Antibodies form more commonly after administration of beef lung heparin, and are 8–10 times more likely to develop using unfractionated heparin than low-molecular-weight heparin.

2. **Diagnostic considerations.** Type 2 HIT is diagnosed by the combination of thrombocytopenia and the presence of heparin antibodies. These are most reliably identified by a serologic test (enzyme-linked immunosorbent assay [ELISA]) that detects the presence of heparin-PF4 antibodies (although it may be positive in patients without clinical HIT), and by the serotonin release assay (SRA). Both of these tests have greater than 90% sensitivity, although the SRA is more specific. The heparin-induced platelet aggregation (HIPA) test is less sensitive.

3. **Clinical patterns of type 2 HIT**

   a. The platelet count declines by 50% or more starting about 5–10 days after the initiation of heparin therapy, but may occur within 10 hours if the patient had received heparin within the past 100 days.[39] This is due to the presence of antibodies in the serum, rather than an amnestic response. In approximately 30% of patients, HIT will not occur until there is a heparin rechallenge when it may develop very abruptly.

   b. Thrombocytopenia usually occurs when the patient is still receiving heparin, since the antibody must bind to the heparin-PF4 complex. However, there are reports of delayed cases of HIT occurring several days after the heparin infusion has been stopped.

   c. Approximately 50% of patients will develop HIT antibodies after cardiac surgery, although type 2 HIT occurs in only about 2%. Nonetheless, due to the high morbidity and mortality of HIT, progressively falling platelet counts should always raise the suspicion of type 2 HIT, prompting appropriate diagnostic testing and therapy, as delineated below.

   d. Because HIT antibodies are so common and are usually not associated with thrombocytopenia (serologic HIT), their mere presence is of unclear significance. It is not known whether the development of HIT antibodies subsequent to catheterization has any clinical relevance at the time of cardiac surgery. Theoretically, these patients would be more susceptible to HIT with a heparin rechallenge at surgery, but this has not been confirmed. One study reported that 22% of patients developed antibodies after catheterization, which were primarily low-titer IgM antibodies; in fact, 61% developed antibodies after surgery, yet HIT did not develop in any patient.[40] In another study, antibodies were detected by ELISA in 19% of patients prior to cardiac surgery (in 35% who received heparin during that hospital stay) and in 51% after surgery, yet there was no difference in platelet count between those with positive antibodies and those without.[41] Because of the high incidence of positive tests for low-titer antibodies in the absence of thrombocytopenia, there is no indication for preoperative HIT testing after prior heparin exposure unless thrombocytopenia is also present.

   e. Heparin antibodies usually clear within 120 days and usually do not reform upon heparin rechallenge. Thus, if a patient with HIT does not require urgent surgery, it is best to wait until the antibody is no longer detectable.

4. **Management** of type 2 HIT requires removal of all heparin from the patient (including heparin flushes and heparin-coated pulmonary artery catheters) and administration of alternative anticoagulation. These measures should minimize the risk of thrombotic events and also provide anticoagulant protection for the process for which heparin was initially indicated.

   a. Warfarin should not be started immediately, because tissue necrosis from microvascular thrombosis may occur due to depletion of the vitamin K-dependent natural anticoagulant protein C.[42] This has been noted in patients who rapidly develop a supratherapeutic international normalized ratio (INR) due to reduced protein C levels. Warfarin can be safely started after the platelet count reaches 100,000 μg/dL.

   b. Platelets should not be administered because they may promote thrombosis.

   c. **Lepirudin** is a direct thrombin inhibitor that is the first choice of therapy, although it must be used cautiously in patients with renal dysfunction. It is given as a 0.4 mg/kg load, followed by a continuous infusion of 0.15 mg/kg/h. It is monitored by the PTT, aiming for 1.5–2.5 times baseline.[43]

   d. **Argatroban** is a synthetic direct thrombin inhibitor that is preferred in patients with renal dysfunction because it undergoes hepatic metabolism. It is given starting at a dose of 2 μg/kg/min once heparin effect has been eliminated (usually 4 hours for unfractionated heparin and 12 hours after the last dose of low-molecular-weight heparin). It is monitored by the PTT, aiming for 1.5–3 times baseline. Conversion of argatroban to warfarin can be somewhat problematic because both affect the INR. Generally, warfarin should be given in doses of 2.5–5 mg for 5 days of overlapping treatment. Once the platelet count exceeds 100,000 and the INR is > 4, the argatroban should be stopped. The INR should be rechecked in 4–6 hours. If the INR drops below 2.0, the argatroban should be restarted.[43]

   e. **Bivalirudin** is a direct thrombin inhibitor that produces reversible binding to thrombin and has a short half-life of only 25 minutes. Although FDA-approved only for coronary interventions in patients with unstable angina as of late-2004, bivalirudin has been used as the preferential anticoagulant for on- and off-pump coronary surgery in many centers for patients with type II HIT. Advantages include 80% enzymatic metabolism (although some modification is indicated in patients with renal dysfunction), nonimmunogenicity, and no effect on the INR. Thus, bivalirudin may be useful in the treatment of HIT although dosing levels need to be defined. One recommended dose is approximately 2 mg/kg/h to achieve a PTT of 1.5–2.0 times baseline.[44] Dosing for CPB and off-pump surgery is discussed on page 156.

   f. **Danaparoid** is a heparinoid that has a low degree of reactivity with heparin antibodies. It is given in a bolus dose of 2250 U anti-Xa, followed by 400 U/h × 4 hours, then 300 U/h × 4 hours, then a maintenance infusion of 150–200 U/h. It is monitored by anti-Xa levels, with the goal of achieving a level of 0.5–0.8 U/mL.[45] It is no longer available in the United States.

   g. Recommendations for anticoagulation for CPB are presented on pages 154–156.[46]

D. **Coronary bypass surgery.** Antiplatelet therapy is recommended for 1 year to increase saphenous vein graft patency. Aspirin is given by nasogastric tube

Table 13.2 • Recommended Anticoagulation Regimens for Prosthetic Heart Valves

	Warfarin	Antiplatelet Drugs
AVR-mechanical	Target INR of 2.5 (2.0–3.0) indefinitely (increase to 3.0 if high risk*)	Aspirin 75–100 mg qd if high risk*
AVR-tissue	Target INR of 2.5 (2.0–3.0) for 3 months or none if aspirin used	Aspirin 75–100 mg qd
MVR-mechanical	Target INR of 3.0 (2.5–3.5) indefinitely	Aspirin 75–100 mg qd if high risk*
MVR-tissue or MV repair	Target INR of 2.5 (2.0–3.0) for 3 months; continue for 1 year if history of systemic embolism; indefinitely if atrial fibrillation and left atrial thrombus at time of surgery	Aspirin 75–100 mg qd after 3 mos
AVR-MVR-mechanical	Target INR of 3.0 (2.5–3.5) indefinitely	Aspirin 75–100 mg qd
AVR-MVR-tissue	Target INR of 2.5 (2.0–3.0) for 3 months	Aspirin 75–100 mg qd after 3 mos
Atrial fibrillation with any of above	Continue warfarin indefinitely	Aspirin 75–100 mg qd

AVR = aortic valve replacement; MVR = mitral valve replacement
*High risk = atrial fibrillation, myocardial infarction, enlarged left atrium, endocardial damage, low ejection fraction, or history of systemic embolism despite therapeutic anticoagulation

starting 6 hours postoperatively and then taken orally in a dose of 75–325 mg qd. Aspirin 75–162 mg qd should be given indefinitely to all patients, including those receiving only arterial conduits, because of its beneficial effect on the secondary prevention of coronary events.[21] Warfarin should be considered to improve graft patency when an extensive coronary endarterectomy has been performed, although there is little evidence that this is actually beneficial. Aspirin should be given in low doses along with warfarin because of its antiplatelet effects.

E. **Prosthetic heart valves** (Table 13.2). Heart valves are more susceptible to thromboembolic complications during the first 3 months after implantation, during which time warfarin is generally recommended. It is then continued indefinitely for mechanical valves and converted to aspirin for tissue valves. Warfarin is continued indefinitely if AF is present.[47]

1. **Tissue valves**

   a. **Aortic valves:** The American College of Chest Physicians (ACCP) 2004 guidelines suggest that warfarin should be used for 3 months (target INR 2.5, range 2.0–3.0) to reduce the incidence of thromboembolism and should then be converted to aspirin 75–100 mg qd. However, numerous studies have shown that aspirin is just as effective as warfarin, and most surgeons follow the alternative recommendation of aspirin 80–100 mg/day following surgery.[47–49]

b. **Mitral valves:** Warfarin should be given for 3 months to achieve a target INR of 2.5 (range 2.0–3.0) and should then be converted to aspirin 75–100 mg qd if the patient is in sinus rhythm. Warfarin should be continued indefinitely in high-risk patients with AF, an enlarged left atrium (>50 mm in diameter), or a history of thromboembolism. The decision to initiate heparin if the INR is not therapeutic by the 4th or 5th postoperative day must be individualized.

c. **Mitral rings:** Warfarin is commonly used after mitral valve repairs with ring annuloplasties, but aspirin may suffice.

2. **Mechanical valves**

a. Aortic valves: Patients receiving current-generation tilting-disc (Medtronic-Hall) or bileaflet valves should receive warfarin indefinitely to achieve an INR of 2.5 (range 2.0–3.0).

b. Mitral valves: Patients receiving current-generation mechanical valves should receive warfarin indefinitely to achieve a target INR is 3.0 (range 2.5–3.5).

c. A target INR of 3.0 with the addition of aspirin 75–100 mg is recommended for any patient with a mechanical valve and additional risk factors. These include AF, MI, an enlarged left atrium, endocardial damage, a low EF, or if systemic embolism occurs despite the recommended regimen.

d. Patients with double valves or Bjork-Shiley or Starr-Edwards valves in either position should receive warfarin to achieve an INR of 3.0 (range 2.5–3.5) in combination with aspirin 75–100 mg/day.

e. The threshold for initiating postoperative heparin when the INR is not therapeutic is lower for mechanical valves, especially when AF is present. Most surgeons start heparin on POD #4, but they should remain cognizant of the potential risks of aggressive postoperative anticoagulation, especially delayed tamponade. Patients can usually be discharged when the INR approaches the therapeutic range (1.8 for AVR and 2.0 for MVR). To expedite discharge of patients at higher risk of thromboembolism, low-molecular-weight heparin 1 mg/kg SC can also be given for a few days.

3. **Dosing and overanticoagulation.**[50] The dosing of warfarin should be carefully individualized to avoid rapid overanticoagulation. An initial dose of 5 mg is given to most patients. However, 2.5 mg should be given to small elderly women, patients with hepatic dysfunction, patients with chronic illness, and those receiving antibiotics or amiodarone. Potential dangers of overanticoagulation include cardiac tamponade from intrapericardial bleeding, and gastrointestinal, intracranial, or retroperitoneal hemorrhage.

a. If the patient is bleeding with an elevated INR, fresh frozen plasma is indicated. If the INR is significantly elevated, vitamin K 5–10 mg IV should be given slowly and repeated q12h.

b. If the patient has no evidence of bleeding, general recommendations for treatment of the overanticoagulated patient are as follows:

      i. INR >10: hold warfarin, give vitamin K 3–5 mg PO (INR should fall within 24–48 hours) and consider fresh frozen plasma.

      ii. INR of 5–9: hold warfarin for 1–2 days and restart when INR is < 4; alternatively, one dose of warfarin may be omitted and 1–2.5 mg of vitamin K may be given orally.

      iii. INR of 4–5: omit one dose or reduce the dose of warfarin for a few days.

  c. Vitamin K given in small oral doses can reduce the INR to a therapeutic level within a few days and is usually the best approach when withholding of warfarin does not reduce the INR. Large doses of IV vitamin K will produce more rapid reversal of the INR, but may lead to warfarin resistance and should be avoided. Nonetheless, if the INR becomes subtherapeutic (which is usually safer than a markedly elevated INR), heparin can be given until the INR rises to the therapeutic range.

VIII. Wound Care and Infectious Complications

A. General Comments

  1. Prophylactic antibiotics should be given for 36–48 hours starting just before surgery. First- or second-generation cephalosporins (cefazolin or cefamandole) are commonly used because of their effectiveness against gram-positive cocci. Vancomycin is substituted if there is a penicillin allergy. Even though vancomycin is probably the most effective antibiotic in preventing sternal wound infections, its use should be confined to patients receiving prosthetic material (valves, grafts) because of its added cost and the risk of promoting the growth of resistant organisms (i.e., vancomycin-resistant enterococci).[51,52]

  2. Antibiotics can be stopped if chest tubes, the endotracheal tube, Foley catheter, or even an IABP remain in place. Prolonging antibiotic therapy for several days while an IABP is in place does not reduce the risk of infection.[53]

  3. Wounds closed with subcuticular sutures and covered with 2-octylcyanoacrylate adhesive (Dermabond) at the conclusion of surgery do not require dressing coverage. Otherwise, the wound should be cleansed and covered with a dressing every day for the first three postoperative days. Subsequent coverage is not necessary unless drainage is noted. All drainage should be cultured and sterile occlusive dressings applied.

B. Nosocomial infections develop in 10–20% of patients undergoing cardiac surgery. Such infections may produce bacteremia, but most commonly affect the surgical sites as well as the respiratory and urinary tracts. They commonly increase the length of stay and, because of their association with multisystem organ failure, they increase operative mortality by 4–5 fold.[54–57]

  1. Risk factors include:

    a. Comorbidities: older age, females, diabetes, obesity

    b. Nasal carriage of *Staphylococcus aureus*

    c. Operative factors:
- Long complex operations
- Urgent surgery
- Reoperations

    d. Postoperative factors:
- Prolonged mechanical ventilation (predisposes to pneumonia, which occurs in about 5% of patients)[55]

- Prolonged duration of indwelling Foley catheter (UTI)
- Empiric use of broad-spectrum antibiotics (pneumonia)
- Low cardiac output syndrome
- Postoperative stroke
- Hyperglycemia
- Requirement for blood transfusions (pneumonia) [58–60]

2. **Preventive measures** that may reduce the incidence of nosocomial infections include:[61,62]

   a. Hand washing by the health care team.

   b. Chlorhexidine gluconate 0.12% oral rinse: one study showed that perioperative use of this solution reduced the incidence of nosocomial respiratory infections by 70% and also reduced mortality rate in cardiac surgical patients.[63]

   c. Early removal of invasive catheters, especially central lines, upon suspicion of infection.[1]

   d. Avoidance of empiric use of broad-spectrum antibiotics and prolonged use when no longer necessary. One study showed that early postoperative pneumonia was usually caused by organisms that colonized the respiratory tract prior to surgery. However, prolonged use of antibiotics was ineffective in reducing the incidence of pneumonia.[64]

   e. Aggressive ventilatory weaning protocols to reduce the duration of mechanical ventilation and other steps to avoid ventilator-associated pneumonia (see pages 320–321). Selective decontamination of the gut has arguably been effective in reducing this problem.

   f. Raising the threshold for blood transfusions (transfuse if HCT < 26%)

3. The **treatment** of a nosocomial infection requires appropriate antibiotic selection for the organism involved and also a recognition of the appropriate time course of treatment. Prolonged treatment is often unnecessary and may lead to the development of resistant strains or fungal infections, and not infrequently to hepatic or renal dysfunction. When a gram-positive bacteremia occurs in a patient with a prosthetic heart valve, a 6-week course of treatment for presumed endocarditis may be indicated. In complex situations, infectious disease consultation is essential.

C. **Sepsis**

1. **Clinical features.** Sepsis resulting in hemodynamic compromise and multisystem organ failure is a very uncommon, yet highly lethal, complication of cardiac surgery. It is usually noted in critically ill patients who remain in the ICU with multiple invasive monitoring lines, have respiratory complications, and preexisting or imminent renal dysfunction. It may complicate the delayed diagnosis of a sternal wound infection.

2. **Management.** Aggressive ICU-directed, goal-oriented therapy may be able to reduce the high mortality associated with sepsis.[65] Important features of this approach include:

   a. Optimization of hemodynamics with early aggressive fluid resuscitation, inotropic support, and selective use of vasoconstrictors (initially α-agents, and then vasopressin if necessary). This should be assessed by adequate hemodynamic monitoring (PA catheter and central or mixed venous oxygen saturations aiming for an oxygen saturation > 70%).

   b. Initiation of broad-spectrum antibiotic coverage after panculturing with prompt modification to cover the specific organism isolated.

   c. Low tidal volume ventilation if ARDS develops; minimizing sedation to promote early extubation.

   d. Early aggressive use of renal replacement therapies (CVVH).

   e. Tight control of blood sugars (in the 100–120 mg/dL range).

   f. Adequate nutrition, preferably by the enteral route.

   g. DVT prophylaxis (pneumatic compression devices, possibly SC heparin).

   h. Stress ulcer prophylaxis (sucralfate, proton pump inhibitors).

   i. Low-dose stress steroids may be considered in patients with documented inadequate response to an ACTH challenge.

   j. Recombinant activated protein C (drotrecogin alfa [Zigris]) has reduced mortality in patients with severe sepsis associated with organ system dysfunction by modulating the inflammatory and fibrinolytic responses to sepsis. It should only be considered in severely ill patients after infectious disease consultation.

D. Sternal wound infections complicate about 1% of cardiac surgical procedures performed via a median sternotomy and are associated with significant mortality (>20%). Coagulase-negative *Staphylococcus* and *S. aureus* are the most common pathogens encountered despite the use of prophylactic antibiotics specifically directed at these organisms. Sternal infections are a major source of physical, emotional, and economic stress, although advances in plastic surgical coverage techniques have improved results dramatically.

   1. Risk factors. Several risk models have been devised to predict the risk of developing mediastinitis (Society of Thoracic Surgeons [STS], Northern New England Cardiovascular Study Group; see page 116).[66, 67] Among the risk factors identified in these and other studies are the following:[66–74]

   a. Comorbidities: obesity, diabetes, COPD, renal dysfunction, peripheral vascular disease (PVD), older age, impaired nutritional status (low serum albumin)

   b. Surgical considerations
   • Emergency surgery
   • Reoperations
   • Bilateral ITA use in diabetics (controversial)[75–78]
   • Prolonged duration of bypass or surgery

   c. Postoperative complications
   • Excessive mediastinal bleeding, reexploration for bleeding, multiple transfusions
   • Prolonged ventilatory support (usually in patients with COPD who are actively colonized)
   • Low cardiac output states
   • Prolonged ventilatory support
   • Poorly controlled blood sugars in the ICU[36]

   2. Prevention. Several measures can be taken to reduce the risk of infection.[79–83]

   a. Preoperative measures
      i. Identify and manage preexisting infections (pneumonia, urinary tract, skin)
      ii. Hibiclens wash several times the night before surgery.[80]

    iii. Hair clipping just prior to surgery.[81]

    iv. Administer an adequate dose of antibiotics prior to skin incision. Commonly used antibiotics include cefazolin 1 g (2 g may be preferable in larger patients) or vancomycin 15 mg/kg.[82,83]

    v. Intranasal mupirocin to reduce nasal carriage of staphylococcal organisms.[84]

  b. Intraoperative measures

    i. Ensure a midline sternotomy and provide secure sternal closure.

    ii. Be selective in use of bilateral ITAs in diabetic patients. Skeletoning the ITA may be helpful, but avoidance of bilateral use in patients with other risk factors, such as severe obesity and COPD, is prudent.[78]

    iii. Meticulous surgical technique with respect for tissues and adequate hemostasis to minimize mediastinal bleeding.

    iv. Avoid bone wax.[79]

    v. Use subcuticular sutures rather than skin staples and seal wound with a topical adhesive (Dermabond).

  c. Postoperative measures

    i. Maintain blood sugars < 180–200 mg/dL during surgery and the early postoperative course.[35]

    ii. Raise the threshold for administering blood products during and after surgery.

3. Presentation of a mediastinal wound infection can be overt or occult, and often depends on the infectious agent.[85,86] For example, *S. aureus* infections tend to be virulent and present within the first 10 days of surgery. In contrast, coagulase-negative staphylococcal infections tend to present late in an indolent fashion with an insidious onset.[87,88]

  a. Minor/superficial infections usually present with local tenderness, erythema, serous drainage, or a localized area of wound breakdown with purulent drainage. The sternum is usually stable.

  b. Major/deep incisional infections (deep subcutaneous, osteomyelitis, mediastinitis) may have any of the above but usually present with significant purulent drainage, often with an unstable sternum. The patient commonly has fever, chills, lethargy, and chest wall pain. Leukocytosis is invariably present. Sternal instability may be noted when mediastinitis is present, but in the absence of other clinical evidence may represent a sterile dehiscence.

  c. Inexplicable chest wall pain or tenderness, fever, gram-positive bacteremia, or leukocytosis should raise suspicion of a major sternal wound infection. Sternal wound infections account for more than 50% of postoperative gram-positive bacteremias. Occult infections are particularly common in diabetic patients who often mount a very poor inflammatory response and may present several weeks after surgery with extensive purulent mediastinitis but few systemic signs.

  d. A chronic draining sinus tract is a common delayed presentation of chronic osteomyelitis.

4. Evaluation

  a. Assessment of the degree of sternal instability is important in deciding how to proceed with the workup. If the sternum is unstable, operative exploration is indicated. If it is stable, further diagnostic testing is warranted in order to identify a deep infection.[86]

b. Culture of purulent drainage may identify the organisms and direct appropriate antibiotic therapy.

c. Wound aspiration ("sternal puncture") may diagnose an infection when purulent drainage is not present.[89]

d. Chest CT may be beneficial if the sternum is stable. It may help identify a deep infection if there is loss of the integrity of retrosternal soft-tissue fat planes or an undrained retrosternal abscess with air.[89] Although there are reports that CT is quite sensitive and specific for diagnosing wound infections,[90] one must be cautious in its interpretation because hematoma formation and fibrin tracts commonly seen in the postoperative chest may be interpreted as infection.[91,92] Clinical correlation and usually a wound aspirate are necessary before exploring a patient.

e. White cell scanning, using indium or technetium labeling, or ^{99m}Tc-labeled monoclonal granulocyte antibody scintigraphy are among the radionuclide tests that have been helpful in identifying the presence and/or location of infections.[93-95]

f. Occasionally, the infection "declares itself" by spontaneous drainage when diagnostic techniques are inconclusive but the clinical suspicion remains high.

5. **Management of minor infections**

a. Minor infections usually respond to intravenous antibiotics, opening of the wound, and local wound care. Persistence of a sinus tract or presence of multiple areas of recurrent breakdown suggests a more deep-seated infection, often involving the sternal sutures. This usually requires surgical exploration rather than dressing changes *ad infinitum*. It may respond to simple wire removal and curetting of the involved bone with a 6-week course of antibiotics.

b. If the sternal wires or the bone are exposed at an early stage, a deeper infection must be ruled out and mediastinal exploration is indicated. This may introduce infection into the mediastinum from the superficial tissues but may allow for primary reclosure over drains depending on the extent of infection.

6. **Management of major infections.** Major infections require mediastinal exploration for debridement of infected tissues, removal of foreign bodies, drainage, and elimination of dead space. Antibiotic therapy is generally recommended for 6 weeks.

a. The closed method entails primary sternal reclosure with wires and placement of substernal drainage catheters for postoperative antibiotic irrigation (usually 0.5% povidone-iodine). This may be successful if performed within 2–3 weeks of surgery if there is a sterile dehiscence, minimal purulence, a healthy-appearing sternum, and mediastinal tissues that are pliable enough to eliminate dead space.[86,96] However, this technique is associated with a significant failure rate (as high as 90%) if not used in patients who satisfy these criteria.[96-98] Primary closure is probably best avoided in patients with ITA grafting, which produces some degree of devascularization of the sternum.

i. If there is a substantial amount of dead space behind the sternum, but minimal infection and a healthy bone, omental transposition beneath the bone (especially over prosthetic material or exposed grafts) can be considered.[99]

ii. If the sternum requires any debridement, rewiring may not provide for adequate bony union of the remaining chest wall and may predispose the patient to chronic osteomyelitis. In cases of sterile dehiscence with an unreconstructable bone, immediate muscle flap coverage is recommended.

iii. Small redon catheters placed behind the sternum and attached to strong negative suction have been used successfully in managing infections even beyond the 3-week period. However, methicillin-resistant *S. aureus* (MRSA) infections should be managed with aggressive debridement and muscle flaps.[100,101]

b. The open method is used for severe mediastinitis, chronic osteomyelitis, recalcitrant infections, or extensive subcutaneous involvement that extends down to the sternum and contaminates the sternal wires. Sternal debridement with placement of muscle flaps (pectoralis major or rectus abdominis) or omentum after several days of dressing changes to clean up the wound is very successful in managing these infections.[99,102] One disadvantage of leaving the wound open for dressing changes is the risk of right ventricular rupture, especially if sternal debridement has been inadequate and the right ventricle has not been mobilized from the back of the sternum.[103] If the sternum is left open, it is imperative that the patient remain intubated and sedated to prevent chest wall motion that could contribute to this problem. Early flap coverage is then recommended.[104] It is important to augment the patient's nutritional status to ensure a satisfactory result from flap coverage.

c. Vacuum-assisted closure (VAC) has been used in recent years to expedite the healing process, either as a bridge to muscle flap coverage or to achieve delayed secondary healing.[105–107] This system consists of a polyurethane ether foam with an evacuation tube that drains into an effluent canister connected to negative suction. The wound is covered with an adhesive drape to create a closed system. The VAC system produces arteriolar dilatation and improves microcirculatory flow, which encourages granulation tissue formation and accelerates wound healing. At the same time, it reduces wound edema and reduces bacterial colonization. It has also been suggested that by stabilizing the remaining sternal halves, VAC systems may help to prevent right ventricular rupture.[107]

d. An interesting concept that has been around for years is the use of granulated sugar to control recurrent staphylococcal mediastinitis. A contemporary study reported earlier healing and a reduced mortality in very high-risk patients with use of granulated sugar dressings compared with muscle flap surgery.[108]

e. The **prognosis** after development of a wound infection is poor, with a mortality around 20%, usually from multisystem organ failure. Early aggressive intervention may decrease the length of stay in the ICU and the requirement for mechanical ventilation, and may improve short- and long-term results.[67]

E. **Leg wound** complications are noted in 10–20% of patients having saphenous vein harvesting via the open technique.[109] Patients at higher risk include those with severe PVD and female patients with diabetes and obesity. Most complications are related to poor surgical technique with creation of flaps, failure to eliminate dead space, use of excessive suture material, or hematoma formation. Endoscopic vein harvesting has become more commonplace over the past few years and has reduced the incidence of complications to less than 5%. Nonetheless, the potential still exists for hematoma formation within the endoscopic tract and for infection to occur in the small incision near the knee. With the technique of multiple skip incisions, infections can also occur in a similar fashion to open incisions, especially because this technique may be accompanied by significant tissue trauma from retraction of the tissues for visualization.

1. **Presentation**
   a. Cellulitis
   b. Wound breakdown with purulent drainage
   c. Skin necrosis from thin flaps or a large subcutaneous hematoma; formation of eschar
   d. Warm, indurated wound overlying an endoscopic tract, often with accompanying hematoma or skin ecchymosis

2. **Prevention**
   a. Use careful surgical technique: avoid tissue trauma, minimize flap formation, obtain meticulous hemostasis, avoid excessive suture material and tissue strangulation, especially in the small knee incision for endoscopic harvesting.
   b. Use antibiotic wound irrigation prior to closure.
   c. Use a sponge to decompress an endoscopic tunnel and evacuate blood that may accumulate during heparinization.
   d. Place a suction drain to eliminate dead space and evacuate venous bleeding within endoscopic tunnels or underneath flaps.
   e. Ace wrap the leg at the conclusion of surgery.

3. **Treatment** requires antibiotics, drainage, and potentially debridement. If a large hematoma or necrotic skin edges are present, early return to the operating room should be considered to evacuate the hematoma and close the leg primarily. Infections in endoscopic tunnels may require opening of the skin, but often can be managed by opening the skin incision and placing a Blake drain for antibiotic irrigation.[110]

F. There is little information on the prevalence of forearm infections after radial artery harvesting. Hemostasis during harvesting and prior to a layered closure that leaves the fascia open should prevent hematoma formation. Cellulitis is the most common manifestation and responds to antibiotics. Rarely, a purulent infection may occur that requires further drainage.

G. **Antibiotic prophylaxis** for dental or surgical procedures is mandatory for all patients with prosthetic valves and grafts. The American Heart Association (AHA) recommendations published in 1997 for prevention of bacterial endocarditis are shown in Table 13.3.[111]

Table 13.3 • Antibiotic Prophylaxis to Prevent Endocarditis in Adult Patients

Dental/oral/respiratory/esophageal procedures

Standard regimen	Amoxicillin 2.0 g PO 1h before procedure
Unable to take PO medications	Ampicillin 2.0 g IV/IM within 30 min of starting procedure
Penicillin allergic	Clindamycin 600 mg, cephalexin 2 g, or clarithromycin 500 mg PO 1h before surgery
PCN allergic and unable to take PO	Clindamycin 600 mg or cefazolin 1 g IV within 30 min of starting procedure

GI/GU procedures

High risk	Ampicillin 2 g IM/IV plus gentamicin 1.5 mg/kg IV/IM within 30 min of starting procedure; then ampicillin 1 g IM/IV or amoxicillin 1 g PO 6h later
High risk but ampicillin/amoxicillin allergic	Vancomycin 1 g IV over 1–2 h plus gentamicin 1.5 mg/kg IV within 30 min of starting procedure
Moderate-risk	Amoxicillin 2 g PO 1 h before procedure or ampicillin 2 g IM/IV within 30 min of starting procedure
Mod-risk but ampicillin/amoxicillin allergic	Vancomycin 1 g IV over 1–2 h within 30 min of starting procedure

1. High risk: prosthetic heart valves (including homografts), history of endocarditis, prosthetic intravascular grafts
2. Moderate risk: valvular heart disease, hypertrophic cardiomyopathy, mitral valve prolapse with valvular regurgitation and/or thickened leaflets
3. Not required: pacemakers, implantable defibrillators, transesophageal echocardiography
Dajani AS, Taubert KA, Wilson W, et al. Prevention of bacterial endocarditis. Recommendations by the American Heart Association. JAMA 1997;277:1794–1908; Circulation 1997;96:358–66.

IX. Neurologic Complications

Neurologic complications are dreaded sequelae of cardiac surgical procedures. In one often quoted study, type 1 (focal) neurologic events were noted to complicate approximately 3% of coronary bypass operations performed on-pump with an additional 3% suffering type 2 (neurocognitive) deficits.[112] Although the degree of cerebral embolization may be less during off-pump surgery, reduction in both types of deficits has not been unequivocally demonstrated in numerous comparative studies.[113-120] The risk is greater in patients undergoing valve surgery and may be expected to increase as older patients with more advanced atherosclerosis undergo more complex surgical procedures.

A. Central nervous system deficits

1. **Risk factors** have been identified in multiple studies[120-126] and a risk model has been devised by the STS and the Northern New England Cardiovascular Disease Study Group (Table 3.9).[66,126]

   a. Preoperative factors
   - Prior stroke. One study reported that 44% of patients with a history of stroke developed a focal neurologic deficit after surgery. Of these, 8.5% were new, 27% represented reappearance of an old deficit, and 8.5% were worsening of the old deficit.[127]
   - Cerebrovascular disease, including the presence of carotid bruits and/or the documentation of carotid stenosis
   - Increasing age (risk of up to 10% in patients > age 75)
   - Comorbidities, including diabetes, smoking, hypertension, PVD, and renal dysfunction
   - Poor LV function
   - Reoperative surgery
   - Urgent/emergent surgery

   b. Intraoperative/postoperative findings/events
   - Ascending aortic and arch atherosclerosis and calcification[128,129]
   - LV mural thrombus
   - Opening of a cardiac chamber during surgery
   - Long duration of CPB
   - Perioperative hypotension or cardiac arrest
   - Postoperative AF

2. **Mechanisms**

   a. Particulate embolism from the aorta is the most common cause of stroke. Transcranial Doppler studies have demonstrated an association between cerebral complications and the number of microemboli detected during surgery.[130] Sources may be as follows:
   - Atherosclerotic aorta (during cannulation or clamping, and especially unclamping)
   - Solid or gaseous microembolism from the extracorporeal circuit
   - Air embolism
   - Left atrial or LV thrombus
   - Platelet-fibrin debris from carotid ulceration

   b. Cerebral hypoperfusion may be the result of systemic hypotension or impaired cerebral flow from intra- or extracranial carotid disease.
   - Systemic hypotension is common during CPB, although cerebral autoregulation can maintain cerebral blood flow down to a mean pressure of 40 mm Hg. However, this compensatory mechanism may not be operative in diabetic, hypertensive patients, and blood pressure usually must be raised to provide adequate cerebral flow independent of the systemic flow rate.[131,132] Interestingly, there is the suggestion that cerebral microembolization may impair cerebral autoregulation, thus confounding the precise mechanism of neurologic dysfunction.[133]

- The blood pressure may be compromised during off-pump surgery during manipulation of the heart, and is usually reduced pharmacologically during construction of proximal anastomoses, when a side clamp in placed on the ascending aorta.
- The potential exists for cerebral hypoperfusion during an episode of postoperative hypotension. This may result in a watershed infarct, especially in patients with uncorrected carotid disease.

3. **Presentation** depends primarily on the site and extent of the cerebral insult. The vast majority of deficits occur during surgery and will be evident within the first 24–48 hours. A few patients appear to awaken without a deficit and then develop one later during the hospital stay, usually as a result of postoperative hemodynamic instability or AF. Because intraoperative embolization is the most common cause of stroke, multiple infarcts are a common finding on brain CT or magnetic resonance imaging (MRI). Common presentations include:

   a. Focal deficits that most commonly produce hemiparesis/hemiplegia, aphasia, or dysarthria. Visual deficits may occur as the result of retinal embolization, occipital lobe infarction, or anterior ischemic optic neuropathy.[134] The latter is more common in patients with long pump runs with extreme hemodilution.[135] One study found that posterior strokes involving the posterior cerebral artery and cerebellum were the most common type of stroke, although embolization to the middle cerebral artery was also encountered in about 50% of patients, since multiple emboli were commonly noted.[136]

   b. Transient ischemic attacks or reversible neurologic deficits

   c. Severe confusion or delirium

   d. Coma

4. **Prevention** of neurologic complications requires the identification and appropriate management of potential precipitating factors.

   a. Preoperative **evaluation for extracranial carotid disease** should be considered in any patient with current or remote neurologic symptoms or the presence of a carotid bruit. Noninvasive studies followed by magnetic resonance angiography, if indicated, may identify significant carotid disease. The approach to symptomatic carotid disease invariably involves a preliminary carotid endarterectomy (CEA) or simultaneous CABG-CEA procedure. The management of high-grade asymptomatic carotid disease at the time of cardiac surgery is controversial, and general recommendations are presented on page 103.[137]

   b. Intraoperative epiaortic echocardiography can be used to identify aortic atherosclerosis that might alter cannulation and clamping techniques to prevent manipulation of a diseased ascending aorta.[138] Use of off-pump surgery can provide a "no touch" technique using the ITAs as inflow vessels to avoid aortic manipulation and may reduce the incidence of stroke.[116] In patients with severe aortic calcification requiring CPB, circulatory arrest may be indicated to avoid aortic cross-clamping.

   c. Other measures that can reduce the risk of embolic stroke are meticulous valve debridement and irrigation and complete removal of air from the left heart after intracardiac procedures, which can be very difficult during minimally invasive surgery. Use of a single aortic cross-clamp technique to avoid application of a partial-exclusion clamp is also beneficial. Particulate emboli can be captured by use of the Embol-X intraaortic filter (Edwards Lifesciences) at the time of unclamping.[139]

   d. Use of a higher mean arterial pressure during CPB may be beneficial to patients with hypertension or known intracranial vascular disease.

   e. Transcranial Doppler can be used to identify cerebral embolization during surgery, but has not achieved widespread usage. Cerebral oximetry is beneficial in assessing the adequacy of cerebral oxygenation during periods of low flow, but is unable to detect embolization.[140]

5. **Evaluation** requires an assessment of the degree of functional impairment by careful neurologic examination and identification of the anatomic extent of cerebral infarction by CT or MRI. The latter can be logistically difficult to obtain in critically ill patients on a ventilator and multiple infusion pumps. Particular attention should be paid to evidence of hemorrhage, which might alter therapy. Evaluation should also be undertaken to search for a possible source of the stroke that might require additional attention (echocardiogram, carotid noninvasive studies). An initial CT scan may not show evidence of a fresh nonhemorrhagic infarction that may be present on follow-up studies. Studies comparing diffusion-weighted MRI with CT have shown that MRI is more sensitive to ischemic changes and commonly shows multiple embolic infarcts.[141]

6. **Treatment**

   a. Heparin is generally recommended for an embolic stroke once a CT or MRI scan has demonstrated no evidence of intracranial hemorrhage. However, the possibility of subsequent hemorrhage into an infarct zone should be weighed when deciding if heparinization is indicated. Heparin may be beneficial to improve cerebral microcirculatory flow or prevent propagation of an intracardiac thrombus, but is of unclear benefit in preventing further aortic atheroembolism from dislodged plaque.

   b. Standard measures to reduce intracranial pressure, including diuresis, mannitol, and steroids, may be indicated depending on the extent of cerebral infarction.

   c. CEA may be considered in patients with severe carotid stenosis and postoperative transient neurologic deficits or small strokes.

   d. Early institution of physical therapy is important.

7. **Prognosis** is favorable for patients with small or temporary deficits. The mortality rate in the STS database for patients suffering permanent strokes is around 25%. The outlook for comatose patients is extremely poor with over 50% dying or remaining in a vegetative state. A long-term follow-up study from Johns Hopkins University showed that the survival of stroke patients was less than 50% at 5 years, with moderate-severe disability in nearly 70% of patients. A worse survival was predictably noted in patients who took longer to awaken from surgery, developed renal dysfunction, or had longer ICU stays.[142] With such a dismal prognosis, any steps that can possibly be taken to reduce the incidence of stroke must be entertained.

B. **Encephalopathy and delirium** represent an acute change in a patient's mental status that is associated with a global impairment in cognitive function. These problems are fairly common after open-heart surgery, with an incidence of approximately 8–10%. The mechanism is frequently not clear. It may result from microembolization associated with use of CPB and the associated aortic manipulations, an etiology common to patients suffering both stroke and neurocognitive dysfunction.[143] It may also be related to mild cerebral hypoperfusion. It is usually transient and has a fluctuating course, but it can be very disturbing to the patient and his or her family.

1. **Risk factors**[144,145]
   a. Older age
   b. Recent alcoholism
   c. Preoperative organic brain disease (mild degrees of cognitive dysfunction or dementia)
   d. Severe cardiac disease and high-risk status at the time of surgery (cardiogenic shock, urgent status, severe LV dysfunction)
   e. Multiple associated medical illnesses (especially diabetes, cerebrovascular and peripheral vascular disease) and poor nutritional status (including amino acid disturbances)
   f. Complex and prolonged surgical procedures on CPB, especially valve procedures

2. **Common contributing causes**
   a. Medication toxicity (including benzodiazepines and analgesics)
   b. Metabolic disturbances
   c. Alcohol withdrawal
   d. Low cardiac output syndromes
   e. Periods of marginal cerebral blood flow during bypass that are just above the threshold for cerebral infarction
   f. Hypoxia
   g. Sepsis
   h. Recent/new stroke

3. **Manifestations**
   a. Disorientation, confusion, attention deficit, memory loss, disturbed sleep-wake cycle
   b. Lethargy or agitation
   c. Paranoia and hallucinations

4. **Evaluation**
   a. Review of current medications and drug levels.
   b. Identify possible history of recent alcoholism or substance abuse.
   c. Neurologic examination, often with brain CT or MRI.
   d. ABGs, electrolytes, BUN, creatinine, CBC, magnesium, calcium, cultures.

5. **Management**
   a. Use soft restraints and side rails.
   b. Correct metabolic abnormalities.
   c. Stop inappropriate medications.
   d. The occurrence of delirium may be related to the type of sedative used in the ICU. One study showed that the incidence of delirium was significantly reduced after open-heart surgery using propofol rather than midazolam.[146]
   e. Select the appropriate medication to control agitation and the delirious state.
      i. Haloperidol 2.5–5.0 mg PO/IM/IV q6h is the most commonly prescribed medication for delirium. One should always be aware of the risk of torsades de pointes in patients receiving IV haloperidol.[147]

ii. Although benzodiazepines, such as lorazepam (Ativan), have been recommended to control delirium, they are often poorly tolerated in elderly patients, exacerbating confusion and producing either agitation or stupor. However, olanzapine (Zyprexa), a thienobenzodiazepine, has been used successfully in delirious critically ill patients and has been associated with fewer side effects than haloperidol.[148] It is given in a dosage of 5–10 mg PO qd.

iii. Ondansetron (Zofran), which is a 5-HT_3 receptor antagonist that counteracts activation of the serotoninergic system, has been used successfully in the management of postcardiotomy delirium without major side effects. It is given in a dose of 4–8 mg IV or PO.[149] A similar medication, dolasetron (Anzemet) 12.5–25 mg IV, can also be used. These medications are usually prescribed for control of postoperative nausea.

f. Manage suspected alcohol withdrawal:[150]

i. Benzodiazepines (lorazepam, diazepam, or chlordiazepoxide) are indicated in this situation for several days and should then be gradually tapered. Patients often require a few additional days of ventilatory support during a period of sedation to avoid agitation and self-destructive behavior. Reintubation may be necessary when symptoms develop after early extubation has been accomplished.

ii. Thiamine 50–100 mg IM bid and folate 1 mg qd.

iii. Propofol can be used for refractory delirium tremens.[151]

g. Psychotherapy: reassurance and support

C. Seizures may accompany cerebral insults from hypoxia, or air and particulate emboli. However, they can also result from medication overdoses (e.g., lidocaine). Contributing factors should be addressed and the patient evaluated by a neurologist. A CT scan, EEG, or anticonvulsant therapy with phenytoin should be considered based on advice from the neurologist.

D. Neurocognitive dysfunction is extremely common after surgery, being noted in at least 20% of patients. The extent and variability of dysfunction depend on the nature of the neuropsychological tests performed. To some patients, the degree of dysfunction is immediately obvious; in others, it can only be detected by comparison of pre- and postoperative studies.

1. Risk factors include older age, diabetes, aortic atherosclerosis, cerebrovascular disease, and PVD.[152–154] Cognitive decline has been noted more commonly in patients with preexisting dementia or cognitive dysfunction, chronic disabling neurologic disease, or a history of anxiety/depression; those living alone; and patients suffering any postoperative complication. It is also inversely related to educational level. It has been suggested that patients with less cognitive reserve are inclined to note more disabling cognitive dysfunction.[155] The correlation between the duration of CPB and cognitive dysfunction has not been consistently reported.[152,155] Furthermore, although off-pump surgery might be associated with less immediate decline in function,[156] follow-up studies have shown no difference at 12 months.[157]

2. Mechanisms. Cerebral microembolization is believed to be the most likely source of cognitive decline, although cerebral hypoperfusion may also be a factor.[143] It has been proposed that early deficits may arise from either cause; intermediate cognitive symptoms, particularly memory problems, are usually the result of multiple emboli, and late cognitive effects, usually pertaining to visuospatial abilities, may be related to hypoperfusion or the combination of hypoperfusion and microemboli.[153]

3. **Prevention.** Steps mentioned above that might reduce cerebral embolization might reduce the risk of neurocognitive dysfunction. Maintenance of a higher perfusion pressure might also be helpful.[158] Other recommended strategies include alpha stat pH regulation (see page 192) and better control of intraoperative glucose levels.[152]

4. **Evaluation.** MRI often shows multiple infarctions, although such findings are also common in patients who are asymptomatic.[159] Brain SPECT studies have shown worse cerebral perfusion at baseline and during surgery in patients with cognitive decline after surgery.[160]

5. **Natural history.** The extent and duration of cognitive decline has been variable in numerous studies. One study reported that there was no impact of CABG on cognitive function at one year, either with on-pump or off-pump techniques.[161] Yet another important study of CABG patients found that 53% of patients had cognitive decline at hospital discharge, which decreased to 24% at 6 months, but then increased to 42% at 5 years.[162] Another study found an improvement in baseline tests up to one year but a subsequent decline up to 5 years.[163] These results suggest that, after early improvement, late decline is most likely due to the presence of poorly controlled risk factors for cerebrovascular disease, including hypertension and diabetes.

E. **Psychiatric problems** are fairly common in patients undergoing open-heart surgery. Anxiety and depression occur frequently in patients with known psychiatric disorders but are also noted in patients who have lost family members due to coronary disease. The occurrence of these symptoms after surgery is associated with a less favorable outcome.[164,165] Exacerbation of preexisting disorders, such as affective (bipolar) and personality disorders is also not unusual. A psychiatrist with an interest in postoperative problems is invaluable in helping patients resolve distressing psychiatric symptoms and in providing advice on the appropriate use of psychotropic medications.

F. **Critical illness polyneuropathy** is a syndrome of unknown cause that complicates the course of sepsis and multisystem organ failure, especially respiratory and renal failure. Because of its association with such critical illness, it is associated with a mortality rate greater than 50%. It usually presents as failure to wean from the ventilator due to weakness of the diaphragm and chest wall muscles. Axonal degeneration of motor and sensory fibers is the underlying pathologic process and is manifested by proximal muscle atrophy and paresis, decreased deep tendon reflexes, and, in some cases, laryngeal and pharyngeal weakness, with resultant swallowing difficulties. It may produce motor and sensory deficits and can be diagnosed by electromyography and nerve conduction studies. The syndrome is self-limited and has no specific treatment other than supportive care (ventilatory support and physical therapy). It must be distinguished from other causes of postoperative muscle weakness, such as medications, nutritional deficiency, disuse atrophy, and other neuromuscular disorders.[166]

G. **Brachial plexus injuries**

1. **Etiology and prevention.** Stretch of the inferior cords of the brachial plexus by lateral sternal retraction or asymmetric elevation during ITA harvesting is the most likely cause of brachial plexus injury. The incidence may be minimized by cautious and limited asymmetric retraction for ITA takedown; ensuring a

midline sternotomy; using caudad placement of the retractor, opening it only as much as necessary for adequate exposure; and maintaining a neutral head position.[8] The incidence may also be lessened by positioning the patient in the "hands up" position.[167] Despite taking all of these precautions, a small number of patients will still develop a brachial plexus stretch injury, most probably related to their individual chest wall architecture. First rib fractures are often noted by bone scan, although they are frequently missed by routine chest x-rays.

2. **Presentation.** Sensory changes, including numbness, paresthesias, and occasionally sharp pains, are common in the ulnar nerve distribution (T8–T1), which affects the fourth and fifth fingers. Weakness of the interosseous muscles is commonly noted. In more extreme forms, the median or radial nerve distribution may be involved. Radial nerve deficits are more likely to be caused by direct arm compression by retraction bars used for the ITA takedown.

3. **Evaluation.** Electromyography, motor and sensory conduction velocities, and somatosensory evoked potentials can be used to assess changes in nerve function, but their significance is not clear. They may be useful in assessing the extent of the deficit and the return of function.

4. **Treatment.** Symptoms resolve in more than 95% of patients within a few months. Rarely, recovery may take up to a year, and some patients may have persistent, bothersome symptoms. Physical therapy is essential to maintain motor tone. If the patient has significant pain, amitriptyline (Elavil) 10–25 mg qhs or gabapentin (Neurontin) starting at 300 mg qd may be helpful.

H. **Paraplegia** is a very rare complication of open-heart surgery. It may occur as the result of an aortic dissection or as a complication of an IABP, presumably on the basis of atherosclerotic plaque or cholesterol embolism to the spinal cord. When it occurs after an isolated CABG, it is invariably associated with a period of hypotension in a patient with preexisting hypertension and severe vascular disease that compromises spinal cord perfusion.[168,169]

I. **Saphenous neuropathy** is caused by damage to small branches of the saphenous nerve that lie adjacent to the saphenous vein in the lower leg. It causes sensory changes along the medial side of the calf and foot to the level of the great toe and is fairly common after open vein harvesting. Vein dissection from the ankle up is more likely to cause this problem than dissection from top down. It is proposed that the former is more likely to cause avulsion of the pretibial or infrapatellar branches of the nerve.[8] Neuropathy is also more common when an open incision is closed in two layers, producing neuropraxis from too tight a closure. These symptoms are much less frequent when the vein is harvested endoscopically.

J. **Recurrent laryngeal nerve** neuropathy may contribute to vocal cord dysfunction and hoarseness.[8,170] Damage may occur during ITA mobilization at the apex of the chest, from intubation or line placement. Aside from hoarseness, it may be suspected if the patient has ventilatory problems and an ineffective cough, and it may lead to aspiration pneumonia. Diagnosis can be made by laryngoscopy. Symptomatic improvement may take up to one year, but if problems persist, Teflon cord injection or arytenoidectomy may be necessary.

K. **Phrenic nerve palsy** (see pages 519–520)

L. **Pituitary apoplexy** (see page 500)

X. Gastrointestinal Complications

Gastrointestinal complications develop in 1–2% of patients undergoing open-heart surgery. Because they frequently occur in critically ill patients, they are associated with a significant mortality rate (25–75%).[171–177] The common pathophysiologic mechanism is a low cardiac output state, which produces sympathetic vasoconstriction, hypoperfusion, and hypoxia of the splanchnic bed.[178] Inadequate tissue perfusion contributes to mucosal ischemia and the so-called acute GI focal necrosis syndrome. Changes that are seen may include stress ulceration, mucosal atrophy, bacterial overgrowth from stress ulcer prophylaxis, and loss of barrier function with increased permeability. These changes may potentially lead to bacterial translocation, sepsis, and multiorgan failure.[179] Use of preventive measures and prompt, aggressive surgical intervention are necessary to decrease the mortality associated with these complications. The incidence of GI complications and their associated mortality has been reported to be comparable with on- and off-pump surgery. However, GI bleeding is more common after off-pump surgery, whereas visceral ischemia is more common after on-pump surgery. Nonetheless, splanchnic vasoconstriction may be a common mechanism.[173,180]

A. **Routine care and common complaints.** Most patients have a nasogastric tube inserted in the operating room before heparinization or after its reversal by protamine. This maintains gastric decompression during positive-pressure ventilation, removes gastric contents to minimize the risk of aspiration, decreases gastric acidity, and allows for the administration of oral medications and antacids in the ICU. The tube is usually removed after extubation if bowel sounds are present. An oral diet is then advanced from clear liquids to a regular diet.

1. Anorexia, nausea, and a distaste for food are fairly common complaints after surgery and may be attributable to the side effects of medications (narcotics, morphine, type IA antiarrhythmics), and possibly to mineral deficiency (especially zinc). Bothersome nausea can be managed by a number of medications that have fairly comparable efficacy, but significantly variable cost. In decreasing order of cost-effectiveness, these include:

   a. Droperidol 0.625–2.5 mg IV. This medication, like haloperidol, may occasionally be associated with QT prolongation and the risk of torsades de pointes.[181]

   b. Metoclopramide (Reglan) 10–20 mg IM qid. This may also stimulate gastrointestinal motility and decrease the incidence of distention.

   c. The 5-HT$_3$ antagonists are powerful antiemetic medications, although they are significantly more expensive.[182] They also may also be associated with a proarrhythmic effect from QT interval prolongation.

      i. Dolasetron (Anzemet) 12.5 mg IV

      ii. Ondansetron (Zofran) 4 mg IV

      iii. Granisetron (Kytril) 1 mg IV/PO bid

2. Pharyngeal dysfunction with dysphagia and difficulty swallowing liquids or solids has been noted in 1–3% of patients undergoing CABG and can lead to silent or overt aspiration pneumonia.[183,184] It is more common in older patients, insulin-dependent diabetics, and patients with COPD, CHF, renal dysfunction, or a history of stroke. It is also fairly common after prolonged intubation, and has been associated with intraoperative TEE.[185,186] Because TEE is routine in most institutions, one must be alert to this problem in the early postoperative period if the patient has impaired pharyngeal sensation or coughing at the time of initial oral intake. The occurrence of pharyngeal dysfunction in patients who have not had

intraoperative TEE has been ascribed to intraoperative cerebral injury and is often associated with other neurologic deficits. Thus, a full neurological evaluation with CT or MRI may be indicated to identify the causative mechanism.

   a. If there are clinical concerns about aspiration, a modified barium swallow using videofluoroscopy may be indicated before the patient is allowed to eat.[187]

   b. The management of patients with pharyngeal dysphagia may include dietary modification, postural adjustments, and working with speech therapists on swallowing maneuvers.

3. Constipation is a common problem after surgery. Preoperative enemas are usually not given, narcotics are used for analgesia, and elderly patients are often poorly mobilized for several days. Milk of magnesia, bulk laxatives (e.g., Metamucil), or stool softeners (e.g., Colace) may be helpful in older patients.

B. Differential diagnosis of acute abdominal pain

  1. Manifestations. Detection of an acute intraabdominal process in critically ill patients in the ICU setting can be difficult. It is frequently suggested by the presence of fever, an elevation in WBC count, marked tenderness to abdominal palpation, hemodynamic evidence of sepsis, or positive blood cultures. Arriving at the appropriate diagnosis can be even more challenging.

  2. Etiology

    a. Cholecystitis (acalculous or calculous)

    b. Perforated viscus (gastric or duodenal ulceration, diverticulitis)

    c. Gastritis

    d. Pancreatitis

    e. Visceral ischemia (mesenteric ischemia or ischemic colitis)

    f. *Clostridium difficile* colitis

    g. Severe paralytic ileus (occasionally idiopathic [Ogilvie's syndrome], but frequently associated with an acute inflammatory process or colitis)

    h. Small bowel or colonic obstruction

    i. Retroperitoneal bleeding

    j. Severe constipation

    k. UTI

    l. Bladder distention

  3. Risk factors

    a. Preoperative factors: New York Heart Association class IV or CHF, older age, chronic renal failure, poor nutritional status

    b. Intraoperative factors: long duration of CPB, valve surgery, emergency surgery

    c. Postoperative factors

      i. Low cardiac output or hypotension, frequently requiring vasopressors or an IABP (usually starting at the termination of CPB and then continuing into the ICU)

      ii. Sepsis

      iii. Prolonged ventilatory support

      iv. Postoperative acute tubular necrosis

      v. Blood transfusions and reexploration for bleeding

  4. Evaluation

    a. Review of preexisting conditions

    b. Serial abdominal examinations

    c. Laboratory tests: KUB (for obstruction or ileus), semiupright chest x-ray (for free air under the diaphragm), liver function tests (LFTs), serum amylase and lipase, *C. difficile* titer if diarrhea is present.

    d. An upper abdominal ultrasound or HIDA scan should be obtained if biliary tract obstruction is suspected.

    e. Abdominal CT, peritoneal lavage, or laparoscopy may be helpful in making the diagnosis.[188]

    f. A mesenteric arteriogram should be obtained if mesenteric ischemia is suspected.

  5. Treatment. General surgery consultation should be obtained from the outset because early exploration may reduce the high mortality associated with the development of GI complications. Laparoscopy is very sensitive in evaluating the nature of the problem, but an exploratory laparotomy may be necessary to further assess and potentially manage the problem. Although many patients with these complications are very ill and often septic, they are usually better able to tolerate exploration after cardiac surgery than they had been before.

C. Paralytic ileus occasionally persists for several days after surgery. It is frequently a benign, self-limited problem of undetermined cause, but occasionally it may reflect sepsis or a severe intraabdominal pathologic process.

  1. Contributing factors

    a. Gastric distention (possibly related to vagal injury)

    b. Congestion of the hepatic or splanchnic bed (from poor venous drainage during surgery or systemic venous hypertension)

    c. Inflammatory processes (e.g., cholecystitis, pancreatitis)

    d. Retroperitoneal bleeding (from groin catheterization, but occasionally spontaneously in an anticoagulated patient)

    e. *Clostridium difficile* colitis

    f. Mesenteric ischemia

    g. Drugs (narcotics)

  2. Evaluation

    a. Serial patient examinations for inflammatory signs, distention, return of bowel sounds.

    b. Laboratory tests: KUB, CBC, amylase, LFTs, *C. difficile* titers.

    c. "Pseudo-obstruction" is suggested by documentation of cecal dilatation to 9 cm. Perforation is more likely to occur when the diameter reaches 12 cm, although it may be related more to the rate of dilatation than the absolute size of the bowel.

  3. Management

    a. Decompression of the bowel is accomplished by keeping the patient NPO with nasogastric suction. This should prevent gastric distention until peristaltic activity returns. A rectal tube may also be beneficial when colonic distention is marked.

    b. Total parenteral nutrition should be started.

    c. Medications that can impair colonic motility must be stopped. This includes narcotics, calcium channel blockers, and anticholinergic drugs.

    d. All metabolic disturbances must be corrected and therapy directed at any identifiable precipitating problem.

   e. Decompressive colonoscopy is indicated when the colonic diameter reaches 12 cm. If dilatation persists or worsens, urgent surgery is indicated.

   f. Neostigmine 1 mg IV has been reported to produce rapid colonic decompression of "pseudo-obstruction."[189]

D. Cholecystitis

  1. Etiology. Cholecystitis is noted more commonly in older patients and those with prolonged pump times, suggesting that hypoperfusion is a contributing factor. Other risk factors include vascular disease, reexploration for bleeding, prolonged ventilation, bacteremia, and nosocomial infections.[190] Fasting, parenteral nutrition, and narcotics can decrease gallbladder contractility and produce biliary stasis. Acalculous rather than calculous cholecystitis is usually present.

  2. Evaluation

   a. Serial abdominal examinations may draw attention to an inflammatory process in the right upper quadrant.

   b. Liver function tests (ALT, AST, bilirubin, alkaline phosphatase) may suggest extrahepatic biliary obstruction.

   c. Right upper quadrant ultrasound or HIDA scan can identify a dilated gallbladder and biliary obstruction.

  3. Treatment

   a. Percutaneous cholecystostomy is often recommended in critically ill patients, but it is not adequate treatment when gangrene is present.

   b. Cholecystectomy (open or laparoscopic) is the preferred procedure unless the patient is considered too ill to tolerate the procedure.

E. Upper GI bleeding

  1. Etiology. Upper GI bleeding is one of the most common GI complications encountered after both on- and off-pump surgery and usually results from stress ulceration.[180] The causative mechanism is usually decreased blood flow, mucosal ischemia, and hypoperfusion/reperfusion injury that may be exacerbated by increased gastric acidity.[191] A thorough preoperative history and physical examination (stigmata of liver disease, stool guaiac) may identify patients at increased risk of developing postoperative GI bleeding.

  2. Risk factors[191–193]

   a. Preoperative: older age, preexisting gastritis or ulcer disease

   b. Intraoperative: long duration of CPB, valve operations, reoperations

   c. Postoperative risk factors: low cardiac output, respiratory failure, anticoagulation

  3. Prophylaxis. Any patient with a history of ulcer disease or gastritis should receive medications in the ICU to prevent stress-related mucosal damage and potentially GI bleeding. In addition, any patient on prolonged ventilatory support, with sepsis, or with a coagulopathy should receive stress ulcer prophylaxis. Although routine prophylaxis may not be necessary in patients at low risk, there is little downside to using sucralfate during the early postoperative period of intubation when the patient may have marginal cardiac output, visceral hypoperfusion, and some coagulopathy.[194]

   a. Sucralfate 1 g q6h can be given orally or by nasogastric tube. It does not raise the gastric pH (which increases gastric bacterial colonization) and may reduce the incidence of nosocomial pneumonia associated with medications that raise the gastric pH.

  b. Proton pump inhibitors and H_2 blockers are effective in raising the gastric pH and in preventing stress ulceration. Pantoprazole 40 mg IV/PO, omeprazole 20 mg qd, or ranitidine 150 mg PO bid are common medications that are used for prophylaxis.

  4. **Manifestations.** Drainage of bright red blood through a nasogastric tube or vomiting of blood is an overt sign of upper GI bleeding. Slow bleeding usually produces melena, but very rapid bleeding may produce bloody stools. Attention should be drawn to potential GI bleeding in the critically ill or heparinized patient with an unexplained fall in HCT or progressive tachycardia or hypotension. If GI bleeding cannot be documented, a retroperitoneal bleed should be entertained as a possible diagnosis and evaluated by abdominal CT.

  5. **Evaluation and treatment.** Bleeding that persists despite correction of coagulation abnormalities and intensification of a medical regimen requires further evaluation. Bleeding during anticoagulation is commonly associated with an underlying pathologic process.

    a. The proton pump inhibitors are superior to the H_2 blockers in controlling and preventing recurrent bleeding.[195] A daily 40-mg dose of pantoprazole IV is effective in raising and maintaining the gastric pH > 6, which may account for its superiority over the H_2 blockers in maintaining clotting.[192]

    b. Ranitidine can be given as a continuous infusion (6.25 mg/h) to maintain the gastric pH > 4, but tolerance may develop.

    c. Upper GI endoscopy should be performed to identify the site of bleeding and can be used therapeutically with laser bipolar coagulation to control hemorrhage. It can achieve hemostasis in > 90% of patients.[193]

    d. Since surgery has traditionally been reserved for patients with unremitting hemorrhage, it has been associated with a mortality rate of about 50%. If the patient requires anticoagulation indefinitely following surgery (i.e., for a mechanical prosthetic valve), a definitive procedure must be performed.

F. **Lower GI bleeding** may be manifested by bright red blood per rectum, blood-streaked stool, or melena and must be differentiated from upper GI bleeding by passage of a nasogastric tube.

  1. **Etiology**

    a. Mesenteric ischemia or ischemic colitis caused by periods of prolonged hypoperfusion.

    b. Antibiotic-associated colitis (usually *C. difficile*).

    c. Bleeding from colonic lesions (polyps, tumors, diverticular disease) may be precipitated by anticoagulation.

    d. Colonic angiodysplasia. This is termed Heyde's syndrome when associated with aortic stenosis. It abates after aortic valve replacement with a tissue valve.

  2. **Evaluation.** Once an upper GI source has been ruled out, sigmoidoscopy or colonoscopy can be performed. A bleeding scan may identify the bleeding source. Mesenteric arteriography should be considered if bleeding persists.

  3. **Treatment** involves correction of any coagulopathy and elimination of precipitating causes. Antibiotics (metronidazole 500 mg PO q8h or vancomycin 500 mg

PO q6h) can be used for *C. difficile* colitis. Mesenteric angiography with infusion of vasopressin (0.1–0.4 U/min) or injection of autologous clot or Gelfoam may be considered.[196] Octreotide (50 μg over 30 minutes) or somatostatin (50 μg bolus followed by an infusion of 250 μg/h) decreases splanchnic blood flow and may be beneficial. Surgical intervention is rarely required for persistent bleeding.

G. **Mesenteric ischemia** is usually noted in elderly patients with prolonged low cardiac output states requiring pharmacologic or mechanical support.

   1. **Etiology.** Nonocclusive mesenteric ischemia is the most common etiology resulting from splanchnic hypoperfusion from a low cardiac output state or a long pump run. Atherosclerotic embolism from an IABP or mesenteric thrombosis occurs less commonly.

   2. **Presentation.** Typical manifestations are a profound ileus or abdominal pain out of proportion to physical findings. The diagnosis can be very difficult to make in the critically ill patient who is frequently ventilated and heavily sedated. Sepsis, lactic acidosis, respiratory distress, GI bleeding, or diarrhea is often present as well. The diagnosis is typically made about 5–10 days after surgery.

   3. **Diagnosis** may be suggested by the association of the clinical picture just mentioned with severe acidosis, an ileus on KUB, or evidence of free abdominal fluid. Endoscopy may be helpful in documenting colonic ischemia. Biphasic CT or mesenteric CT angiography may show evidence of pneumatosis intestinalis, venous gas, bowel wall thickening, arterial occlusion, or venous thrombosis.[197] Standard mesenteric arteriography may identify thromboembolism but most commonly demonstrates vasoconstriction of the peripheral mesenteric vessels. Unfortunately, the diagnosis is frequently made at surgery when irreversible changes have occurred. Early suspicion of mesenteric ischemia, based on a persistent paralytic ileus, no bowel movement in several days despite laxatives, and a borderline or elevated lactate level, may allow for earlier successful intervention with vasodilator infusion.[198]

   4. **Treatment.** Early diagnosis and treatment are essential to lower the mortality rate of mesenteric ischemia, which generally exceeds 50%. If mesenteric vasoconstriction is identified, an infusion of papaverine 0.7 mg/kg/h for up to 5 days may be helpful, especially at an early stage of ischemia.[198] When ischemia is prolonged, irreversible intestinal necrosis may occur within hours. Emergency abdominal exploration is indicated if bowel necrosis is suspected and can rule out other intraabdominal pathology. Although a limited bowel resection can be performed, a more likely finding is multiple areas of ischemic bowel that prohibit extensive bowel resection. A second-look operation is indicated if the viability of the bowel is in doubt.

H. **Diarrhea** developing in a patient in the ICU setting is often an ominous sign because it may result from bowel ischemia caused by a low flow state. However, it is frequently caused by a manageable problem, such as:

   1. Side effects from medications

      a. Antibiotics have been implicated in causing diarrhea from *C. difficile*. Titers should be sent in triplicate and metronidazole 500 mg PO q8h or vancomycin 500 mg PO qid should be given for 7–10 days if titers are high. Rarely a subtotal colectomy is required for severe colitis.

b. Quinidine is infrequently used today for AF because of its proarrhythmic effects and because it causes diarrhea in nearly every patient.

2. GI bleeding

3. Intolerance of hyperosmolar tube feedings. Dilute with more water and start at a slower infusion rate.

I. **Hepatic dysfunction,** manifested by a transient low-grade elevation in LFTs, including ALT, AST, bilirubin, and alkaline phosphatase, is not uncommon after open-heart surgery. About 20% of patients develop transient hyperbilirubinemia, but fewer than 1% of patients have evidence of significant hepatocellular damage that may progress to chronic hepatitis or liver failure.[199,200]

1. **Etiology.** Significant hepatic dysfunction may result from either reduced hepatic perfusion or systemic congestion. It is more common in patients with underlying liver disease that occasionally may be undetected by normal preoperative LFTs, but often suggested by impaired synthetic function (low albumin, high INR). Other predisposing factors include CHF, diabetes, and hypertension. Patients with preoperative cardiogenic shock (acute MI, papillary muscle rupture, valve thrombosis) often show evidence of a "shock liver" before surgery and are at particularly high risk for developing hepatic and multisystem organ failure after salvage open-heart surgery.

   a. Hepatocellular necrosis
      i. Low cardiac output states usually requiring inotropic and/or vasopressor support
      ii. Right heart failure or severe tricuspid regurgitation (chronic passive congestion)
      iii. Posttransfusion hepatitis C or cytomegalovirus infection (late)
      iv. Drugs (acetaminophen, quinidine)
   b. Hyperbilirubinemia
      i. Hemolysis (paravalvular leak, long pump run, sepsis, multiple transfusions, drugs)
      ii. Intrahepatic cholestasis (hepatitis, hepatocellular necrosis, benign postoperative cholestasis, parenteral nutrition, bacterial infections, medications)
      iii. Extrahepatic obstruction (biliary tract obstruction)

2. **Manifestations** depend on the specific diagnosis. Jaundice is a common accompaniment of hepatocellular damage or cholestasis. Severe liver failure may result in a coagulopathy, refractory acidosis, hypoglycemia, renal failure, or encephalopathy.

3. **Evaluation.** The specific LFT abnormalities usually indicate the nature of the problem. Additional tests may include those that detect hemolysis (lactate dehydrogenase, reticulocyte count), assess cardiac and valvular function (echocardiography), identify a biliary pathologic process (right upper quadrant ultrasound or HIDA scan), or detect hepatitis (HBV, HCV serologies).

4. **Treatment**
   a. An elevated bilirubin is usually a benign and self-limited postoperative occurrence. Bilirubin levels gradually return to normal when hemodynamics improve unless there is evidence of severe underlying liver pathology. In this situation, progressive and irreversible hepatic dysfunction may result, leading to multisystem organ failure and death.

   b. Coagulopathy with "autoanticoagulation" may occur during a period of hepatic dysfunction because of the impaired capacity of the liver to produce clotting factors. In patients requiring anticoagulation, small doses of warfarin should be used to prevent the INR from becoming elevated to dangerous levels. If this occurs, the patient may develop cardiac tamponade or GI bleeding. In addition, the doses of medications that undergo hepatic metabolism must be altered.

   c. Stress ulcer prophylaxis should be considered using one of the proton pump inhibitors (pantoprazole 40 mg IV/PO qd).

   d. Hyperammonemia and encephalopathy can be managed with:[201]
      i. Dietary protein restriction
      ii. Lactulose 30 mL qid with sorbitol
      iii. Oral neomycin 6 g daily
      iv. Zinc sulfate 600 mg qd

   e. Blood glucose should be carefully monitored to prevent hypoglycemia.

   f. Lactic acidosis may result from impaired lactate metabolism rather than lactate generation from impaired tissue perfusion. Partial correction with sodium bicarbonate or Tris buffer (THAM), if renal function is adequate, should be considered if the base deficit exceeds 10.

J. Hyperamylasemia is noted in a substantial number (35–65%) of patients in the early postbypass period but is associated with clinical pancreatitis in only about 1–3% of patients. Isolated hyperamylasemia, not associated with clinical symptoms or an elevated lipase level, most commonly arises from a nonpancreatic source, such as the salivary glands, or from decreased renal excretion. Subclinical pancreatitis is suggested by the presence of mild symptoms (anorexia, nausea, ileus) with elevation of serum lipase levels. A brief period of bowel rest may be beneficial for these patients, but no specific treatment is indicated unless there is clinical evidence of overt pancreatitis or GI tract dysfunction.[202]

K. Overt pancreatitis is noted in about 1% of patients undergoing cardiac surgery, but is a serious problem associated with a significant mortality rate. Pancreatic necrosis has been noted in 25% of patients dying from multisystem organ failure after cardiac surgery.[203,204]

   1. Etiology. Pancreatitis usually represents an ischemic, necrotic injury resulting from a low cardiac output state and hypoperfusion. Potential contributing factors during surgery include hypothermia and nonpulsatile perfusion during bypass, systemic emboli, and venous sludging. A persistent low-output state requiring vasopressors is usually noted in patients developing overt pancreatitis.

   2. Presentation is atypical and relatively nonspecific. Fever, elevated WBC, paralytic ileus, and abdominal distention occur first, with abdominal pain, tenderness, and hemodynamic instability representing late manifestations.

   3. Diagnosis is suggested by the association of abdominal pain with hyperamylasemia, although most patients with fulminant pancreatitis do not have markedly elevated amylase levels. Abdominal ultrasound or CT may demonstrate a pancreatic phlegmon or abscess.

   4. Treatment should begin with nasogastric drainage and antibiotics. Exploratory laparotomy with debridement and drainage is usually performed as a desperate measure but may be the only hope for survival in patients with aggressive necrotizing pancreatitis.[204]

XI. Nutrition

A. Reversal of the catabolic state with adequate nutrition is important during the early phase of postoperative convalescence. The diet must provide enough calories to allow wounds to heal and to maintain immune competence. Although limitations in salt content, fluids, and cholesterol intake are important, overly strict control should be secondary to providing tasty, high-calorie foods that stimulate the patient's appetite. Too frequently, the combination of anorexia, nausea, and an unpalatable diet prevents the patient from achieving satisfactory nutrition.

B. If caloric intake is not satisfactory but the GI tract is functioning well, a nasogastric feeding tube should be placed and tube feedings initiated after confirming the position of the catheter in the stomach or, preferably, in the small bowel. Use of metoclopramide 20 mg IV along with erythromycin 200 mg IV (in 50 mL NS through central line or 200 mL peripherally) to stimulate gastric motility aids in the placement of these tubes. If the GI tract cannot be used, total parenteral nutrition provided through a central line may be necessary.

C. Most patients who require tracheostomy for prolonged ventilatory support will benefit from the placement of a feeding tube. If there is no evidence of gastroesophageal reflux, a percutaneous gastric feeding tube can be placed. If reflux is present, a feeding jejunostomy tube can be placed at the time of the tracheostomy.

D. Total caloric intake should be 25 kcal/kg/day. General nutritional requirements for adult patients include 1 mL/kg/day of water, 2–5 g/kg/day of glucose, 1.2–1.5 g/kg/day of protein, and 1.2–1.5 g/kg/day of fat, half of which should be omega-6 polyunsaturated fatty acids.[205] Specific considerations in critically ill patients include the following:

1. Multisystem organ failure increases total caloric requirements by about 10–20%. It is associated with protein catabolism and requires an increase in protein intake to 1.5–2 g/kg/day. Hyperglycemia may necessitate a reduction in glucose loads and use of IV insulin. Triglyceride intolerance often necessitates a reduction in glucose and fat intake. Increased macro- and micronutrient loss necessitates monitoring and replacement of potassium, zinc, magnesium, calcium, and phosphates, as needed.

2. Patients with respiratory failure must not be overfed. A respiratory quotient greater than 1 indicates excessive CO_2 production. In this situation, a specially formulated low-carbohydrate tube feeding should be used.

3. Protein intake should be optimized to promote nitrogen retention while avoiding protein overload. Protein should not be restricted in patients with acute renal dysfunction. In patients with chronic renal insufficiency, protein intake should be reduced to 0.5–0.8 g/kg/day. In contrast, protein intake should be increased for patients on dialysis, since hemodialysis or hemofiltration removes 3–5 g/h of protein. A tube feeding formulated for patients with renal failure that contains high levels of protein and low levels of potassium should be used.

4. Monitoring of visceral protein levels (transferrin and prealbumin) may indicate the adequacy of nutrition, but levels have not been shown to correlate with improved outcomes.

XII. Valve-Associated Problems

A. Careful follow-up is required for all patients receiving a prosthetic valve because of the risk of developing valve-related complications, including thromboembolism, endocarditis, anticoagulant-related hemorrhage, and valve degeneration.[206] It has been aptly stated that the use of a prosthetic valve replaces "one disease with another."

B. Thromboembolism. The annual risk of thromboembolism averages 1–2% for aortic valves and 2–4% for mitral valves, with a slightly higher incidence in patients with mechanical valves taking warfarin than in those with bioprosthetic valves taking only aspirin. The recommended regimens for tissue and mechanical valves are summarized in Table 13.2 on page 532.[46,47,207]

C. Valve thrombosis may occur with a mechanical valve, even during therapeutic anticoagulation. It is very rare with a bioprosthetic valve. Suspicion of mechanical valve thrombosis is raised by loss of valve clicks on auscultation and confirmed by fluoroscopy or two-dimensional echocardiography (see Figure 2.8). Although thrombolytic therapy can be used in selected circumstances, an immediate operation to replace the valve is usually required.[208]

D. Pregnancy poses a serious problem for the woman with a prosthetic valve. The incidence of fetal wastage is 60% if warfarin is used during the first trimester, and there is a significant incidence of other congenital defects if pregnancy is completed ("coumadin embryopathy"). Tissue valves have been used for women of childbearing age, acknowledging the limited durability of valves in this age group. Cryopreserved homograft valves or a pulmonary autograft (Ross procedure) can be considered for women undergoing aortic valve replacement. One recommended anticoagulation regimen for women with mechanical valves who desire to become pregnant is as follows:[209]

1. Stop warfarin before conception.

2. Alternatives during pregnancy:

    a. Adjusted-dose unfractionated heparin (UFH) throughout pregnancy to achieve a PTT of 2 times control (usually around 10,000 units SC q12h)

    b. Adjusted-dose low molecular weight heparin (LMWH) SC q12h throughout pregnancy to maintain a 4–6-hour postinjection antifactor Xa heparin level >0.5 U/mL.

    c. Either UFH or LMWH as above until the 13th week of pregnancy, then warfarin with a target INR of 2.5–3.0 until the middle of the third trimester, followed by UFH or LMWH (often up to 20,000 U SC q12h) until delivery.

    d. Aspirin may be added to any of these regimens.

3. Before delivery, initiate intravenous heparin.

4. With the onset of labor, give heparin 5000 U SC q8h.

5. Resume warfarin after delivery.

E. Anticoagulant-related hemorrhage is a major source of morbidity in patients receiving warfarin, especially in patients over the age of 65. It is absolutely critical that careful follow-up be arranged for any patient discharged on warfarin. The INR must remain in the therapeutic range to avoid valve thrombosis or bleeding problems.

F. Prosthetic valve endocarditis may develop at any time during the life span of a prosthetic valve with an annual risk of approximately 1–2%.[210, 211] Early endocarditis (within 60 days of surgery) most commonly results from infection with staphylococci (coagulase negative > *aureus*), fungi, gram-negative organisms, and enterococci. This carries a significantly higher mortality than late prosthetic valve endocarditis. The latter is most commonly caused by coagulase-negative *Staphylococcus* and *Streptococcus viridans*. Clinical manifestations may include recurrent fevers, valve dysfunction with regurgitation and heart failure, cerebral or peripheral embolization, and, most ominously, the development of conduction defects resulting from a periannular abscess. It is critical that the patient understand the need for prophylactic antibiotics when any dental or other surgically invasive procedure is performed. The AHA recommendations detailed on page 541 should be followed.[111]

G. **Hemolysis** usually reflects the development of a paravalvular leak and is often worse when the leak is small due to increased turbulence. It may also result from transvalvular leaks resulting from pannus ingrowth or thrombus formation that restricts leaflet movement and may keep one leaflet in a partially open fixed position (Figure 2.8). Subclinical hemolysis is noted by elevation of lactate dehydrogenase and the reticulocyte count. The patient may also develop mild jaundice or persistent anemia necessitating transfusion. Valve re-replacement is indicated for severe hemolysis or a significant paravalvular leak.

H. **Valve failure** is defined as a complication necessitating valve replacement. Mechanical valve failure is usually caused by thrombosis, thromboembolism, endocarditis, or anticoagulation-related bleeding, and rarely by structural failure. In contrast, primary tissue failure is the most common cause of bioprosthetic dysfunction necessitating valve replacement. Porcine mitral valves not treated with any anticalcification agents or treated with high- or low-pressure fixation degenerate more rapidly than valves processed with improved technology, especially in young patients. Structural valve deterioration necessitating reoperation occurs in only about 10% of patients with aortic pericardial valves at 20 years, suggesting that pericardial valves may fare better than porcine valves in the mitral position as well. Nonetheless, earlier failure can occur and constant vigilance and careful follow-up examinations are essential. Fortunately, surgery for bioprosthetic valve failure can usually be performed on an elective basis at low risk in contrast to the high-risk emergency surgery required for catastrophic mechanical valve failure.

XIII. Discharge Planning

A. As the length of hospital stay continues to decrease, appropriate discharge planning is essential to ensure a smooth convalescence after hospital discharge. Patients requiring additional subacute care may be transferred to rehabilitation hospitals or skilled nursing facilities for several days before going home. Even when patients are well enough to be cared for at home, it is not uncommon for separation anxiety to develop, with both patients and family members experiencing difficulty handling minor problems.

B. Appropriate discharge planning should involve the patient, family members, dietitians, nurses, physician assistants, nurse practitioners, and physicians. Patients must be given explicit instructions as to how they will feel, how fast they should anticipate recovery, what they must do, what they should look for, and when to contact the hospital. Several manuals are available that discuss expectations and the reestablishment of standard routines at home. Phone contact from the doctor's office is very beneficial in allaying patients' fears, answering routine questions, and dealing appropriately with potential problems. Since the definition of operative mortality extends to 30 days after surgery, it is imperative for appropriate outcomes analysis that patients be contacted at this time to see whether they have been readmitted and see how they are faring.

C. Most patients should have an available family member or friend at home for the first week after discharge. This provides reassurance for the patient who may not yet be able to care for himself or herself, and it also provides an objective observer who is able to contact the hospital if serious problems arise.

D. **Medications.** The patient should be provided with a list and schedule of all medications. The reason each medication has been prescribed as well as possible side effects and interactions with other medications should be discussed. If the patient is receiving an anticoagulant such as **warfarin,** it is **absolutely imperative that follow-up be arranged** for prothrombin times (INR) and regulation of drug dosage. The adverse influence of alcohol and other medications and certain foods on the level of anticoagulation must be emphasized.

E. **Prophylactic antibiotics.** Any patient who has received prosthetic material (valves or grafts) must be aware of the necessity of prophylactic antibiotics if dental work or other surgical procedures are contemplated. Patients should be told to inform their physician or dentist accordingly and follow the AHA guidelines for antibiotic prophylaxis delineated on page 541.[111]

F. **Diet.** Dietitians should meet with patients before discharge to discuss the particular dietary restrictions for their cardiac disease. This entails discussions of the significance of low-cholesterol or low-salt diets and the provision of appropriate dietary plans. Appropriate management of hypercholesterolemia involves use of a "statin" medication to reduce cholesterol, stabilize coronary plaque, and perhaps prevent progression of disease.[212,213]

G. The patient must participate in self-evaluation at home. A daily assessment of pulse rate, oral temperature, and weight should be performed, and all incisions should be inspected for redness, tenderness, or drainage. Patients should be instructed to contact the physician's office if any abnormalities are noted.

H. Patients should be encouraged to gradually increase their activity as tolerated. Patients with a median sternotomy incision should be discouraged from lifting objects heavier than 10–15 pounds because it puts strain on the healing sternum. Driving should be avoided for 6 weeks. In contrast, there are few physical limitations on patients who have small thoracotomy incisions for minimally invasive surgery.

I. The long-term care of the patient after coronary bypass surgery entails use of aspirin indefinitely to improve vein graft patency and for the primary and secondary prevention of myocardial infarction. In addition, control of all modifiable risk factors (obesity, smoking, hyperlipidemia, diabetes, hypertension) with medications, changes in lifestyle, and involvement in cardiac rehabilitation programs are essential to optimize the surgical result.[214]

References

1. McGee DC, Gould MK. Preventing complications of central venous catheterization. N Engl J Med 2003;348:1123–33.
2. Tripp HF, Bolton JW. Phrenic nerve injury following cardiac surgery: a review. J Card Surg 1998;13:218–23.
3. Dimopoulou I, Daganou M, Dafni U, et al. Phrenic nerve dysfunction after cardiac operations. Electrophysiologic evaluation of risk factors. Chest 1998;113:8–14.
4. Canbaz S, Turgut N, Halici U, Balci F, Ege T, Duran E. Electrophysiological evaluation of phrenic nerve injury during cardiac surgery: a prospective, controlled, clinical study. BMC Surg 2004;4:2.
5. Mills GH, Khan ZP, Moxham J, Desai J, Forsyth A, Ponte J. Effects of temperature on phrenic nerve and diaphragmatic function during cardiac surgery. Br J Anaesth 1997;79:726–32.
6. Deng Y, Byth K, Paterson HS. Phrenic nerve injury associated with high free right internal mammary artery harvesting. Ann Thorac Surg 2003;76:459–63.
7. Tripp HF, Sees DW, Lisagor PG, Cohen DJ. Is phrenic nerve dysfunction after cardiac surgery related to internal mammary harvesting? J Card Surg 2001;16:228–31.
8. Sharma AD, Parmley CL, Sreeram G, Grocott HP. Peripheral nerve injuries during cardiac surgery: risk factors, diagnosis, prognosis, and prevention. Anesth Analg 2001;91:1358–69.
9. Yamazaki K, Kato H, Tsujimoto S, Kitamura R. Diabetes mellitus, internal thoracic artery grafting, and the risk of an elevated hemidiaphragm after coronary artery bypass surgery. J Cardiothorac Vasc Anesth 1994;8:437–40.
10. Cruz-Martinez A, Armijo A, Fermoso A, Moraleda S, Mate I, Marin M. Phrenic nerve conduction study in demyelinating neuropathies and open-heart surgery. Clin Neurophysiol 2000; 111:821–5.
11. Katz MG, Katz R, Schachner A, Cohen AJ. Phrenic nerve injury after coronary artery bypass grafting: will it go away? Ann Thorac Surg 1998;65:32–5.
12. Huttl TP, Wichmann MW, Reichart B, Geiger TK, Schildberg FW, Meyer G. Laparoscopic diaphragmatic plication: long-term results of a novel surgical technique for postoperative phrenic nerve palsy. Surg Endosc 2004;18:547–51.
13. Shammas NW. Pulmonary embolus after coronary artery bypass surgery: a review of the literature. Clin Cardiol 2000;23:637–44.
14. Mariani AM, Guy J, Boonstra PW, Grandjean JG, Van Oeveren W, Ebels T. Procoagulant activity after off-pump coronary operation: is the current anticoagulation adequate? Ann Thorac Surg 1999;68:1370–5.
15. Goldhaber SZ, Schoepf J. Pulmonary embolism after coronary artery bypass grafting, Circulation 2004;109:2712–5.
16. Ramos R, Salem BI, De Pawlikowski MP, Coordes C, Eisenberg S, Leidenfrost R. The efficacy of pneumatic compression stockings in the prevention of pulmonary embolism after cardiac surgery. Chest 1996;109:82–5.
17. Carman TL, Deitcher SR. Advances in diagnosing and excluding pulmonary embolism: spiral CT and D-dimer measurement. Cleve Clin J Med 2002;69:721–9.
18. Cho KJ, Dasika NL. Catheter technique for pulmonary embolectomy or thrombofragmentation. Semin Vasc Surg 2000;13:221–35.
19. Glikson M, Dearani JA, Hyberger LK, Schaff HV, Hammill SC, Hayes DL. Indications, effectiveness, and long-term dependency in permanent pacing after cardiac surgery. Am J Cardiol 1997;80:1309–13.
20. Baerman JM, Kirsh MM, de Buitleir M, et al. Natural history and determinants of conduction defects following coronary artery bypass surgery. Ann Thorac Surg 1987;44:150–3.
21. Stein PD, Schunemann HJ, Dalen JE, Gutterman D. Antithrombotic therapy in patients with saphenous vein and internal mammary artery grafts. The Seventh ACCP conference on antithrombotic and thrombolytic therapy. Chest 2004;126:600S–8S.
22. Kimmelstiel CD, Udelson JE, Salem DN, Bojar R, Rastegar H, Konstam MA. Recurrent angina caused by a left internal mammary artery-to-pulmonary artery fistula. Am Heart J 1993;125:234–6.
23. Kuvin JT, Harati NA, Pandian NG, Bojar RM, Khabbaz KR. Postoperative cardiac tamponade in the modern surgical era. Ann Thorac Surg 2000;74:1148–53.

24. Tsang TS, Barnes ME, Hayes SN, et al. Clinical and echocardiographic characteristics of significant pericardial effusions following cardiothoracic surgery and outcomes of echo-guided pericardiocentesis for management: Mayo Clinic experience, 1979–1998. Chest 1999;116: 322–31.

25. Malouf JF, Alam S, Gharzeddine W, Stefadouros MA. The role of anticoagulation in the development of pericardial effusion and late tamponade after cardiac surgery. Eur Heart J 1993;14: 1451–7.

26. Niva M, Biancari F, Valkama J, Juvonen J, Satta J, Juvonen T. Effects of diclofenac in the prevention of pericardial effusion after coronary artery bypass surgery. A prospective, randomized study. J Cardiovasc Surg (Torino) 2002;43:449–53.

27. Kuvin JT, Khabbaz K, Pandian NG. Left ventricular apical diastolic collapse: an unusual echocardiographic marker of postoperative cardiac tamponade. J Am Soc Echocardiogr 1999;12: 218–20.

28. Lindenberger M, Kjellberg M, Karlsson E, Wranne B. Pericardiocentesis guided by 2-D echocardiography: the method of choice for treatment of pericardial effusion. J Intern Med 2003;253: 411–7.

29. Horneffer PJ, Miller RH, Pearson TA, Rykiel MF, Reitz BA, Gardner TJ. The effective treatment of postpericardiotomy syndrome after cardiac operations. A randomized placebo-controlled trial. J Thorac Cardiovasc Surg 1990;100:292–6.

30. Kocazeybek B, Erenturk S, Calyk MK, Babacan F. An immunological approach to postpericardiotomy syndrome occurrence and its relation to autoimmunity. Acta Chir Belg 1998;98:203–6.

31. Hoffman M, Fried M, Jabareen F, et al. Anti-heart antibodies in postpericardiotomy syndrome: cause or epiphenomenon? A prospective, longitudinal pilot study. Autoimmunity 2002;35:241–5.

32. Finkelstein Y, Shemesh J, Mahlab K, et al. Colchicine for the prevention of postpericardiotomy syndrome. Herz 2002;27:791–4.

33. Kurth T, Glynn RJ, Walker AM, et al. Inhibition of clinical benefits of aspirin on first myocardial infarction by nonsteroidal anti-inflammatory drugs. Circulation 2003;108:1191–5.

34. Matsuyama K, Matsumoto M, Sugita T, et al. Clinical characteristics of patients with constrictive pericarditis after coronary bypass surgery. Jpn Circ J 2001;65:480–2.

35. Kerr KJ, Furnary AP, Grunkemeier GL, Bookin S, Kanhere V, Starr A. Glucose control lowers the risk of wound infection in diabetics after open heart operations. Ann Thorac Surg 1997;63: 356–61.

36. Latham R, Lancaster AD, Covington JF, Pirolo JS, Thomas CS. The association of diabetes and glucose control with surgical-site infections among cardiothoracic surgery patients. Infect Control Hosp Epidemiol 2001;22:607–12.

37. Furnary AP, Gao G, Grunkemeier GL, et al. Continuous insulin infusion reduces mortality in patients with diabetes undergoing coronary artery bypass grafting. J Thorac Cardiovasc Surg 2003;125:1007–21.

38. Shorten GD, Comunale ME. Heparin-induced thrombocytopenia. J Cardiothorac Vasc Anesth 1996;10:521–30.

39. Warkentin TE, Kelton JG. Temporal aspects of heparin-induced thrombocytopenia. N Engl J Med 2001;34:1286–92.

40. Visentin GP, Malik M, Cyganiak KA, Aster RH. Patients treated with unfractionated heparin during open heart surgery are at high risk to form antibodies reactive with heparin:platelet factor 4 complexes. J Lab Clin Med 1996;128:376–83.

41. Bauer TL, Arepally G, Konkle BA, et al. Prevalence of heparin-associated antibodies without thrombosis in patients undergoing cardiopulmonary bypass surgery. Circulation 1997;95: 1242–6.

42. Srinivasan AF, Rice L, Bartholomew JR, et al. Warfarin-induced skin necrosis and venous limb gangrene in the setting of heparin-induced thrombocytopenia. Arch Intern Med 2004;164: 66–70.

43. Warkentin TE. Management of heparin-induced thrombocytopenia: a critical comparison of lepirudin and argatroban. Thromb Res 2003;110:73–82.

44. Francis JL, Drexler A, Gwyn G. Bivalirudin, a direct thrombin inhibitor, is a safe and effective treatment for heparin-induced thrombocytopenia. Blood 2003;102:abstract 571.

45. Tardy-Poncet B, Tardy B, Reynaud J, et al. Efficacy and safety of danaparoid sodium (ORG 10172) in critically ill patients with heparin-associated thrombocytopenia. Chest 1999;115:1616–20.

46. Warkentin TE, Greinacher A. Heparin-induced thrombocytopenia and cardiac surgery. Ann Thorac Surg 2003;76:2121–31.

47. Salem DN, Stein PD, Al-Ahmad A, et al. Antithrombotic therapy in valvular heart disease—native and prosthetic. The Seventh ACCP conference on antithrombotic and thrombolytic therapy. Chest 2004;126:457S–82S.

48. Blair KL, Hatton AC, White WD, et al. Comparison of anticoagulation regimens after Carpentier-Edwards aortic or mitral valve replacement. Circulation 1994;90(part 2):II-214–9.

49. Orszulak TA, Schaff HV, Mullany CJ, et al. Risk of thromboembolism with the aortic Carpentier-Edwards bioprosthesis. Ann Thorac Surg 1995;59:462–8.

50. Hirsh J, Fuster V, Ansell J, Halperin JL. American Heart Association/American College of Cardiology Foundation guide to warfarin therapy. Circulation 2003;41:1633–52.

51. Finkelstein R, Rabino G, Mashiah T, et al. Vancomycin versus cefazolin prophylaxis for cardiac surgery in the setting of a high prevalence of methicillin-resistant staphylococcal infections. J Thorac Cardiovasc Surg 2002;123:326–32.

52. Kreter B, Woods M. Antibiotic prophylaxis for cardiothoracic operations. Meta-analysis of thirty years of clinical trials. J Thorac Cardiovasc Surg 1992:104:590–9.

53. Niederhauser U, Vogt M, Vogt P, Genoni M, Kunzli A, Turina MI. Cardiac surgery in a high-risk group of patients: is prolonged postoperative antibiotic prophylaxis effective? J Thorac Cardiovasc Surg 1997;114:162–8.

54. Kollef MH, Sharpless L, Vlasnik J, Pasque C, Murphy D, Fraser VJ. The impact of nosocomial infections on patient outcome following cardiac surgery. Chest 1997;112:666–75.

55. Rebollo MH, Bernal JM, Llorca J, Rabasa JM, Revuelta JM. Nosocomial infections in patients having cardiovascular operations: a multivariate analysis of risk factors. J Thorac Cardiovasc Surg 1996;112:908–13.

56. Gol MK, Karahan M, Ulus AT, et al. Bloodstream, respiratory, and deep surgical wound infections after open heart surgery. J Card Surg 1998;13:252–9.

57. Spelman DW, Russo P, Harrington G, et al. Risk factors for surgical wound infection and bacteraemia following coronary artery bypass surgery. Aust N Z J Surg 2000;70:47–51.

58. Leal-Noval SR, Marquez-Vacaro JA, Garcia-Curiel A, et al. Nosocomial pneumonia in patients undergoing heart surgery. Crit Care Med 2000;28:935–40.

59. Chelemer SB, Prato BS, Cox PM Jr, O'Connor GT, Morton JR. Association of bacterial infection and red blood cell transfusion after coronary artery bypass surgery. Ann Thorac Surg 2002; 73:138–42.

60. Leal-Noval SR, Rincon-Ferrari MD, Garcia-Curiel A, et al. Transfusion of blood components and postoperative infection in patients undergoing cardiac surgery. Chest 2001;119:1461–8.

61. Dagan O, Cox PN, Ford-Jones L, Posonby J, Bohn DJ. Nosocomial infection following cardiovascular surgery: comparison of two periods, 1987 vs. 1992. Crit Care Med 1999;27:104–8.

62. Koleff M. Prevention of ventilator-associated pneumonia. N Engl J Med 1999;340:627–34.

63. DeRiso AJ II, Ladowski JS, Dillon TA, Justice JW, Peterson AC. Chlorhexidine gluconate 0.12% oral rinse reduces the incidence of total nosocomial respiratory infection and nonprophylactic systemic antibiotic use in patients undergoing heart surgery. Chest 1996;109:1556–61.

64. Carrel TP, Eisinger E, Vogt M, Turina MI. Pneumonia after cardiac surgery is predictable by tracheal aspirates but cannot be prevented by prolonged antibiotic prophylaxis. Ann Thorac Surg 2001;72:143–8.

65. Dellinger RP. Cardiovascular management of septic shock. Crit Care Med 2003;31:946–55.

66. Shroyer ALW, Coombs LP, Peterson ED, et al. The Society of Thoracic Surgeons: 30-day mortality and morbidity risk models. Ann Thorac Surg 2003;75:1856–64.

67. Braxton JH, Marrin CAS, McGrath PD, et al. Mediastinitis and long-term survival after coronary artery bypass graft surgery. Ann Thorac Surg 2000;70:2004–7.

68. Gummert JF, Barten MJ, Hans C, et al. Mediastinitis and cardiac surgery: an updated risk factor analysis in 10,373 consecutive adult patients. Thorac Cardiovasc Surg 2002;50:87–91.

69. Trick WE, Scheckler WE, Tokars JI, et al. Modifiable risk factors associated with deep sternal site infections after coronary artery bypass grafting. J Thorac Cardiovasc Surg 2000;119:108–14.

70. Olsen MA, Lock-Buckley P, Hopkins D, Polish LB, Sundt TM, Fraser VJ. The risk factors for deep and superficial chest surgical-site infections after coronary artery bypass graft surgery are different. J Thorac Cardiovasc Surg 2002;124:136–45.

71. Zacharias A, Habib RH. Factors predisposing to median sternotomy complications. Deep vs superficial infection. Chest 1996;110:1173–8.

72. Stahle E, Tammelin A, Bergstrom R, Hambreus A, Nystrom SO, Hans HE. Sternal wound complications—incidence, microbiology, and risk factors. Eur J Cardiothorac Surg 1997;11: 1146–53.

73. Abboud CS, Wey SB, Baltar VT. Risk factors for mediastinitis after cardiac surgery. Ann Thorac Surg 2004;77:676–83.

74. Lu JCY, Grayson AD, Jha P, Srinivasan AK, Fabri BM. Risk factors for sternal wound infection and mid-term survival following coronary artery bypass surgery. Eur J Cardiothorac Surg 2003;23:943–9.

75. Lev-Ran O, Mohr R, Amir K, et al. Bilateral internal thoracic artery grafting in insulin-treated diabetics: should it be avoided? Ann Thorac Surg 2003;75:1872–7.

76. Hirotani T, Nakamichi T, Munakata M, Takeuchi S. Risks and benefits of bilateral internal thoracic artery grafting in diabetic patients. Ann Thorac Surg 2003;76:2017–22.

77. Matsa M, Paz Y, Gurevitch J, et al. Bilateral skeletonized internal thoracic artery grafts in patients with diabetes mellitus. J Thorac Cardiovasc Surg 2001;121:668–74.

78. Sofer D, Gurevitch J, Shapira I, et al. Sternal wound infections in patients after coronary artery bypass grafting using bilateral skeletonized internal mammary arteries. Ann Surg 1999;229: 585–90.

79. Baskett RJF, MacDougall CE, Ross DB. Is mediastinitis a preventable complication? A 10-year review. Ann Thorac Surg 1999;67:462–5.

80. Kaiser AB, Kernodle DS, Barg NL, Petracek MR. Influence of preoperative showers on staphylococcal skin colonization: a comparative trial of antiseptic skin cleansers. Ann Thorac Surg 1988;45:35–8.

81. Ko W, Lazenby WD, Zelano JA, Isom OW, Krieger KH. Effects of shaving methods and intraoperative irrigation on suppurative mediastinitis after bypass operations. Ann Thorac Surg 1992;53:301–5.

82. Fellinger EK, Leavitt BJ, Hebert JC. Serum levels of prophylactic cefazolin during cardiopulmonary bypass surgery. Ann Thorac Surg 2002;74:1187–90.

83. Lehot JJ, Reverdy ME, Etienne J, et al. Cefazolin and netilmicin serum levels during and after cardiac surgery with cardiopulmonary bypass. J Cardiothorac Anesth 1990;4:204–9.

84. Cimochowski GE, Harostock MD, Brown R, Bernardi M, Alonzo N, Coyle K. Intranasal mupirocin reduces sternal wound infection after open heart surgery in diabetics and nondiabetics. Ann Thorac Surg 2001;71:1572–9.

85. El Oakley RM, Wright JE. Postoperative mediastinitis: classification and management. Ann Thorac Surg 1996;61:1030–6.

86. Francel TJ, Kouchoukos NT. A rational approach to wound difficulties after sternotomy: the problem. Ann Thorac Surg 2001;72:1411–8.

87. Tegnell A, Aren C, Ohman L. Coagulase-negative staphylococci and sternal infections after cardiac operation. Ann Thorac Surg 2000;69:1104–9.

88. Mossad SB, Serkey JM, Longworth DL, Cosgrove DM III, Gordon SM. Coagulase-negative staphylococcal sternal wound infections after open heart operations. Ann Thorac Surg 1997; 63:395–401.

89. Benlolo S, Mateo J, Raskine L, et al. Sternal puncture allows an early diagnosis of poststernotomy mediastinitis. J Thorac Cardiovasc Surg 2003;125:611–7.

90. Gur E, Stern D, Weiss J, et al. Clinical-radiological evaluation of poststernotomy wound infections. Plast Reconstr Surg 1998;101:348–55.

91. Bitkover CY, Cederlund K, Aberg B, Vaage J. Computed tomography of the sternum and mediastinum after median sternotomy. Ann Thorac Surg 1999;68:858–63.

92. Misawa Y, Fuse K, Hasegawa T. Infectious mediastinitis after cardiac operations: computed tomographic findings. Ann Thorac Surg 1998;65:622–4.

93. Liberatore M, Fiore V, D'Agostini A, et al. Sternal wound infection revisited. Eur J Nucl Med 2000;27:660–7.

94. Bitkover CY, Gardlund B, Larsson SA, Aberg B, Jacobsson H. Diagnosing sternal wound infections with 99mTc-labeled monoclonal granulocyte antibody scintigraphy. Ann Thorac Surg 1996;62:1412–6.

95. Oates E, Payne DD. Postoperative cardiothoracic infection: diagnostic value of indium-111 white blood cell imaging. Ann Thorac Surg 1994;58:1442–6.

96. Satta J, Lahtinen J, Raisanen L, Salmela E, Juvonen T. Options for the management of poststernotomy mediastinitis. Scand Cardiovasc J. 1998;32:29–32.

97. Rand RP, Cochran RP, Aziz S, et al. Prospective trial of catheter irrigation and muscle flaps for sternal wound infection. Ann Thorac Surg 1998;65:1046–9.

98. Levi N, Olsen PS. Primary closure of deep sternal wound infection following open heart surgery: a safe operation? J Cardiovasc Surg (Torino) 2000;41:241–5.

99. Shrager JB, Wain JC, Wright CD, et al. Omentum is highly effective in the management of complex cardiothoracic surgical problems. J Thorac Cardiovasc Surg 2003;125:526–32.

100. Kirsh M, Mekontso-Dessap A, Houel R, Giroud E, Hillion ML, Loisance DY. Closed drainage using redon catheters for poststernotomy mediastinitis: results and risk factors for adverse outcome. Ann Thorac Surg 2001;71:1580–6.

101. Berg HF, Brands WGB, van Geldorp TR, Kluytmans-VandenBergh MFQ, Kluytmans JAJW. Comparison between closed drainage techniques for the treatment of postoperative mediastinitis. Ann Thorac Surg 2000;70:924–9.

102. Castello JR, Centella T, Garro L, et al. Muscle flap reconstruction for the treatment of major sternal wound infections after cardiac surgery: a 10-year analysis. Scan J Plast Reconstr Surg Hand Surg 1999;33:17–24.

103. Cartier R, Diaz OS, Carrier M, Leclerc Y, Castonguay Y, Leung TK. Right ventricular rupture. A complication of postoperative mediastinitis. J Thorac Cardiovasc Surg 1993;106:1036–9.

104. De Feo NM, Renzulli A, Ismeno GM, et al. Variables predicting adverse outcome in patients with deep sternal wound infection. Ann Thorac Surg 2001;71:324–31.

105. Tang AT, Ohri SK, Haw MP. Novel application of vacuum assisted closure techniques to the treatment of sternotomy wound infection. Eur J Cardiothorac Surg 2000;17:482–4.

106. Fleck TM, Fleck M, Moidl R, et al. The vacuum-assisted closure system for the treatment of deep sternal wound infections after cardiac surgery. Ann Thorac Surg 2002;74:1596–600.

107. Luckraz H, Murphy F, Bryant S, Charman SC, Ritchie AJ. Vacuum-assisted closure as a treatment modality for infections after cardiac surgery. J Thorac Cardiovasc Surg 2003;125:301–5.

108. De Feo M, De Santo LS, Romano G, et al. Treatment of recurrent staphylococcal mediastinitis: still a controversial issue. Ann Thorac Surg 2003;75:538–42.

109. Athanasiou T, Aziz O, Skapinakis P, et al. Leg wound infections after coronary artery bypass grafting: a meta-analysis comparing minimally invasive versus conventional vein harvesting. Ann Thorac Surg 2003;76:2141–6.

110. Allen KB, Fitzgerald EB, Heimansohn DA, Shaar CJ. Management of closed space infections associated with endoscopic vein harvest. Ann Thorac Surg 2000;69:960–1.

111. Dajani AS, Taubert KA, Wilson W, et al. Prevention of bacterial endocarditis. Recommendations by the American Heart Association. JAMA 1997;277:1794–1801 and Circulation 1997; 96:358–66.

112. Roach GW, Kanchuger M, Mangano CM, et al. Adverse cerebral outcomes after coronary bypass surgery. N Engl J Med 1996;335:1857–63.

113. Lund C, Hol PK, Lundblad R, et al. Comparison of cerebral embolization during off-pump and on-pump coronary artery bypass surgery. Ann Thorac Surg 2003;76:765–70.

114. Bucerius J, Gummert JE, Borger MA, et al. Stroke after cardiac surgery: a risk factor analysis of 16,184 consecutive adult patients. Ann Thorac Surg 2003;75:472–8.

115. Lee JD, Lee SJ, Tsushima WT, et al. Benefits of off-pump bypass on neurologic and clinical morbidity: a prospective randomized trial. Ann Thorac Surg 2003;76:18–25.

116. Leacche M, Carrier M, Bouchard D, et al. Improving neurologic outcome in off-pump surgery: the "no touch" technique. Heart Surg Forum 2003;6:169–75.

117. Scarborough JE, White W, Derilus FE, Mathew JP, Newman MF, Landolfo KP. Neurologic outcomes after coronary artery bypass grafting with and without cardiopulmonary bypass. Semin Thorac Cardiovasc Surg 2003;15:52–62.

118. Hirose H, Amano A. Stroke rate in off-pump coronary artery bypass: aortocoronary bypass versus in-situ bypass. Angiology 2003;54:647–53.

119. Patel NC, Deodhar AP, Grayson AD, et al. Neurological outcomes in coronary surgery. Independent effect of avoiding cardiopulmonary bypass. Ann Thorac Surg 2002;74:400–5.

120. Trehan N, Mishra M, Sharma OP, Mishra A, Kasliwal RR. Further reduction in stroke after off-pump coronary artery bypass grafting: a 10-year experience. Ann Thorac Surg 2001;72: S1026–32.

121. John R, Choudhri AF, Weinberg AD, et al. Multicenter review of preoperative risk factors for stroke after coronary artery bypass grafting. Ann Thorac Surg 2000;69:30–6.

122. McKahnn GM, Goldsborough MA, Borowicz LM Jr, et al. Predictors of stroke risk in coronary artery bypass patients. Ann Thorac Surg 1997;63:516–21.

123. Almassi GH, Sommers T, Moritz TE, et al. Stroke in cardiac surgical patients: determinants and outcome. Ann Thorac Surg 1999;68:391–8.

124. Ascione R, Reeves BC, Chamberlain MH, Ghosh AK, Lim KH, Angelini GD. Predictors of stroke in the modern era of coronary artery bypass grafting: a case control study. Ann Thorac Surg 2002;74:474–80.

125. Puskas JD, Winston AD, Wright CE, et al. Stroke after coronary artery operation: incidence, correlates, outcome, and cost. Ann Thorac Surg 2000;69:1053–6.

126. Likosky DS, Leavitt BJ, Marrin CAS, et al. Intra- and postoperative predictors of stroke after coronary artery bypass grafting. Ann Thorac Surg 2003;76:428–35.

127. Redmond JM, Greene PS, Goldsborough MA, et al. Neurologic injury in cardiac surgical patients with a history of stroke. Ann Thorac Surg 1996;61:42–7.

128. Goto T, Baba T, Matsuyama K, Honma K, Ura M, Koshiji T. Aortic atherosclerosis and postoperative neurological dysfunction in elderly coronary surgical patients. Ann Thorac Surg 2003; 75:1912–8.

129. van der Linden J, Jadjinikolaou L, Bergman P, Lindblom D. Postoperative stroke in cardiac surgery is related to the location and extent of atherosclerotic disease in the ascending aorta. J Am Coll Cardiol 2001;38:131–5.

130. Clark RE, Brillman J, Davis DA, Lovell MR, Price TRP, Magovern GJ. Microemboli during coronary artery bypass grafting. Genesis and effect on outcome. J Thorac Cardiovasc Surg 1995;109:249–58.

131. Schwartz AE, Sandhu AA, Kaplon RJ, et al. Cerebral blood flow is determined by arterial pressure and not cardiopulmonary bypass flow rate. Ann Thorac Surg 1995;60:165–70.

132. Croughwell N, Lyth M, Quill TJ, et al. Diabetic patients have abnormal cerebral autoregulation during cardiopulmonary bypass. Circulation 1990;82(suppl):IV-407–12.

133. Sungurtekin H, Boston US, Orszulak TA, Cook DJ. Effect of cerebral embolization on regional autoregulation during cardiopulmonary bypass in dogs. Ann Thorac Surg 2000;69:1130–4.

134. Kalyani SD, Miller NR, Dong LM, Baumgartner WA, Alejo DE, Gilbert TB. Incidence of and risk factors for perioperative optic neuropathy after cardiac surgery. Ann Thorac Surg 2004; 78:34–7.

135. Nuttall GA, Garrity JA, Dearani JA, Abel MD, Schroeder DR, Mullany CJ. Risk factors for ischemic optic neuropathy after cardiopulmonary bypass: a matched case/control study. Anesth Analg 2001;93:1410–6.

136. Barbut D, Grassineau D, Lis E, Heier L, Hartman GS, Isom OW. Posterior distribution of infarcts in strokes related to cardiac operations. Ann Thorac Surg 1998;65:1656–9.

137. Zacharias A, Schwann TA, Riordan CJ, et al. Operative and 5-year outcomes of combined carotid and coronary revascularization: review of a large contemporary experience. Ann Thorac Surg 2002;83:491–8.

138. Wilson MJ, Boyd SYN, Lisagor PG, Rubal BJ, Cohen DJ. Ascending aortic atheroma assessed intraoperatively by epiaortic and transesophageal echocardiography. Ann Thorac Surg 2000; 70:25–30.

139. Banbury MK, Kouchoukos NT, Allen KB, et al. Emboli capture using the Embol-X intraaortic filter in cardiac surgery: a multicentered randomized trial of 1,289 patients. Ann Thorac Surg 2003;76:508–15.

140. Stump DA, Jones TJJ, Rorie KD. Neurophysiologic monitoring and outcomes in cardiovascular surgery. J Cardiothorac Vasc Anesth 1999;13:600–13.

141. Wityk RJ, Goldsborough MA, Hillis A, et al. Diffusion- and perfusion-weighted brain magnetic resonance imaging in patients with neurologic complications after cardiac surgery. Arch Neurol 2001;58:571–6.

142. Salazar JD, Wityk RJ, Grega MA, et al. Stroke after cardiac surgery: short- and long-term outcomes. Ann Thorac Surg 2001;72:1195–202.

143. Stump DA, Rogers AT, Hammon JW, Newman SP. Cerebral emboli and cognitive outcome after cardiac surgery. J Cardiothorac Vasc Anesth 1996;10:113–9.

144. van der Mast RC, van den Broek WW, Fekkes D, Pepplinkhuizen L, Habbema JD. Incidence of and preoperative predictors for delirium after cardiac surgery. J Psychosom Res 1999;46:479–83.

145. Bucerius J, Gummert JF, Borger MA, et al. Predictors of delirium after cardiac surgery: effect of beating-heart (off-pump) surgery. J Thorac Cardiovasc Surg 2004;127:57–64.

146. Maldonado JR, van der Starre PJ, Wysong A. Post-operative sedation and the incidence of ICU delirium in cardiac surgery patients. Presented at the American Society of Anesthesiologists Annual Meeting, San Francisco, October 2003.

147. Hassaballa HA, Balk RA. Torsade de pointes associated with the administration of intravenous haloperidol: a review of the literature and practical guidelines for use. Expert Opin Drug Saf 2003;2:543–7.

148. Skrobik YK, Bergeron N, Dumont M, Gottfried SB. Olanzapine vs haloperidol: treating delirium in a critical care setting. Intensive Care Med 2004;30:444–9.

149. Bayindir O, Akpinar B, Can E, Guden M, Sonmez B, Demiroglu C. The use of the 5-HT$_3$-receptor antagonist ondansetron for the treatment of postcardiotomy delirium. J Cardiothorac Vasc Anesth 2000;14:288–92.

150. Kosten TR, O'Connor PG. Management of drug and alcohol withdrawal. N Engl J Med 2003;348:1786–95.

151. McCowan C. Refractory delirium tremens treated with propofol: a case series. Crit Care Med 2000;28:1781–4.

152. Arrowsmith JE, Grocott HP, Newman NF. Neurological risk assessment, monitoring and outcome in cardiac surgery. J Cardiothorac Vasc Anesth 1999;13:736–43.

153. Selnes OA, Goldsborough MA, Borowicz LM Jr, Enger C, Quaskey SA, McKhann GM. Determinants of cognitive change after coronary artery bypass surgery: a multifactorial problem. Ann Thorac Surg 1999;67;1669–76.

154. Van Dijk D, Keizer AMA, Diephius JC, Durand C, Vos LJ, Hijman R. Neurocognitive dysfunction after coronary artery bypass surgery: a systematic review. J Thorac Cardiovasc Surg 2000; 120:632–9.

155. Ho PM, Arciniegas DB, Grigsby J, et al. Predictors of neurocognitive decline following coronary artery bypass graft surgery. Ann Thorac Surg 2004;77:597–603.

156. Diegeler A, Hirsch R, Schneider R, et al. Neuromonitoring and neurocognitive outcome in off-pump versus conventional coronary bypass operation. Ann Thorac Surg 2000;69:1162–6.

157. Van Dijk D, Jansen EWL, Hijman R, et al. for the Octopus Study Group. Cognitive outcome after off-pump and on-pump coronary artery bypass graft surgery: a randomized trial. JAMA 2002;287:1405–12.

158. Gold JP, Charlson ME, Williams-Russo P, et al. Improvement of outcomes after coronary artery bypass. A randomized trial comparing intraoperative high versus low mean arterial pressure. J Thorac Cardiovasc Surg 1995;110:1302–14.

159. Goto T, Baba T, Honma K, et al. Magnetic resonance imaging findings and postoperative neurologic dysfunction in elderly patients undergoing coronary artery bypass grafting. Ann Thorac Surg 2001;72:137–42.

160. Hall RA, Fordyce DJ, Lee ME, et al. Brain SPECT imaging and neuropsychological testing in coronary artery bypass patients. Ann Thorac Surg 1999;68:2082–8.

161. Keizer AMA, Hijman R, van Dijk D, Kalkman CJ, Kahn RS. Cognitive self-assessment one year after on-pump and off-pump coronary artery bypass grafting. Ann Thorac Surg 2003;75:835–9.

162. Newman MF, Kirchner JL, Phillips-Bute B, et al. Longitudinal assessment of neurocognitive function after coronary artery bypass surgery. N Engl J Med 201;344:395–402.

163. Selnes OA, Royall RM, Grega MA, Borowicz LM Jr, Quaskey S, McKhann GM. Cognitive changes 5 years after coronary artery bypass grafting. Is there evidence of late decline? Arch Neurol 2001;58:598–604.

164. Pignay-Demaria V, Lesperance F, Demaria RG, Frasure-Smith N, Perrault LP. Depression and anxiety and outcomes of coronary artery bypass surgery. Ann Thorac Surg 2003;75:314–21.

165. Peterson JC, Charlson ME, Williams-Russo P, et al. New postoperative depressive symptoms and long-term cardiac outcomes after coronary artery bypass surgery. Am J Geriatr Psychiatry 2002;10:192–8.

166. Piper SN, Koetter KO, Triem JG, et al. Critical illness polyneuropathy following cardiac surgery. Scand Cardiovasc J 1998;32:309–12.

167. Jellish WS, Blakeman B. Warf P, Slogoff S. Hands-up positioning during asymmetric sternal retraction for internal mammary artery harvest: a possible method to reduce brachial plexus injury. Anesth Analg 1997;84:260–5.

168. Thomas NJ, Harvey AT. Paraplegia after coronary bypass operations: relationship to severe hypertension and vascular disease. J Thorac Cardiovasc Surg 1999;117:834–6.

169. Geyer TE, Naik MJ, Pillai R. Anterior spinal artery syndrome after elective coronary artery bypass grafting. Ann Thorac Surg 2002;73:1971–3.

170. Hamdan AL, Moukarbel RV, Farhat F, Obeid M. Vocal cord paralysis after open-heart surgery. Eur J Cardiothorac Surg 2002;21:671–4.

171. D'Ancona G, Baillot R, Poirier B, et al. Determinants of gastrointestinal complications in cardiac surgery. Tex Heart Inst J 2003;30:280–5.

172. Zacharias A, Schwann TA, Parenteau GL, et al. Predictors of gastrointestinal complications in cardiac surgery. Tex Heart Inst J 2000;27:93–9.

173. Poirier B, Baillot R, Bauset R, et al. Abdominal complications associated with cardiac surgery. Review of a contemporary surgical experience and a series done without extracorporeal circulation. Can J Surg 2003;46:176–82.

174. Byhahn C, Strouhal U, Martens S, Mierdl S, Kessler P, Westphal K. Incidence of gastrointestinal complications in cardiopulmonary bypass patients. World J Surg 2001;25:1140–4.

175. Fitzgerald T, Kim D, Karakozis S, Alam H, Provido H, Kirkpatrick J. Visceral ischemia after cardiopulmonary bypass. Am Surg 2000;66:623–6.

176. Sakorafas FH, Tsiotos GG. Intra-abdominal complications after cardiac surgery. Eur J Surg 1999;165:820–7.

177. Simic O, Strathausen S, Hess W, Ostermeyer J. Incidence and prognosis of abdominal complications after cardiopulmonary bypass. Cardiovasc Surg 1999;7:419–24.

178. Kumle B, Boldt J, Suttner SW, Piper SN, Lehmann A, Blome M. Influence of prolonged cardiopulmonary bypass times on splanchnic perfusion and markers of splanchnic organ function. Ann Thorac Surg 2003;75:1558–64.

179. Baue AE. The role of the gut in the development of multiple organ dysfunction in cardiothoracic patients. Ann Thorac Surg 1993;55:822–9.

180. Sanisoglu I, Guden M, Bayramoglu Z, et al. Does off-pump CABG reduce gastrointestinal complications? Ann Thorac Surg 2004;77:619–25.

181. White PF. Droperidol: a cost-effective antiemetic for over thirty years. Anesth Analg 2002; 95:789–90.

182. Hill RP, Lubarsky DA, Phillips-Bute B, et al. Cost-effectiveness of prophylactic antiemetic therapy with ondansetron, droperidol, or placebo. Anesthesiology 2000;92:958–67.

183. Ferraris VA, Ferraris SP, Moritz DM, Welch S. Oropharyngeal dysphagia after cardiac operations. Ann Thorac Surg 2001;71:1792–6.

184. Harrington OB, Duckworth JK, Starnes CL, et al. Silent aspiration after coronary artery bypass grafting. Ann Thorac Surg 1998;65:1599–603.

185. Hogue CW Jr, Lappas GD, Creswell LL, et al. Swallowing dysfunction after cardiac operations. Associated adverse outcomes and risk factors including intraoperative transesophageal echocardiography. J Thorac Cardiovasc Surg 1995;110:517–22.

186. Rousou JA, Tighe DA, Garb JL, et al. Risk of dysphagia after transesophageal echocardiography during cardiac operations. Ann Thorac Surg 2000;69:486–9.

187. Partik BL, Scharitzer M, Schueller G, et al. Videofluoroscopy of swallowing abnormalities in 22 symptomatic patients after cardiovascular surgery. Am J Roentgenol 2003;180:987–92.

188. Hackert T, Keinle P, Weitz J, et al. Accuracy of diagnostic laparoscopy for early diagnosis of abdominal complications after cardiac surgery. Surg Endosc 2003;17:1671–4.

189. Ponec RJ, Saunders MD, Kimmey MB. Neostigmine for the treatment of acute colonic pseudoobstruction. N Engl J Med 1999;341:137–41.

190. Rady MY, Kodavatiganti R, Ryan T. Perioperative predictors of acute cholecystitis after cardiovascular surgery. Chest 1998;114:76–84.

191. Fennerty MB. Pathophysiology of the upper gastrointestinal tract in the critically ill patient. Rationale for the therapeutic benefits of acid suppression. Crit Care Med 2002;30(suppl): S351–5.

192. Conrad SA. Acute upper gastrointestinal bleeding in critically ill patients: causes and treatment modalities. Crit Care Med 2002;30(suppl):S365–8.

193. Steinberg KP. Stress-related mucosal disease in the critically ill patient: risk factors and strategies to prevent stress-related bleeding in the intensive care unit. Crit Care Med 2002;30(suppl): S362–4.

194. Van der Voort PHJ, Zandstra DF. Pathogenesis, risk factors, and incidence of upper gastrointestinal bleeding after cardiac surgery: is specific prophylaxis in routine bypass procedures needed? J Cardiothorac Vasc Anesth 2000;14:293–9.

195. Lau JYW, Sung JJY, Lee KKC, et al. Effect of intravenous omeprazole on recurrent bleeding after endoscopic treatment of bleeding peptic ulcers. N Engl J Med 2000;343:310–6.

196. Darcy M. Treatment of lower gastrointestinal bleeding: vasopressin infusion versus embolization. J Vasc Interv Radiol 2003;14:535–43.

197. Kirkpatrick ID, Kroeker MA, Greenberg HM. Biphasic CT with mesenteric CT angiography in the evaluation of acute mesenteric ischemia: initial experience. Radiology 2003;229:91–8.

198. Klotz S, Vestring T, Rotker J, Schmidt C, Scheld HH, Schmid C. Diagnosis and treatment of nonocclusive mesenteric ischemia after open heart surgery. Ann Thorac Surg 2001;72:1583–6.

199. Wang MJ, Chao A, Huang CH, et al. Hyperbilirubinemia after cardiac operation. Incidence, risk factors, and clinical significance. J Thorac Cardiovasc Surg 1994;108:429–36.

200. Raman JS, Kochi K, Morimatsu H, Buxton B, Bellomo R. Severe ischemic early liver injury after cardiac surgery. Ann Thorac Surg 2002;74:1601–6.

201. Riordan SM, Williams R. Treatment of hepatic encephalopathy. N Engl J Med 1997;337:473–9.

202. Ihaya A, Muraoka R, Chiba Y, et al. Hyperamylasemia and subclinical pancreatitis after cardiac surgery. World J Surg 2001;25:862–4.

203. Lonardo A, Grisendi A, Bonilauri S, Rambaldi M, Selmi I, Tondelli E. Ischaemic necrotizing pancreatitis after cardiac surgery. A case report and review of the literature. J Gastroenterol Hepatol 1999;31:872–5.

204. Baron TH, Morgan DE. Acute necrotizing pancreatitis. N Engl J Med 1999;340:1412–6.

205. Cerra FB, Benitez MR, Blackburn GL, et al. Applied nutrition in ICU patients. A consensus statement of the American College of Chest Physicians. Chest 1997;111:769–78.

206. Vesey JM, Otto CM. Complications of prosthetic heart valves. Curr Cardiol Rep 2004;6:106–11.

207. Vink R, Van Den Brink RB, Levi M. Management of anticoagulation therapy for patients with prosthetic heart valves and atrial fibrillation. Hematalogy 2004;9:1–9.

208. Rinaldi CA, Heppell RM, Chambers JB. Treatment of left-sided prosthetic valve thrombosis: thrombolysis or surgery? J Heart Valve Dis 2002;11:839–43.

209. Ginsberg JS, Chan WS, Bates SM, Kaatz S. Anticoagulation of pregnant women with mechanical heart valves. Arch Intern Med 2003;163:694–8.

210. Vlessis AA, Khaki A, Grunkemeier GL, Li HH, Starr A. Risk, diagnosis, and management of prosthetic valve endocarditis: a review. J Heart Valve Disease 1997;6:443–65.

211. Gordon SM, Serkey JM, Longworth DL, Lytle BW, Cosgrove DM III. Early onset prosthetic valve endocarditis: the Cleveland Clinic experience 1982–1987. Ann Thorac Surg 2000; 69:1388–92.

212. Werba JP, Tremoli E, Masironi P, et al. Statins in coronary bypass surgery: rationale and clinical use. Ann Thorac Surg 2003;76:2132–40.

213. Lazar HL. Role of statin therapy in the coronary bypass patient. Ann Thorac Surg 2004;78:730–40.

214. Charlson ME, Isom OW. Care after coronary-artery bypass surgery. N Engl J Med 2003;348: 1456–63.

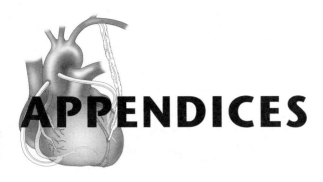

APPENDICES

Typical Preoperative Order Sheet

1. Admit to: _____
2. Surgery date: _____
3. Planned procedure: _____
4. Laboratory tests:
   - ☐ CBC with differential
   - ☐ PT/INR   ☐ PTT
   - ☐ Electrolytes, BUN, creatinine, blood sugar
   - ☐ Bilirubin, AST, ALT, alkaline phosphatase, albumin
   - ☐ Urinalysis
   - ☐ Electrocardiogram
   - ☐ Chest x-ray PA and lateral
   - ☐ Antibody screen   ☐ Crossmatch: ___ units PRBC
   - ☐ Other:
5. Treatments/Assessments
   Admission vital signs
   Obtain room air O_2 by pulse oximetry; ABG if < 90%
   Measure height and weight
   NPO after midnight except sips of water with meds
   Shave/Hibiclens scrub to chest and legs
   Incentive spirometry teaching
6. Medications
   - ☐ Peridex gargle on-call to OR
   - ☐ Cefazolin 1 gm IV to OR with patient
   - ☐ Vancomycin 15 mg/kg = ____ g IV to OR with patient
   - ☐ Discontinue aspirin, clopidogrel, NSAIDs immediately
   - ☐ Stop heparin at _____
   - ☐ Continue heparin drip into OR
   - ☐ Discontinue low-molecular-weight heparin after AM dose on _____
   - ☐ Stop IIb/IIIa inhibitors at _____
   - ☐ Other:

Typical Orders for Admission to the ICU

1. Admit to ICU
2. Procedure: _____
3. Condition: _____
4. Vital signs q15 min until stable, then q30 min
5. Continuous ECG, arterial, PA tracings, Sao_2 on bedside monitor
6. Cardiac output q15 min × 1h, then q1h × 4 h, then q2–4h when stable
7. Chest tubes to chest drainage system with 20 cm H_2O suction; record hourly
8. Urinary catheter to gravity drainage and record hourly
9. Elevate head of bed to 30 degrees
10. Hourly I&O
11. Daily weights
12. Advance activity after extubation (dangle, out of bed to chair)
13. GI/nutrition:
    - ☐ NPO while intubated
    - ☐ Nasogastric tube to low suction
    - ☐ Clear liquids as tolerated 1h after extubation and removal of NG tube
14. Ventilator settings _____
    - Fio_2: _____ in SIMV mode
    - IMV rate: _____ breaths/min
    - Tidal volume: _____ mL
    - PEEP: _____ cm H_2O
    - Pressure support: ____ cm H_2O
15. Respiratory care
    - ☐ Endotracheal suction q4h, then prn
    - ☐ Wean ventilator to extubate per protocol
    - ☐ O_2 via face mask with Fio_2 0.6–1.0 per protocol
    - ☐ O_2 via nasal prongs @ 2–6 liters/min to keep $Sao_2 > 95\%$
    - ☐ Incentive spirometer q1h when awake
16. Laboratory tests
    - ☐ STAT ABGs, CBC, electrolytes, glucose
    - ☐ STAT PT, PTT, platelet count if chest tube output > 100/h
    - ☐ STAT chest x-ray
    - ☐ STAT ECG
    - ☐ ABGs 4 h after arrival, prior to weaning and prior to extubation
    - ☐ HCT, K^+ every 4–6 h and prn
    - ☐ In morning of POD #1: ECG, CXR, electrolytes, BUN, creatinine, CBC

(continued)

17. Pacemaker settings: Mode: ☐ Atrial ☐ VVI ☐ DVI ☐ DDD

                    Atrial output: ___ mA Ventricular output ____ mA

                    Rate: ___ min AV interval: ___ msecs

                    ☐ Pacer attached but off

18. Notify MD/PA for:

    a. Systolic blood pressure < 90 or > 140 mm Hg

    b. Cardiac index <1.8 liters/min/m^2

    c. Urine output <30 mL/h × 2 h

    d. Chest tube drainage >100 mL/h

    e. Temperature >38.5°C

19. Medications

Allergies _____

    a. IV drips

        ☐ Dextrose 5% in 0.45 NS 250 mL via Cordis/triple lumen at KVO

        ☐ Arterial line and distal Swan-Ganz port: heparin 250 U/250 mL NS at 3 mL/h

        ☐ Epinephrine 1 mg/250 mL D5W: _____ µg/min to maintain cardiac index >2.0

        ☐ Milrinone 20 mg/100 mL NS: _____ µg/kg/min

        ☐ Norepinephrine 8 mg/250 mL D5W: _____ µg/min to keep systolic BP >100

        ☐ Phenylephrine 40 mg/250 mL D5W: _____ µg/min to keep systolic BP >100

        ☐ Nitroprusside 50 mg/250 mL D5W: _____ µg/kg/min to keep systolic BP <130

        ☐ Nitroglycerin 100 mg/250 mL D5W: _____ µg/kg/min

        ☐ Lidocaine 2 g/250 mL D5W: _____ mg/min IV; wean off at 06:00 POD #1

        ☐ Diltiazem: 100 mg/100 mL D5W: _____ mg/h

        ☐ Other: _____

        ☐ Other: _____

    b. Antibiotics

        ☐ Cefazolin 1 g IV q8h for 6 doses

        ☐ Vancomycin 1 g IV q12h for 4 doses

    c. Sedatives/analgesics

        ☐ Propofol infusion 10 mg/mL: 25–50 µg/kg/min per protocol

        ☐ Midazolam 2 mg IV q2h prn agitation; stop after extubation

        ☐ Morphine sulfate 25 mg/100 mL D5W: 0.01–0.02 mg/kg continuous IV infusion; supplement with 2–5 mg IV q1–2h prn for breakthrough pain; discontinue in AM POD #1

        ☐ Meperidine 25 mg IV prn shivering

        ☐ Ketorolac 15–30 mg IV q6h prn for breakthrough pain; d/c after 72 h

(*continued*)

d. Other medications

- ☐ Metoprolol 25 mg PO/per NG tube starting 8 h after arrival, then q12h; hold for HR <60 or SBP <100
- ☐ Digoxin 0.25 mg IV q6h × 2 doses starting 8 h after arrival; then 0.25 mg PO q6h × 2 doses, then 0.25 mg PO qd; hold for HR <60
- ☐ Magnesium sulfate 2 g IV on POD #1 in AM
- ☐ Sucralfate 1 g per NG tube q6h until NG tube removed
- ☐ Pantoprazole (Protonix) 40 mg PO qd
- ☐ Aspirin ☐ 325 mg ☐ 81 mg PO qd (starting 6 hours after arrival); hold for platelet count <75,000 or chest tube drainage >50 mL/h
- ☐ Warfarin _____ mg starting _____ ; check with HO for daily dose

e. PRN medications

- ☐ Acetaminophen 650 mg PO/PR q4h prn temp > 38.5°C
- ☐ Droperidol 0.625–1.25 mg IV q6h prn nausea
- ☐ Ondansetron 4 mg IV prn nausea
- ☐ KCl 80mEq/250 mL D5W via central line to keep K⁺ > 4.5 meq/liter:

    K⁺ 4.0–4.5 KCl 10 mEq over 30 min

    K⁺ 3.5–3.9 KCl 20 mEq over 60 min

    K⁺ < 3.5   KCl 40 mEq over 90 min

- ☐ Initiate hyperglycemia protocol if BS >240 mg/dL on admission or >180 mg/dL 8 h after admission
- ☐ Other

Transfer Orders from the ICU

ALLERGIES:

1. Transfer to _____
2. Procedure: _____
3. Condition: _____
4. Vital signs q4h × 2 days, then qshift
5. ECG telemetry
6. I&O q8h
7. Daily weights
8. Foley catheter to gravity drainage; D/C at _____ ; due to void in 8 h
9. Spo$_2$ q8h and 1 time before and after ambulation
10. Chest tubes to –20 cm H$_2$O suction
11. Diet
    - □ NPO
    - □ Clear liquids/no added salt (NAS)
    - □ Full liquids/NAS
    - □ NAS, low fat, low cholesterol diet
    - □ Fluid restriction ___ mL per 24 hours (IV + PO)
    - □ _____ cal ADA, NAS low cholesterol diet, if diabetic
12. Activity
    - □ Bed rest
    - □ OOB and ambulate with assistance per protocol
13. Elastic antiembolism (TEDs) stockings
14. Dry sterile dressing changes qd until POD #4
15. Temporary pacemaker settings:
    - □ Pacemaker on: Mode: □ Atrial □ VVI □ DVI □ DDD
      Atrial output ____ mA   Ventricular output ____ mA
      Rate ___ /min   AV interval: ____ msecs
    - □ Pacer attached but off
    - □ Detach pacer but keep at bedside
16. Respiratory care
    - □ Oxygen via nasal prongs at 2–6 L/min to keep Spo$_2$ >92%
    - □ Incentive spirometer q1h when awake
17. Wire and wound care per protocol

(continued)

18. Laboratory studies
   □ Chest x-ray after chest tube removal
   □ Daily PT, PTT if on heparin/warfarin
   □ Daily platelet count if on heparin
   □ Glucose via fingerstick/glucometer AC and qHS in diabetics
   □ Chest x-ray, ECG, CBC, electrolytes, BUN, creatinine day prior to discharge

MEDICATIONS:

1. Antibiotics
   □ Cefazolin 1 g IV q8h for ____ more doses (6 doses total)
   □ Vancomycin 1 g IV q12h for ___ more doses (4 doses total)
2. Cardiac medications
   □ Metoprolol __ mg PO q12h. Hold for HR <60 and SBP <100
   □ Digoxin 0.25 mg PO qd. Hold for HR <60
   □ Antihypertensives:
   □ Diltiazem 100 mg/100 mL NS @ ___ mg/h × 24 h, then 30 mg PO qid (radial artery grafts)
3. Anticoagulants/antiplatelet agents
   □ Enteric-coated aspirin 325 mg PO qd (coronary bypass patients); hold for platelet count <75,000
   □ Enteric-coated aspirin 81 mg (if on warfarin)
   □ Heparin 25,000 U/500 mL D5W at _____ U/h starting on _____ (per protocol)
   □ Coumadin ___ mg PO qd starting on ____ ; daily dose check with HO
4. Pain medications
   □ Morphine sulfate via PCA pump or 10 mg IM q3h prn severe pain
   □ Ketorolac 15–30 mg IV q6h prn pain, D/C after 72 hours
   □ Acetaminophen with oxycodone (Percocet) 1 tab PO q4h prn pain
   □ Acetaminophen with codeine (Tylenol #3) 1–2 tabs PO q4h prn pain
5. GI medications
   □ Pantoprazole (Protonix) 40 mg PO qd
   □ For nausea:
      □ Metoclopramide 10 mg IV/PO q6h prn
      □ Prochlorperazine 10 mg PO/IM q6h prn
   □ Milk of magnesia 30 mL PO qhs prn
   □ Metamucil 12 g in H_2O qd prn constipation
   □ Docusate (Colace) 100 mg PO bid
   □ Dulcolax suppository PR qd prn constipation

(continued)

6. Diabetic patients

☐ Oral hypoglycemic: _____

☐ ____ units regular Humulin insulin SC ____ qAM ____ qPM

☐ ____ units NPH Humulin insulin SC ____ qAM ____ qPM

☐ Sliding scale: treat fingerstick/glucometer BS according the following scale at 06:00, 11:00, 15:00, and 20:00

    161–200, give ___ units regular Humulin insulin SC

    201–250, give ___ units regular Humulin insulin SC

    251–300, give ___ units regular Humulin insulin SC

    >300, call house officer

7. Other medications

☐ Acetaminophen 650 mg PO q3h prn temp >38.5°C

☐ Chloral hydrate 0.5–1.0 g PO qhs prn sleep

☐ Furosemide ____ mg IV/PO q ____ h

☐ Potassium chloride ____ mEq PO bid (while on furosemide)

☐ Albuterol 2.5 mg/2.5 mL NS via nebulizer q6h prn

☐ Other medications:

8. Saline lock, flush q8h and prn

Typical ICU Flowsheet

Tufts-New England Medical Center
**ADULT CARDIOTHORACIC ICU
PATIENT CARE RECORD**

DATE: ___/___/___   POD # _____   SURGEON: _____
PAGE # _____   PROCEDURE: _____

VITAL SIGNS

TIME	T	RHY/RATE	BP	CVP	PAD/PCW	CO/CI	SVR/SV	IABP Ratio	RIKER	PAIN
1										
2										
3										
4										
5										

IV INFUSIONS

mL	DOSE	mL	DOSE	mL	DOSE

IV INFUSIONS

mL	DOSE	mL	DOSE	mL	DOSE

MEDICATIONS

NAME/DOSE ROUTE

COMMENTS

COLLOID

TYPE   AMOUNT

FEEDS

URINE

AMT	NG	OTHER
TOTAL		

CHEST TUBES

AMT	AMT	AMT
TOTAL	TOTAL	TOTAL

PULSES

	LEFT	RIGHT	OTHER
	DP PT	DP PT	

VENTILATION

Vent Mode	FiO2/PEEP	TV/Rate	Pt's Rate	Press Supp

BLOOD GASES

pH	pCO2	pO2	HCO3	O2 Sat

OTHER

Hct	Plts	Pt		
Hgb	WBC	PTT		

HEMATOLOGY/CHEMISTRY

Na	K	BUN	BS	iCa	Mg	OTHER
INR	Cr		TCa	phos		

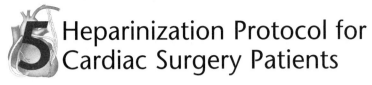

Heparinization Protocol for Cardiac Surgery Patients

Indication: _____

1. Patient weight: ___ kg
2. PT, PTT, CBC and platelet count prior to starting heparin
3. Initial PTT 6 h after starting infusion (4 h if a bolus is given)
4. Recheck PTT after changing infusion rate per chart
5. Daily PTT in AM
6. Check platelet count daily if < 100,000 and qod if > 100,000 while on heparin
7. Guaiac all stools
8. Notify house officer for any bleeding, PTT < 35 or > 100 seconds
9. Discontinue all previous heparin orders. Hold heparin bolus and drip for 12 h after last dose of low-molecular-weight heparin
10. Heparin bolus
    □ No bolus
    □ Give IV bolus of 80 units/kg = _____ units (round to nearest 100)
11. Heparin infusion 25,000 units/250 mL D5W @ _____ units/h
    * 15 units/kg for unstable angina, atrial fibrillation, prosthetic heart valves (therapeutic range 50–70 seconds)
    * 18 units/kg for deep venous thrombosis or pulmonary embolism (therapeutic range 60–85 seconds)
12. Heparin adjustment schedule (for postoperative AF or prosthetic heart valves)

PTT	Infusion Rate	Next PTT
< 40	Bolus with 40 units/kg and increase drip by 4 units/kg/h	4 h
41–50	Bolus with 25 units/kg and increase drip by 2 units/kg/h	6 h
51–70	No change	Daily once 2 PTTs 6 h apart are in therapeutic range
71–80	Reduce by 1 unit/kg/h	6 h
81–90	Reduce by 2 units/kg/h	6 h
91–100	Stop for 1 h and reduce by 3 units/kg/h	4 h
> 100	Stop for 2 h & reduce by 4 units/kg/h	4 h

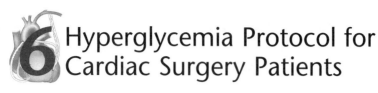

Hyperglycemia Protocol for Cardiac Surgery Patients

Goal: to maintain blood sugar (BS) between 110 and 180 mg/dL after surgery

1. Check glucometer BS q2h; increase to q1h during rapidly changing conditions and decrease to q4h if no changes in insulin drip rate for 6 h and serum BS < 180 on 3 consecutive measurements
2. Correlate glucometer BS to serum BS daily
3. Maintain serum potassium > 4 mEq/L
4. Page house officer for BS < 90 or > 320
5. Initiate protocol for BS > 240 on admission to ICU or BS > 180 at 8 h

BS	Regular Insulin IV Bolus	Infusion Rate*
181–200	No bolus	0.5 unit/h
201–240	3 units	1 unit/h
241–280	5 units	1 unit/h
281–320	10 units	2 units/h

*Regular humulin insulin 100 units in 100 mL NS

6. Adjustment protocol of insulin infusion

<95	IV bolus with 12.5 g (25 mL) of 50% dextrose and lower infusion by 1 unit/h
96–110	Lower infusion by 0.5 unit/h
111–180	No change in infusion rate
181–225	Increase infusion rate by 0.5 unit/h
226–250	IV bolus with 5 units and increase infusion by 0.5 unit/h
251–320	IV bolus with 10 units and increase infusion by 1 unit/h
>320	Page house officer

7. Transitioning from infusion to SC insulin:

24 h requirement in units divided by 8 = × units = _____ units

Give first SC dose 30 min before stopping insulin infusion

BS adjustment to insulin regimen

≤ 80	Page house officer
81–120	Give ___ units SC q6h (× – 4 units)
121–160	Give ___ units SC (× – 2 units)
161–200	Give ___ units SC q6h (× units)
201–240	Give ___ units SC q6h (× + 2 units)
> 240	Page house officer

Doses of Parenteral Medications Commonly Used in the ICU and Their Modifications in Renal Failure

Drug Class	Usual Dosage	Route of Elimination*	Adjustment in Moderate Renal Failure
Analgesics			
Fentanyl	50–100 µg IV → 50–200 µg/h	H	No change
Ketorolac	30–60 mg IV q6h (×72 h)	R	Reduce
Meperidine	50–100 mg IM q3h	H	Use with caution
Morphine	2–10 mg IV/IM q2–4h	H	No change
Antacids			
Pantoprazole (Protonix)	40 mg IV over 15 min	H	No change
Ranitidine (Zantac)	50 mg IV q8h or 6.25 mg/h	R	Reduce
Antianginals			
Esmolol	0.25–0.5 mg/kg IV → 0.05–0.2 mg/kg/min IV	M	No change
Metoprolol	5 mg IV q15 min × 3	H	No change

(*continued*)

Drug Class	Usual Dosage	Route of Elimination*	Adjustment in Moderate Renal Failure
Antiarrhythmics (see also Table 11.12, pages 443, 444–449)			
Amiodarone	150 mg IV → 1 mg/min × 6 h → 0.5 mg/min × 18 h, then 1 g/day	H	No change
Digoxin	0.125–0.25 mg IV qd	R	Reduce
Lidocaine	1 mg/kg IV → 1–4 mg/min	H	No change
Procainamide	10 mg/kg IV → 1–4 mg/min	R > H	Reduce
Antibiotics (Prophylactic Doses)			
Cefamandole	1 g IV q4–6h	R	Reduce
Cefazolin	1 g IV q8h	R	Reduce
Ceftriaxone	1 g IV q24h	R	Reduce
Vancomycin	15 mg/kg IV, then 1 g IV q8–12h	R	Reduce
Antiemetics			
Dolasetron (Anzemet)	12.5 mg IV	H/R	No change
Droperidol (Inapsine)	0.625–1.25 mg IV	H	No change
Granisetron (Kytril)	1 µg/kg IV	H	No change
Metoclopramide (Reglan)	10–20 mg IM/IV qid	R > H	Reduce

(continued)

Drug Class	Usual Dosage	Route of Elimination*	Adjustment in Moderate Renal Failure
Antiemetics (*cont.*)			
Ondansetron (Zofran)	4–8 mg IV	H	No change
Prochlorperazine (Compazine)	5–10 mg IM q4h	H	No change
Antihypertensives (see Table 11.5, page 391)			
Diuretics			
Acetazolamide (Diamox)	250–500 mg IV q8h	R	Use with caution
Bumetanide	1–5 mg IV q12h 0.5–2 mg/h drip	R > H	Use with caution
Chlorothiazide	500 mg IV qd	R	Use with caution
Ethacrynic acid	50–100 mg IV q6h	H > R	Use with caution
Furosemide	10–500 mg IV q6h (10–40 mg/h) drip	R > H	Use with caution
Inotropic Agents (see Table 11.4, page 360)			
Paralytic Agents (see Table 4.3, page 147)			
Atracurium	0.4–0.5 mg/kg IV → 0.3 mg/kg/h	M	No change
Doxacurium	0.06 mg/kg → 0.005 mg/kg q30 min	R	Reduce
Pancuronium	0.1 mg/kg IV → 0.01 mg/kg q1h or 2–4 mg/h	R > H	No change

(continued)

Drug Class	Usual Dosage	Route of Elimination*	Adjustment in Moderate Renal Failure
Paralytic Agents (*cont.*)			
Vecuronium	0.1 mg/kg IV → 0.01 mg/kg q30–45 min or 2–6 mg/h	H	No change
Rocuronium	0.6–1.2 mg/kg IV	H	No change
Psychotropics/Sedatives			
Dexmedetomidine (Precedex)	1 µg/kg load, then 0.2–0.7 mg/kg/h	H	No change
Haloperidol (Haldol)	1–5 mg IM/IV q6h	H	No change
Lorazepam (Ativan)	1–2 mg IV/2–4 mg IM q6h	H	No change
Midazolam (Versed)	2.5–5 mg IV q1–2h	H	No change
Propofol (Diprivan)	25–50 µg/kg/min	M	No change
Other			
Aminophylline	5 mg/kg IV load → 0.2–0.9 mg/kg/h	H	No change
Flumazenil	0.2 mg over 30 sec, then 0.3 mg, then 0.5 mg up to 3 mg max/h	H	No change
Naloxone	0.4–2 mg IV	H	No change

* Medications metabolized by the liver do not require reduction in dosage for renal failure; medications metabolized by the kidneys must be adjusted according to the serum creatinine or, more precisely, by the glomerular filtration rate (creatinine clearance). The reader should refer to the *Physicians' Desk Reference* for complete prescribing information.

H = hepatic metabolism; R = renal elimination; M = metabolized in the bloodstream.

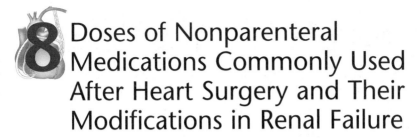

Doses of Nonparenteral Medications Commonly Used After Heart Surgery and Their Modifications in Renal Failure

Drug Class	Usual Dosage	Route of Elimination	Adjustment in Moderate Renal Failure
Analgesics			
Acetaminophen	650 mg PO q4h	R	Reduce
Ketorolac (Toradol)	20 mg PO → 10 mg q4–6h	R	Reduce
Ibuprofen	400–800 mg PO tid	R	Reduce
Oxycodone[a]	4.5 mg PO q6h	H	No change
Antacids/antireflux medications			
H₂ blockers			
Famotidine (Pepcid)	20–40 mg PO HS	R > M	Reduce
Nizatidine (Axid)	150 mg PO bid or 300 mg HS	R	Reduce
Ranitidine (Zantac)	150 mg PO bid	R	Reduce

(continued)

Drug Class	Usual Dosage	Route of Elimination	Adjustment in Moderate Renal Failure
Proton-pump inhibitors			
Pantoprazole (Protonix)	40 mg PO qd	H	No change
Omeprazole (Prilosec)	20 mg PO qd	H	No change
Others			
Sucralfate (Carafate)	1 g PO qid	R	Reduce
Antianginals[b]			
β-Blockers			
Atenolol	25–50 mg PO qd	R	Reduce
Metoprolol	25–100 mg PO bid	H	No change
Calcium channel blockers			
Diltiazem	30–60 mg PO tid	H	No change
Nicardipine	20–40 mg PO tid	H	No change
Nifedipine	10–30 mg PO/SL tid	H	No change
Verapamil	80–160 mg PO tid	H	No change
Nitrates			
Isosorbide dinitrate	5–40 mg PO tid	H	No change
Isosorbide mononitrate	20 mg PO bid (7 h apart)	–	No change
Nitropaste	1–3" q4h	H	No change

(continued)

Drug Class	Usual Dosage	Route of Elimination	Adjustment in Moderate Renal Failure
Antiarrhythmics (see Table 11.12, page 443, 444–449)			
Amiodarone	400 mg tid weaned to 200 mg qd	H	No change
Digoxin	0.125–0.25 mg qd	R	Reduce
Procainamide	Procan SR 500–1000 mg q6h Procanbid 500–1000 mg bid 375 mg PO q3–4h	R > H	Reduce
Sotalol	80 mg bid	R	Reduce
Antibiotics			
Cephalexin	500 mg PO qid	R	Reduce
Ciprofloxacin	500 mg PO bid	R	Reduce
Antidiabetic Drugs (oral hypoglycemics)			
Chlorpropamide (Diabinese)	250 mg qd	R	Avoid
Glipizide (Glucotrol)	5 mg qAM	H	No change
Glyburide (Micronase, DiaBeta)	2.5–5 mg qAM	H = R	Use with caution
Metformin (Glucophage)	500–1000 mg bid	R	Avoid
Pioglitazone (Actos)	15–30 mg qd	H	No change
Rosiglitazone (Avandia)	4–8 mg qd	H	No change

(continued)

Drug Class	Usual Dosage	Route of Elimination	Adjustment in Moderate Renal Failure
Antiemetics			
Dolasetron (Anzemet)	100 mg PO	H/R	No change
Metoclopramide (Reglan)	10–20 mg PO qid	R > H	Reduce
Ondansetron (Zofran)	8–16 mg PO	H	No change
Prochlorperazine (Compazine)	5–10 mg PO q6h	H	No change
Antihypertensives			
Angiotensin-converting enzyme (ACE) inhibitors			
Captopril (Capoten)	6.25–50 mg PO bid	R	Avoid
Enalapril (Vasotec)	2.5–5 mg PO qd	R	Avoid
Lisinopril (Zestril)	10 mg PO qd	R	Avoid
Quinapril (Accupril)	10 mg PO qd	R	Avoid
Angiotensin II receptor blockers (ARBs)			
Candesartan (Atacand)	8–32 mg PO qd or in 2 divided doses	H	No change

(continued)

Drug Class	Usual Dosage	Route of Elimination	Adjustment in Moderate Renal Failure
Angiotensin II receptor blockers (ARBs) (cont.)			
Irbesartan (Avapro)	150–300 mg PO qd	H	No change
Losartan (Cozaar)	25–100 mg PO qd or in 2 divided doses	H	No change
Valsartan (Diovan)	80–160 mg PO qd	H	No change
β-blockers (see also antianginals)			
Labetalol (Trandate, Normodyne)	100–400 mg PO qid	H	No change
Calcium channel blockers (see also antianginal medications)			
Amlodipine (Norvasc)	2.5–10 mg PO qd	H	No change
Nicardipine (Cardene)	20–40 mg PO tid	H	No change
Others			
Clonidine (Catapres)	0.1–0.3 mg PO bid	R	Reduce
Doxazosin (Cardura)	1–8 mg PO qd	H	No change
Prazosin (Minipress)	1–7.5 mg PO bid	H	No change

(continued)

Drug Class	Usual Dosage	Route of Elimination	Adjustment in Moderate Renal Failure
Cholesterol-lowering medications			
Atorvastatin (Lipitor)	10 mg PO qd	H	No change
Ezetimibe (Zetia)	10 mg PO qd	H	No change
Fluvastatin (Lescol)	20–40 mg PO qd	H	No change
Lovastatin (Mevacor)	20–40 mg PO qd	H	No change
Pravastatin (Pravachol)	10–20 mg PO qd	H	No change
Rosuvastatin (Crestor)	10–20 mg PO qd	H	No change
Simvastatin (Zocor)	5–10 mg PO qd	H	No change
Diuretics			
Acetazolamide (Diamox)	250–500 mg PO qid	R	Reduce
Furosemide (Lasix)	10–200 mg PO bid	R > H	No change
Hydrochlorothiazide (Hydrodivril)	50–100 mg PO qd	R	No change
Metolazone (Zaroxolyn)	5–20 mg PO qd	R	No change
Diuretics (Potassium Sparing)			
Amiloride (Midador)	5–10 mg PO qd	R	Avoid

(continued)

Drug Class	Usual Dosage	Route of Elimination	Adjustment in Moderate Renal Failure
Diuretics (Potassium Sparing) (*cont.*)			
Spironolactone (Aldactone)	25 mg qd	R	Avoid
Eplerenone (Inspra)	25–50 mg qd	H	No change
Psychotropics/Sedatives/Antidepressants			
Alprazolam (Xanax)	0.25–0.5 mg PO tid	H, R	Reduce
Amitriptyline (Elavil)	10–20 mg qhs or bid	H	No change
Bupropion (Wellbutrin)	100 mg PO bid	H	No change
Buspirone (Buspar)	7.5 mg PO bid	?	No change
Citalopram (Celexa)	20 mg PO qd	H	No change
Chlordiazepoxide (Librium)	5–25 mg PO tid	?	No change
Diphenhydramine (Benadryl)	50 mg PO HS	H	No change
Fluoxetine (Prozac)	20–40 mg PO qd	H	No change
Haloperidol (Haldol)	0.5–2.5 mg PO tid	H	No change
Lorazepam (Ativan)	1–2 mg PO bid or HS	H	No change

(*continued*)

Drug Class	Usual Dosage	Route of Elimination	Adjustment in Moderate Renal Failure
Psychotropics/Sedatives/Antidepressants (*cont.*)			
Paroxetine (Paxil)	20–50 mg PO qd	H/R	Reduce
Sertraline (Zoloft)	50–200 mg PO qd	H	No change
Venlafaxine (Effexor)	25 mg PO bid or tid	R	Reduce
Sleep Medications			
Chloral hydrate	500–1000 mg PO HS	H	No change
Diphenhydramine	25–50 mg PO HS	H	No change
Temazepam (Restoril)	15–30 mg PO HS	H	No change
Triazolam (Halcion)	0.125–0.25 mg PO HS	H	No change
Zaleplon (Sonata)	5–10 mg PO HS	H	No change
Zolpidem (Ambien)	10 mg PO HS	H	No change
Other			
Carbamazepine (Tegretol)	200 mg bid	H	No change

(*continued*)

Drug Class	Usual Dosage	Route of Elimination	Adjustment in Moderate Renal Failure
Other (*cont.*)			
Gabapentin (Neurontin)	300 mg qd–600 mg tid	R	Reduce
Theophylline (Theo-Dur)	300 mg PO bid	H	No change

Medications metabolized by the liver do not require reduction in dosage for renal failure; medications metabolized by the kidneys must be adjusted according to the serum creatinine, or more precisely, by the glomerular filtration rate. The reader should refer to the *Physicians' Desk Reference* for complete prescribing information

[a] = Usually given with acetaminophen 325 mg (Vicodin or Percocet).

[b] = Antianginal medications given four times a day (qid) are usually taken 4 h apart during the daytime. Other medications should generally be taken at equally spaced intervals.

H = hepatic metabolism; R = renal elimination; M = metabolized in bloodstream.

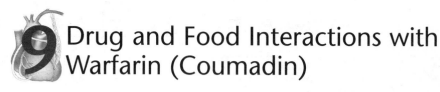 Drug and Food Interactions with Warfarin (Coumadin)

Potentiation (Increase INR)	Inhibition (Decrease INR)	No Effect
Acetaminophen	Azathioprine	Alcohol (if no liver disease)
Alcohol (if liver disease)	Barbiturates	Antacids
Amiodarone	Carbamazepine	Atenolol
Anabolic steroids	Chlordiazepoxide	Bumetanide
Cefamandole	Cholestyramine	Diltiazem
Cefazolin	Cyclosporine	Famotidine
Chloral hydrate	Dicloxacillin	Fluoxetine
Cimetidine	Multivitamins	Ibuprofen
Clofibrate	Nafcillin	Ketoconazole
Erythromycin	Phenytoin	Ketorolac
Floxin-antibiotics	Rifampin	Metoprolol
Fluconazole	**Sucralfate**	Nizatidine
Isoniazid	Trazodone	Ranitidine
Lovastatin		Vancomycin
Metronidazole	Alfalfa	
Omeprazole	Avocado	
Phenylbutazone	Green leafy vegetables	
Propranolol	Green tea	
Quinidine	Parsley	
Sulfamethoxazole/	Soybean oil	
Trimethaprim (Bactrim)		
Tamoxifen		
Garlic		
Ginger		
Ginkgo Biloba		
Grapefruit juice		

Reprinted in part from Hirsh J, Dalen JE, Anderson DR, et al. Oral anticoagulants mechanism of action, clinical effectiveness, and optimal therapeutic range. Chest 2001;119:8S–21S.

Definitions from the STS Data Specifications (2004)

Preoperative Conditions

1. **Chronic lung disease**
   a. Mild: FEV_1 60–75% of predicted, and/or on chronic inhaled or bronchodilator therapy
   b. Moderate: FEV_1 50–59% of predicted, and/or on chronic steroid therapy aimed at lung disease
   c. Severe: FEV_1 <50% of predicted, and/or room air pO_2 <60 torr or pCO_2 >50 torr

2. **Peripheral vascular disease:**
   a. Claudication either with exertion or at rest
   b. Prior amputation for arterial insufficiency; aortoiliac occlusive disease reconstruction; peripheral vascular bypass surgery, angioplasty, or stent; documented AAA, AAA repair, or stent
   c. Positive noninvasive testing documented
   d. Does **NOT** include carotid disease or procedures originating above the diaphragm

3. **Cerebrovascular disease:** any of the following:
   a. Unresponsive coma >24 h
   b. CVA (symptoms >72 h after onset)
   c. Reversible ischemic neurologic deficit (RIND) (recovery within 72 h after onset)
   d. Transient ischemic attack (TIA) (recovery within 24 h)
   e. Noninvasive carotid test with >75% occlusion
   f. Prior carotid surgery

4. **Diabetes:** history of diabetes, regardless of duration of disease or need for antidiabetic agents

5. **Renal failure:** documented history of renal failure and/or history of creatinine >2.0

6. **Hypercholesterolemia:** any of the following: total cholesterol >200, LDL >130, HDL < 30, or triglycerides >150 mg/dL

7. **Hypertension:** history of hypertension diagnosed and one of the following:
   a. Treated with medications, diet, and/or exercise
   b. BP >140 systolic or >90 diastolic on at least two occasions
   c. Currently on antihypertensive therapy

8. **Congestive heart failure** as evidenced within the preceding two weeks by: presence of paroxysmal nocturnal dyspnea, dyspnea on exertion, pulmonary congestion on CXR, or pedal edema/dyspnea and receiving diuretics or digoxin

9. **Stable angina:** angina controlled by oral or transcutaneous medication. May be pain free with/without medication but with a history of angina.

10. **Unstable angina:** angina that necessitates the initiation, continuation, or increase of angina control therapies that may include a nitroglycerin drip, heparin drip, or IABP placement. It may be characterized by any of the following:

  a. Rest angina

  b. New-onset exertional angina of at least CCS class III

  c. Recent acceleration of pattern and increase of one CCS class or to at least CCS class III

  d. Variant angina

  e. Non–Q-wave infarction

  f. Postinfarction angina

11. **Urgency**

  a. Emergent salvage: patient is undergoing CPR en route to the OR or prior to anesthesia induction

  b. Emergency: patient's clinical status includes any of the following:

   i. Ischemic dysfunction: (1) ongoing ischemia including rest angina despite maximal medical therapy, (2) acute evolving MI within 24 h before surgery, or (3) pulmonary edema requiring intubation

   ii. Mechanical dysfunction with shock with or without circulatory support

  c. Urgent: all of the following:

   i. Not elective or emergent

   ii. Procedure required during same hospitalization in order to minimize chance of further clinical deterioration

   iii. Any of the following may be included: worsening or sudden chest pain, CHF, acute MI, compelling anatomy, IABP, unstable angina with IV NTG or rest angina

  d. Elective: the patient's cardiac function has been stable for days or weeks prior to the operation. The procedure could be deferred without increased risk of compromised cardiac output.

Postoperative Complications

1. **Operative mortality:** death occurring during the hospitalization in which the operation was performed (even if after 30 days) or death occurring after hospital discharge, but within 30 days, unless the cause of death is clearly unrelated to the operation.

2. **Stroke**

  a. Permanent: central neurologic deficit persisting postoperatively for >72 h

  b. Transient: neurologic deficit lasting <24 h (TIA) or <72 h (RIND)

3. **Renal failure:** worsening of renal function with increase in serum creatinine to >2.0 and $2 \times$ the most recent preoperative creatinine level; new requirement for dialysis

4. **Prolonged ventilation:** the patient has pulmonary insufficiency requiring mechanical ventilatory support for >24 h postoperatively

5. **Myocardial infarction**

  a. Within 24 h of surgery: CK-MB >5 times upper limit of normal with or without new Q waves in two or more contiguous leads

b. After 24 h:
    i. Evolutionary ST-segment elevation
   ii. Development of new Q waves in two or more contiguous leads
  iii. New left bundle branch block on ECG
   iv. CK-MB > 3 times upper limit of normal
6. **Deep sternal wound infection**: infection involving muscle, bone, and/or mediastinum requiring operative intervention with all of the following:
    a. Wound opened with excision of tissue or reexploration of mediastinum
    b. Positive culture
    c. Treatment with antibiotics

Technique of Thoracentesis

A. The level of the fluid should be determined on chest x-ray and confirmed by dullness to percussion. The skin is prepped and draped. One percent lidocaine is used for local anesthesia of the skin. A 22-gauge needle is passed to the upper border of the rib, and the periosteum is anesthetized. The needle is then passed over the rib into the pleural space.

B. When the pleural space has been entered, fluid should be aspirated to confirm that the effusion has been located. A larger "intracatheter" needle is then passed into the pleural cavity, the plastic catheter advanced, and the metal needle withdrawn to prevent injury to the lung as it expands to appose the parietal pleura. The fluid is then aspirated into collection bottles.

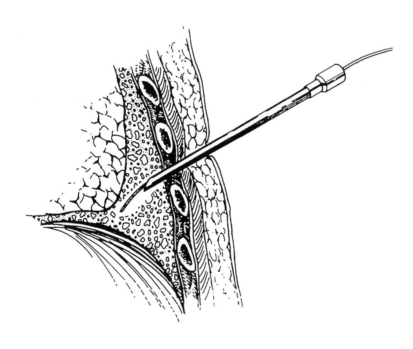

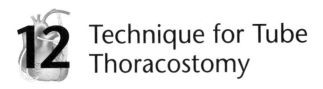

Technique for Tube Thoracostomy

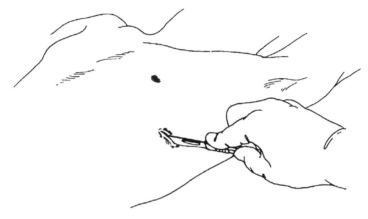

Skin incision. One percent lidocaine is used for local anesthesia. A subcutaneous wheal is raised over the fifth or sixth intercostal space in the midaxillary line. The needle is passed to the upper border of the rib and the periosteum is anesthetized. Fluid should be aspirated from an effusion to confirm its location. A 1-cm incision is then made.

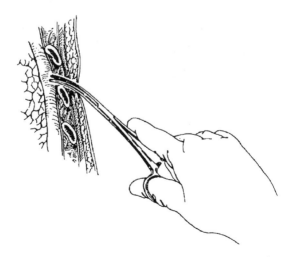

Pleural entry. The dissection is carried down to and through the intercostal muscles with a Kelly clamp, the parietal pleura is penetrated, and the pleural cavity is entered. Finger dissection should be used only if loculations are known to be present.

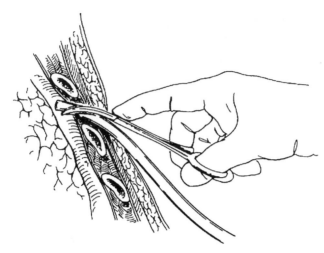

Chest tube placement. The chest tube is inserted and directed towards the apex for air and posteriorly for fluid. The tube should be clamped during insertion if fluid is being drained. The tube is then secured with a 2-0 silk suture. A trocar can be used as a stent to advance the tube but should **never** be used to penetrate the pleura.

Technique for Insertion of Percutaneous Tracheostomy Tube

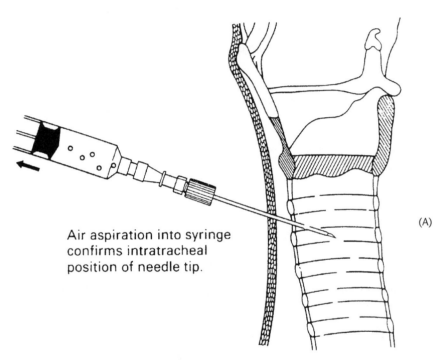

Air aspiration into syringe
confirms intratracheal
position of needle tip.

(A)

This procedure should be performed with the assistance of an individual trained in airway management and bronchoscopy. The diagrams represent an overview of the procedure derived from the package insert for the Ciaglia percutaneous tracheostomy set manufactured by Cook Critical Care. *(Reproduced with permission from Cook Critical Care.)*

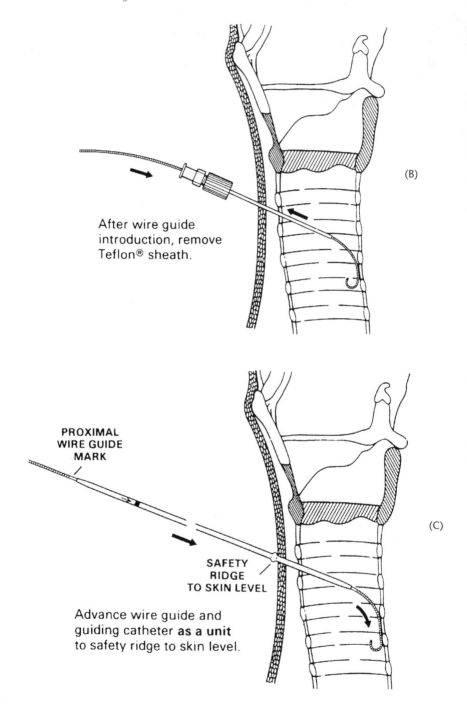

(B)

After wire guide
introduction, remove
Teflon® sheath.

**PROXIMAL
WIRE GUIDE
MARK**

(C)

**SAFETY
RIDGE
TO SKIN LEVEL**

Advance wire guide and
guiding catheter **as a unit**
to safety ridge to skin level.

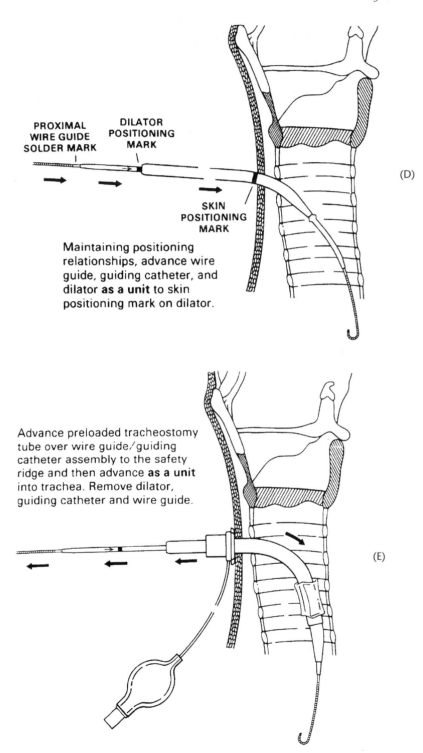

PROXIMAL WIRE GUIDE SOLDER MARK

DILATOR POSITIONING MARK

SKIN POSITIONING MARK

(D)

Maintaining positioning relationships, advance wire guide, guiding catheter, and dilator **as a unit** to skin positioning mark on dilator.

Advance preloaded tracheostomy tube over wire guide/guiding catheter assembly to the safety ridge and then advance **as a unit** into trachea. Remove dilator, guiding catheter and wire guide.

(E)

Body Surface Area Nomogram for Adults

Height	Body Surface Area	Weight

Height

cm 200 ┬ 79 in
      ├ 78
195 ┼ 77
      ├ 76
190 ┼ 75
      ├ 74
185 ┼ 73
      ├ 72
180 ┼ 71
      ├ 70
175 ┼ 69
      ├ 68
170 ┼ 67
      ├ 66
165 ┼ 65
      ├ 64
160 ┼ 63
      ├ 62
155 ┼ 61
      ├ 60
150 ┼ 59
      ├ 58
145 ┼ 57
      ├ 56
140 ┼ 55
      ├ 54
135 ┼ 53
      ├ 52
130 ┼ 51
      ├ 50
125 ┼ 49
      ├ 48
120 ┼ 47
      ├ 46
115 ┼ 45
      ├ 44
110 ┼ 43
      ├ 42
105 ┼ 41
      ├ 40
cm 100 ┴ 39 in

Body Surface Area

2.80 m²
2.70
2.60
2.50
2.40
2.30
2.20
2.10
2.00
1.95
1.90
1.85
1.80
1.75
1.70
1.65
1.60
1.55
1.50
1.45
1.40
1.35
1.30
1.25
1.20
1.15
1.10
1.05
1.00
0.95
0.90
0.86 m²

Weight

kg 150 ┬ 330 lb
145 ┼ 320
140 ┤ 310
135 ┤ 300
130 ┤ 290
125 ┤ 280
120 ┤ 270
115 ┤ 260
        250
110 ┤ 240
105 ┤ 230
100 ┤ 220
95 ┤ 210
90 ┤ 200
85 ┤ 190
80 ┤ 180
        170
75 ┤ 160
70 ┤ 150
65 ┤ 140
60 ┤ 130
55 ┤ 120
50 ┤ 110
        105
45 ┤ 100
        95
40 ┤ 90
        85
35 ┤ 80
        75
        70
kg 30 ┴ 66 lb

Index

Note: Page numbers with an *f* indicate figures; those with a *t*, tables; those with a *b*, boxes; those with an *a*, appendices.